Clinicians and researchers working with children frequently encounter problems in multiple domains, including language, learning, and behavior, and recent studies show that as many as one-third of children seen in psychiatric clinics for behavioral and learning problems may also have underlying language disorders. Language as a connecting bridge between learning disability and psychiatric disorder is the unifying theme of this wide-ranging book.

In a combination of review chapters and research reports on major studies such as the Connecticut Longitudinal Study, and the Colorado Reading Project, the distinguished international contributors cover many important neuropsychiatric disorders of childhood. Particular prominence is given to attention deficit hyperactivity disorder, dyslexia, and autistic disorder. Explanations for the comorbidity of psychiatric and language disorder are sought in developmental, cognitive, and biological fields, the contribution of new imaging modalities is considered, and implications for etiology, treatment, and rehabilitation are explored. Topical issues such as syndrome definition in dyslexia, acquired memory disorder in childhood, and biology-behavior correspondence are well covered, as are a range of treatment options. A final section is devoted to outcome studies.

Enlivened with case vignettes, and offering insights into the range of current thinking on language and behavior, this book is a rich resource for professionals and advanced students concerned with child health and development, offering ideas for a unified view of language, learning, and behavior problems.

T0318556

Language, learning, and behavior disorders

ABOUT THE EDITORS

Joseph H. Beitchman, MD
Professor of Psychiatry and Preventive Medicine and Biostatistics, University of Toronto
Head, Child and Family Studies Centre, Clarke Institute of Psychiatry, Toronto

Dr. Beitchman has published and presented widely in the fields of psychiatric epidemiology and particularly on speech and language disorders and developmental psychopathology. He has edited two books in child psychiatry and is currently Chairperson of the Language/Cognition group in the Division of Child Psychiatry at the University of Toronto.

Nancy J. Cohen, PhD
Associate Professor and Director of Research, C.M. Hincks Institute, Toronto

Dr. Cohen has published extensively in a variety of topics related to the psychopathologies of childhood. The focus of most of her research efforts, however, has been the area of language and communication impairments in a variety of psychopathological conditions of childhood.

M. Mary Konstantareas, PhD
Professor of Psychology, University of Guelph, Ontario
Professor of Psychiatry, University of Toronto

Dr. Konstantareas has worked with diverse populations of children and adolescents and their families over a twenty-year period. She has an extensive publication record and has authored or edited a number of volumes. Her main area of interest is pervasive developmental disorder.

Rosemary Tannock, PhD
Assistant Professor of Psychiatry, University of Toronto
Scientist, The Hospital for Sick Children, Toronto

The two major foci of Dr. Tannock's research and publications are language intervention for preschool children with developmental disorders and mechanisms of action of stimulant medication on cognitive function in children with attention hyperactivity disorder.

Language, learning, and behavior disorders

Developmental, biological, and clinical perspectives

Edited by

JOSEPH H. BEITCHMAN

Clarke Institute of Psychiatry, Toronto

NANCY J. COHEN

University of Toronto

M. MARY KONSTANTAREAS

University of Guelph, Ontario

ROSEMARY TANNOCK

University of Toronto

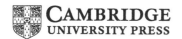
CAMBRIDGE
UNIVERSITY PRESS

CAMBRIDGE UNIVERSITY PRESS
Cambridge, New York, Melbourne, Madrid, Cape Town, Singapore, São Paulo

Cambridge University Press
The Edinburgh Building, Cambridge CB2 2RU, UK

Published in the United States of America by Cambridge University Press, New York

www.cambridge.org
Information on this title: www.cambridge.org/9780521472296

© Cambridge University Press 1996

First published 1996
This digitally printed first paperback version 2006

A catalogue record for this publication is available from the British Library

Library of Congress Cataloguing in Publication data

Language, learning, and behavior disorders: developmental,
    biological, and clinical perspectives / edited by Joseph H.
    Beitchman . . . [et al.].
        p.   cm.
    ISBN 0-521-47229-6 (hc)
    1. Language disorders in children.   2. Learning disabilities.
3. Behavior disorders in children.   I. Beitchman, Joseph H.
[DNLM: 1. Child Behavior Disorders.   2. Language Disorders.
3. Learning Disorders.   4. Mental Disorders—in infancy & childhood,
WS 350.6 L287 1996]
RJ496.L35L.368   1996
618.92′855—dc20
                                                              95-37659
                                                                  CIP

ISBN-13 978-0-521-47229-6 hardback
ISBN-10 0-521-47229-6 hardback

ISBN-13 978-0-521-03133-2 paperback
ISBN-10 0-521-03133-8 paperback

Contents

Part IV: Biological considerations

Part V: Intervention

Part VI: Outcome studies

Contributors to this volume

Joseph H. Beitchman
Clarke Institute of Psychiatry, Toronto, Ontario, Canada

Ursula Bellugi
The Salk Institute for Biological Studies, La Jolla, California, USA

Joseph Biederman
Massachusetts General Hospital, Boston, Massachusetts, USA

Amy Bihrle
The Salk Institute for Biological Studies, La Jolla, California, USA

E.B. Brownlie
Clarke Institute of Psychiatry, Toronto, Ontario, Canada

Rochelle Caplan
University of California, Los Angeles, California, USA

Peter Chaban
Sunnybrook Health Services Centre, Toronto, Ontario, Canada

Nancy J. Cohen
C.M. Hincks Treatment Centre/Institute, Toronto, Ontario, Canada

Patricia M. Crittenden
Family Relations Institute, Miami, Florida, USA

Philip S. Dale
University of Washington, Seattle, Washington, USA

J.C. DeFries
University of Colorado, Boulder, Colorado, USA

Rita S. Eagle
Surrey Place Centre, Toronto, Ontario, Canada

Stephen V. Faraone
Massachusetts General Hospital, Boston, Massachusetts, USA

Jack M. Fletcher
University of Texas Medical School, Houston, Texas, USA

Tanya M. Gallagher
McGill University, Montreal, Quebec, Canada

Jeffrey M. Halperin
Queens College of the City University of New York, Flushing, New York, USA

Deborah A. Hayden
The PROMPT Institute, Santa Fe, New Mexico, USA

Lily Hechtman
Montreal Children's Hospital, Westmount, Quebec, Canada

Wendy Jones
The Salk Institute for Biological Studies, La Jolla, California, USA

Kathleen Kiely
Massachusetts General Hospital, Boston, Massachusetts, USA

Edward S. Klima
The Salk Institute for Biological Studies, La Jolla, California, USA

M. Mary Konstantareas
University of Guelph, Guelph, Ontario, Canada

Joan Kouri
Montreal Children's Hospital, Westmount, Quebec, Canada

Penelope Krener
University of California Davis, Sacramento, California, USA

Jacquelyn G. Light
University of Michigan, Ann Arbor, Michigan, USA

William J. Logan
Hospital for Sick Children, Toronto, Ontario, Canada

Sherri MacKay
Clarke Institute of Psychiatry, Toronto, Ontario, Canada

Rob McGee
University of Otago Medical School, Dunedin, New Zealand

Carol Musselman
Ontario Institute for Studies in Education, Toronto, Ontario, Canada

Jeffrey H. Newcorn
Mount Sinai School of Medicine, New York, USA

Margit Pukonen
Speech Foundation of Ontario, Toronto Children's Centre, Toronto, Ontario, Canada

Chava Respitz
Montreal Children's Hospital, Westmount, Quebec, Canada

Michael Rossen
University of Rochester Medical Center, Rochester, New York, USA

Russell Schachar
The Hospital for Sick Children, Toronto, Ontario, Canada

Debbie C. Schachter
Clarke Institute of Psychiatry, Toronto, Ontario, Canada

Vanshdeep Sharma
Mount Sinai School of Medicine, New York, USA

Bennett A. Shaywitz
Yale University School of Medicine, New Haven, Connecticut, USA

Sally E. Shaywitz
Yale University School of Medicine, New Haven, Connecticut, USA

Bryna Siegel
Langley Porter Psychiatric Institute, San Francisco, California, USA

Linda S. Siegel
Ontario Institute for Studies in Education, Toronto, Ontario, Canada

Jim Stevenson
University of Southampton, Southampton, UK

Rosemary Tannock
The Hospital for Sick Children, Toronto, Ontario, Canada

Sandra E. Trehub
University of Toronto, Toronto, Ontario, Canada

Margaretha C. Vandervelden
Ontario Institute for Studies in Education, Toronto, Ontario, Canada

Sheila Williams
University of Otago Medical School, Dunedin, New Zealand

Beth Wilson
Clarke Institute of Psychiatry, Toronto, Ontario, Canada

Preface

The theme of this book is the interrelation between language, learning, and behavior. The idea for the volume arose from discussions at monthly meetings of a multidisciplinary language/cognition group organized in an attempt to focus a university community working on different aspects of the association between language and behavior. In the not too distant past, speech/language pathologists refused to work with children who had behavioral problems, maintaining that these needed to be addressed before language therapy began. Likewise, mental health professionals ignored language and learning problems as less critical to a child's mental well-being than intrapsychic or family problems. The relative isolation and limited communication between clinicians and researchers was something we felt the need to overcome by bringing together our experiences and sharing ideas. In the process of engaging in this exercise, we came to see how crucial it was to pull together information on assessment and classification, notions on etiology and intervention, and efforts to look at clinical course and outcome. Although coming from diverse backgrounds and disciplines, studying different populations, and relying on different clinical and research methodologies, we were impressed by the many common threads that run across the apparent diversity in our perspectives and interests.

The concept that language is a connecting bridge between learning disabilities and psychiatric disorders serves as a unifying theme of this book. This volume represents an attempt to explore the links in all directions, between language and behavior disorders, language and learning disabilities and, in some cases, between all three. It covers a wide range of disorders. We opted for this heterogeneity with the purpose of examining commonalities that may underlie the diversity in conditions associated with language and learning problems.

The authors come from diverse backgrounds and disciplines, have studied different populations, and have used a variety of clinical and research methodologies. Nevertheless, there are several recognizable themes. First, for instance, there is general agreement that adopting a developmental perspective is fundamental to any study of children and adolescents. When the focus has been on cross-sectional data, without regard to examining developmental trajectories, it has sometimes been less well appreciated that symptoms identified at one age may appear different at a later age. In this way, manifestations of similar underlying processes may be mistakenly thought of as due to different disorders, when they may actually represent a common underlying process. We believe that our attempt to highlight normal developmental processes as a backdrop against which abnormal behavior should be assessed brings some clarity to the different conditions being considered.

A second theme that runs through the chapters is the need to expand our view of language, and to go beyond examining language structure to consider the broader communicative components of language in the social context, or pragmatics. Understanding the pragmatic or social function of language seems particularly pertinent for understanding the links of language with behavior disorder.

Third, we also found that questions of comorbidity inevitably arise and, likewise, the debate of discrete versus dimensional views of language, learning, and behavior disorder. We are gratified that for the first time the overlap between language, learning, and behavior, as comorbid conditions, has been given formal and long overdue recognition in the new DSM-IV classification system. Healthy tension between the dimensional view versus the discrete view is evident as a recurring theme throughout the book.

Some issues have been introduced because they are topical, timely, and represent new ideas of relevance to our concerns. For example, rapid technological advances in biological methodologies have inspired hope that brain functioning can be correlated with language and behavior, such as through brain imaging. However, as the technology has advanced, new conceptualizations have emerged, that confirm the previously acquired wisdom that structure and function are not always well correlated. Instead, our current understanding is that the brain is organized into neuronal networks, such that disruption at any point in the chain can lead to functional change. This has vastly complicated the task of demonstrating the brain correlates of behavioral, language, and learning disorders. To complicate this task even further, there is little consensus about how the boundaries between and among these conditions should be drawn.

We were struck by the implications of the multidimensionality of the language, learning, and behavioral conditions for strategies of intervention. The complex interplay of biological, intrapersonal, and interpersonal forces that appear to shape the expression of the various language and communication impairments and behavior disorders has given a renewed impetus to the need to employ multimodal strategies in intervention, as well as to refine focused strategies for use with particular populations.

The chapters in this volume are organized into six groupings. The papers in the various parts, although not always easy to classify, reflecting as they do a diversity of viewpoints and perspectives, nevertheless do fall into distinct sections. We have provided short introductory sections that bind the proffered material and simultaneously offer the highlights of each chapter. Part I sets the groundwork by examining normal and atypical developmental processes, contributing to links between language and communicative development and psychiatric disorder. Part II examines comorbidity of language impairment with a broad range of psychiatric conditions, including conduct disorder, internalizing disorders such as depression and anxiety, attention deficit hyperactivity disorder (ADHD), schizophrenia, and autism. Part III tackles issues related to the definition of learning disabilities and the delineation of meaningful subgroups and syndromes. Researchers continue to struggle with the question of whether learning disabilities represent categorical or dimensional constructs and with the complex relation between conditions that overlap with learning disabilities such as language and communicative disorders and ADHD. Part IV reviews advances in biological methodologies that have opened new avenues for exploration of language, learning, and behavior disorders. Part V describes approaches to intervention in children with these conditions. Finally, in Part VI, the last section of this volume, long-term outcome studies are reviewed.

Although intended for a knowledgeable readership of both clinicians and researchers in the general areas of language, communication impairment, behavior, and psychopathological conditions, the book could also serve as a text for advanced undergraduate and graduate students. Many disciplines are represented here, from academic psychology and psycholinguistics, to psychiatry, pediatrics, speech pathology, nursing, epidemiology, genetics, and medicine as well as child care, occupational therapy, and social work. This is not surprising in view of the fact that language and communication is the central dimension around which human cultures have revolved since their earliest origins.

This book brings together common trends into a unified body of literature. We offer it as a means of familiarizing others with the key issues in this general area. We hope it will stimulate collaborative work, particularly on issues of syndrome definition, comorbidity, and biology-behavior correspondence, and facilitate the translation of research into practice.

J.H.B.

N.J.C.

M.M.K.

R.T.

PART I

DEVELOPMENTAL PERSPECTIVE

Introduction

NANCY J. COHEN

The chapters in this part all discuss developmental processes associated with the interrelation of language, cognition, and behavior. In most of the chapters the perspective of developmental psychopathology is applied to highlight the ways that growth or retardation in one aspect of development can have profound implications for other aspects.

In the first two chapters, Dale and Chaban examine normal developmental processes that may underlie the relation between cognitive, language, and emotional development. The central thesis of Philip Dale's Chapter 1 is that language is a complex tool that is used for emotional and cognitive self-regulation as well as for social communication. Dale begins his chapter by delineating the qualities of language important for socioemotional development that begin to emerge at an early age. These include use of language for categorization, displacement of events from the here-and-now, productivity or creativity, and for intrapersonal and interpersonal functions. Whereas these qualities of language have been accepted as being associated with cognitive development for some time, it is only more recently that their importance for affective functioning has been acknowledged. In particular, current functional theories of emotion have led to a shift away from the view of language and affect as incompatible systems to a view that they are integrated and that language is essential to express and regulate internal states ("internal state language"). Dale also outlines trends in research that have elucidated the developmental sequence of components of internal state language and factors that influence it. By way of illustration, Dale considers the implications of a functional developmental framework in relation to three disorders of development that vary in organismic and environmental etiology: autism, childhood maltreatment, and language and learning disabilities. The chapter ends by raising some issues for consideration in research on intervention.

In Chapter 2, Chaban provides a much needed overview of the development of communication. Going beyond the simple language structures that children normally develop by the age of 3, Chaban traces the growth of pragmatic abilities and the underpinnings of specific pragmatic constructs within various social contexts. Pragmatic abilities are broadly defined as the ability to use language appropriately within a specified social, situational, and communicative context. These abilities depend on higher order cognitive processes, in particular, executive function or metacognitive abilities, as well as social and linguistic knowledge. Through his explanation of pragmatic constructs such as turn-taking, speech acts, topic maintenance, and cohesion, Chaban illustrates how problems in language usage may reflect either metacognitive or linguistic problems or both. This chapter serves as a useful reference for terminology adopted in other chapters in this volume that address causes, effects, and remediation of pragmatic deficits (see chapters by Caplan, Cohen, Gallagher, Hayden and Pukonen, Tannock and Schachar).

Turning to atypical populations, Siegel's Chapter 3 describes a developmental model for systematically observing growth in children with neuropathological conditions. Her working hypothesis is that disability in any single developmental domain will affect relatively intact functions from other domains to compensate for or potentiate disability. Siegel distinguishes between primary or innate signs which are a direct expression of the neuropathological disorder from secondary or virtual signs of a disorder that represent an adaptation to it and tertiary or epiphenomenal signs that represent a failure in coping with the disorder. She illustrates the use of this developmental approach by mapping the emergence of symptoms, their earliest manifestations, and their later transformations in children with autistic spectrum disorders, attention deficit hyperactivity disorder, learning disabilities, mental retardation, and language disorders. Siegel argues that it is important to adopt a developmental rather than a medical model to chart the simultaneous progression of normal and atypical development. By doing so, early emerging innate signs can be separated from later emerging virtual and epiphenomenal signs, which is critical for early identification and intervention.

Crittenden's Chapter 4 presents the thought provoking view that caregiver–child relationships can have an impact on mental processing of affective and cognitive information, and ultimately on the representational models of reality. In her chapter she explores individual differences in brain structure and maturation and in the process of children's learning to use their minds as that process is inferred from language use in interpersonal relationships. Integrating research on memory systems, she postulates that insecurely attached children, who do not obtain accurate information from their attachment figures, can learn to distrust language. Crittenden illustrates how the child's expressive and receptive language can come to reflect this distortion in relationships, such as by using language to hide feelings or to lie about them. This is contrasted to the situation for securely attached children who can mentally integrate affective and cognitive information. In their day-to-day life securely attached children use language to express feelings, to plan for the future, and to negotiate and reach satisfying compromises. Throughout the chapter, Crittenden's integrative theoretical view is applied to the analysis of numerous samples of dialogues between mother–child dyads from the preschool years through adolescence.

In the final chapter in this section, Stevenson steps back to take a broad view of the complex transactions between biology, and individual and familial factors to show the bidirectional effects that contribute to behavior disorders. He first discusses the strength and specificity of the relations between language impairments, verbal and nonverbal learning disabilities and behavior disorders, and then considers the nature of the underlying causal mechanisms for the associations. Throughout Chapter 5, Stevenson provides evidence for developmental changes in the relation between the type of behavior problem and language impairment. Accordingly, he proposes that the importance of various mechanisms will likely change with age. The chapter concludes with a preliminary developmental model of mechanisms linking language development and behavior which Stevenson offers for empirical validation.

1 Language and emotion: a developmental perspective

PHILIP S. DALE

Many of the chapters in this volume document a strikingly high, yet less than perfect, comorbidity of language and learning disabilities with a range of behavioral and emotional disturbances. The present chapter, like others in this first part, is addressed to constructing a developmental framework to illuminate this connection, and by extension, the relationship between language and socioemotional development in all children. In particular, the chapter reflects the perspective of a developmental psycholinguist fascinated by a unique and complex component of language, the language of internal states and emotions. It is not a comprehensive review of research in this area, but rather an overview of some key questions, findings, and theories.

For better and for worse, language stands near the core of both psychiatry and developmental psychology. There are a good many reasons for this. Probably the most important is the highly public nature of language, unique among human cognitive functions. Because we can, and do, talk about nearly every aspect of our experience, our lives are permeated with language. Language also serves a central methodological role in both fields, in introspection, in research, and in therapy. Sometimes this misleads us. As Fred Pine (1985) has noted, the overwhelming emphasis on oedipal-level pathology in classical psychoanalytic theorizing is probably due in large part to the fact that at this level and beyond, language is central to the child's mental and social life. Similarly in cognitive psychology, the availability of language for observation and experimentation for a long time blinded us to the extent and importance of spatial and other nonverbal processes. Nevertheless, language is a crucial aspect of human experience, and the focus of this chapter.

THE PUBLIC AND PRIVATE FACES OF LANGUAGE

What *is* language? What aspects of this universal communicative system are distinctively human and distinctively significant for socioemotional development? Four characteristics are most important. The first is that language is a system of *categorization*. Word meanings, grammatical rules, all linguistic structures function as categories that can be used to go "beyond the information given" (Bruner, 1973). This is obvious for the categories that correspond to nouns, such as *dog* or *woman*, but it is equally valid for verbs (e.g., *walk* and *love*), prepositions (e.g., *in* and *to*), and adjectives (e.g., *green* and *good*). Categories provide us a basis for acting in the future on the basis of the past, even though the past never repeats itself exactly. The challenge for the child learner of language is to perform a leap of induction for each word, a leap from a few examples (a few dogs, a few shades of green, etc.) to a general concept, and to do this 6000 times by the age of 6 (Carey, 1978).

A second distinctive quality of language is *displacement*; we are not limited to the here-and-now, but can talk about persons, objects, and events not present. In this way language unites past, present, and future. A third essential property of language is *productivity*, or creativity. The overwhelming majority of utterances we produce and hear are novel. When we encounter new situations, or have new meanings to convey, we can construct new sentences with reasonable hope that we will be understood by our listeners (or readers). This is possible because among the categories we have acquired in learning language are the patterns, or rules, for constructing and decoding sentences.

Finally, language has both a public and a private face. That is, language has an interpersonal function – as an instrument of social interaction – and an intrapersonal function – as an instrument of cognitive functioning – without any distinct formal marking to distinguish them. This view of language has a long intellectual heritage, but in psychology today is most associated with the name of the great Russian psychologist Lev Vygotsky (1986), whose rediscovery by English-speaking psychologists in the 1960s (Vygotsky died very young, in 1934) transformed cognitive and developmental psychology. Vygotsky emphasized the private, cognitive function of language, and proposed a developmental model of the relationship between the two faces of language. Somewhat oversimplified, his model runs as follows. Cultures transmit tools from generation to generation; not just physical tools such as fire and the wheel, but cognitive tools such as number systems, and above all, language. There is a developmental shift from interpersonal to intrapersonal functioning in the use of these tools. The child can first use language for problem-solving, for example, under direct stimulation from a more competent adult; later he/she can function in this way independently, but necessarily overtly; still later he/she can use language internally. It was Vygotsky who first coined the term "inner speech," and characterized it as an abbreviated streamlined version of language, a form of cognition which is thinking in pure word meanings. The process of learning new tools at first involves a kind of "scaffolding" (Ninio & Bruner, 1978; Rogoff, 1990) in which adults simplify and structure the problem so that the child can make the small advance necessary to solve it. Vygotsky coined the term "zone of proximal development" to capture the idea that beyond what a child can do on his/her own is a range of problems which can be solved *with* adult assistance.

Now the interesting thing about this set of four distinctive qualities of language is that they have been well accepted for some time for cognitive functioning, that is, for representation and communication about the nonsocial physical world. But the validity of this characterization of language for affective functioning has been much more slowly acknowledged. The growth of this approach is one of the most exciting and fruitful developments in psychology today. It is one component of a "sea-change" in psychology over the past 20 years. Previously there has been an all too strong tendency in psychology, as in our culture more generally, to see affect and cognition, feeling and knowing, as not only distinct, but having nothing to do with each other, except possibly get in each other's way. Which certainly happens. But the parallels and interconnections between affect and cognition are much clearer now, and this makes it possible to understand the parallel roles of language in the two domains.

FUNCTIONALIST THEORIES OF EMOTION, AND THE ROLE OF LANGUAGE

An understanding of these parallels and connections has emerged in several fields, and with differing terminologies. But one particularly useful perspective is provided by functionalist theories of emotion (Bretherton et al., 1986). Like language, emotions have both an interpersonal and an intrapersonal function. Bretherton et al. (1986) characterize this approach on the basis of three fundamental postulates. First, emotions have evolved as adaptive, survival-promoting processes with intrapsychic and interpersonal functions. Second, emotions have major intrapsychic regulative functions: categorizing and evaluating the meaning of events, and motivating and guiding subsequent behavior. Third, emotions have interpersonal regulative functions, including gaining indirect access to another's emotional states, predicting future behavior, and masking emotional expression.

Perhaps the most important consequence of such a viewpoint, emphasizing as it does the parallels and potential connections among systems previously viewed discretely, is to identify the integration of cognitive, language, and emotional systems as a fundamental challenge of human development. A vivid example is provided by the research of Bloom and her associates (Bloom & Capatides, 1987; Bloom & Beckwith, 1989). On the basis of observational research on young children's communication, they have posited a shift from language and affect as incompatible systems to an integrated system. Children in the second year of life can express positive and negative emotions directly, as in laughter and crying, or they can communicate in words when in a neutral emotional state, but they can neither communicate under conditions of emotional arousal nor communicate in words *about* emotions. Furthermore, rate of early language development is correlated with the amount of time spent in *neutral* affect expression; both positive and negative affect displays

Table 1.1. *A model of the stages of developmental integration*

1. *Infancy* (Birth to 18 months)
    Emotion = communication
    Arousal and desire = behavior
2. *Toddlerhood* (18 months to 36 months)
    Language supplements emotion = communication
    Very initial development of emotional labeling
    Arousal and desire = behavior
3. *Preschool Years* (3 to 6 years)
    Language develops powerful role in communication
    Child can recognize/label basic emotions
    Arousal and desire > symbolic mediation > behavior
    Development of role-taking abilities
    Beginning of reflective social planning and problem-solving
4. *School Years* (6 to 12–13 years)
    Thinking in language has become habitual
    Increasing ability to reflect on and plan sequences of action
    Developing ability to consider multiple consequences of action
    Increasing ability to take multiple perspectives on a situation
5. *Adolescence*
    Utilize language in the service of hypothetical thought
    Ability to simultaneously consider multiple perspectives

Source: Adapted from Greenberg & Kusché (1993).

are negatively correlated with development. Thus language learning is at first incompatible with the expression of affect.

Thus the developmental task is not simply to manage both systems; it is to integrate them. The potential of integration for the child's emotional life has been captured eloquently by Pine:

As the child learns speech, he can begin to express in a "cooler" medium, in general, what before could be expressed only in action, image, or affectivity (p. 163).

Words provide a moment of recognition and delay in which discomfort over feeling might have a chance of being handled in ways other than denial or immediate discharge through action. Words facilitate coping ... (p. 139)

Similarly, Kopp (1989) proposed that language plays an important role in helping young children understand emotions, especially for negative emotional regulation.

With language, children can state their feelings to others, obtain verbal feedback about the appropriateness of their emotions, and hear and think about ways to manage them ... Especially in pretend play, children use language to describe feelings and share them with others, to sharpen their understanding of feelings, and to act out ways of regulating feelings without fear of sanctions. (p. 349)

Kopp also poses a crucial question, to which we return later: What are the relative roles of caregivers and peers in fostering emotion regulation?

The ideas of Vygotsky, Freud, Pine, and others have been integrated by Greenberg & Kusché (1993) into their "Affective-Behavioral-Cognitive-Dynamic Model" (the ABCD model), which provides a useful organizing framework (see Table 1.1). Like Vygotsky, Greenberg and Kusché assume that the emergence of new skills is largely dependent on adult–child interactions in which the child can develop a growing sense of self-confidence. The two factors which contribute most to this confidence are first, being able to successfully take increasing responsibility for more complex plans of behavior, and secondly, being able to utilize language to express internal states of being (cf. quotation above from Pine, 1985).

THE LANGUAGE OF EMOTIONS AND OTHER INTERNAL STATES

The language of emotions has most often been studied as part of a larger subset of language, typically referred to as "internal state language." Table 1.2, based on the work of Bretherton and others, illustrates the subcategories of internal state language most frequently studied.

Some investigators have focused exclusively on the emotion lexicon (Ridgeway, Waters, & Kuczaj, 1985), or on the lexicon of desire (subset of volition and ability), feeling (positive and negative emotion), and mental state (Brown & Dunn, 1991), or other subsets. These semantic subcategories are quite heterogenous, and all findings must be interpreted in the context of the specific definitions used.

Many words of English which can refer to emotions or other internal states have multiple meanings, only some of which are relevant here. For example, the word *like* may refer to an emotional state or a judgement of similarity; the word *blue* to an emotional state or a color; and the word *can* to ability/permission or to a container. For this reason, observational studies of internal state language require careful examination of potential internal state words in context, and parental checklists require the specification of the relevant meaning.

Although the vocabulary of emotions and other internal states is extensive and distinctive, these words have no distinctive grammatical correlate (they include nouns, verbs, adjectives, and adverbs) or pronunciation. Thus this aspect of language is not specifically marked in any way for children, despite the very considerable challenge such words pose. These words are relatively abstract: most of them do not have a clear, consistent, visible referent. Even in those cases which do have a visible referent, such as *happy* and *mad*, it is transitory and somewhat idiosyncratic across individuals. Furthermore, the essence of each word is a categorization across the internal state of other persons as well as the self. Such an act of categorization would appear to

Table 1.2. *Representative subcategories and examples of internal state vocabulary*

Subcategory	Example items
Sensory perception:	see, taste, hot, ...
Physiology:	sleepy, hungry, sick, ...
Emotion-positive:	love, good, happy, ...
Emotion-negative:	bad, mad, yucky, ...
Affect expression:	cry, kiss, smile, ...
Volition and ability (includes desire words):	wanna, hard, need to, ...
Cognition (mental state):	know, think, wish, ...
Moral judgement and obligation:	should, bad, naughty

require a high degree of nonegocentrism on the part of the child to infer an internal state for another. Research on internal state language did not begin until relatively recently, in part because of the assumption that such non-egocentrism would not be reliably established until the concrete operational period, i.e., the early school years. Finally, the processes that have been posited to enable children to master an enormous vocabulary in the preschool years have little to offer in this area of learning. For example, the taxonomic constraint has been proposed as a pre-existing bias to apply labels to categories of similar objects, and the principle of mutual exclusivity has been proposed as a bias to assume that a new label refers to a new object or set of objects (Markman & Wachtel, 1988). Neither appears to be particularly relevant for internal state language.

Nevertheless, despite these challenges children do learn internal state language, and they begin surprisingly young. Numerous studies, using both direct observation and parent report (Bretherton & Beeghly, 1982; Ridgeway et al., 1985; Bretherton et al., 1986; Brown & Dunn, 1991) have confirmed that emotion and other internal state language emerges late in the second year of life, and undergoes a major expansion during the third year. Ridgeway et al. (1985) have provided norms for 125 emotion-descriptive adjectives for children between 18 and 71 months. Bretherton et al. (1986) provide a set of illuminating examples of internal state language drawn from observational records; most of the examples cited below are taken from this source.

Four particularly interesting trends are apparent in this research. The first concerns the relative order of emergence of the various subcategories of internal state words. Physiological and emotion labels are relatively early to appear, whereas mental state words are among the latest. For example, Ridgeway et al. (1985) report that just seven words are reported to be understood by at least 50% of 18–23-month-olds: *sleepy, hungry, good, happy, clean, tired,* and *sad.* Mental state words, e.g., *know, think, guess,* have the least in the way of physical correlates. It has also been argued, as will be discussed below, that these words require a particular level of cognitive development which is late developing.

A second trend of interest concerns the application of these labels to the self as opposed to others. In the earliest stages of production of internal state language, children speak more frequently about their own states than others. As mothers are more likely to be referring to the child's internal state than to their own, this finding may reflect the role of imitation on the part of the children. However, toddlers' ability to label and discuss emotions develops rapidly, and by the middle of the third year, reference to self and others are both common (Bretherton & Beeghly, 1982; Brown & Dunn, 1991; Muchmore, Greenberg, & Crnic, unpublished). Bretherton & Beeghly (1982) traced the emergence of individual emotion words, and observed that production of a given word for self *and* other did not lag far behind production for self *or* other. Such a correlation in emergence is consistent with the view that the concepts of self and other are mutually interdependent, that a conscious sense of self is only possible in alliance with a conscious sense of other. The correlation also highlights the nature of vocabulary learning as categorization across self and other.

A third, related dimension of development was first identified by Brown & Dunn (1991). They distinguished *immediate self-interest* from *sophisticated* utterances concerning desire, feeling, or mental state. The *immediate self-interest* utterances did not imply knowledge of another's internal state; e.g., "want that kitty" and "need another green one." In contrast, *sophisticated* utterances did imply knowledge of another's internal state, typically in the context of attempting to influence or manipulate; e.g., "it's right here, just pretend." Both Brown & Dunn (1991) and Muchmore et al. (unpublished) noted a substantial development from primarily immediate self-interest use of internal state language to sophisticated use between 24 and 36 months.

The emergence of sophisticated use of internal state language strongly suggests an awareness on the part of quite young children that emotions are part of a larger system that includes behavior as well; in short, a simple functionalist theory of emotions. This is confirmed by the results of one of the most striking analyses of Bretherton & Beeghly (1982; also summarized in Bretherton et al., 1986). Twenty-eight-month-old children produced numerous examples of utterances reflecting a causal role for emotion, including

- Antecedents of motion:
    "I give a hug. Baby be happy."
    "Me fall down. Me cry."
- Interventions motivated by a negative state:
    "No cry, Mama. It will be all right."
    "Wash my hands. They're messy."
- Behavioral correlates of emotion:
    "I not cry now. I happy."
    "I laugh at funny man."

Children's understanding of emotions as evaluations and motivations for behavior, and of expressive behavior as the correlate of emotion, is not limited to their own emotions and actions. There are many examples which are focused on other persons, including the third example above. Brown & Dunn (1991) also observed a substantial increase from 24 to 36 months in reference to the causes and consequences of inner states. Clearly 3-year-old children do not have a fully developed theory of emotion and action; there are many developments to come. Understanding sarcasm, for example, requires the ability to register and relate two superficially contradictory expressions of a single internal state of another person, and appears to be a late elementary school age acquisition (Capelli, Nakagawa, & Madden, 1990). But young children are surprisingly sophisticated.

SOURCES AND INFLUENCES FOR THE DEVELOPMENT OF INTERNAL STATE LANGUAGE

Recent research has demonstrated clearly that despite the challenge posed by internal state vocabulary, children begin learning it early and progress rapidly. How is this possible? Five potentially important factors will be discussed here. They include maternal language to young children, the nature of the attachment bond between mother and child, the role of siblings and friends, the child's own cognitive development, and the child's language learning ability and style.

Children's earliest, and for several years the most frequent, exposure to emotion and other internal state language is from their primary caregiver, most often the mother. Reference both to emotions and other internal states is frequent in maternal speech. Although the frequency of occurrence increases over the second year of life (Beeghly, Bretherton, & Mervis, 1986), it is high and relatively stable during the third year of life. For example, Muchmore et al. (unpublished) observed mothers produce a mean of 40 internal state words to 2-year-olds and a mean of 32 to 3-year-olds during a 10-minute play period. Over this period there were no changes in the proportion of various internal state words, nor in the proportion of use to control behavior or simply comment. The only significant change was a decrease in the proportion of reference to the child's internal state, a decrease which has been noted by several other investigatiors, e.g., Brown & Dunn (1991). Muchmore et al. noted very few correlations between maternal and child use of internal state language, and in particular, no predictive correlations from mother's use of specific categories of words to child's use at a later time point. Thus during the third year of life, mothers provide a rich dataset of examples of internal state language, but frequency of such use does not have significant implications for the child's acquisition. Dunn, Bretherton, & Munn (1987) did observe a positive correlation between references to feeling states by mothers at child age 18 months and children's speech about feeling states at 24 months. Thus there is a mixed pattern of results concerning a possible correlation between maternal frequency of use and children's acquisition. However, even significant positive correlations are not easily interpreted. Parental speech to young children is very likely to be influenced by the child's comprehension ability (or the parent's estimate thereof), and thus the correlation may be child driven. This interpretive caution is especially relevant for one of Dunn et al.'s (1987) most intriguing findings: mothers and older siblings mentioned feeling states more frequently to girls than to boys at 18 months, and by 24 months the girls themselves referred to feeling states more often. In any case, research on maternal speech cannot provide an explanation for the relatively late acquisition of mental state terms, since mothers use them at a high and stable rate from age 2 on.

Conversations between mothers and children are just one facet of the relationship between these two persons. A tantalizing possibility is that the affective quality of this relationship, i.e., attachment, is closely connected to the development of language about emotions and other internal states. Although some correlations have been reported for internal state language use and attachment classification, these studies have focused on atypical, high risk children, and have drawn their language samples from the actual attachment paradigm, the Strange Situation, which may have produced a spurious correlation. Muchmore et al. (unpublished) have provided the first evaluation of the relationship between attachment status and internal state language for a normal, low risk sample, using language derived independently of the Strange Situation. Their findings are quite surprising. Two-year-old children were classified as very secure, moderately secure, or insecure. More feeling words were produced by both mothers and children for the insecure group than in the very secure and moderately secure groups. The finding runs counter to the more general finding of a positive correlation of security of attachment with general language measures (Cicchetti & Beeghly, 1987), and points to a special status for internal state language. The insecure group also showed a higher level of conversational discontinuities – nonresponsiveness, irrelevant replies, etc. – than the other groups, confirming a lack of harmony between the two partners in the dyad. Muchmore et al. proposed several nonexclusive explanations for the negative correlation between attachment and internal state language. The frequency or intensity of emotion may simply be higher in the environment of children rated as insecure, and this saliency of emotion may lead to an increase in talk about feelings. Alternatively, insecure children and their mothers may be less skillful at interpreting nonverbal information and therefore need to resort to language more frequently.

A somewhat contrary finding is reported by Denham, Cook, & Zoller (1992), who evaluated emotion language produced by 33 to 56-month-old children during joint picture examination and discussion between mother and child, using photographs of infants showing intense emotional states. Denham et al. also observed children's emotional displays during free play in the classroom and on the playground. They found modest but significant correlations between children's reference to emotions while looking at photographs, and their "affective balance" at play (happy displays minus angry displays). Thus Denham et al. observed a positive relation between child emotional state and feeling language, a finding which seems somewhat inconsistent with the first of the two explanations offered by Muchmore et al. However, the ages, situations, and measures used in the two studies are far from directly comparable, and no firm conclusion can be drawn at this time.

Like much of developmental psychology, the theorizing above rests on the commonplace assumption that parents provide the most important, perhaps only, significant environment for young children. Yet it is clear from both cross-cultural research and research on the changing nature of families in our own culture that many other persons play a role in the young child's development. Judy Dunn (1985) and her colleagues have called attention to the important role played by siblings, and sibling relationships, in emotional development. Even toddlers (18 to 36-month-olds) receive much input concerning feeling states from their preschool-aged older siblings (Dunn et al., 1987; Brown & Dunn, 1991), and this input shares many qualities with that provided by mothers, such as an initial focus on the young child's internal state. Thus it is not surprising that as later-born children enter the preschool period, their conversations about feelings are increasingly likely to be with siblings (Brown & Dunn, 1992). Brown & Donelan-McCall (1993) recorded conversations of 4-year-olds with older siblings, friends, and mothers. Reference to mental state was more frequent with siblings than with mothers, and most often with friends. In addition, reference to other's or shared mental states was more common with siblings and friends than with mothers. It has often been noted (even by Piaget, 1959) that the quality of relationships with other children is fundamentally different from those with adults due to perceived similarity with other children, which elicits more cooperation *and* more conflict. It is an open question whether children with siblings differ from singletons in rate or quality of development of emotion and internal state language.

We turn now from external, social influences on the development of internal state language to the internal factors of cognitive and language development. As discussed early in this chapter, internal state words pose a cognitive challenge to the young learner, given their abstractness and the need to generalize across the unobservable internal states of others. It seems highly likely that there is a cognitive requirement for development in this area. Mental state words (*know, understand, guess*, etc.) have received special attention in this regard, due to their lateness of acquisition despite frequent use by mothers. Effective production and comprehension of these terms appears to require an ability to represent the existence and content of other persons' cognition, i.e., a "theory of mind" (Leslie, 1992). The False Belief Task (Wellman & Bartsch, 1988) is often used to index the emergence of such representations. An object is hidden in one of two locations while a confederate watches. The confederate leaves the room, and the experimenter changes the location of the hidden object. The subject is then asked where the confederate will look when he/she returns. A correct response requires the child to maintain, in addition to his own representation of the current location of the object, a representation of the confederate's now false belief. Brown & Donelan-McCall (1993) found a significant positive relationship between performance on the false belief task (data collected somewhat earlier, at 40 months) and the frequency (at 4 years) of reference to mental states in conversation with friends and siblings. Thus the ability to label mental states appears to require a representational advance, not a specific change in linguistic input by the mother. Further evidence for the linkage of reference to mental states to an ability to represent other persons' cognition is provided by the very specific deficit of autistic children in this area, discussed below.

Emotion and other internal state vocabulary are a part of language. We turn, finally, to a consideration of the relationship between development in this area specifically and language development more generally. Is mastery of these words, despite their specific difficulties, simply another manifestation of the extraordinarily rapid vocabulary growth of the toddler and preschool years (Fenson et al., 1994), or do these words pose a special challenge? Muchmore et al. obtained moderate correlations between measures of internal state language use and Peabody Picture Vocabulary Test-Revised scores (a measure of receptive vocabulary) and MLU (mean length of utterance – a measure of expressive syntax) for 2-year-olds, though not for 3-year-olds. Nevertheless, the correlations were not large (0.46–0.55) and they were smaller than other estimates of the intercorrelations among various linguistic categories (Fenson et al., 1994), suggesting that these words pose a somewhat distinct problem to young children.

A rather different linkage to language development is suggested by the results of Toth-Sadjadi's (1993) investigation of internal state language in a group of linguistically precocious toddlers. The children had been selected at 20 months on the basis of language development at least two standard deviations above the mean on one or more standardized measures. Even at 20 months, these toddlers frequently referred to internal states, and they did so equally for their own and other's states. At 24 months, reference to cognitions (mental states) was one of their most frequent categories, in contrast to the late emergence of this category in other populations of children. Without a measure such as the False Belief task, it is not possible to confirm the plausible suggestion that these children were also precocious in developing a "theory of mind." Like Muchmore et al., Toth-Sadjadi found a moderate positive correlation with MLU (but not for PPVT-R). The most striking finding of Toth-Sadjadi's results was the correlation with a measure of language-learning style. As first noted by Bloom, Lightbown, & Hood (1975), children differ in their earliest approach to syntax. Some children primarily use nouns in early word combinations, whereas others use pronouns. Nouns are highly specific, but a large number is required for effective communication; a smaller number of pronouns will suffice, but the child and conversational partner must rely on the social context to make the meaning clear. The nominal-pronominal dimension of individual differences is moderately related to an earlier difference in early vocabulary, the so-called referential-expressive dimension (Nelson, 1981). Referential vocabularies are made up primarily of nouns; expressive vocabularies include many nouns but also other categories, such as personal-social words (*yes, thank you*, etc.). Together, these differences suggest that some children's early language is primarily object-oriented, whereas other children's language is more socially-oriented. Toth-Sadjadi observed a significant positive correlation between internal state language and a measure of pronominal orientation at 20 months. Internal state language, therefore, may lie more on the social-orientation side of language than the object-mapping side.

The available research is far too limited at present to make a comparative evaluation of the role of these external and internal factors in the development of internal state language. At most we can conclude that all of them appear to play some role. Research designs which incorporate several of them in a single study are much needed, as are designs which more carefully distinguish the acquisition of these words from their frequency of use in specific contexts.

WHEN THINGS GO WRONG: LANGUAGE AND EMOTIONAL DISTURBANCE

If the ideas sketched above are even approximately valid, the development of emotional and behavioral self-regulation is a long and complex process, with all too many places where things can go wrong. The initial cause may well be organismic or environmental or a combination of both. As Pine (1985) suggests, the sources of psychopathology include "failed very early development, destructive parental inputs, and the absence of a solid base of quiet pleasure." Because of the importance of language for both cognitive development and social relationships, it is likely to cause, reflect, and/or exacerbate behavioral and emotional problems, as shown in the chapters in the first section of this book.

Consider three quite different disorders of development: autism (largely organismic), childhood maltreatment (largely environmental), and language and learning disabilities (an unknown combination, but probably more organismic). Language, cognitive, and emotional disorders constitute the core definition of childhood autism, but only recently has the specificity of interconnection among them become clear. On the cognitive side, autistic children are selectively impaired, even relative to age- and language-matched children with Down syndrome, on a variety of versions of the false belief task discussed earlier (Leslie, 1992; Tager-Flusberg, 1992). They are far less impaired on other tasks that require visual perspective taking, such as Piaget's three-mountain task. There is something special about tasks which require an awareness of the mental states of others. Leslie (1992) summarizes research demonstrating that autistic children can arrange sequences of pictures that depict physical-causal sequences, but are far less able to sequence events that require consideration of the mental states of the participants. This and similar research with a variety of ages and populations has stimulated the hypothesis that an essential part of development is the emergence of a "theory of mind" on the part of the child. The distinctive cognitive profile of the autistic child is, in Leslie's phrase, a *metarepresentational deficit*, not a more general cognitive or affective disorder. On the language side, Tager-Flusberg compared the spontaneous speech produced by autistic and age- and language-matched Down syndrome. She found few differences for most categories of internal state words, but much less language to call for attention or to refer to cognitive mental states. Thus there are uneven profiles in both the cognitive and language domains, but these uneven profiles match up in a fashion which is highly consistent with an impaired ability to reflect on their own and other people's minds. The enormous obstacle this places in the development of social relationships is both obvious, and well-documented.

Childhood maltreatment – a term used here to include both abuse and neglect – contrasts with autism in both cause and language outcome (Cicchetti & Beeghly, 1987). Although some characteristics of children put them at higher risk than others for maltreatment, the primary causal factor is environmental. Abusive and neglecting mothers interact with their young children less; they are less likely to play with their children or talk with them, and more likely to ignore verbal messages from their children. Not surprisingly, maltreated infants are more likely to form insecure attachments with their primary caregivers. Thus, both directly, via reduced communication from their mothers, and indirectly, via higher risk of insecure attachment, maltreated children are at risk for communication disorders. Nevertheless, in a study of Gersten and others (reported in Cicchetti & Beeghly, 1987), a group of 25-month-old maltreated children showed no significant differences from a matched non-maltreated group on a variety of measures of language development. The authors suggest that early language development may be highly canalized, that is, buffered against wide variation in environment. Later stages may be more sensitive to input. Gersten and others did observe a strong correlation between attachment security and language performance at 25 months. They hypothesized that the effects of maltreatment on language would be more evident later. Coster et al. (1989) therefore examined the language of a (separate) group of 31-month-old maltreated children. At 31 months, maltreated toddlers had smaller expressive vocabularies and shorter MLU than the matched nonmaltreated group. Their discourse skills were also affected, particularly in the frequency of talking about their own activities, requesting information, and using decontextualized speech, i.e., references to persons and events outside the here and now. Most relevant for the current discussion, the maltreated children had mastered fewer internal state words (assessed from parent report) and produced fewer such words in conversation (from observations) than the nonmaltreated group. On the whole, the types of internal state language produced were quite similar in the groups, with the exception that the maltreated children were less likely to refer to physiological stages (hunger, thirst, sleepiness) and negative affect (hate, disgust, anger) than the nonmaltreated group. This pattern might be an early signal of difficulty in negative emotion regulation.

A plausible explanation for the contrasting results at 25 months and 31 months is that they reflect the emergence of a stage-specific deficit in language due to maltreatment. However, longitudinal research will be necessary to confirm this explanation. It would be particularly interesting to know if it is the insecurely attached toddlers at 25 months who develop language disorders later.

Finally, we consider the relation of language and learning disabilities, and behavior/conduct problems. In both domains, along with much controversy, there is a long history of theorizing which places self-regulation at the core of the problem and which utilizes language as a primary intervention medium, e.g., Meichenbaum (1977) and Feuerstein et al. (1980). As Rutter (1972) pointed out, it is unlikely that the behavioral disturbance is a major cause of the language disorder, as the onset of the language disorder occurs earlier. However, this still leaves open two possibilities. First, the language disfunction may be the cause of the behavioral problem, mediated by impaired social relationships with both parents and peers due to communication deficits, as well as by educational failure. Alternatively, language and behavioral problems may both reflect a common underlying factor, such as brain disfunction, family discord, or specific cognitive skills such as categorization or self-regulation. Sorting out these two possibilities is an underlying theme of the present book. For the present discussion, we will simply focus on the evidence for the role of language in self-regulation.

Functioning in a social world requires a responsivity to the actions of others. Neither children nor adults can completely control the actions of other people, but they must interpret the actions of others and respond appropriately. This conception of the nature of social interaction is a highly cognitive one, and reflects the emergence of information processing models of social competence (Dodge et al., 1986). Their model includes five separable and sequential steps for social interaction:

1. encoding social cues or stimuli, e.g., perceiving facial expressions or gestures;
2. interpretation of those cues; e.g., recognizing an expression of anger;

3. response search; e.g., generating possible actions under the circumstances, such as grabbing, or turn-sharing;
4. response evaluation; e.g., considering the likelihood of various responses by the other person to each of the child's possible responses; and
5. enactment; e.g., producing an effective request for turn-sharing.

Language may play a role in all of these, but is especially likely to be important for numbers 2, 4, and 5. In other research, Dodge and his colleagues have found evidence for deficits in each of these areas for children with poor social competence (Crick & Dodge, 1994).

A re-examination of Table 1.1, will illustrate the similarity of the ABCD model of Greenberg & Kusché (1993), especially for the preschool and school years, to that of Dodge et al. On the basis of this model, Greenberg & Kusché developed the PATHS (Promoting Alternative Thinking Strategies) curriculum for school-aged children. The curriculum was first developed by Greenberg for hearing-impaired children. The majority of hearing-impaired children are born to hearing parents. Due to the limited efficacy of oral approaches and the limited ability of parents to learn sign language, communication between hearing-impaired children and their parents is often severely limited. Greenberg hypothesized that limitations in language, especially for emotion and other internal states, might be a cause for social difficulties for many hearing-impaired children and adolescents. The success of the PATHS curriculum led Greenberg & Kusché to elaborate the curriculum for use with a wider range of children at risk for behavior problems and conduct disorders.

The PATHS curriculum is designed to be utilized in three 20–25 minute lessons per week for 24 weeks. Lessons focus on recognition and understanding of social problems, recognition and labeling of emotion and other cues, generating alternative responses and evaluation of those alternatives, using role-playing and other techniques. For hearing-impaired students, total communication (signing and speech) is used to maximize communication.

Greenberg et al. (1995) report the results of three studies of the effectiveness of PATHS: one with deaf and hearing-impaired students, one with children in regular education, and one with children in special education (including a large proportion with learning disabilities). In each case there was a well-matched control group. In all three studies, use of the curriculum led to improvements in the ability to understand social problems and to develop effective alternative solutions, decreases in the percentage of aggressive/violent solutions, and increased understanding and recognition of emotions. All these results were based on children's response to hypothetical social problems such as being teased or being rejected from a game. In addition, teachers reported significant improvements in self-control, emotional understanding, thinking before acting, and other skills targeted by PATHS. In the study of children in special education, teachers reported improvement in the ability to tolerate frustration and to carry on positive peer relations. Strikingly

– given the general emphasis on externalizing conduct problems in this area – both children and teachers reported a decrease in children's sadness and depression.

The PATHS curriculum is a substantial and complex one, and it is not possible to identify the contribution of each component. But if the models discussed in this chapter are correct, *all* the components are essential.

CONCLUSION

The central idea of this chapter is that language is a tool for emotional and cognitive self-regulation as well as for social communication. It is a complex tool, not "all of a piece," and it is essential to look at some of the specific components of language, such as emotion and internal state vocabulary to understand the role of language in cognitive and social functioning.

The tool metaphor has much validity. Just as a physical tool, such as a saw, requires an intelligent hand to guide it, language requires intelligence to put it to work effectively. That intelligence has its sources partly within the developing human being, e.g., the cognitive requirements for use of mental state words, and partly outside the individual, in the experience provided by other people, both parents and peers.

Current research has demonstrated that children begin to learn some relevant components of language at a remarkably early age, though it is less clear why some children do this more rapidly and effectively than others. Still less is known about the development of the skills to use these socially acquired elements as a tool of self-regulation. More focused analysis of the linguistic interactions between children and their parents and peers, for a variety of populations, is needed to discover the most important kinds of modeling and scaffolding that make the remarkable transfer from public to private use of language possible.

REFERENCES

Bartsch, K. & Wellman, H. (1989). Young children's attribution of action to beliefs and desires. *Child Development*, **60**, 946–964.

Beeghly, M., Bretherton, I., & Mervis, C.B. (1986). Mothers' internal state language to toddlers. *British Journal of Developmental Psychology*, **4**, 247–260.

Bloom, L. & Beckwith, R. (1989). Talking with feeling: integrating affective and linguistic expression in early language development. *Cognition and Emotion*, **3**, 313–342.

Bloom, L. & Capatides, J.B. (1987). Expression of affect and the emergence of language. *Child Development*, **58**, 1513–1522.

Bloom, L., Lightbown, L., & Hood, L. (1975). Structure and variation in child language. *Monographs of the Society for Research in Child Development*, **40** (Serial No. 160).

Bretherton, I. & Beeghly, M. (1982). Talking about internal states: the acquisition of an explicit theory of mind. *Developmental Psychology*, **18**, 906–921.

Bretherton, I., Fritz, J., Zahn-Waxler, C., & Ridgeway, D. (1986). Learning to talk about emotions: a functionalist perspective. *Child Development*, **57**, 529–548.

Brown, J.R. & Donelan-McCall, N. (March, 1993). Mental states in daily conversations: children, siblings, mothers, and friends. Society for Research in Child Development, New Orleans, LA.

Brown, J.R. & Dunn, J. (1991). "You can cry, mum": The social and developmental implications of talk about internal states. *British Journal of Developmental Psychology*, **9**, 237–256.

Brown, J.R. & Dunn, J. (1992). Talk with your mother or your sibling? Developmental changes in early family conversations about feelings. *Child Development*, **63**, 336–349.

Bruner, J.S. (1973). *Beyond the Information Given: Studies in the Psychology of Knowing*. New York: Norton.

Capelli, C.A., Nakagawa, N., & Madden, C.M. (1990). How children understand sarcasm: the role of context and intonation. *Child Development*, **61**, 1824–1841.

Carey, S. (1978). The child as word learner. In M. Halle, J. Bresnan, & G.A. Miller (eds) *Linguistic Theory and Psychological Reality*. Cambridge: MIT Press (pp. 264–293).

Cicchetti, D. & Beeghly, M. (1987). Symbolic development in maltreated youngsters: an organizational perspective. *New Directions for Child Development*, No. 36, 47–68.

Coster, W.J., Gersten, M.S., Beeghly, M., & Cicchetti, D. (1989). Communicative functioning in maltreated toddlers. *Developmental Psychology*, **25**, 1020–1029.

Crick, N.R. & Dodge, K.A. (1994). A review and reformulation of social information-processing mechanisms in children's social adjustment. *Psychological Bulletin*, **115**, 74–101.

Denham, S.A., Cook, M., & Zoller, D. (1992). "Baby looks *very* sad": Implications of conversations about feelings between mother and preschooler. *British Journal of Developmental Psychology*, **10**, 301–315.

Dodge, K.A., Pettit, G.S., McClaskey, C.L., & Brown, M.M. (1986). Social competence in children. *Monographs of the Society for Research in Child Development,* **56** (Serial No. 213).

Dunn, J. (1985). *Sisters and Brothers*. Cambridge: Harvard University Press.

Dunn, J., Bretherton, I., & Munn, P. (1987). Conversations about feeling states between mothers and their young children. *Developmental Psychology*, **23**, 132–139.

Fenson, L., Dale, P.S., Reznick, J.S., Bates, E., Thal, D., & Pethick, S.J. (1994). Variability in early communicative development. *Monographs of the Society for Research in Child Development*, **59** (Serial No. 242).

Feuerstein, R., Rand, Y., Hoffman, M.B., & Miller, R. (1980). *Instrumental Enrichment: An Intervention Program for Cognitive Modifiability*. Baltimore, MD: University Park Press.

Greenberg, M.T. & Kusché, C.A. (1993). *Promoting Social and Emotional Development in Deaf Children: The PATHS Project*. Seattle, WH: University of Washington Press.

Greenberg, M.T., Kusché, C.A., Cook, E.A., & Quamma, J. (1995). Promoting emotional competence in school-aged children: The effects of the PATHS Curriculum. *Development and Psychopathology*, **7**, 117–136.

Kopp, C.B. (1989). Regulation of distress and negative emotions: a developmental view. *Developmental Psychology*, **25**, 343–354.

Leslie, A.M. (1992). Pretense, autism, and the theory-of-mind module. *Current Directions in Psychological Science*, **1**, 18–21.

Markman, E.M. & Wachtel, G.F. (1988). Children's use of mutual exclusivity to constrain the meanings of words. *Cognitive Psychology*, **20**, 121–157.

Meichenbaum, D. (1977). *Cognitive-behavior Modification: An Integrative Approach*. New York: Plenum.

Nelson, K.E. (1981). Individual differences in language development: Implications for development and language. *Developmental Psychology*, **17**, 170–187.

Ninio, A. & Bruner, J. (1978). The achievement and antecedents of labelling. *Journal of Child Language*, **5**, 1–15.

Piaget, J. (1959). *The Language and Thought of the Child*, 3rd edn. London, Routledge.

Pine, F. (1985). *Developmental Theory and Clinical Process*. New Haven, CT: Yale University Press.

Ridgeway, D., Waters, E., & Kuczaj, S.A. (1985). Acquisition of emotion-descriptive language: receptive and productive vocabulary norms for ages 18 months to 6 years. *Developmental Psychology*, **21**, 901–908.

Rogoff, B. (1990). *Apprenticeship in Thinking*. New York: Oxford University Press.

Rutter, M. (1972). *The Child with Delayed Speech*. Philadelphia, PA: Lippincott.

Tager-Flusberg, H. (1992). Autistic children's talk about psychological states: Deficits in the early acquisition of a theory of mind. *Child Development*, **63**, 161–172.

Toth-Sadjadi, S. (April, 1993). The development of internal state language in linguistically precocious toddlers. In E.V. Clark (ed.) *Proceedings of the Twenty-fifth Annual Child Language Research Forum*. Stanford, CA: Center for the Study of Language and Information (pp. 271–279).

Vygotsky, L.S. (1986). *Thought and Language* (revised edition). Cambridge: MIT Press.

Wellman, H.M. & Bartsch, K. (1988). Young children's reasoning about beliefs. *Cognition*, **30**, 239–277.

2 Understanding language dysfunction from a developmental perspective: an overview of pragmatic theories

PETER CHABAN

INTRODUCTION

Over the last decade there has been a shift in focus concerning the clinical view of language usage by children and adolescents. Traditionally, children's language has been described in terms of phonology (i.e. sounds), lexis (i.e. words) and syntax (i.e. sentences). Morphological rules explained the use of inflections and grammar rules the appropriate word orders, while semantics primarily gave the referential meanings for individual words or sentences. Psychologically and biologically, language was perceived as hard-wired (Pinker & Bloom, 1990). This meant that it was linked to a specific region of the brain (the left hemisphere) and that every child had an innate predisposition to acquire language skills. These language skills were further seen as developmental rather than random. This meant that each skill has been clearly marked out in terms of building blocks or stages from first phonemes to lexical classes and degrees of syntactic complexity. The failure to achieve certain levels of speech and language proficiency by a specified age usually signalled the possibility of a language disability. Disabilities were generally divided into two categories. They were either receptive problems (i.e. understanding language) or expressive problems (i.e. formulating and producing language). Both receptive and expressive language disabilities could be further identified as either phonological, lexical or syntactic problems.

Though many children with speech and language problems benefited from intensive remediation, there was also a group who either continued to have problems using language or developed problems after appropriate acquisition of speech and language. The problems usually involved the application of language in social or learning situation, the use of language for problem solving or in expressing affect. These problems were not language specific; that is they did not involve phonological, lexical or syntactic problems. Instead, they were language related problems. They involved the use of language in specialized situations. Known as communication problems, they were represented by different cognitive difficulties, rather than speech and language disorders. Here the psychological factors shifted from perceptual and short-term memory problems to higher order cognitive problems hampering language performance. These could include attentional problems in the area of control and self-analysis (Alexander, Benson, & Stuss, 1989) or problems allocating cognitive resources to memorize and recall complex behavioral scripts (Montgomery, 1992) or the inability to integrate visual-spatial information with linguistic information (Bruder et al., 1992). As well, evidence from head injury patients and imaging data began to suggest that these were not left hemisphere problems, but rather they were the result of insults to the right hemisphere of the brain (Chapman, Culhane, & Levin, 1992).

Though the traditional linguistic categories were able to describe speech and language disabilities, they fell short in explaining more complicated communication problems evident in right brain dysfunctions. As a result researchers and clinicians began to look for alternative language models that would work as adjuncts to the more structural models. Two approaches were found. One came from a linguistic background and was called "functional linguistics," while the other came from a philosophical background and was called "pragmatics" (Levinson, 1983). The traditional models of language were generally concerned with describing the form and its meaning in language. Pragmatics and functional linguistics introduced context as a third dimension into the communication process. It had been evident to many researchers that the same "form" could alter its "meaning" based on the "context" used for the "form." This can be shown in the following example:

Speaker A: That's a Yankee's cap you're wearing.
Speaker B: No its not. Its mine.

This example is taken from a conversation between an adult and a mentally handicapped youngster. The youngster has interpreted the language form's literal meaning, yet he has failed to comprehend the contextual (pragmatic) meaning. He has failed to integrate linguistic information with subtle contextual information.

Introducing context into the language equation brings with it a variety of new questions. The first one is, how do you define context. Since it is everything outside of the actual form of the language, its scope initially appears to defy systemization. This is why some linguistic models (i.e. transformational-generative) do not believe context has a place in linguistics. The second question is, what is the connection between the organization of contextual information and the ability of the brain's cognitive systems to process that information. It has been argued that context is a cultural phenomena and therefore not to be equated with biologically based behaviors, yet a certain proportion of people with specific neurological abnormalities are unable to integrate contextual cues with language in order to generate appropriate conversations. In this chapter, I would like to review some approaches to pragmatics, first from a philosophical and then from a linguistic point of view. In describing these two approaches, hopefully we can begin to refine the scope of contextualization and explore the connections between pragmatic behavior and cognitive correlates.

PHILOSOPHY'S APPROACH TO PRAGMATICS

Prior to the influence of pragmatics, the study of meaning in language had generally focused on what was known as "reference" theory. This was the belief that words and their arrangement into sentences mapped the complete meaning. This could in turn be checked by testing the truth-value (logic) of the proposition. In philosophy this thinking was supported by the logical positivist school. Wittgenstein, in his early work adhered to this, but later realized that it did not apply to everyday conversational language. He would later state: "Don't ask for the meaning, ask for the use of a word" (Cranston 1969, p. 39). Wittgenstein was proposing that meaning not be defined in terms of decontextualized meaning, but rather in terms of the speaker's overall intentions towards his or her audience. The speaker-listener perspective was one of the first to be examined by philosophers. Interest was directed towards the speaker's intentions and the listeners expectations within a conversation. This required examining social norms that both speaker and a listener shared during a conversation.

H.P. Grice (1975) was one of the first to set out co-operative principles for conversations. Grice believed that much of the decoding done by the listener in a conversation depended not on their ability to pick up the referential meaning, but rather the ability to read the inferential meaning coming out of a conversation. To do this, it was necessary to establish socially accepted ground rules for conversations. Grice developed four "maxims" necessary for conversations to be understood by both participants. The first was the maxim of Manner, which stated that a speaker must be perspicuous by avoiding obscurity and ambiguity, while being brief and orderly. Next, was the maxim of Relation which stated that a speaker's contribution to a conversation must be relevant to the topic at hand. Third, was the maxim of Quality, which required that a speaker state what he believes to be true and that he supports it with evidence. The fourth maxim is that of Quantity which required that a speaker contributes no more than is necessary to a conversation.

These maxims allowed both the speaker and listener to assume that a conversation was functioning within the contextual boundaries established by these principles. For example:

Speaker A: How was your day?
Speaker B: At least it didn't rain today.
Speaker A: That Bad.
Speaker B: You Bet.

It is difficult to deduce, based solely on referential meaning, that B's response has anything to do with A's question. Yet, A is able to draw a meaning from B's utterance. As Levinson (1983, p. 103) has pointed out, it is not that the speakers always adhere to these maxims, but that the listener always tries to interpret conversational information in terms of Grice's maxims. This is what A has done by interpreting B's reply. A has assumed that B's response was to his question (relation and quality maxims). Once speaker A has interpreted A's obtuse reply, he signals that he understands B's statement. It then becomes B's responsibility to confirm A's inference. Though all four utterances lack any referential connection, they make sense to the conversants based on their mutual knowledge of the co-operative principles for conversation. It is not unusual to find Gricean Maxims not being applied when examining pragmatic problems associated with certain insults to the brain, like those associated with head injury. In such cases it is often the maxims of Manner and Quantity that are ignored. Buckingham (see Schwartz, 1982) has also suggested that the failure to comprehend schizophrenic discourse may in part be due to the consistent failure of schizophrenic speakers to respect conversational maxims, especially those of Quality and Relation. This in turn results in the listener's inability to draw out the implications of the speaker's intent.

Whereas, Grice's "Maxims" presented a kind of Queensbury rules for shared knowledge in conversations, "Speech Act Theory" which was developed by Austin (1962) and refined by Searle (1969, 1975) looked specifically at the results in terms of speaker's intent and the realized effect on the listener.

Austin recognized that when we speak, we do much more than just describe the world around us. In interacting with others, we also convey our feelings, our beliefs as well as our wishes through conversation. Austin differentiated this dichotomy of information into constative and performative statements. Constative statements were descriptive utterances and could be analyzed in terms of their referential meaning. Performative statements on the other hand, carried speaker intentions in being uttered. For example, the statement, "I haven't eaten all day," has a constative meaning which is exactly the above statement, but it also has a performative meaning which could be, "When do we eat?" or "Please, feed me." Austin recognized that a single utterance could convey information, express a speaker's intentions and affect a listener's behavior. He proposed the following three speech acts occurred simultaneously when we spoke:

1. a *Locutionary Act*: This is the actual production of the words used. It is the "form" and "referential meaning."
2. an *Illocutionary Act*: This is the utterance having an actual function (force), such as apologizing, requesting, demanding, informing, etc. This could be described as part of the "pragmatic" meaning.
3. a *Perlocutionary Act*: This refers the listener's response, either verbally or behaviorally to the speaker's locutionary act and its illocutionary force (e.g. the listener's reaction to a speaker's demands).

These three acts combine to create a speech act. The "locutionary act" by itself represents a decontextualized look at language form. It tells us nothing of the full meaning of the utterance. The illocutionary force and its perlocutionary effect represent the pragmatic meaning and they require contextual knowledge by the participants in order to generate the pragmatic meaning. The three acts taken together represent the form, the semantic and pragmatic meaning as well as the context as defined in terms of the speaker, listener, and social situation.

John Searle, who had been a student of Austin's further refined Austin's speech act theory. He replaced Austin's three speech acts with a single illocutionary act consisting of the illocutionary force and the propositional content. He also suggested that there were five basic types of action or illocutionary acts that a speaker could convey (Searle, 1976). These were "representatives" (i.e. assertions, conclusions, etc.), "directives" (i.e. requests and questions), "commissives" (i.e. promises, offerings, etc.), "expressives" (i.e. apologies, thanking, etc.) and "declarations" (i.e. christening, marriage vows, etc.) (Levinson, 1983, p. 240). Coulthard (1977) has also pointed out that though Searle continued Austin's work, there was one important difference. Searle viewed illocutionary force as the result of the listener's interpretation, rather than the speaker's intention (Coulthard, 1977, p. 24). Searle recognized that listeners had to be especially vigilant in understanding conversational information, especially in casual conversation because much of the information was through indirect directives. He categorized six primary indirect directives in speech acts that listener's need to be able to decode. These examples are from Coulthard (1977, p. 25):

1. Sentences concerning listener's ability: "Can you pass the salt?"
2. Sentences concerning listener's future action: "Will you pass the salt?"
3. Sentences concerning wish or want: "I would like (you to pass) the salt."
4. Sentences concerning listener's desire or willingness: "Would you mind passing the salt?"
5. Sentences concerning reasons for action: "It might help if you passed the salt."
6. Sentences embedding either one of the above or explicit performative: "Can I ask you to pass the salt?"

Searle's work on refining speech act theory, especially in the area of indirect directives has found useful application in researching pragmatic difficulties in right-brain damaged individuals (for a summary of studies, see Stemmer, 1994).

The work done on conversational co-operation and speech act theory can be seen as a necessary knowledge or metadiscourse knowledge required to ensure successful conversations. But, there is also interest in the specific organization of conversations. This is often called conversation analysis. It is also a diverse field of study with a variety of approaches and theories. I would like to focus on three constructs that are often discussed. They are "turn taking," "adjacency pairs" and "overall organization" (Levinson, 1983).

Turn taking initially studied by sociologists Sacks, Schegloff, & Jefferson (1974) describes the processes involved in conversational exchanges between speakers. Smith & Leinonen (1992, p. 71), identify five essential areas of interest in studying turn taking:

1. how the speaker indicates to the listener that he or she wants to yield the floor;
2. how the change of role of speaker/listener proceeds;
3. how silence is dealt with;
4. how overlap is dealt with;
5. how interruptions are dealt with.

The ability to manage these five "hows" becomes essential to successful communication. For example, Scallon & Scallon (1981) show how the difference in pause time between English and Athabaskan can lead to failed conversations as well as biased impressions. English has a pause time of about maximum one second. If the listener does not take his turn in that one-second pause, the speaker takes that as a cue to continue his discourse. Athabaskan has a pause time of one and a half seconds. As a result of this variation in pause time, English speakers feel that native Athabaskans have nothing to say because the English speaker cannot wait that extra half-second for the Athabaskan's reply and Athabaskans believe that English speakers never stop talking and have no desire to listen to other people's ideas because they are unable to pause for that extra half-second. The result is failed communication as well as stereotyped impressions of different cultures.

Adjacency pairs identify the different types of initiation-response types in a conversation. The first part of the pair is able to predict the second member of the pair. For example, a question will predict an answer. The taxonomy of adjacency pairs is not a closed class since the number of performatives has yet to be quantified. As a result, adjacency pairs will vary from researcher to researcher. Common adjacency pairs include: question–answer, offer–acceptance, greeting–greeting, complaint–apology, etc. Olson, Bell, & Torrance (1983) in their study of discourse in first graders set up the following adjacency pairs:

- if comment, then acknowledgments
- if directives, then compliance
- if turnabouts, then compliance

Comments included the following: assertions, acknowledgments, responses, and rhetorical questions. Directives included: genuine questions, indirect questions, clarifications, requests for action and suggestions. Turnabouts were comments followed with directives. The point to be made here is that the construct of adjacency pairs is not a closed class, but rather defined according to one's area of interest.

The third construct for speech analysis is that of overall organization (Levinson, 1983). Levinson sees this as a type of recurrent sequencing evident in specific kinds of conversation (p. 309). These are conversations that have set moves, such as a telephone conversation, job interview or polite greeting. Ruqaiya Hasan has suggested that there is an organizational model for everyday reasoning (personal communication). In Ruqaiya's model of conversational reasoning she identifies a four-step process used by a speaker trying to make a point. The first step is the Claim. This can be either an assertion or a command. It is followed by Reason, which either characterizes the claim as part of a class or a consequence of the claim. This is followed by stating a Principle which is a universal domain and finally the reasoning is Grounded by defining the universal domain. She gives as an example the following comment by a mother to her child:

> Claim: don't shake that juice about
> Reason: it will spill and you'll get it over me
> Principle: you know liquids spill, if shaken about
> Grounding: this is a law of nature.

Co-operative principles, speech acts, and conversational analysis represent three components of pragmatics that make minimal reference to linguistic structures. This has to do with two phenomena in conversational language. The first is the stretch of language that is being described. The larger the stretch of language, the less predictable the linguistic choices. As a result it becomes very difficult to draw up rules. The second problem concerns the dependency on context to derive meaning from utterances. Linguistic description has traditionally been concerned with describing decontextualized language. Models for contextualized linguistics are not common in North American scholarship. In the next section I will look at approaches to contextualized linguistics also known as functional linguistics.

LINGUISTIC APPROACH TO PRAGMATICS

The last 20 years have seen linguistic theory divided into two camps; those who see language in terms of universal properties and these who see language in terms of its functional properties. According to universal theory, because of cognitive homogeneity in the human species, all languages share the same infrastructures. These models are usually "idealized models" that do not explain language behavior beyond the sentence. Their phonology, syntax, and semantics are highly rule-governed and formalized. Functional theory, on the other hand, does not begin with the cognitive-language dynamic. Instead, it sees language as a tool for communication and communication as a primary part of social interaction, with all that socialization entails in the human species.

In devising a grammar, linguists have to deal with the relationship between form and meaning (referential and contextual). Universal grammars tend to put more emphasis on form, therefore developing abstract and usually very parsimonious formalizations of language. These grammars tend to be syntagmatic, that is they look at the relationships between words, but they shy away from explaining why these forms are able to represent meanings and when they are to be used. Functional grammars tend to put less description into form and more description into meaning. They tend to be more paradigmatic, emphasizing the relationship between user choices and language operations (Halliday, 1985). The challenge in a functional model is to identify the categories of meaning that the grammar can describe within specific situations. When looking at functional grammars, there are two important distinctions to note. First, the primary unit of study is the text which can be realized through sentences and their related components. Secondly, the text's meaning is dependent on the context it is used in. Thus, it is necessary to identify different contexts and how they alter text meaning.

Halliday, working in the Firthian tradition had identified three types of meaning or metafunctions as he calls them, that language realizes through its grammar. These metafunctions were initially called the ideational, interpersonal and textual functions (in the 1985 Functional Grammar, these were changed to representation, exchange, and message). These metafunctions are carried by stretches of language identified as units. These units ranked from largest size are sentence, clause, word group, word, morpheme, and phoneme. Each unit can realize a metafunction, though only the sentence will realize all three metafunctions at once. Halliday identified that each metafunction has specific systems that operate within any rank and are used to achieve meaning. These systems represent a speaker's possible choices within the grammar. One can see why these grammars are called "chain and choice," "systemic" and finally "functional" based on the primary operators within the grammar.

In functional linguistics the primary unit of study is the clause, which carries within its grammatical structure the potential for realizing metafunctions (Halliday, 1985, p. 37). But the expression of thoughts and ideas consists of stretches of language larger than clauses. Halliday identified systems that work within each metafunction to build a cohesive and coherent text. Within the textual metafunction, three systems work to organize the discourse into a unified thought. Halliday identified these as theme, information and cohesive systems. The theme system represents the internal organization of a clause. Theme represents the most important information in a statement and as such always comes first in the English clause. It is followed by the rheme which is the elaboration of the theme. The information system does not correspond to clause structure, but in spoken language it is identified through tone groups. The use of tonality not only reveals speaker affect, but it also differentiates new and given (old) information in a text. Because of limited cognitive capacity, discourse has built in redundancy (previously given information) in order to contextualize new information. When we speak, we always give tonic prominence to the introduction of new information. The following example shows both the theme and information systems in operation.

A: Are **you** coming back to work?

theme	rheme
new	given

B: | don't **know** yet.

theme	rheme
given	new

In theme and information systems it can be seen how phonology and grammar function to connect information.

The third system is that of cohesion. Initially introduced in 1976 (Halliday & Hasan), it was further refined in Halliday's *Introduction to Functional Grammar* (1985). Four cohesive devices were identified. They were Reference, Ellipsis/Substitution, Conjunction and Lexical Cohesion. Cohesive Reference entails using one word to point to another word in the discourse (known as endophoric reference) or to point to an entity outside the discourse, but part of the situation (known as exophoric reference). The three types of cohesive reference include personal pronouns, demonstrative pronouns and comparative references. The personal and demonstrative pronouns are able to show both endophoric and exophoric relationships, while the comparative references express only endophoric relationships. The following are examples of Cohesive Reference:

1. Personal Pronouns: John is absent. **He** is ill.
2. Demonstrative Pronoun: **This** goes over **there**.
3. Comparative: John ate **more than you**.

The second cohesive device is ellipsis/substitution. Ellipsis involves the omission of text with the assumption that the listener can infer what has been omitted. It occurs in nominal and verbal positions, as well as with whole clauses. For example:

A: "Who is going to the game?"
B: "John (is going to the game), but Mary can't." (go to the game)

Ellipsis is one of the most common devices in everyday speech, yet it is one of the most difficult to recognize for people with pragmatic problems. It is very dependent on memory skills, since the listener must carry information to fill the gaps and it is dependent on implicature knowledge since the listener must also infer meaning based on his or her understanding of the speaker's intent. Substitution involves slotting either "do," "one," "so," or "the same" in the nominal, verbal or clausal position. The following example is of substitution:

A: "Which sandwich would you like?"
B: "I'll have that **one**."
C: "And I'll have **the same**."

The third cohesive device is conjunction. Halliday (1985) sees cohesive conjunctions as the logical-semantic organization of propositions within a discourse. It allows the speaker to set up relationships between ideas. Halliday has identified three relational categories which he calls elaboration, extension and enhancement (1985, pp. 302–10). Lexical Cohesion is the fourth type of cohesion. This involves the use of repetition, synonyms, superordinates and collocations (thematic relations) to unify a text. For example:

John heard the sound of a bear. The noise of the bear was subtle, but this animal was not to be judged by his level of expression.

Repetition: bear; Synonymy: sound, noise; Superordinate: animal, bear; Collocation: subtle, level of sound.

Rochester & Martin (1979) used Halliday's Cohesion and Information systems to show how schizophrenic discourse breaks down. Among the things they identified was the over-dependency on lexical cohesive ties, specifically repetition to hold an extended stretch of thoughts together and failure to use the context. The following example, is that of a 17-year-old male (from data collected at Sunnybrook Health Science Centre's Adolescent Psychiatric Unit) diagnosed with schizophrenia who had disordered thoughts at the time of this sample:

1. Okay, here I go
2. I like this form of writing
3. think now
4. it is changing
5. I could write a bit on people with guns who shoot
6. everyone is nice but the sheriff knows everyone
7. he is mean and he loves flowers
8. keep on ticking

In reading these eight sentences, it becomes evident that the text does not hold together. Sentences 1 and 2 are unified by the personal pronoun "I." Sentence 3, we can assume refers to the speaker, since no new person has been introduced into the text. The text begins to fall apart in sentence 4 when "it" is presented without an antecedent ("it" turned out to be a reference to the clock on the wall). Both sentence 4 and 8 also introduce new information without any given information. Sentence 5 ends with an odd ellipsis. It also appears that the conjunctions in 6 and 7 would function with more clarity if they were reversed. In fact, what we are looking at in this sample is not disordered thought, but problems with language usage. This sample can easily be corrected once the cohesive and informational dysfunctions are identified.

1. Okay, here I go
2. I like this form of writing
3. think now
4. the clock is changing and I haven't much time
5. I could write a bit on people with guns who shoot each other
6. everyone in this town is nice and the sheriff knows everyone
7. he is mean, but he loves flowers
8. I better hurry, the clock keeps ticking

The work on cohesion and information systems helps to explain how language is able to chain thoughts into a unified whole. This type of context between clauses and larger stretches of meaning is often referred to as contextual organization. Contextual organization leads to the formation of discourse which functions according to internal textual organization, but also according to its usage within specified situations.

An interesting development in the systemic-functional tradition over the last decade has been the development of a model known as "communication linguistics." Developed by Michael Gregory and his colleagues, this model has attempted to account for language as context sensitive social behavior and as the mechanism for organizing knowledge structures. The elegance of this model is its ability to show an interactive relationship between situation, discourse structures and the language code (phonology-morphosyntax-semantics). Like Halliday's Functional Linguistic model, it uses systemic grammar, but it also sets out an elaborate description of situational domains, where specific language strategies are applied.

Gregory proposes that to communicate, we require both a knowledge of the world and a knowledge of language. He identifies these as "planal knowledge" and "stratal knowledge" respectively (Gregory, 1986). When we look at language as behavior, we identify three planes of knowledge, which are situation, discourse and manifestation. The situational plane accounts for cultural attitudes, staged events and incidents; the discourse plane is the linguistic encoding of the message and the manifestation plane is the substance (phonic or graphic) realization of the message (Gregory, 1982). When we look at language as code, we describe three strata; semology which involves conceptual and propositional relationships, morphosyntax which involves words and their arrangements, and phonology concerns the nature and patterning of sounds (1982, p. 5).

Because language is a behavior that varies according to situations, it is necessary to define situational constructs that predict language varieties. Two such constructs are the speech community context and the generic situation. The speech community context is a type of macro-setting. It is defined in terms of the speaker's temporal, geographic, social and individual provenances (Gregory, 1986). These are mirrored in the discourse plane as temporal, geographic, social and individual dialects. Temporal dialects would best be described as diachronic language features. Geographic dialect features capture regional differences in language variety. Social dialects reflect education and economic based variations, while individual dialect features would represent a person's idiosyncratic language qualities. The second construct is the generic situation. It is a micro-setting or an archetypal setting, such as a visit to the doctor, a school, a restaurant, and so on. Generic situations require knowledge about appropriate interactional behavior, experience around the sequence of events and the relationship between channel (medium) and the content of expression. The ability to select and use this knowledge manifests itself in the discourse plane as register. Register is the appropriate use of language within a specific situation. For example we will shift our register from casual to formal discourse depending on who we are speaking to and in what situation. Friends usually are addressed in a casual register, whereas strangers or people in authority are addressed in a formal register.

Both dialect and register (Gregory, 1967) features are represented in discourse. As mentioned earlier, dialect can be described in terms of *temporal, geographic, social,* and *individual* qualities. Register on the other hand is represented by the concurrence of *field, mode,* and *tenor* of discourse (Gregory & Carroll, 1978). These three features of register are the linguistic reflection of the speaker's purpose within a situation (Gregory, 1967, pp. 186–8).

The *field* of discourse relies to a great extent on the ideational metafunction (see Halliday's metafunctions) of language according to Gregory. As such, the *field* of discourse draws on the linguistic resources associated with the ideational metafunction. These may include transitivity, adjunctivization, tense, aspect, and lexical taxonomies (Gregory, 1986). *Tenor,* which is subdivided into personal and functional tenor, is the speaker's acknowledgment of the interpersonal nature of discourse. It is realized through the interpersonal metafunction and draws from the mood and modal system in the grammar, and the lexical use of attitudinals. Finally, the *mode* of discourse is dependent on the choice of presentation of information. In the most general sense, written and spoken discourse are two separate *modes* and within these two categories there are many subcategories. An example of how these two *modes* differ is in their respective use of words and sentences. Written language carries a higher lexical density with simpler sentence structures than spoken language (Halliday, 1985). The recognition of this type of distinction in language variety is represented within the textual metafunction and expresses itself with cohesion, theme, and information (new and given) systems. The failure to heed the importance of *mode* in discourse often leads to stilted discourse. This is sometimes evident in the presentation of seminars, which are often written to be read rather than to be spoken. As a result, the short syntax and nominal density leads to excessive information being presented too quickly for the audience to assimilate.

The clinical uses for "communication linguistics" are vast, both diagnostically and in treatment for communication disorders. One possible approach may be to take a closer look at the difference between discourse register (language variety according to use) and discourse dialect (language variety according to user) (Halliday, McIntosh, & Strevens, 1964). If the communication dysfunction is dialectal, then it may reflect limited or misused language behavior for a generic situation. If the dysfunction is with discourse register, then the issue may not be language based, but rather the failure to understand the different situations and the need for alternative varieties of language usage.

CONCLUSION

Communication appears to be a three-part process involving biology, language, and behavior. The biological nature of communication is evident in that children are able to acquire complex language skills by the age of three without any formal instruction. In the early stages of language development, these structures are simple because the needs of the child are simple. As the demands of the world increase, so does the size and complexity of the information one carries. These demands outstrip the capacity of the child's memory and attentional systems. As we grow older, we overcome these limitations by learning to use language structures in a variety of different ways. Single words develop multiple meanings, sentences develop ways of saying more with less, and discourses are able to compress both descriptive and emotional information into the same utterance. As well, we are able to process vast amounts of complex information by chunking it into categories, concepts, taxonomies, and other knowledge structures. These abilities are designated as metacognitive, metalinguistic or executive functions. They are skills that utilize language as a cognitive and social tool. This ability is called pragmatics. It involves the ability to use language not only to convey information, but to participate in the community and to learn. When pragmatic skills fail to develop, the implications are far-reaching, from failure in the school system to social and cultural exclusion. It is for these reasons that a systemized pragmatics needs to be developed that can characterize language performance in any situation.

REFERENCES

Alexander, M.P., Benson, D.F., & Stuss, D.T. (1989). Frontal lobes and language. *Brain and Language*, **37**, 656–691.

Austin, J.L. (1962). *How to do Things with Words*. Cambridge, MA: Harvard University Press.

Benson, J.D. & Greaves, W.S. (eds) (1985). *Systemic Perspectives on Discourse, Vol. 1, Selected Theoretical Papers from the 9th International Systemic Workshop*. Norwood, NJ: Ablex.

Benson, J.D., Cummings, M., & Greaves, W.S. (eds) (1988) *Linguistics in a Systemic Perspective*. Amsterdam: John Benjamins.

Berry, M. (1975). *Introduction to Systemic Linguistics, Vol. 1, Structures and Systems*. New York: St Martin's Press.

Berry, M. (1976). *Introduction to Systemic Linguistics, Vol. 2, Levels and Links.* New York: St Martin's Press.

Brown, G. & Yule, G. (1983). *Discourse Analysis.* Cambridge University Press.

Bruder, G., Stewart, J., Towey, J., et al. (1992). Abnormal cerebral laterality in bipolar depression: convergence of behavioral and brain event-related potential findings. *Biological Psychiatry,* **32**, 33–47.

Chapman, S., Culhane, K., & Levin, H. (1992). Narrative discourse after closed head injury in children and adolescents. *Brain and Language,* **43**, 42–65.

Coulthard, M. (1977). *An Introduction to Discourse Analysis.* London: Longman.

Cranston, M. (1969). *Philosophy and Language.* Toronto: CBC Publications.

de Beaugrande, R. & Dressler, W. (1981). *Introduction to Text Linguistics.* London: Longman.

Gregory, M. (1967). Aspects of variety differentiation. *Journal of Linguistics,* **3**, 177–198.

Gregory, M. (1982). *Notes on Communication Linguistics* (with the assistance of K. Malcolm, L. Asp, D. Watt, & J. Dill). Toronto: Glendon College Mimeo.

Gregory, M. (1985). Towards communication linguistics: a framework. In J.D. Benson & W.S. Greaves (eds) (1985) pp. 119–134.

Gregory, M. (1986). Generic structure and register: a functional view of communication. In J. D. Benson et al. (eds) (1988).

Gregory, M. & Carroll, S. (1978). *Language and Situation: Language Varieties and Their Social Context.* London: Routledge & Kegan Paul.

Grice, H.P. (1975). Logic and conversation. In P. Cole & J. Morgan (eds) *Syntax and Semantics 3: Speech Acts.* New York: Academic Press (pp. 41–58).

Halliday, M.A.K. (1985). *An Introduction to Functional Grammar.* Sevenoaks: Edward Arnold.

Halliday, M.A.K. & Hasan, R. (1976). *Cohesion in English.* London: Longman.

Halliday, M.A.K., McIntosh, A., & Strevens, P. (1964). *The Linguistic Science of Language Teaching.* London: Longman.

Hudson, R.A. (1980). *Sociolinguistics.* Cambridge: Cambridge University Press.

Katz, J. (1977). *Propositional Structure and Illocutionary Force.* Cambridge, Mass.: Harvard University Press.

Levinson, S. (1983). *Pragmatics.* Cambridge: Cambridge University Press.

Montgomery, J. (1992). Easily overlooked language disabilities during childhood and adolescence. *Pediatric Clinics of North America,* **39**, 513–524.

Olson, D., Bell, B., & Torrance, N. (1983). Discourse cohesion in first grade children's conversations. Paper presented at H.A. Gleason Retirement Symposium, University of Toronto.

Piaget, J. (1959). *The Language and Thought of the Child.* New York: Meridian.

Pinker, S. & Bloom, P. (1990). Natural language and natural selection. *Behavioral and Brain Sciences,* **13**, 707–784.

Rochester, S. & Martin, J.R. (1979). *Crazy Talk: A Study of the Discourse of Schizophrenic Speakers.* New York: Plenum Press.

Sacks, H., Schegloff, E.A., & Jefferson, G. (1974). The simplest systematics for the organization of turn-taking in conversation. *Language,* **50**, 696–735.

Sampson, G. (1980). *Schools of Linguistics.* Stanford: Stanford University Press.

Scallon, R. & Scallon, B. (1981). *Narrative, Literacy and Face in Interethnic Communication.* Norwood: Ablex.

Schegloff, E. (1972). Sequencing in conversational openings. In John Gumperz and

Dell Hymes (eds) *Directions in Sociolinguistics*. New York: Holt, Rinehart & Winston.

Schwartz, S. (1982). Is there a schizophrenic language? *Behavioral and Brain Sciences*, **5**, 576–626.

Searle, J.R. (1969). *Speech Acts*. London: Cambridge University Press.

Searle, J.R. (1975). Indirect speech acts. In P. Cole & J.L. Morgan (eds) *Syntax and Semantics 3: Speech Acts*. New York: Academic Press (pp. 59–82).

Searle, J.R. (1976). The classification of illocutionary acts. *Language in Society*, **5**, 1–24.

Smith, B.R. & Leinonen, E. (1992). *Clinical Pragmatics*. London: Chapman & Hall.

Stemmer, B. (1994). A pragmatic approach to neurolinguistics: Requests (re)considered. *Brain and Language*, **46**, 565–591.

Young, L. (1990). *Language as Behaviour, Language as Code*. Amsterdam: John Benjamins.

3 Atypical ontogeny: atypical development from a developmental perspective*

BRYNA SIEGEL

A child with a neuropsychiatric or learning disorder naturally grows and matures, but the normal processes of growth and development are subject to limitations defined by some sort of neuropathology. This chapter provides a model for systematically observing growth in such children. The model distinguishes among symptoms that result directly from neuropathology, symptoms that are adaptations to the neuropathology, and symptoms that result when the adaptations are inadequate. The model is designed to help efforts at prevention, early identification and treatment planning for neuro-psychiatric and learning disorders, and also to help investigators seeking correlations between etiologic risk factors and the most likely, direct manifestations of those risk factors.

ATYPICAL ONTOGENY

From the developmental perspective, behavioral change is viewed as "ontogeny" – a natural, upward, successively more integrated, intra-organismic evolution. From the medical-psychiatric perspective behavioral change is viewed as "morbidity" – an organic, downward, successively less well-integrated, intra-organismic devolution. These diametrically opposed concepts apply simultaneously when studying the emergence of neurodevelopmental disorders in children. Biologically based forms of atypical development in children consist of a decalage of normal ontogeny with increasing morbidity for the characteristics of the disorder that a child will eventually acquire.

Presented here is a model for characterizing *atypical ontogeny*, the process by which normal and atypical development proceeds simultaneously and interactively. Atypical ontogeny is defined as being present in those children who have some type of innate neurological dysfunction, whether or not specific, that results in neurologically based psychiatric and learning disorders.

* Parts of this chapter were presented at Society for Research in Child Development, New Orleans, LA, March, 1993; the International Association for Child and Adolescent Psychiatry, San Francisco, CA, July, 1994; and the American Academy of Child and Adolescent Psychiatry, New York, NY, October, 1994.

The term "neuropsychiatric" will be used to refer to specific disorders with psychiatric features such as autism or attention deficit disorder, and the broader term "neurodevelopmental" will also be used to refer to neuropsychiatric and other childhood-onset disorders of learning with a biological basis. Examples of atypical ontogeny will be drawn from the developmental histories of children with autistic spectrum disorders, attention deficit hyperactivity disorder, learning disabilities, mental retardation, and language disorders. Signs of atypical ontogeny also exist in some cases of other childhood onset neuropsychiatric disorders. These may include obsessive compulsive disorder, mood disorders, and childhood-onset schizophrenia, or other apparently developmental disorders where there is evidence for a significant heritable or other organic component. The present work focuses on understanding developmental trajectories in behaviorally disordered children where the dominant etiology is *not* environmental compromise, but rather compromise that starts with neurodevelopmental suboptimality. The working model presented in this chapter starts at the level of post-natal behavioral development, but is also complementary to studies of biological homologies of functional equivalents on the genetic, neurodevelopmental, and morphological levels (cf., Gottlieb, 1991; Striedter & Northcutt, 1991; Morgane et al., 1993).

The working hypothesis about atypical ontogeny is that disability in any single domain of development will systematically alter the way stimuli may be fully processed in other domains. Further, functional limitation in any one domain of development will affect the way in which intact (or relatively intact) functions from other domains of development may be deployed to compensate for, or to potentiate residual function in the more debilitated domain(s) of disability. Via this mechanism, atypical ontogeny – some innate and automatic compensation that moves the child in the direction of achievement of the original developmental potential – will have been attempted, but will have been achieved with only partial success depending on the severity of the original impairment, and the presence of concomitant impairments in other domains of development. Thus, development in a domain unaffected by disability may proceed normally – but only to the point at which some efferent input from the domain of disability might typically be expected to interdigitate with the unaffected domain of development. Subsequently, development in the area where development was previously normal will become atypical too. Development then proceeds via compensatory relationships formed among domains of development, restricted by the matrix of disability.

"Atypical ontogeny" versus "developmental psychopathology"

The term "atypical ontogeny" is used to refer to atypical development to emphasize that atypical development is the product of an interaction between

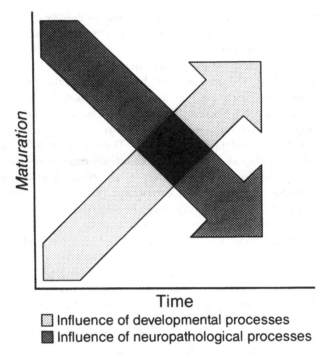

Time

Influence of developmental processes

Influence of neuropathological processes

Figure 3.1. Atypical ontogeny: interaction of maturation and morbidity.

atypical processes in some domains of development with more normal development proceeding in other domains of development. The study of "atypical ontogeny" can be distinguished from the study of "developmental psychopathology," a term most often used to refer to the study of psychopathology in children. "Developmental psychopathology" does not specifically refer to the natural history of development in such children. The term "developmental psychopathology" is not usually used to refer to studies of *how* atypical neurodevelopmental processes many begin to influence more unaffected domains of development; or how neurodevelopmental disorders are expressed with increasing specificity, finally reaching the point where they can be recognized as constituting discrete disorders. The central feature of studying atypical ontogeny in children is examining how the developmental trajectory of such children is an interaction between expected, normal ontogenetic processes and atypical features that are direct or adaptive products of brain dysfunction. Another way in which the study of atypical ontogeny can be contrasted to the study of developmental psychopathology is that the former implies a biological basis for dysfunction, while the latter may or may not include the study of behavioral disorders that have a biological basis.

In developmental neuropsychiatry, "maturational change" and "morbidity of the disease process" are basically seen as separate, coexisting phenomena, rather than as interdependent phenomena, even though both are seen as neurobiologically driven, and proceeding simultaneously. The concept of atypical ontogeny is employed here to emphasize that maturational change and morbidity are indeed interdependent phenomena (see Figure 3.1).

In Greek mythology, the goddess of wisdom, Athena, is born by emerging as a full-grown woman from the forehead of her father Zeus. Unlike Athena, children with neurodevelopmental disorders do not appear at birth to have the characteristics of their later disorders – these develop gradually. Autistic children are not born flapping their hands; nor are children with obsessive compulsive disorder born washing theirs. Instead, neurodevelopmental symptoms in children metamorphize over time, and in predictable ways that can be characterized by examining how functional aspects of developmental processes interact during both pre-morbid and clinical stages of a neurodevelopmental disorder.

DEVELOPMENTAL AND PSYCHIATRIC MODELS OF BEHAVIOR CHANGE IN CHILDREN

A main impetus for the conceptual framework for studying atypical ontogeny comes from a comparative analysis and synthesis of the developmental and medical models of clinical-behavioral change. Much of what is being studied as developmental neuropsychiatry or developmental psychopathology follows from a medical model of disease rather than from developmental theories that emphasize the dynamic, step-wise, or stage-wise behavioral changes in children.

Nomenclature

Models of behavioral disorders in children characterized by the developmental psychology and by the medical taxonomy of child psychiatry differ in characterization of action. In developmental psychology, "behavior" is studied, with behaviors being actions that can change in form, function, and frequency. In the more medical, child psychiatric model, behavioral signs of neuropsychiatric disorders are studied as "symptoms," mainly in terms of severity and duration. Developmental theory regards much behavioral change as "maturation," which quantitatively is usually best described as ordinal; that is, occurring in steps, stages, or other transformations that lead between one set of behaviors, and another set that it functionally subsumes (e.g., Pinard, 1975; Burger, 1977). The medical-psychiatric model, using the concept of morbidity to characterize change essentially focuses on a nondevelopmental, nominal relationship – that of the "pre-morbid" state, versus the later fully morbid state. (There is also talk of "subclinical" disorders, but no developmental progression is necessarily implied there either.) Thus, growth of a neuropsychiatric disorder is not so much seen as growth, but as a black and white classification. Clinically, the stance is not to characterize a child as "developing" a case of attention deficit hyperactivity disorder (ADHD) or becoming increasingly schizophrenic, but rather that the child may "meet full criteria for" (i.e., cross the threshold into) ADHD or schizophrenia in the future. Stages or steps to reaching such a threshold tend to be poorly characterized, since the clinical implication is to determine whether or not the disorder is present, and if so, to treat it. The medical model can conceptualize "residual" states of a disorder, but similarly, without any real developmental model for predicting how behavior may have become reintegrated so as to no longer constitute a fully expressed case of a particular disorder.

Form, function, and frequency of behaviors

In neuropsychiatric studies of children, some attention may be given to how symptoms change in form (i.e., severity) and some to changes in frequency (i.e., alleviation of symptoms), but less attention is paid to function. Sometimes symptoms are even referred to as "signs" which further denotes the emphasis on the static way in which symptomatic behavior may be viewed. In the medical model, it is taxonomically precise to be able to say that a symptom exists as a discrete entity that can be reliably measured without having to also describe its environmental antecedents or behavioral consequences. Thus "frequently speaking out of turn" for an ADHD child, or "unusual insistence on routines" for an autistic child is a symptom that exists *sui generis* – we do not have to understand where it came from or why the child does it except in a tautological way (i.e., he talks out of turn because he's hyperactive) in order to accept its role in characterizing the disorder.

It can be argued that the medical model is limited when studying the development of neuropsychopathology in children because of this lack of emphasis on function. Analyses of function are needed to comprehend how behaviors emerge in the first place and why. From a developmental perspective, a newly emerged behavior is seen as the dynamic result of assimilating or accommodating existing mental structures with new experience.

"INNATE," "VIRTUAL," AND "EPIPHENOMENAL" SIGNS OF ATYPICAL ONTOGENY

Signs of atypical ontogeny in a given disorder may be classifiable in one of three hierarchically ordered ways. These will be described as primary, *innate* signs; secondary, *virtual* signs; and tertiary *epiphenomenal* signs. The application of this three-level taxonomy may be helpful in analyzing the emergence of neurodevelopmental disorders in children, and in tracing the possible function of symptoms as they emerge.

First, some signs of atypical ontogeny are direct expressions of an inborn neurological defect, and can be thought of as the primary or innate signs of a disorder. This would include any clinical manifestation that is a direct result of the underlying defect, such as the impression of deafness in a child with a severe receptive language disorder, grimacing in a child with a movement disorder, or spontaneous laughing or crying in a young child with an incipient mood disorder.

The second form of atypical ontogeny is attempts made via remaining intact developmental processes to compensate for the inborn defect. Such forms of atypical development can be classified as secondary, or the virtual signs of a disability, meaning that they directly arise from the presence of the defect, but constitute an automatic self-adaptation to it. Thus, virtual signs of a receptive language disorder include echolalia (an attempt to use good auditory memory to hold on to in-coming language to allow more time for central processing); and the semantic-associational reading errors of a dyslexic (e.g., "car" for "jar" – another noun) as an attempt to use anticipated meaning in place of faulty visual perception. For an individual with a vocal tic due to Tourette's disorder, a virtual sign of disability might be the development of meta-cognitive strategies to temporarily mask the expression of involuntary tics with spontaneous laughing, or clowning behavior that apparently gives context to the odd noises. In any case, a virtual sign would be one where functionally, the behavior arises as a (partial) adaptation to neurodevelopmental defect. To the extent that such automatic adaptations are successful, the presence of a neurodevelopmental disorder may never be clinically detected, or never questioned until adulthood, when an individual may come to appreciate qualitative differences between his or her own mental processes and those of others (Denckla, 1993).

The third form of atypical ontogeny is the child's responses to trying, but failing to cope adequately given his inborn defect, which can be thought of as a tertiary, epiphenomenal sign of atypical ontogeny. Epiphenomena frequently encompass what are most likely to be thought of as the comorbid psychiatric manifestations of a developmental disorder. So for example, a child who has receptive language problems may come to be viewed as negativistic and often "not listening." A child with a movement disorder may become withdrawn in response to being taunted about tics or his attempts to cover them up. A child with an incipient mood disorder may be seen as unpredictable and uncaring because his affective responses appear out of proportion to how others react to the same situation. Epiphenomena therefore, are symptoms that emerge as people around a child react to his or her virtual disabilities that have developed as automatic means to cope with the underlying innate defect.

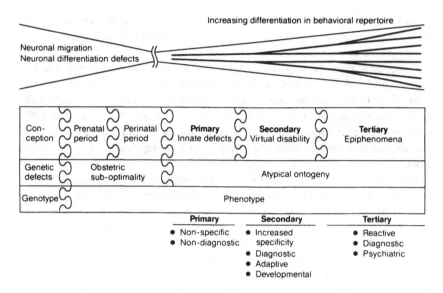

Figure 3.2. Developmental schema for atypical ontogeny.

It is probably also true that the earlier the innate disability interfered with normal development, the earlier virtual disabilities would have begun to emerge. At earlier stages the child's resources to formulate automatic compensations are likely to have been less well organized (as fewer mental resources would have been developed), and therefore the magnitude of overall later disability, both virtual disability as well as epiphenomena, would likely be relatively more prominent compared to when innate disability does not interfere until later in development.

In summary, from a developmental perspective, primary innate signs would develop at the earliest ages. These would be followed by the emergence of automatic attempts at self-generated adaptation – from which would arise secondary virtual signs of a disorder. Finally, tertiary epiphenomena of the disorder would emerge as a result of failures to adapt well enough.

Speculation: types of primary innate signs of neurodevelopmental disorders in children

The present model is intended to imply that understanding primary, innate signs of neurodevelopmental disorders in children is central to investigations that plan to link the continuum of reproductive casualty, or range of phenotypic expression to a particular clinical trait. Therefore it is useful to begin to generate a glossary of primary, innate signs that may be posited as central to a number of early arising neurodevelopmental disorders. Innate signs include a variety of phenomena that may be best measured on a psychophysiological level but that also have strong behavioral correlates, as will be described.

One innate sign of atypical ontogenetic processes is behaviors related to defects in *arousal regulation*, operationally defined as the child's ability to fully process all kinds of sensory stimulation without threshold malfunction. Manifestations of poor arousal regulation can include hyper- and hypo-responsitivity to sensory stimuli as commonly associated with autism and with mental retardation syndromes (cf., Ornitz & Ritvo, 1968). For example, dysfunction in visual arousal regulation could be manifested in visual over-attention to detail, viewing objects along a particular discrete axis or out of peripheral vision. Dysfunction in auditory arousal regulation could be manifested as seeming deafness (hypoacussis), or covering the ears in response to certain kinds of sounds (hyperacussis). Dysfunction in tactile and kinesthetic arousal regulation could be manifest by tactile scrutiny of certain textures, or a diminished pain reaction. Dysfunction in vestibular arousal regulation could be manifest in over- or under-responsiveness to movement stimulation such as swings, escalators, elevators, or a seeming inability to "get dizzy."

On a more cognitive level, deficits in *attention-habituation*, and *response to novelty* can be classified as innate signs of neurodevelopmental disorders. These areas of dysfunction are ones most often associated with attention deficit disorder and the physical hyperactivity that often accompanies a pattern of attention deficit. The constant draw to novel stimuli, the inability to attend for average durations, and the rapid rate of habituation to stimuli and subsequent rapid onset of boredom could all be considered innate phenomena that constitute maladaptive functions, leading to virtual signs of neuro-developmental disorders such as fidgetiness, constant movement, and other pathognomonic traits of ADHD (cf., Barkley, 1990).

A closely related cluster of innate signs of neurodevelopmental disorders include perseveration and failure to adapt to change. In severely cognitively impaired children perseveration is characterized by repetitive motor move-ments or perseverative activity. In children with more mild impairments (which may or may not be biologically homologous), there may be a compulsion to repetitively do things a certain way although there is no functional reason to persist in the pattern as is seen mainly in children with early onset OCD, and some children with autism.

Another possible innate deficit associated with neurodevelopmental dis-orders is an apparent lack of *reinforcer saliency*. Specifically, some children seem innately nonresponsive to contingent positive response to typically salient reinforcers such as positive social appraisal, or even foods. While lack of responsiveness to specific reinforcers can unquestionably be acquired through experience, clinically, there seems to be substantial individual differences among infants with neurodevelopmental disorders in terms of how readily re-sponsive they may be to common motivators. Infant stimulators working with neurodevelopmentally impaired infants are familiar with those for whom no social, food or other material reinforcer seems to have sustaining appeal.

Another type of innate phenomenon associated with neurodevelopmental disorders is *processing speed*. This is described last, because it is probably superordinate rather than unique, affecting the expression of many other types of innate defects across domains of development. The rate at which a child is able to integrate any type of sensory, cognitive or affective input probably has a primary and direct effect on the range of adaptations that may subsequently develop.

APPLICATIONS FOR THE STUDY OF ATYPICAL ONTOGENY

There are two major reasons to delineate the atypical ontogeny of neurodevelopmental disorders. First, by studying the natural history of neurodevelopmental disorders, we can parcel out earlier-emerging primary, innate signs that most likely relate to the disorder's biological origins from later-emerging virtual and epiphenomenal signs that are a result of the child's developmental and behavioral attempts to adapt to having some faulty apparatus. Thus, applying the taxonomy of innate versus virtual and epiphenomenal signs is useful for advancing investigations that examine the influence of reproductive casualty, or the developmental neurogenetics of manifestations of childhood neuropsychiatric and neurodevelopmental disorders. Second by studying the order in which signs of a disorder emerge, which is facilitated by hierarchically classifying signs as innate, virtual or epiphenomenal, it becomes possible to develop more prophylactic clinical interventions for neurodevelopmental disorders by preferentially treating primary, innate signs as they emerge, and providing the neurodevelopmentally compromised infant or toddler with means to make better adaptive accommodations that help circumvent the emergence of secondary, virtual signs.

In order to characterize the atypical ontogeny of each neurodevelopmental disorder and to document the progression of the various pre-morbid and fully expressed symptoms of the disorder, it is necessary to examine developmental trajectories for separate domains of development that are and are not innately affected — according to the specific nature of the disorder. In constructing the natural history of a disorder, it is necessary to know which earlier symptoms led to which later ones. Such a natural history later becomes a map for tracing a disorder's atypical ontogenetic processes.

Once a natural history is broken into its primary, secondary and tertiary constituent parts, each may be used for different sorts of studies or interventions: studies of innate signs are likely to be more elucidating in investigations on etiological factors than the study of virtual or epiphenomenal signs. A study of virtual signs may be most helpful in unraveling maladaptive patterns of learning and in creating new, highly tailored clinical interventions that can result in better adaptations to innate defects. Studying the presence of epiphenomenal characteristics of a disorder after understanding underlying innate and virtual characteristics of the disorder should be helpful in estimating the relative contribution of biology versus environment (i.e., adaptive or maladaptive learning) that is likely to occur in a particular disorder.

Each neurodevelopmental disorder of childhood can be described in terms of how early it is first manifest, and the extent to which the constituent symptoms are viewed as organic rather than as primarily environmentally induced. It can be postulated that disorders that are primarily organic in etiology will be represented by a heavier mix of innate or virtual signs, and that disorders with a relatively small biological component will be characterized primarily by some level of virtual disability, and later, by marked epiphenomena.

ATYPICAL ONTOGENY: APPLICATIONS FOR STUDYING THE ETIOLOGY OF NEURODEVELOPMENTAL DISORDERS

Presently, there are broadly accepted assumptions (and some data) that support an understanding that subtle neurogenetically regulated structural or chemical alterations in the brain are likely to be etiologically highly significant in the expression of specific neurodevelopmental disorders (Striedter & Northcutt, 1991; Morgane et al., 1993). Thus, the two areas of research where it can be heuristically useful to consider atypical ontogeny, and in particular, the concept of innate defects are: (1) studies of obstetric suboptimality and neuropsychiatric disorder, and (2) studies of the behavioral genetics of neuropsychiatric disorders in children. Figure 3.2, presented above, shows a hypothetical relationship between etiologic factors for neurodevelopmental disorders and subsequent innate, virtual, and epiphenomenal signs of those disorders.

Reproductive casualty continuum and atypical development

It has been shown that it is an over-simplification to hypothesize a one-to-one correspondence between specific pre- or peri-natal suboptimal events and subsequent specific developmental abnormalities (cf., Finegan & Quarrington, 1979, Deykin & MacMahon, 1980, for studies on autism; Goodman & Stevenson, 1989, Chandola et al., 1992, for studies of ADHD). Most infants and toddlers judged to show signs of neurological dysfunction have no or nonspecific neurological findings even when specific signs of neurodevelopmental maldevelopment (like not learning to walk by 18 months of age) are present. Obstetric suboptimality leading to atypical development appears to result from a continuum of reproductive casualty that implies increased *risk* for various types of atypical development rather than predicting *specific* domains in which developmental damage will most likely become evident. Conversely, some children with specific and observable brain damage subsequently develop normally (Shaffer, Chadwick, & Rutter, 1975; Rutter, Chadwick, Shaffer, & Brown, 1980), further supporting the idea that brain insults in young children have far less specificity when experienced early on in behavioral development. In both cases, knowledge about early brain plasticity and transferability of function as well as our understanding of the continuum of reproductive casualty suggest that direct predictive links between atypical brain structure and function, and atypical behavioral development will probably continue to be weakly linked. It therefore seems more logical that from the perspective of trying to understand neurodevelopmental disorders developmentally, the starting point should be observable post-natal behavior.

Innate signs of atypical ontogeny and phenotypic expression

The first task in studying atypical ontogeny is to better characterize early, premorbid signs (specifically, innate defects). Knowing more about which earlier and less specific behaviors (innate defects) lead to later, more specific, more diagnostic behaviors (specicifally, virtual disabilities) should help ferret out which basic neurogenetic, neuroanatomical, or neurochemical processes may be malfunctioning by identifying initial manifestations of inborn defects. However, as is the case in studies of obstetric suboptimality where it would be conceptually most parsimonious to assume that a structural agenesis in the brain results in a corresponding behavioral agenesis in some specific developmental function, it is probably also inaccurate to expect any one-to-one genotype-phenotype correlations. Such a formulation can only be derived from an over-simplified view of behavioral genetics. In reality, variability in behavior is likely partly attributable to variable penetrance resulting in a range of phenotypic expression. In addition, any model for the genetics of a childhood neuropsychiatric disorder is usually further complicated by the fact that as a syndrome, a polygenetic origin may be hypothesized (e.g., Feldman et al., 1993, in studies of dyslexia; Sprich-Buckminster et al., 1993, Gross-Tour, Shalev, & Amir, 1991, in studies of ADHD; Goodman & Stevenson, 1989, in studies of hyperactivity; Tallal et al., 1991, Beitchman, Hood, & Inglis, 1992, in studies of language impairment; and Folstein & Piven, 1991, and Smalley, Asarnow, & Spence, 1988, in studies of autism).

How, then, does one delineate clinical signs that may be most directly influenced genetically from those that correlate more strongly with environmental factors that have interacted with a genetic predisposition? Current behavioral genetics clinical research designs might be enhanced by taxonomizing signs of a neurodevelopmental disorder by whether a particular sign is likely an innate, virtual, or epiphenomenal manifestation of a child's neurodevelopmental disorder. This accomplished, it becomes possible to narrow the field of candidate behaviors to those which represent innate defects as they may most directly demonstrate a gene's functional significance of a clinical level. By definition, those manifestations of a disorder that appear earliest and are displayed without precipitation by a pattern of learning are innate signs of the disorder, as has already been described. By applying criteria to determine whether a clinical sign is a primary (innate) one, it is possible to hypothesize that one is targeting clinical phenomena most likely to correlate highly with the presence or absence of a particular genetic defect. Of course, behavioral genetics studies that measure virtual or epiphenomenal manifestations of the same defect may correlate too, but weaker correlations would be expected. For example, if a gene marker unique to pedigrees of autistic probands was found, and most of these autistic probands had the trait of echolalia, one *might* suggest that the gene regulated the expression of echolalia. Could there be a gene for echolalia? Probably not. Using the present taxonomy, we would suggest that the gene might influence the most basic language processing trait – faulty auditory processing which would be designated as a primary, innate sign. Affected autistic probands might be at high risk to develop echolalia, but a small percentage might have automatically developed some other adaptation, or received some sort of early treatment that resulted in a different profile of subsequent virtual disability that did not include echolalia. Therefore, delayed echolalia, immediate echolalia, and even mutism might all be variable expressions (i.e., virtual disabilities that could have resulted from different developmental attempts to self-compensate for faulty auditory processing through whatever means was available). Consequently, when thinking in terms of behavioral genetics, the concept of "virtual disability" corresponds broadly to the concept of "a range of phenotypic expression." Therefore, it would be reasonable to search for genetic homologies in other non-autistic neurodevelopmentally impaired populations that share the same innate, primary trait (e.g., faulty auditory processing) with autistic probands who are echolalic or mute as these could be individually with the homologous genetic defects.

Mechanisms affecting variable expression of virtual disabilities

The secondary or virtual signs of a disorder can be expected to vary from one neuropsychiatric disorder to another even if primary, innate signs of the disorder are similar. This could be due to other features of the particular disorder that would determine what were other areas of intact or impaired function, and therefore, the availability of other means to compensate. So, using the example above, an autistic child with faulty auditory processing would also have social impairments, and would not be likely to use exaggerated amounts of gestural communication to compensate. However, another child with faulty auditory processing who has no social impairment, might show a great deal of compensatory gestural communication in his attempt to compensate. Thus, excessive levels of gestural communication would be seen as a secondary, virtual sign of an expressive language disorder. In the case of autism, it has been established that there is, in fact, an increased incidence of language disorders (without autism) in siblings of autistic probands (Bartak, Rutter, & Cox, 1975). This suggests that a shared gene(s), (and a shared innate defect) may be the same in each affected sibling in the sibship, but without the additional insults (possibly additional defective genes) associated with autism, the automatic accommodations made by the language-disordered siblings may be relatively more successful because of the greater range of automatic accommodations available to them.

Neuroanatomical and neurochemical markers and innate defects

It has just been suggested that the strongest correlation between a gene marker for a neuropsychiatric disorder and observable behavior should occur when the behavior represents an innate defect. An innate defect is the closest behavioral representation to the causative pathology. Similarly, studies that identify neuroanatomical differences or neurochemical differences between children with neurodevelopmental disorders and their controls might also expect to find the strongest correlations to observable psychopathology by examining behaviors that represent innate defects.

ATYPICAL ONTOGENY: APPLICATIONS FOR STUDYING THE TREATMENT OF NEURODEVELOPMENTAL DISORDERS

The second reason for studying atypical ontogeny is that clinically, understanding precursor manifestations (innate signs) of neurodevelopmental symptoms seen in infants and toddlers should be helpful in designing more prophylactic approaches to intervention in somewhat older children with more fully fulminant symptoms, that is, the virtual or epiphenomenal signs of their disorders. It should be easier and more efficient to intervene behaviorally (and perhaps more effective psychopharmacologically as well) at the developmental stage where there is a more primary manifestation of a symptom, than later, when teaching a more adaptive behavior, may mean not only teaching something new, but having to help the child extinguish or unlearn a maladaptive pattern of functioning (i.e., a poor automatic self-accommodation) that may have been created to deal with the primary innate deficit. Taking the echolalia example further, it can be argued that it is preferable to intervene before echolalia develops as a compensation. An echolalic child *can* be trained not to use echolalia via modeling of appropriate semantic structures and differential reinforcement of nonecholalic utterances, but this involves undoing a partially adaptive function that echolalia serves (Prizant & Rydell, 1984) that has already been adopted to help digest incompletely processed language. However, if intervention were to begin after identification of the primary innate defect (i.e., an auditory processing problem) and *before* development of secondary signs (i.e., the echolalia), there is no behavioral pattern to extinguish. In fact, to the extent that echolalia has been a helpful strategy to a particular child, it should be even more difficult to extinguish. However, an intervention that involves directly addressing auditory processing problems by teaching language in small segments, with slowed input, and high repetition, and so on, might result in a by-pass of an echolalic "compensation" stage entirely.

Other examples of innate, virtual, and epiphenomenal signs

Auditory processing and echolalia comprise just one example of how behavioral manifestations of neuropathology in children can be classified into innate signs versus virtual signs of a disorder such as autism or a receptive language disorder for the purposes of better understanding etiology and treatment of neuropsychiatric disorders in children. Similar taxonomies can be devised for other disorders. In the case of ADHD, difficulties in modulating perception of stimulus intensity resulting in a short attention span (an innate sign) might lead to impaired retention of content of spoken language (a virtual sign), and later to a diagnosis of conduct disorder (an epiphenomena) because of poor cooperation and high non-compliance. In children with obsessive-compulsive features, an early innate sign may be high anxiety in the face of novelty. As an adaptation, repetitions to create familiarity could be seen as a secondary, virtual sign. Later, a meta-cognitive, ego-dystonic sense of being trapped by the need to repeat; or anxiety when a routine or ritual is interfered with, would be an epiphenomena. In each of these cases the relative specificity of the primary, innate signs will determine the likelihood that the disorder can be accurately identified early.

Understanding how virtual signs of the disorder are likely to emerge may help in early recognition of the forme fruste of certain childhood neuro-psychiatric disorders, and thereby result in initiation of earlier interventions, or in earlier clinical referral for genetic diagnoses once markers are established. In essence, this type of model is already implicit in the formulation of psychopharmacological treatments for childhood neuropsychiatric disorder, where for example, an epiphenomenal sign of a disorder such as non-compliance is historically traced back to determine if it might have origins in a mood disturbance or and anxiety disorder in order to select a specific medication.

ATYPICAL ONTOGENY, ATYPICAL DEVELOPMENT, AND DELAYED DEVELOPMENT

Thus far in illustrating the concept of atypical ontogeny, it has been formulated that virtual signs of a disorder arise from automatic processes whereby mental processes originating from (more) intact domains of development compensate for weaker ones. The concept of atypical ontogeny has been defined to imply development that results from interdependence among domains of development where some domains are neurobiologically constrained. Atypical ontogeny begins as two or more domains of development interact to create a neurobiologically constrained decalage. The term "decalage" is used here in the Piagetian sense to refer to a coming together of heterogeneously staged abilities from different domains of development that together represent developmental functions that cannot be wholly characterized as fitting one stage of development or another (cf., Piaget & Inhelder, 1969).

Prior to the onset of atypical ontogenetic processes, development in a particular domain may be truly delayed. In some cases, development in a particular domain is simply slower in maturing (e.g., due to individual differences), but finally catches up. Most often, true delay, where the ultimate behavioral development is normal, is found in children with more mild neurodevelopmental compromise. For example, the degree of delay typically seen in many pre-term infants has led to the concept of "corrected age," where a simple subtraction of the pre-term interval from chronological age yields a good clinical estimate of expected developmental level across a number of domains.

In contrast, atypical development begins at the point when there is enough of a delay that the "handshake" (to borrow an analogy from the field of computer science) between two or more domains of development fails to take place because mental faculties in one of the domains is not yet sufficiently mature. For example, in earlier work (Siegel, Detmers, & Schuler, 1991), we have hypothesized that there is a "handshake" failure in toddlers who develop single-word speech and then lose most or all speech for a time, before finally gaining atypical, echolalic language. Early one-word speech may arise typically as more of "reflexive" process; and then, when the stage for developing more semiotic, semantic functions should occur, speech may be lost because higher order processes governing language understanding are not yet sufficiently developed to "handshake" with the mechanisms governing more semiotic verbal production, resulting in an atypical developmental phenomenon – atrophy of speech. Thus, if delay goes on long enough, it is likely to no longer be "delay," but truly atypical development, as lack of normal integration with related developmental functions fails to occur. At this point, when the "handshake" fails to take place, the compensatory abilities that may be brought to bear begin to create an atypical profile.

Clinical confusion between delayed and atypical development

Even without explicit criteria, clinicians can often sense when "delayed" development becomes "atypical," i.e., when delays are so persistent, or of a sufficient magnitude that it becomes possible to prognosticate that age appropriate development in a particular domain of development (e.g., arithmetic, reading) is likely never to be achieved. Psychologically, for many clinicians working with parents of young developmentally disabled children, the term "delay" may be easier to deliver than the terms "disorder," "disability," or "dysfunction," precisely for this reason. Parents told that their child's development is "delayed" can feel it is like a train that is delayed – and that it will arrive at a metaphorical hour – one, two, or three years behind schedule. While clinicians may feel it is kinder to talk to parents of "delay" (with implications of later "arrival"), it obfuscates the fact that the clinician can (and should) be looking for how the child is (or might) compensate for his disability by relying on more intact abilities from another domain.

Even areas where development is not delayed may become atypical as developmental milestones that integrate abilities across domains fail to emerge because required resources for one of the domains is missing. A good clinical example is a child with a severe language disorder: non-verbal intelligence may appear normal for a while, even in the complete absence of spoken language. But eventually, internalized language bolstered by expressive practice needs to exist too, if nonverbal problem solving is still going to be normal at the eight year developmental level because internalized language of an increasingly sophisticated nature will be needed to represent action and plans.

In clinically analyzing children with neurodevelopmental disorders, it can be very useful to conceptualize development as existing at several "ages" at the same time. For example, a child may have one receptive language age, another expressive language age; nonverbal intelligence may be at another "age," and so on. Drawing upon such a framework sets up a basis for understanding where development may emerge atypically.

ATYPICAL ONTOGENY AND THE CONCEPT OF DECALAGE

In cases of genetically based or acquired neurodevelopmental disability, neurobiology becomes a rate limiting factor that may distort, in some systematic way, the acquisition of subsequently emerging behaviors in a developmental sequence. The working model for atypical ontogeny postulates that the child automatically begins to form compensations in areas of limitation on his or her own (i.e., the virtual signs of a disorder). When this begins, domains of development not directly affected by the disability become woven into the fabric of the disability as they are drawn upon to form compensations. This can result in either positive or negative decalage.

Positive decalage

Positive decalage can be defined as when specialized abilities in one domain develop particularly well as a result of weakness in another domain. Positive decalage can be thought of as optimizing ability in an intact domain of development because of an acquired preference to develop skills in domains not constrained by neurobiological insult. In essence, positive decalage may be thought of as virtual "talent" – the converse of virtual disability – which has already been discussed. So, for example, a child with mild cerebral palsy may show disability in non-verbal problem-solving because of lack of physical exploratory capacity (if for example he has a truncal hypotonia), or because of lack of fine motor skill (if he has a fine motor palsy). Although such a child may have the cognitive capacity to engage normally in nonverbal problem solving, he may develop a "virtual" or secondary disability in nonverbal problem solving tasks that involves physical manipulation of smaller objects (even if the criterion test is one where performance speed is discounted). This assumes that the child has fewer experiences (and feedback, and learning) with fine-motor tasks because they are avoided since they are relatively difficult to master. It is also possible that such a child, if otherwise cognitively intact, may prefer to focus on developmental accomplishments in the verbal domain (like memorizing, or reading at a high level for chronological age) since these skills may be more readily mastered. This pattern of positive decalage has been anecdotally described in sensorially handicapped children such as the musicality of blind children. Using the concept of positive decalage, it would be posited, not that blind children on average have greater musical talent, but that it is more rewarding to attend to stimuli that can be most meaningfully processed, and thus more effort is expended developing such ability. Another clinical example of positive decalage may be found in the use of gestural communication by mute children with severe expressive language disorders. Many use vivid gestures, almost a natural sign language to communicate, thus showing a highly differentiated use of nonverbal communication – more differentiated, and more frequently used than if spoken language was present. Thus, positive decalage is one type of atypical development that may occur when abilities in one domain have become especially well developed because of maldevelopment in another domain.

Negative decalage

In most cases, virtual disabilities would be expressed as *negative decalage* – when behavioral development in one domain lags because it lacks integration (a "handshake") with closely allied aspects of cognition that are needed for further developmental milestones to be reached. In the preceding example of a child with cerebral palsy and fine motor tremor, poor nonverbal performance would be an example of negative decalage – a failure of cognitive and motor functions to become integrated in the expected manner. Instead, more primitive aspects of development from one domain (e.g., fine motor – immature grasp) combine with more normal development from another domain (e.g., visual-spatial skills) resulting in a partial accommodation – a virtual disability such as slowed performance time on tasks that combine fine motor skill with visual-spatial analysis. A slightly different example of negative decalage can be given from a developmental pattern that is typical for children with ADHD. Many children with ADHD are described as having a high drive for affiliation with peers (because they seek constant novelty – an innate defect), but also have a relatively poor ability to read nonverbal and other more subtle social cues that might indicate whether the peer wishes to respond in kind or not. This result is the virtual, secondary symptom frequently seen in children with ADHD – poor peer relationships. Poor peer relationships would be an example of a negative decalage arising when deficits in attention and the drive for social affiliation fail to achieve a "handshake" and form a new area of developmental competency.

Designing clinical interventions and the concept of decalage

Clinically, the most ready way to conceptualize developmental age is by examining age equivalent scores on a developmental test that breaks abilities into various domains. In a very gross way, possible patterns of decalage may be represented by scores in domains that are somewhere between the highest and lowest domains. "Intermediate" levels of functioning in certain domains may be a decalage of abilities from disabled and intact domains. This pattern of findings may be helpful in alerting a clinician to relative strengths and weaknesses. It may be possible to tailor interventions that mimic the automatic self-accommodations the child seems most able to make. An example of this is teaching sign language to a nonverbal child who compensates with exaggerated natural gesture. Conversely, the child's development may be increasingly limited by the automatic accommodations he or she makes, and the clinician can intervene by introducing further accommodations that in the long run will facilitate more mature competencies. For example, a nonverbal child who compensates through the use of gesture may retreat from trying to make him or herself understood by poorly articulated verbalizations.

However, if an intervention pairs the child's use of pictures along with the poorly articulated verbalizations, the verbalizations will more likely be understood, reinforced, and with successive modeling, improved in clarity.

On a very basic level, interventions for the atypically developing child can be geared to mental age – with different aspects of intervention geared to different developmental levels in each affected domain of development. So for example, a 5-year-old hyperlexic child with a language disorder may have a 3-year-old vocabulary and a fifth grade reading level. One "developmental" model would be to challenge him by giving him 4-year-old tasks in semantic language use – and sixth grade reading books. A better integrated approach would be to introduce tasks that bring together the high and low abilities so that the child can compensate for the decalage. Having the child read, and then demonstrate comprehension by matching written words to illustrations would be an example of such an intervention.

Therefore, from a clinical perspective, recognition of patterns of positive and negative decalage are useful for treatment planning. Examples of positive decalage (where innate defects have lead to certain sorts of positive adaptations) can be exploited to give the child further opportunities to make similar adaptations. Another example would be a nonverbal 4-year-old autistic child who lines up magnetic letters to spell the alphabet over and over again may be more readily taught phonics via letter recognition rather than from watching someone's mouth make sounds. Since there is clearly an aversion of people, but an interest and aptitude for ordering, teaching phonics as a visually linked ordering task may exploit a strength and circumvent a weakness. Atypical ontogeny is resolved to the extent that interventions can minimize decalage.

CONCLUSIONS: IMPLICATIONS FOR EARLIER DIAGNOSES AND UNDERSTANDING THE NATURAL HISTORIES OF NEURODEVELOPMENTAL DISORDERS

In various editions of the Diagnostic and Statistical Manual (e.g., DSM-III-R, 1987; DSM-IV, 1994) used to diagnose childhood psychiatric disorders, there are mandatory criteria as to the age at which the signs of the disorder must be in evidence. For most of the diagnostic criteria, few if any guidelines are given for differentiating (let alone diagnosing) a forme fruste or otherwise premorbid expression of the disorder. The DSM-III-R criteria for autistic disorder did make a nod to the need to rate behavior "according to the developmental level" of the patient, but do not operationalize criteria to do it. Since early, less specific, more innate signs of a disorder may not correspond directly to the more specific adaptations that subsequently develop out of the child's own attempts to compensate (i.e., the virtual signs of the disorder), and that are diagnostic of the disorder, early diagnoses are often not made.

Tracing back to very early developmental histories of children with neuro-developmental disorders could improve early diagnosis. However, multi-variate models of clusters of early symptoms would have to be derived in order to identify early patterns that were both sensitive and (more importantly) specific to predicting a later diagnosis. Single early signs tend to be sensitive, but lack specificity unless clustered with other early signs of the same disorder. So for example, early hyporesponsivity to spoken language might be found in children who later develop severe mental retardation, a receptive language disorder or autism, that is, a measure of auditory hyporesponsivity alone would likely be non-specific. However, only when seen in combination with other early innate signs, could we expect that an earlier diagnosis of one of these three disorders might be more reliably established. For diagnostic criteria for neurodevelopmental disorders to be useful for purposes of early identification, a more developmentally sensitive approach to the emergence of signs, their earliest manifestations, and their later transformation by interactions among affected and unaffected domains of development needs to be mapped.

REFERENCES

American Psychiatric Association (1987). *Diagnostic and Statistical Manual*, 3rd edn. Washington, DC: American Psychiatric Association Press.

American Psychiatric Association (1994). *Diagnostic and Statistical Manual*, 4th edn. Washington, DC: American Psychiatric Association Press.

Barkley, R.A. (1990). *Attention Deficit Hyperactivity Disorder: A Handbook for Diagnosis and Treatment*. New York: Guilford Press.

Bartak, L., Rutter, M., & Cox, A. (1975). A comparative study of infantile autism and specific developmental receptive language disorder. I: The children. *British Journal of Psychiatry*, **126**, 127–145.

Beitchman, J.H., Hood, J., & Inglis, A. (1992). Familial transmission of speech and language impairment: a preliminary investigation. *Canadian Journal of Psychiatry*, **37**, 151–156.

Burger, H.G. (1977). Piaget's maturational phases as merely consecutive definitions: the decalage reinterpreted as act-grades. *Communication and Cognition*, **10**, 3–31.

Chandola, C.A., Robling, M.R., Peters, T.J., Melville-Thomas, G., & McGuiffin, P. (1992). Pre- and peri-natal factors and the subsequent risk of referral for hyper-activity. *Journal of Child Psychology and Psychiatry*, **33**, 1077–1090.

Denckla, M.B. (1993). The child with developmental disabilities grown-up: adult residua of childhood disorders. *Neurologic Clinics*, **11**, 105–125.

Deykin, E.Y. & MacMahon, B. (1980). Pregnancy, delivery and neonatal complications among autistic children. *American Journal of Diseases in Children*, **134**, 860–864.

Feldman, E., Levin, B.E., Lubs, H., Rabin, M., Lubs, M.L., Jallad, B., & Kusch, A. (1993). Adult familial dyslexia: a retrospective developmental and psychosocial profile. *Journal of Neuropsychiatry and Clinical Neurosciences*, **5**, 195–199.

Finegan, J. & Quarrington, B. (1979). Pre- and peri- and neonatal factors and infantile autism. *Journal of Child Psychology and Psychiatry*, **20**, 119–128.

Folstein, S. & Piven, J. (1991). Etiology of autism: genetic influences. *Pediatrics*, **87**, 763–767.

Goodman, R. & Stevenson, J. (1989). A twin study of hyperactivity. II: The aetiological role of genes, familial relationships and perinatal adversity. *Journal of Child Psychology and Psychiatry*, **30**, 691–709.

Gottlieb, G. (1991). Behavioral pathway to evolutionary change. *Revista di Biologia*, **84**, 385–409.

Gross-Tour, V., Shalev, R.S., & Amir, N. (1991). Attention deficit disorder: Association with familial genetic factors. *Pediatric Neurology*, **7**, 258–261.

Morgane, P.J., Austin-LaFrance, R., Bronzino, J., Tonkiss, J., Diaz-Cintra, S., Cintra, L., Kemper, T., & Galler, J.R. (1993). Prenatal malnutrition and the development of the brain. *Neuroscience and Biobehavioral Science Reviews*, **17**, 91–128.

Ornitz, E. & Ritvo, E. (1968). Perceptual inconstancy in early infantile autism. *Archives of General Psychiatry*, **18**, 76–98.

Piaget, J. & Inhelder, B. (1969). *Psychology of the Child*. New York: Basic Books.

Pinard, A. (1975). The compatibility of the notions of stage and decalage in Piaget's theory. *Canadian Psychological Review*, **16**, 255–260.

Prizant, B. & Rydell, P.J. (1984). Analysis of functions of delayed echolalia in autistic children. *Journal of Speech and Hearing Research*, **27**, 183–192.

Rutter, M., Chadwick, O., Shaffer, D., & Brown, G. (1980). A prospective study of children with head injury: I. Design and methods. *Psychological Medicine*, **10**, 633–645.

Shaffer, D., Chadwick, O., & Rutter, M. (1975). Psychiatric outcome of localized head injury. In R. Porter & D. FitzSimmons (eds) *Outcome of Severe Damage to the Central Nervous System*. Ciba Foundation Symposium No. 34. Amsterdam: Elsevier.

Siegel, B., Detmers, D., & Schuler, A. (1991). Language loss in autism: Regression or failure to progress? Paper presented at the meeting of the American Academy of Child and Adolescent Psychiatry.

Smalley, S., Asarnow, R., & Spence, A. (1988). Autism and genetics. *Archives of General Psychiatry*, **45**, 953–961.

Sprich-Buckminster, S., Biederman, J., Milberger, S., Faraone, S.V., & Lehman, B.K. (1993). Are perinatal complications relevant to the manifestation of ADD? Issues of co-morbidity and familiarity. *Journal of the American Academy of Child and Adolescent Psychiatry*, **32**, 1032–1037.

Striedter, G.F. & Northcutt, R.G. (1991). Biological hierarchies and the concept of homology. *Brain, Behavior and Evolution*, **38**, 177–189.

Tallal, P., Townsend, J., Curtiss, S., & Wulfeck, B. (1991). Phenotypic profiles of language impaired children based on genetic/familial history. *Brain and Language*, **41**, 81–95.

4 Language and psychopathology: an attachment perspective

PATRICIA M. CRITTENDEN

One of the hallmarks of psychopathology is irrational thinking. Thinking, however, cannot be observed directly; instead, it is inferred from language and behavior. Thus, the pragmatics[1] of language use are tied to disturbances of behavior. The central thesis of this chapter is that, in the context of genetically biased characteristics, humans learn how to use their minds. When the outcome is irrational, the process of learning to mentally integrate information may be presumed to have gone away. This chapter explores individual differences in children's learning to use their minds as that process is inferred from the use of language and expressed as behavior. My focus is exclusively on language tied to interpersonal relationships and, in the extreme, to psychopathologies associated with distorted relationships. Among these are disorders of learning, affect, and behavior. Although no empirical data are analyzed, examples of speech from dyads showing varied patterns are provided.

BRAIN, MIND, AND BEHAVIOR

A new integrative focus

Language is first and foremost a means of representing and communicating information. The nature of that information is, however, determined in part by the structure and maturation of the brain, whereas the specific content is the result of individual experience. I propose that caregiver–child relationships are critical to the nature of this experience, to the language used to encode it, and to the mind's ability to manipulate and integrate it, that is, to think.

The evolved structure of information

The human brain transforms sensory information in several ways. First, it is biased to perceive information from and about humans, especially information

---

[1] Although the term "pragmatics" is laden with special meaning for linguists, only its every day meaning of "practical" or "functional" is intended here.

relevant to protection, in preference to other information (Gallistel, Brown, Carey et al., 1991). Second, the mid-brain has evolved to attribute meaning to the temporal order of motoric events. Specifically, reptilian and higher species modify their behavior, as though presuming causation, on the basis of predictable outcomes (Ornstein & Thompson, 1984; Thompson, 1985). Although this information does not require language (Skinner's pigeons, for example, did not need language to know that certain pecks would "cause" food to appear), nevertheless, language both reflects and facilitates learning about causal relations. It is possible, however, both to mistakenly interpret a relation as causal and also to use language knowingly and falsely, that is, to lie. Thirdly, the limbic system contains genetically transmitted information regarding situations that are potentially too dangerous to risk experiential learning (MacLean, 1973, 1990). Instead, feelings of anxiety are associated with threatening conditions, such as darkness, entrapping conditions, and being alone (Bowlby, 1969/82). Conversely, feelings of comfort accompany the inverse of these conditions, for example, light, openness. Because the presence of even one other person reduces danger, humans feel more comfortable when other humans, especially supportive, wiser, and stronger attachment figures, are nearby (Bowlby, 1969/82). However, feelings of anxiety may occur when there is no actual danger. For simplicity, I am going to call S → R associative learning "cognition" and feelings generated by the limbic system "affect." The function of the maturing cerebral cortex is to carry out increasingly sophisticated integrations of affect with cognition to yield increasingly accurate information about reality and our relation to it.

INFANCY: SENSORIMOTOR FUNCTIONING

Mental processes in infancy

Although human infants lack language, they are born with the innate ability to use lower brain functioning to generate meaningful information about reality. They are attentive to human and protective information, they learn stimulus-response associations and treat them as causal, and they feel and display anxiety and comfort in predictable situations. Adults respond to infants on the basis of their interpretation of the meaning of infants' behavior. These responses provide infants with a first understanding, a sensorimotor understanding, of meaning. Three general possibilities exist (Ainsworth et al., 1978). Adults can respond to infants' affective signals in ways that are predictable and comforting, predictable and distressing, and unpredictable and inconsistent to infants.

As a result of experiencing these patterns of adult response, some infants learn to use feelings to represent and communicate information about their state in ways that lead to predictable and desired outcomes (Crittenden, 1995). These infants, labeled secure (Type B), make meaning from the integration of affect and cognition. Other infants, labeled anxious-avoidant (Type A), learn that expression of feelings leads to uncomfortable outcomes, that is, to parental anger, rejection, or unavailability. These infants learn that affect misleads whereas cognition functions predictably; consequently, they learn to inhibit display of affect. Finally, infants in the third group, labeled anxious-ambivalent (Type C), learn that expression of feelings has no predictable outcome; in this case, neither affect nor cognition is meaningful. Such infants are often highly aroused by feelings of fear, anger, and desire for comfort.

In the absence of language, infants encode information about adult responsiveness as sensorimotor schemata, held in a mental structure labeled "procedural memory" (Tulving, 1985). Based on the content of procedural memory, infants generate sensorimotor expectations, that is, procedural internal representational models, regarding caregivers' behavior (Crittenden, 1990). Memory systems, in other words, are structures that organize information and internal representational models are the means by which that information is applied to new circumstances.

Risks associated with distortions of procedural, sensorimotor memory

There are risks to mental functioning when there are distortions of procedural memory. First, the internal representational models drawn from procedural memory do not fully reflect reality. Instead, infants tend to dichotomize and polarize their representations of mothers (Fischer, 1980). One risk is that they will fail to identify and respond appropriately to less extreme variations among mothers and within a given mother's behavior across time.

Second, in infancy, experiences that are not acted upon have no way of being retained in memory. Thus, for avoidant infants, most negative affect as well as knowledge of the need to inhibit affect may be lost as a result of the inhibition itself. Because negative affect represents evolutionarily selected responses that promote safety and survival (Bowlby, 1980; Darwin, 1872/1965), avoidant (Type A) infants may endanger themselves in circumstances that call for display of affect or the use of affect to predict danger.

Third, the failure of ambivalent (Type C) infants to identify a relation between behavior and outcomes creates risk of intense and unresolvable feelings of fear, anger, and desire for comfort. Because these are displayed as clingy, angry, incessantly demanding behavior, they sometimes elicit aggression from adults.

In all three cases, risk represents the interaction of species specific biases in brain functioning with mental maturity and actual experience. Together, these affect the way infants learn to identify important information and to organize behavioral responses. In other words, infants with differing experiences learn to use their minds differently in the process of extracting meaning from experience and of organizing their interpersonal behavior.

THE PRESCHOOL YEARS: PREOPERATIONAL LOGIC

Maturation and development

Preoperational children represent information linguistically and use language to mediate their relationships with others. They also talk to themselves, thus, expressing their thought processes as private speech. Finally, preschoolers use intuitive logic. Attention to young children's use of language can be informative with respect to their developing mental ability to construct and use models of reality.

Procedural information

Language is used by preschoolers to manage information without having to enact the experience. In particular, language is used to give and receive information about intentions, that is, about what will happen, and to express feelings. In both cases, language gives children the potential for some distance from the material about which they are thinking (Sigel, Stinson, & Flaugher, in press). From an attachment perspective, these functions of language facilitate the development of a goal-corrected partnership with caregivers. Such a partnership allows children to receive information about caregivers' future availability and, thus, to assure themselves of their safety even in the absence of caregivers. Moreover, it allows them to express and have soothed their feelings of fear, anger, and desire for comfort. This, in turn, permits children to explore the world of things and other people with confidence.

Cognitive information about future events

When children cannot obtain accurate information about the future linguistically, they (1) learn to distrust linguistic representations of "cognitive" information about the future, (2) attend excessively to their caregivers' behavior and attempt to elicit attention from their caregivers, and (3) are less free to turn their attention to exploration. This has consequences for both behavior and learning. Let me offer two examples, both from Type C children in the Strange Situation.

Jimmy at 30-months-of-age did not want his mother to leave him even briefly, so as she got up, he rushed to the door with her. There he hung on her leg and begged her to stay in a voice that escalated rapidly toward a tantrum. Recognizing a familiar problem and knowing that there was no easy resolution, Jimmy's mother said enthusiastically, "*Look! Go get the ball!*" Jimmy turned to go and his mother slipped out of the door. If this sort of linguistic sequence is repeated often, Jimmy will learn to doubt the veracity of cognitive explanations. Thus, he will defend against cognition because it often deceives and endangers him.

Heather's mother, in the same situation, spontaneously offered Heather candy if she would let her mother go. Heather acquiesced reluctantly. When her mother returned, Heather went directly to her asking for the candy and reaching in her mother's pocket. There was neither candy nor explanation. Later Heather tried to open the latched door. She asked for her mother's help, but her mother told her to try harder. She appealed again to her mother who, with apparent sincerity, gave Heather more directions. Still the door would not open. Heather told her mother that the door was locked. Instead of telling Heather the truth, her mother continued to pretend to help. Eventually, Heather's mother whined, "*What will you give me?*" Then she offered to open the door if Heather would give her a kiss. Heather did. "*And a hug.*" Heather hugged her very nicely. "*A big hug.*" Heather gave her a really big hug. "*And another.*" Heather complied, but complained. Eventually, Heather pulled and tugged on her immobile mother who just laughed at Heather and did not open the door.

Like Jimmy, Heather was told something about the future that turned out not to be the case. Moreover, in Heather's case, we have two successive examples of bargains in which the promised reward was withheld. Through experiences such as these, both Jimmy and Heather will learn that language can be used to suggest one set of circumstances when, in fact, another is true. Furthermore, they will discover that believing the surface meaning of words leaves them vulnerable to victimization. The very skill that could free them from enactment in the here and now is being distorted such that affect expressed in the here and now becomes the only reliable source of information.

Using language to hide affect

Children and adults who mistrust affect use language differently. Children whose parents are uncomfortable with negative affect learn that positive affect is acceptable, whereas negative affect is not. For example, a parent might say to her crying child, "*Now give me a big smile!*" Children who hear this often will learn to hide, in both display and speech, their true feelings. Although it can be difficult to know when important information about feelings is left unsaid, private, self-speech can sometimes give clues to children's inhibited thoughts.

For example, Karen and a research assistant were playing when there was a knock and Karen's mother left – without comment. The research assistant told Karen that she had drawn a mommy pig. Karen responded, "*And mommies take care of their babies.*" Although an obvious interpretation is that Karen was angry with her mother for not taking care of her and wanted reassurance that she would in fact be cared for, Karen's demeanor was mature and self-reliant. Maybe we read too much into unsaid words. Later, however, Karen and her mother began putting a puzzle together. Again, Karen's mother left saying, "*I'll be back, okay?*" Karen lowered her head as though she could not/would not hear. Her mother repeated, more firmly, "*Okay?*" As she turned her head far away, Karen said softly "*Kay...*" She did not look as her mother went out the door. Then, as she played alone, Karen said, "*I'm angry. I'm angry with my mommy. I'm not angry with my mommy.*" When her mother entered, Karen said nothing of her feelings. In her speech, she was polite, but factual, brief, and distant. The bit of private, self-speech when she perceived herself to be alone is our only sure indication of her underlying internal process of inhibiting affect.

Dalisha and her father show a similar pattern of depersonalization of information, deletion of feelings from communication, and hiding of anger. Dalisha's father asked her to draw a picture. Without much enthusiasm, she did. When her father asked, "*Who's this?*" Dalisha answered, "*Anybody.*" Later, when her father had returned after leaving briefly, he asked, "*What did you do while I was gone?*" "*Nothing.*" Then her father asked for a cup of tea. He was put off with, "*It's not done.*" In spite of repeated requests that included information about his thirst, his desire for sugar and lemon, and his willingness to be patient, Dalisha only nodded, uttered occasional uh-oh's, and kept working (very hard!) to make the tea that she never actually gave to her father. She never refused him, never asked about his departure, and never mentioned her feelings about his absence. In spite of elaborate, extended, and reciprocal communication about the tea, information critical to their relationship was not exchanged. Neither seemed to know what was missing.

In conclusion, both coercive and defended children learn to use language to communicate. In addition, however, they use language to conceal information and, ultimately, to deceive others.

Other memory systems

During the preschool years, children learn to encode two new kinds of information that treat affect and cognition differently (Bowlby, 1980; Tulving, 1972). *Semantic* memory is memory of generalizations regarding the way things are connected to one another. It is, in other words, a verbal expansion of infants' ability to identify contingencies between repeated events. As such, it is "cognitive" in nature. In the preschool years, however, it reflects caregivers' generalizations rather than children's. That is, preschoolers do not yet have either the ability to deduce generalizations from experience or a fund of remembered experiences from which to draw generalizations. Two sorts of generalizations are especially important: those defining contingencies, for example, "If you sneak a cookie, you won't get dinner," and those defining the nature of the self and others, for instance, "*You're a good boy.*" Inaccuracies in adult's generalizations will be reflected in children's earliest semantic models of reality. This distorts both the information available to children and mental processes using the information. Such distortions are, however, not easily discerned by preschool-aged children.

Other young children, often those with inconsistent caregivers, are told contradictory things about reality on different occasions. For example, a boy might hear maternal pride on one occasion when he is told that he is "tough like a man" and then disgust on another occasion when he is admonished for hitting his sister. For such children, semantic memory becomes a confusing and misleading source of information.

Episodic memory consists of memories of specific events that can be expressed verbally. Autobiographical episodes contain information about how the child felt in specific situations and what he did. Although these episodes represent actual events, they are rarely, and possibly never, exact representations of these events. Instead, episodic memories are distorted by omitted, misinterpreted, and forgotten information (Loftus & Hoffman, 1989). Among the most stable aspects of episodic memories is the affect pervading the experience (Bowlby, 1980). Because affect defines the meaning of the episode for the individual, it is essential to the integrity of the memory. Indeed, experiences with complex and conflicting feelings are highly arousing and more likely than ordinary events to have implications for personal safety. Because this increases the probability that important, unresolved events with implications for safety will be available for review on future occasions, it is adaptive that such events are selected for long-term storage.

Caregivers who are uncomfortable with feelings may discourage recitation of memories with negative affect and/or coach children's recitation such that the uncomfortable details are modified, omitted, or replaced by more acceptable feelings of competence. Similarly, such parents may twist children's memories of parents' anger to reflect an emphasis on children's bad behavior. Coercive children, on the other hand, will often be highly aroused by conflicting feelings; memories of these incidents will be retained and elicited when children feel again as they did in the remembered incident. Because the feelings are mixed, current feeling states are likely to elicit a flood of memories. The set of elicited memories may appear disordered in terms of time, characters, or place, but will be connected by the affective logic of related feeling states.

Using procedural, semantic, and episodic memory to regulate behavior

Each memory system contains information that can be used to guide behavior (Crittenden, 1990, 1992b). This guide can be thought of as a "working" internal representational model that captures the meaning of the information in each memory system and applies it to immediate circumstances. Procedural models regulate preconscious behavior in everyday situations. Semantic models regulate problem solving behavior when the outcome of procedural behavior is discrepant with expectations. Episodic models regulate behavior when individuals are too effectively aroused for the "cognitive" problem solving associated with semantic models. Affective resonance is probably the mechanism by which particular memories are selected. Behavior in the memory then becomes the model for what to do at present. In the preschool years, such memories are likely to be invoked directly; later they may be reviewed consciously for applicability and modified prior to enactment.

Evidence of individual differences in preschoolers' use of language

The nature of children's memories and of distortions in them may be important to understanding how children conceptualize reality. These differences can be clustered in terms of the three patterns of procedural functioning described for infancy. The range of subpatterns increases, however, as compared to infants (Crittenden, 1992a). Consequently, the multiple pathways can only be sketched very briefly. More important, however, is recognition that these pathways represent additional "shades of gray" in functioning as opposed to infants' dichotomization of reality.

Secure children have access to both affective and cognitive information which they integrate mentally. They show this in their ability to use language to express feelings, to plan for the future, and to negotiate and reach satisfying compromises.

Defended children omit negative affect from their language. Some defended children, however, distort affect further by pretending to have feelings that are actually the opposite of their true feelings. *Defended compulsive caregiving* children often appear nurturing to withdrawn or helpless appearing parents. Their language contains bids for attention that require little response from adults; to the contrary, they have an entertaining or nurturant quality. For example, Valerie offered her withdrawn mother cups of tea: "*Want some tea, Mommy? Want sugar? Good?*" *Defended compulsive compliant* children are more concerned with rules for behavior. Instead of initiating conversation, they are likely merely to echo the critical part of maternal directives, for example, "*over there?*" "*that one?*"

Coercive children use language and non-verbal communication to establish dominance hierarchies (Anderson, 1984; Sloman et al., 1994). When they accept a submissive position, they elicit nurturance with excessive demands for help, for example, "*Where this go?*" Others simply want to maintain adult attention and accomplish this by negating anything their mothers say, thus, creating an endless, entangling struggle. These verbal struggles often wreck havoc with reality, for instance, Mother: "*See the boy doll?*" Child: "*It is the woman!*" Coercive children in more threatening circumstances find language to be almost meaningless and potentially threatening as a means of interpersonal communication. For example, Gina, a *coercive-aggressive* child, had been extremely upset upon her mother's silent departure in the Strange Situation. She had cried, yelled and hit the door. Upon her mother's entry,

Gina went directly to her with her arms upraised in an infantile pick-up gesture; she then hung against her mother with feigned helplessness. After they were seated, Gina turned to her mother and asked petulantly, "*Why d'you leave me?*" to which her mother replied, "*I didn't leave you.*" They had few more exchanges in which Gina was remonstrative and her mother denied that she had left. Gina leaned against her mother and pouted. When left alone a few minutes later (again without explanation), Gina searched, screamed for her mother, and fell to the floor in a tantrum. When she returned, Gina's mother asked Gina why she had cried. Gina pouted, "*Cause I wanted the stroller!*" Her mother responded, "*No, you didn't; you missed me.*" Gina denied this truth. Soon after, she asked her mother to reach for the microphone hanging from the ceiling. Her mother correctly pointed out that she was not tall enough to reach it. Nevertheless, Gina insisted that she stand up and try. Her mother said that she could not because Gina was on her lap. Gina slipped down and waited. When her mother did not move, Gina complained loudly, "*I knew you wouldn't get up!*" Her mother then stood up, but refused to reach. Gina again complained and her mother protested that she (the mother) was not tall enough. Gina retorted, "*You are so big!*" Suddenly, her mother told Gina to get the microphone, to which Gina retorted, hands on hips, "*I'm too little!*" Her mother responded, "*No, you're not!*" From this complex and twisted dialogue, Gina learned to expect distortions of predictions, to use intense affect to get what she wanted, and to hide or deny some feelings. Her mother's speech provided the model.

THE SCHOOL YEARS: CONCRETE OPERATIONS

Integrating procedural, semantic, episodic memory to regulate behavior

By the beginning of the school years, children experience a second period of rapid neurological growth, one that increases dramatically the ability of their minds to manage information. Specifically, children are able to integrate information from all three memory systems to create sophisticated and increasingly accurate representations of reality. When children lack access to information, integrative explanations become very difficult to generate. For coercive children, this will sometimes lead to illogical explanations and predictions of their own behavior. For example, a boy in a detention facility was asked why he was not participating in recreation. His answer: "*These gunshot wounds got me out of practice.*" His counselor rejoined, "*You been shot lately?*" Although the boy's answer sounded logical, it was neither logical nor accurate. Evasion functions similarly. When others seek confirmation about their future behavior, for example, "*When will you pick up your room?*," coercive children become expert at giving part of what is desired while remaining evasive: "*Soon,*" "*In just a minute...*"

It is paradoxical that distortions of memory are both essential for generalization of what is learned and also the source of irrational thinking and mental disturbance. Specifically, when semantic memory is perfectly coherent, it is meaningless. That is, to be absolutely coherent, the relation between the two conditions of the statement must be invariant. For example, when the statement "*You are a bad girl*" is explained by "*Because I said so*," no meaning is added. Almost any other explanation, such as "*Because you steal*," would permit conditions under which one might not be bad, thus, leading to less than perfect coherence. But less than perfect coherence is (more or less) misleading, that is, a distortion that is itself false.

Similarly, perfect matches between episodic memory and reality are useless and distorted matches are imperfect, that is, not entirely true. In other words, if the memory of an event corresponds in every detail to a specific occasion, the memory cannot fit any other occasion. Because life is made up of infinite variations without exact repetitions, the perfectly remembered episode pertains only to the one experience and cannot be generalized accurately to other occasions. On the other hand, if the memory is distorted by loss of detail, it is both more useful and no longer entirely accurate.

What the mind needs are semantic and episodic memories that are largely accurate, but distorted in ways that make them applicable to future situations without such great distortions that interpretation of the new situation becomes false. Integration of what is known from one imperfect internal representational model from one memory system with what is known from the model from another memory system increases the probability of understanding new circumstances. That is, of course, if the distortions are not too great and the danger of misinterpreting and incorrectly acting upon information is not too severe. When children fear error excessively, exact information is needed; in its absence, children distort information in favor of avoiding the feared risk. Thus, coercive children believe affect, focus on memories of times when affect held the key to safety, and risk cognitive incoherence rather than lose access to attachment figures. Defended children, on the other hand, prefer never to incur caregiver anger or rejection; for them, semantic memory is crucial and conflicting episodic memories are set aside. This leads to a dearth of meaningful generalizations in the speech of coercive children and of episodic detail among defended children.

Linguistic communication

School-aged children use language as their primary means of communication. Consequently, it serves functions that were managed primarily by non-verbal signals in the preschool years. For example, school-aged children use language to establish dominance hierarchies (Ervin-Tripp, O'Connor, & Rosenberg, 1984; Grief & Gleason, 1980; Schieffelin & Ochs, 1983), to sooth, taunt, or hurt feelings, and to convey or hide information. Indeed, the power of language becomes so great that it almost has a life of its own in which words create meanings rather than merely conveying them. Consequently, when children call each other sissies, liars, or scaredy-cats, school-aged children feel that they *are* this thing unless they can win the verbal argument. Name calling, in other words, becomes a defining, literal reality in the school years.

Double meanings

The limited ability of school-aged children to think of language as a symbolic form of communication leads to great attention to determining the actual meaning of words and phrases. This preoccupation can be seen in children's interest in riddles and jokes. Although this newly found type of humor represents an important developmental advance, under it lies the even more important awareness that language can mean more than one thing and that some meanings can be hidden. Depending upon children's experience, these new abilities yield either clearer, more sophisticated communication or communication that creates barriers between people and that distorts children's understanding of reality. For secure/balanced children, the ability of language to convey more than one meaning becomes a source of extending meaning. By adulthood this becomes the humorous and meaningful "double entendre." For coercive children, language's multiple meanings become a way of hiding one's true intent, whereas for defended children, they become a way of expressing true feelings without others' awareness. Among children with low intelligence, the combination of distortions in information plus limited ability to interpret complexity can lead to the limitations of a literal use of language. For example, an autistic child, hearing the request "*Can you pass the salt?*" answers, "*Yes.*"

Semantic rules for behavior

In the school years, semantic memory is developed as a guide to what is permissible, thus becoming the basis for children's emerging conscience (Kohlberg, 1984; Piaget, 1932). Like early internal representational models, early moral understandings tend to be overly dichotomized between good and bad. Although this is common for all school-aged children, it becomes particularly important for defended children to sharply differentiate right from wrong. Coercive children, on the other hand, learn that the appearance of moral reasoning can be used to deceive others.

For example, Kristin and her mother were playing a board game that required joint agreement regarding each move. Kristin's mother promised Kristin that, if she would do as she, the mother, wanted, the mother would then do as Kristin wanted. Instead, Kristin, fearing trickery, insisted that she should have her desire first. Her mother then promised, holding up her fingers in the "Scout's Honor" sign. Kristin, however, accused her of deceiving –

because her feet were crossed. Kristin, in other words, distrusted verbal and cognitive information; she presumed it to be misleading to the point that she sought and found confirming (false) perceptual information of trickery.

Another example demonstrates how the failure of cognitive logic can leave a child with only affective logic, thus, making his communication nearly incomprehensible to others. At age 10, Daryl was a very disturbed boy who told preposterous stories to elicit caregiving and reassurance from others. These stories reached levels that bordered on psychotic when he talked about make-believe monsters (or were they real to Daryl?) *"who attacked me – or you? – am I the monster? did he attack? who?"* The plots twisted until only the themes of rage, aggression, and fear were clear and stable. At night, however, Daryl was alone with his mind and its monsters.

After an explosive outburst of violence at school, Daryl was placed in a detention facility. There he had the following conversation with a therapist. *"I broke lots and lots of windows; that's why my parents won't keep me. They know King Kong breaks windows. Only you can control yourself. Where will you be going once I go home?"* The therapist responded, *"Only you can control yourself?"* to which Daryl replied, *"Where will you be going when I go home? Are you here to see if there is anything I can do?"* Therapist: *"How are you feeling right now?"* Daryl: *"Last year I cut myself right here. I was playing outside. Don't do that because accidents happen."* Therapist: *"What are you feeling now?"* Daryl: *"I had to have stitches. When was the last time you had stitches? When did it happen?"*

There are a number of interesting points to Daryl's dialogue. First, it shows a great deal of cognitive confusion in which reality seems uncertain. Second, the tie between the speakers seems tenuous at best. Daryl seems to be in a private world in which there is no apparent cohesion among ideas and little relation of his speech to the therapist's. The therapist, on the other hand, is following an agenda that we can recognize as coherent, but which, from Daryl's perspective, is not responsive to his communications. Moreover, the therapist's questions ask Daryl to converse through missing and distrusted semantic memory. In the light of the theory presented here, Daryl *is* trying to explain his problems. His theme is clear: "The world is scary and I am scared. Moreover, I can't be sure where the aggression will come from and whether anyone will be here to protect me." Daryl is actually quite direct with the therapist: are you permanent or will you disappear from my life? Is your reality as scary as mine? Can you feel things like I feel them? *Can you understand me?* All of this, however, must be read through episodic memories and distorted episodic stories. Only the logic of affect and, specifically, of anger and fear of abandonment, provides a meaningful pathway through Daryl's speech and thought. Nevertheless, Daryl was unable to articulate his feelings through affect labels. The distance necessary to identify and discuss feelings was unavailable to this intensely anxious and aroused child. Moreover, semantic memory only yielded the information that experience is unpredictable, that "accidents happen."

ADOLESCENCE

Integration

Following the period of rapid neurological change at puberty, adolescents become capable of constructing sophisticated, abstract, and highly differentiated models of reality. Accomplishing this, however, requires access to all memory systems, acceptance of unpleasant information, and toleration of ambiguity. In addition, it becomes necessary for adolescents to distance themselves from information so as to be able to gain balance with regard to feelings and rules. The result is the construction of internal representational models that offer enough shadings of gray that, unlike infants' dichotomous, black-and-white models, they fit reality quite closely.

Humor

Distancing has been treated as an especially important mental function because it enables humans to view their predicament from alternative points of view (Sigel, Stinson, & Flaugher, in press). Humor also serves this function. In the example to follow, humor provided a way out of an unnecessary argument between a secure adolescent and his mother. Bob had taken the car without asking. He and his mother argued until they were each yelling and defending ridiculous positions to each other. In the midst of the rising craziness, Bob suddenly became quiet, cupped his hand to his ear and said, "*Hark! Can you hear the voice of reason calling from afar?!*" Bob and his mother broke into laughter. The struggle was both ended and put in perspective. Bob apologized for what he had done and his mother accepted the apology without need for further admonishment or threats.

In another case, however, Erik was in a fight with his mother over the familiar problem of his breaking his curfew. Mother and son each restated their positions in an escalating match of volume and accusations, each beginning with the phrase "*But you...!*" Suddenly, Erik changed the tenor and process of the dispute by interjecting, "*You know what **you** have forgotten? You must remember, you haven't finished raising me yet!*" Humor and intelligence had combined to save the day. Together, these gave mother and son a little mental distance from the battle and cast it in a different light, one that was humorous. The escalation of angry affect was reversed and in the calm that followed, each could again accept the other. The shift in cognition, however, was less dramatic. Erik had shifted the responsibility for his behavior from himself to his mother in a situation where angry accusations had failed to accomplish this goal. His method of using humor and an appeal to his mother's power not only eased an immediate problem, but created a memory that his mother recalls lovingly years after the event. The charm of the coercive-disarming pattern was integrated with the humor of the school years and formal logic of adolescence to create a more mature concatenation of the pattern, yet one that still disarmed others' anger and elicited nurturance from powerful people.

Balanced speech

Balanced speech is notable for its coherence. Balanced adolescents present information in ways that make their meaning easily accessible to the listener. This meaning provides a reasonable balance of affect and cognition as well as integrative conclusions. In addition, both semantic and episodic probes can be answered easily as can integrative questions. The following examples are drawn from interviews with adolescents. "You said your relationship with your mother was respectful. Can you tell me about that?" "*She's always respected...um, the things that I want to do and also the people I choose to be with. It's always been...um...an issue of how I felt. And she never, she would offer advice, but she would never impose it on me.*" Loving? "*From an early age I could just curl up in her lap...and just understand that she understood me, without ever saying anything.*"

Defensive and coercive patterns

For those adolescents whose reality is too threatening to be acknowledged accurately, distortions of speech become one means of inferring mental processes (Grinder & Bandler, 1976; Main & Goldwyn, 1992). Often verbal distancing enables defended adolescents to avoid feeling affectively aroused. For example, feelings can be nominalized (Bandler & Grinder, 1975): Can you give me an example of when your mother was loving? "*It's just a good feeling she puts on me.*" Many investigators have noted that speech dysfluencies and partial slips of the tongue accompany affectively arousing thoughts: Can you describe your childhood? "*Um...I don't know, I...they brought me up so I, I don't–, I think we're pretty close...um, we always got along...basically. They're strict.*" At other times, the indicators of blocked affect are lack of affect in episodic memories or memories that do not fit semantic generalizations, particularly generalizations that have been distorted into idealized positive or negative models: Which parent did you feel closest to? ......*Probably, my mother. Only because she was home more......'Cause she's always, she's always there...Yeah he's not, I'm not saying he's not a, good dad or anything but he's not at home as much, I mean he does, he helps me with my homework, especially like algebra...so that's like...every time we spend time together, it's like constructive (laugh). Yeah.*" In addition, defended adolescents rely on abstract semantic memory to reconstruct past experiences that can no longer be accessed directly: Can you give me an example of what you would do when you were upset? "*I was probably upset with my parents...so I would go up to my room and cry, sit on my bed (laugh) and cry, and then get over it and it just like, I don't know, cleared my slate or something.*" The words "probably" and "would" suggest the fabricated quality of the memories.

Among *coercive* adolescents, the opposite process is dominant. Thus, episodic memories are recalled with living clarity whereas semantic memory and cognitive generalizations are minimized. In speech, this process may be indicated by organization of discourse around "affective logic": Can you remember your father? "*Well...my mother and father got divorced when I was 7, so I don't remember...the main thing that sticks out in my mind about them...being together like married or whatever, when they were married, was, just the night that he told us he was leaving, that's really all that...sticks out in my mind. So, do you want me to explain that?* [Yes.] *All us kids (mumbles), all us kids were sitting watching a really cool show, and ah, this girl was about to be eaten by a giant rat...: – this is why I remember it, and my father walks in and he shuts it off. And I was so mad at him.......so...and I went to my room and that's why it sticks out in my mind 'cause he shut the TV off. That's the last I really can remember.*"

In addition, there may be uncertainties and inconsistencies with regard to semantic generalizations: Were you ever rejected? "*...Um...no, not really. No. I...um...sometimes with my father. But definitely not with my mother, ever. Sometimes with my father and my sister. She, she, who, she was a killer (laugh). But, yeah, a lotta times with all of them.*" Sometimes there is a complete lack of distancing in which the relation of a past experience is transformed into a re-experiencing of the instance, often indicated by a switch from past to present tense: Describe your mother. "*My mother was overpowering: well, she was always...sh, she always had to give-have control of, of what I am all the time.*"

In spite of their obvious affective arousal, many coercive adolescents are uncertain about precisely what affects they experience. An adolescent in a drug treatment facility demonstrated this. When asked to tell a treatment group how she felt emotionally, Ellen could not identify her feeling. To assist her, the counselor gave her a chart with schematic faces accompanied by affect names. After looking at the pictures for a long time, Ellen said, "*Can I change my choice? **Now** I feel stupid, but before I felt happy.*" She then explained that, without being stoned, she did not recognize the feelings of happiness and comfort. Underlying this anecdote is evidence of (a) the limited access of coercive individuals to the distancing language of semantic memory, (b) their confusing experience of mixed affects in which one or more affects are inhibited while others are exhibited in exaggerated form, with the result that none are readily identified, and (c) their need to experience very intense arousal in order to achieve a single clear feeling state.

Another coercive adolescent exemplifies the false cognition of coercives. Marissa was anorexic. She used her refusal to eat both to punish her mother who offered food as a sign of love and also to keep her family's attention focused on her. Like other extremely punitive adolescents, she was willing to run risks, in this case to her health, and to forego many pleasures in order to maintain the struggle with her parents. After some time in therapy, Marissa, who was by then making some progress in maintaining internal equilibrium, announced, "*I don't have to twist my mother's words to make her hateful anymore.*"

It was a simple statement, but it reflected both her earlier state of false cognition and distorted logic and also her current ability to distance herself so as to engage in self-evaluative, integrative mental activity.

Severe disturbances

Some adolescents who have been avoidant or ambivalent infants, then shifted to the more extreme compulsive caregiving/compliant or punitive/feigned helpless subgroups may shift again to newly forming and more deviant subgroups. Because their minds eliminate and falsify information, such adolescents must negotiate an environment in which important information often does not mean what it appears to mean. Gallows humor is one of the few ways for dealing with awareness of such circumstances: What would you do when you were upset? "*At that time...at that time, oh yeah, I was rrreally suicidal, whenever anybody...made me mad...I'd do something to myself, so...*[like what?] *Cut my wrist and all that stuff, mainly for attention.* [Seriously?] *I mean they weren't so deep, but a couple of them were very deep and ah...my mother taught me how to (laugh). She taught me how to, she said, 'By the way, you don't cut your wrists this way...you cut this way.' I was like, 'Oh, thanks for the tip!' So, I, I, spaz out bad. Now I, I don't try to kill myself because I don't wanna die.*" Were you ever separated from her? "*Nope, I was a lucky kid to have my mother there 24 hours a day.*" Although the ghoulish humor in this answer distances the listener from the underlying tragedy, there are other important features. The adolescent answers in the coercive style of arousing episodes that almost slip into the present tense, while both humor and dismissing phrases, for example, "all that stuff," are used defensively to create distance for the speaker.

Other adolescents escape reality by distorting their thought processes. After an inconclusive trial for date rape, a young man was charged by his new fiancee with battery. His response: "*This is all just a big misunderstanding.*"

Because many very disturbed adolescents fear danger in a wide variety of situations, their distorted mental and behavioral strategies are organized to increase the probability of protection. In addition, unlike more balanced children who trust most information to be accurate, very disturbed adolescents do not have the advantage of a "safety signal." For them, reality gives either clear signals of danger or potentially false signals of safety: Were you ever separated from your parents? "*No, never. My parents still to this day, they don't go away. My parents love us. They just don't leave.*" For this young woman, only the physical presence of loved ones is assurance of their availability. At the other extreme are those who doubt even what they can see. One young man in an explosively violent family claimed, wishfully, "*I can almost tell now when they have and when they haven't* [been drinking]." Another, who had been incarcerated for violent attacks on others, warned, "*If somebody threatens you, don't worry about him; he's warning you. Worry about the guy who gets angry over some little thing and attacks you from behind!"* For such people, information is often false and their minds have few ways to confirm the veracity of information or trustworthiness of individuals. Always, the cost of misplaced trust is greater than the potential reward of reciprocal and intimate relationships.

Karl is an extreme example. Although Karl was a very intelligent young man with an outstanding grasp of quantum physics, nevertheless, he suffered from the severe interpersonal dysfunction of autism. As he put it, everyone thought of him as really weird. Indeed, he thought so too. Exploring this, his therapist asked what made him weird: *"It's hard to say. Other people can't put their finger on it. I have a tendency to look through people, to talk too loud."* The therapist then asked Karl to tell about his development from the beginning: *"Well, first there was the Big Bang. (Laugh). This is a perfect illustration of my theme. I find humor in excessive literalism. (Pause). I was born and raised in Cincinnati..."* Karl's speech has a distancing quality as though he wanted extra time to prepare answers to questions and as though he were watching himself from others' vantage points, seeing and evaluating himself through their eyes. Humor covered this rouse, thus, creating a superficial social persona that eased his social awkwardness.

CONCLUSION

The central thesis of this chapter is that the cortex of the brain integrates information from the lower brain to yield sophisticated models of reality. With maturation, the complexity of these models increases. If, however, some information is found, by experience, to lead to undesired outcomes, that information may come to be distrusted or even falsified. Attachment figures play an important role in teaching children the meaning of information. When information is disregarded or it fails to be integrated, both mental functioning and behavior are affected. Language both gives evidence of the distortion and, through what cannot be said, limits what can be understood.

ACKNOWLEDGMENTS

I wish to thank Kathleen Black, Adela Cammarte, Anne K. Bergeron, Rene Geada, Lothar Krappmann, Kathleen McCartney, and Lucille Moore for the opportunity to discuss cases, view tapes or read transcripts that contributed substantively to my understanding of children's use of language to reflect mental functioning.

REFERENCES

Ainsworth, M.D.S., Blehar, M., Waters, E., & Wall, S. (1978). *Patterns of Attachment: A Psychological Study of the Strange Situation.* Hillsdale, NJ: Erlbaum.

Anderson, E.S. (1984). The acquisition of sociolinguistic knowledge: evidence from children's verbal word play. *Western Journal of Speech Communication,* **48**, 125–144.

Bandler, R. & Grinder, J. (1975). *The Structure of Magic I*. Palo Alto, CA: Science and Behavior Books.

Bowlby, J. (1969/82). *Attachment and Loss. Vol. I: Attachment*. New York: Basic Books.

Bowlby, J. (1980). *Attachment and Loss. Vol. III: Loss*. New York: Basic Books.

Crittenden, P.M. (1990). Internal representational models of attachment relationships. *Infant Mental Health Journal*, **11**, 259–277.

Crittenden, P.M. (1992a). Quality of attachment in the preschool years. *Development and Psychopathology*, **4**, 209–241.

Crittenden, P.M. (1992b). Treatment of anxious attachment in infancy and early childhood. *Development and Psychopathology*, **4**, 575–602.

Crittenden, P.M. (1994). Peering into the black box: an exploratory treatise on the development of self in young children. In D. Cicchetti & S. Toth (eds) *Rochester Symposium on Developmental Psychopathology, Vol. 5. The Self and its Disorders*. Rochester, NY: University of Rochester Press (pp. 79–148).

Crittenden, P.M. (1995). Attachment and psychopathology. In S. Goldberg, R. Muir, & J. Kerr (eds) *Attachment Theory: Social, Developmental, and Clinical Perspectives*. Hillsdale, NJ: The Analytic Press (pp. 367–406).

Darwin, C. (1872/1965). *The Expression of Emotions in Man and Animals*. Chicago, IL: University of Chicago Press.

Ervin-Tripp, S., O'Connor, S., & Rosenberg, J. (1984). Language and power in the family. In M. Schultz and C. Kramerae (eds) *Language and Power*. Belmont, CA: Sage Press (pp. 116–135).

Fischer, K.W. (1980). A theory of cognitive development: The control and construction of hierarchies of skills. *Psychological Review*, **87**, 477–531.

Gallistel, C.R., Brown, A.L., Carey, S., Gelman, R., & Keil, F.C. (1991). Lessons from animal learning for the study of cognitive development. In S. Carey & R. Gelman (eds) *The Epigenesis of Mind: Essays of Biology and Cognition*. Hillsdale, NJ: Lawrence Erlbaum (pp. 3–36).

Grief, E.B. & Gleason, J.B. (1980). Hi, thanks, and goodbye: more routine language in society. *Language in Society*, **9**, 159–166.

Grinder, J. & Bandler, R. (1976). *The Structure of Magic II*. Palo Alto, CA: Science and Behavior Books.

Kohlberg, L. (1984). *Essays on Moral Development. Vol. 1. The Psychology of Moral Development*. San Francisco, CA: Harper & Row.

Loftus, E. & Hoffman, H.G. (1989). Misinformation and memory: the creation of new memories. *Journal of Experimental Psychology*, **118**, 100–104.

MacLean, P.D. (1973). *A Triune Concept of Brain and Behavior*. Toronto: University of Toronto Press.

MacLean, P.D. (1990). *The Triune Brain in Evolution: Role in Paleocerebral Functions*. New York: Plenum Press.

Main, M. & Goldwyn, R. (1992). Adult attachment classification system. Unpublished coding manual, University of California, Berkeley.

Ornstein, R. & Thompson, R.F. (1984). *The Amazing Brain*. New York: Houghton Mifflin.

Piaget, J. (1932). *The Moral Judgment of the Child*. New York: Harcourt, Brace.

Schieffelin, B.B. & Ochs, E. (1983). A cultural perspective on the transition from prelinguistic to linguistic communication. In R.M. Golinkoff (ed.) *The Transition from Prelinguistic to Linguistic Communication*. Hillsdale, NJ: Erlbaum (pp. 115–131).

Sigel, I.E., Stinson, E.T., & Flaugher, J. (in press). The distancing model: A paradigm for studying parental influences on children's cognitive development. In R.J. Sternberg & L. Okagaki (eds) *Directions of Development: Influences on the Development of Children's Thinking.* Hillsdale, NJ: Lawrence Erlbaum.

Sloman, L., Price, J., Gilbert, P., & Gardner, R. (1994). Adaptive function of depression: Psychotherapeutic implications. *American Journal of Psychotherapy,* **48,** 1–13.

Thompson, R.F. (1985). *The Brain: An Introduction to Neuroscience.* New York: W.H. Freeman.

Tulving, E. (1972). Episodic and semantic memory. In E. Tulving & W. Donaldson (eds) *Organization of Memory.* New York: Academic Press.

Tulving, E. (1985). How many memory systems are there? *American Psychologist,* **40,** 385–398.

5 Developmental changes in the mechanisms linking language disabilities and behavior disorders

JIM STEVENSON

INTRODUCTION

This chapter will aim to provide a general overview of the associations between language disabilities and behavior disorders and to attempt to draw some conclusions about the various mechanisms mediating this association and how their importance changes with age. In order to do this I will draw upon empirical studies on a wide range of language disabilities, including specific learning disabilities such as reading disability. I will also discuss disabilities across a wide range of severity from developmental receptive language disorders which may have a profound adverse effect on behavior over the life-span to language delays, which may be of quite limited duration and may be associated with more restricted behavior problems.

There have been few studies designed specifically to investigate the mechanisms linking language impairment and psychopathology and the literature in this field is prone to a number of methodological difficulties (Rutter & Mawhood, 1991). The following problems make the interpretation and synthesis of findings from different studies:

1. heterogeneity in the type and severity of language disorder
2. lack of control of the effects of associated handicaps
3. bias in clinic referred samples
4. lack of standardized measures of behavioral sequelae
5. lack of differentiation between transient and persistent language problems
6. absence of data on control subjects.

A particular difficulty in examining studies for indications of possible mechanisms is the lack of control over the general vulnerabilities to behavior disorders that stem from pervasive factors such as social disadvantage and low IQ. For example, a number of studies indicate that behavioral outcome is worse if language impairment is associated with low IQ (Baker & Cantwell, 1987b; Beitchman et al., 1989; Silva et al., 1984). The mechanisms whereby vulnerabilities to behavior disorders stemming from language impairment interact with those arising from low IQ are simply unexplored.

BEHAVIOR PROBLEMS IN CHILDREN WITH
LANGUAGE IMPAIRMENT

Speech and language delays

A consistent picture has emerged of a greater association between behavior problems and communication disorders that involve language impairment, especially comprehension deficits, than for those concerned with speech disorders. This is illustrated by the findings of Cantwell & Baker (1987a) and Baker & Cantwell (1987a). A sample of 600 children with communication disorders were divided into three groups: those with "pure speech," "speech and language" and "pure language" disorders. A higher rate of both developmental and psychiatric disorders was found in the two groups with language involvement.

Stevenson & Richman (1978) studied a sample of 705 children screened for language delay and found a significant association between behavior problems and language delay. A number of specific behaviors were found to be significantly more common in this group at 3 years of age. They included many items indicative of general immaturity (e.g. soiling, wetting, and dependency) including those associated with a pattern of overactive behavior (e.g. poor concentration and restlessness). This work was based upon a community sample and similar results have been found using clinic referrals. For example, Love & Thompson (1988) found that 75% of children with language delay were also showing attention deficits.

Earlier Beitchman (1985) suggested that expressive language delay was associated with distractibility, impulsivity, and hyperactivity and that receptive language delays have less clear behavioral correlates. He went on to propose that there may be a distinct group of children with language delay and hyperactivity (Beitchman, Tuckett, & Batth, 1987). A group of children with the combined conditions was found to be significantly different on IQ and visual-motor integration from those with hyperactivity alone and a comparison group of nonhyperactive disturbed children. However, with no data on a group of language delayed children without hyperactivity the case for a separate subgroup is incomplete. Indeed, a more parsimonious explanation is that the children with the combined condition are simply more deviant cases with the same mix of aetiological factors as other children but in a more extreme form.

The above studies used questionnaire methods to obtain data on the behavior of language delayed children. There have been fewer attempts to obtain direct observation data. An exception is the study by Caulfield et al. (1989) who observed parent–child interaction in a group of children with expressive language delay and a normal group matched for receptive language and nonverbal IQ. The group with expressive language delay showed more negative behavior than the control group.

In trying to ascertain which children within the language/speech disordered population show behavior problems, Beitchman, Peterson, & Clegg (1988) failed to find any association with family or demographic variables. Social class for example was related to the presence of psychiatric disorder in the normal speech and language group but not within the language disordered sample. This study was impressive in its use of samples obtained by screening a one in three sample of all 5-year-old children (N = 1655). A subsequent study of 142 5-year-old language impaired children (Beitchman, Hood, & Inglis, 1990) showed that the risk for psychiatric disorder was greatest among girls. These findings contrast with Baker & Cantwell (1987b) where psychosocial stresses were related to behavioral disorders within the language delay group.

This issue was also addressed in Stevenson & Richman (1978) by trying to identify factors that differentiated language delayed children with and without behavior problems. There were few differences between the two groups. For example, the children with behavior problems were not those with the more delayed language development.

The findings on the behavior problems found in children with language delay can be summarized under two questions. First, how strong is the association? There is remarkable agreement between studies that significant behavior problems are found in just over half the children with language delay: Baker & Cantwell (1987b) found a rate of 50%; Stevenson & Richman (1978) obtained an estimate of 59% in 3-year-old children; Beitchman, quoted by Baker & Cantwell (1987b), observed 53% of kindergarten children with speech and language delays to show behavior problems. The association therefore is a strong and significant one; behavior disorders are found in children with language delay at about four times the rate in the general population.

Second, how specific is this link? In the young child with language delays the type of behavior problem shown can vary. However, behavioral immaturity (e.g. sphincter control and dependency) and overactivity are particularly common. In older children, more internalizing/neurotic problems are found. These behavior profiles of language delayed children show a limited range of behavior problems and in this sense the association is specific.

Specific language impairments

There are some children who show persistent severe impairments in language which are not associated with low nonverbal IQ (Leonard et al., 1987). A longitudinal study of 156 children with such specific speech and language impairment referred to the Dawn House school was undertaken by Haynes & Naidoo (1991). The measures obtained on these children included teachers' reports on the childrens' behavior. There are no control data for comparison purposes but the study is helpful in identifying trends in the behavior of the children as they moved through the school from age 6 to 11 years. In general, the high rates of behavior indicating frustration and aggression decline quite rapidly while difficulties associated with low self-confidence, low self-esteem and social withdrawal remain. As with other studies, children with speech impairments have fewer behavioral problems than those with language impairment.

Long-term outcome

The evidence considered so far has concerned the *concurrent* association between language impairment and behavior problems. A significant feature of recent research studies has been the identification of adverse outcomes for language delayed children even when the initial language delay has been overcome. It is to this longitudinal data that we will now turn.

Baker & Cantwell (1987b) conducted a follow-up study of the behavior of a group of 202 children referred for communication disorders. They found that four years after initial referral the rates of psychiatric disturbance had increased. Unlike Beitchman, Peterson, & Clegg (1988), they found that they could distinguish those language impaired children with persistent psychiatric disturbance by both the severity of initial language disorders and by psychosocial stress present at follow-up.

There have been three similar longitudinal studies of epidemiological samples of children with preschool language delays. Silva, Williams, & McGee (1987) showed that children with delayed verbal comprehension and general language delay at three years were most at risk for later behavior problems. The Newcastle study found the children with language delays to be more likely to show marked introversion and withdrawal than the control group at follow-up some five years later (Fundudis, Kolvin, & Garside, 1979). The Waltham Forest follow-up study showed there to be a high rate of disturbance in language delayed children at 8-years-of-age (Richman, Stevenson, & Graham, 1982). A control sample matched for a variety of family and child characteristics at age 3 years was used in an attempt to isolate the specific affect of language delay *per se* on later behavior. Neurotic or emotional problems were the most distinctive feature of the behavior of formerly language delayed children. This is confirmed by a variety of other studies. Cantwell & Baker (1987c) found that 30% of their sample of 600 language impaired children had anxiety symptoms with 10% meeting the DSM-III criterion for a diagnosis of anxiety disorder.

In reviewing the link between language delay and *later* psychopathology in children showing language delay in their early years Rutter & Mawhood (1991) conclude: "As judged by all the available data, the main increase in psychopathology seems to be in the domain of anxiety, social relationships and attention-deficit problems rather than in conduct disturbance or antisocial behaviour."

This conclusion gains further support in a follow-up study conducted on children with less severe degrees of language delay (Stevenson, Richman, & Graham, 1985). A sample of 528 children was studied at their third and eighth birthdays. The scores on a simplified version of the structure subscale of the Reynell Developmental Language Scales (Reynell, 1969) (i.e. an index of syntactic complexity of expressive language) were divided at the median to identify children at 3-years-of-age with good and poor expressive language development. The Rutter Teacher Scale (Rutter, 1967) ratings were obtained at age 8 years. The degree of early behavior disturbance was measured using the Behavior Screening Questionnaire (Richman & Graham, 1971). There was no evidence of any specific risk of antisocial behavior problems in the poor language group. At all levels of behavior disturbance at 3-years-old, the children with poor expressive language showed higher levels of neurotic disturbance at 8 years compared to those with good expressive language at 3-years-of-age.

By way of summary, we can ask how strong and specific is the association between early language delay and later behavior problems? The results presented by Baker & Cantwell (1987b) suggest that the association is *even stronger* five years after the children were initially examined. As many as 60% of children with language delay may have enduring or subsequently developing behavior problems. The association is also specific in that at follow-up the most salient behavior problems are introversion/internalizing problems or attention deficits. The specificity of this association is made more striking by the emergence in the general population of sex differences in the rates of behavior problems in middle childhood. In particular antisocial/conduct disorders become more common in boys than in girls by 8-years-of-age (Richman, Stevenson, & Graham, 1982). The majority of children with language delay are boys, which makes the high rate of internalizing problems at this age even more unexpected. These findings indicate that a developmental perspective must be taken if we are to understand the nature of the links between variation in language ability and behavior.

Reading disability

Children with language impairments are at risk of developing reading disability (Mann & Brady, 1988). The study of Bishop & Adams (1990) showed that children with persistent language impairment were particularly prone to reading disabilities and that once non-verbal IQ was controlled, this deficit centered particularly on reading comprehension. This indicates a further set of possible mechanisms for the association between language and behavior. The nature of the associations between reading disability and behavior is not resolved after much extensive research. In particular, it is not clear whether specific reading retardation leads to antisocial behavior or vice versa (Maughan, Gray, & Rutter, 1985; Jorm et al., 1986). It is likely that the effects will be reciprocal but the evidence suggests that poor reading leading to disruptive behavior is the stronger of the two effects (McGee & Share, 1988). However Fergusson and Horwood (1992) have applied structural equation modeling to longitudinal data on a cohort of 1265 children in the Christchurch Child Development Study. They showed that by 12-years-of-age, the predominant direction of effects is from attention deficit disorder to reading achievement. Using this same form of analysis applied to data on 698 children from the Dunedin Multidisciplinary Health and Development Study, Williams and McGee (1994) confirmed the complex transactional effects that link reading attainment and externalizing behaviors. They found that early reading did predict later conduct disorder but at the same time early antisocial behavior had a detrimental effect on later reading. These two studies from New Zealand have provided some of the most sensitive analyses of the mutual influences between reading ability and behavior.

Nonverbal learning disabilities

It has been found repeatedly that children with a history of language impairment are particularly vulnerable to developing behavioral disorders. There are some exceptions. For example in a series of studies Rourke and his colleagues (Rourke & Fuerst, 1991) have suggested that among children with learning disabilities, those with a decrement in performance IQ relative to verbal IQ are more likely to show the most severe psychopathology. Fuerst, Fisk, & Rourke (1990) present data on a sample of 6 to 12-year-old children with learning disabilities. The groups with verbal IQs lower than performance IQ were said to show either normal or mildly disturbed psychosocial functioning. These results are interpreted by Rourke and his colleagues to indicate that children with nonverbal learning disabilities have patterns of severe emotional and behavioral disturbance that are a direct result of their neuropsychological deficits. On the other hand, when children with language based deficits show behavioral disturbance they do so because of the factors that are secondary to their language handicaps.

The conclusions concerning a neuropsychological deficit underlying the behavior disturbance in nonverbal learning disability is not challenged by the studies reviewed in the next section. There is an incompatibility between one aspect of the data from the Fuerst et al. (1990) study and other studies on children with language delay. The behavior of children with verbal deficits is normal for the majority and if abnormal is only mildly so. For these children, unlike other studies, their language deficits are not centrally involved in the behavior problems they show. These inconsistencies might be explained by the use of Personality Inventory for Children (Wirt et al., 1984) by Rourke and colleagues whereas most other research has tended to use behavioral measures such as the Child Behavior Checklist (Achenbach, 1991). Sampling differences and differences in the definition of language disabilities might also be significant. Until more studies are conducted that compare the behavior problems of different types of learning disability this seeming anomaly cannot be resolved.

LANGUAGE ABILITY OF CHILDREN WITH BEHAVIOR DISORDERS

Let us now turn to the language abilities of behaviorally disturbed children. In a series of consecutive referrals to a child psychiatric outpatient clinic of children aged 5 to 12 years, a severe or moderate language disorder was found in 28% of those referred solely for a psychiatric problem (Cohen, Davine, & Meloche-Kelly, 1989; Cohen et al., 1993). These children differed from those referred for both psychiatric and language disorders by being younger and in being more likely to have externalizing behavior problems. Cohen et al. (1989) suggest that routine screening for language impairments should be instigated because such difficulties may be overlooked because of these children's disruptive behavior. Similar findings were reported by Kotsopoulos & Boodoosingh (1987) and by Camarata, Hughes, & Ruhl (1988).

Love & Thompson (1988) found that 65% of the preschool children referred to outpatient psychiatric services showed language disorders. They go as far to suggest that "language disorders are as common among children with psychiatric problems as psychiatric problems are among language disordered children." This conclusion is somewhat distorted by being based on clinic referrals; the situation is different in nonreferred populations. For example, in the Waltham Forest study it was found that 14% of the general population of 3-year-olds showed behavior problems (Richman, Stevenson, & Graham, 1982). Using this same definition 59% of children with language delay showed a behavior problem. Using a definition of language delay that identified 3% of the general population, these language delays were found in 13% of the children with behavior problems.

These results suggest that in population terms a substantial minority of children with behavior problems show language delay. The association appears to be stronger if clinic samples are studied. The specificity of the association is less easy to establish in studies of behavior problem children. However, if referred for language problems and behavior disturbance, children are likely to show internalizing problems; a similar association to that found for children identified by their showing language delay. At the same time children presenting with inattention or conduct disorders may have unsuspected language impairments (Cohen et al., 1993).

CHANGES IN THE PATTERN OF COMORBIDITY BETWEEN LANGUAGE DISORDERS AND BEHAVIORAL DISORDERS WITH AGE

To summarize the evidence reviewed so far. In the preschool period delays in language development and behavior problems are significantly associated.

This is shown particularly by the elevated rates of behavioral immaturity (e.g. sphincter control and dependency) and overactivity. In middle childhood both children with a past history of language delays and those with a concurrent pattern of reading disability are likely to show internalizing or neurotic problems. Later there emerges an association between reading disability and antisocial behavior. It has been found that a history of speech and language delays is associated with specific reading retardation (Rutter & Yule, 1975; Bishop & Adams, 1990). This suggests that with large enough samples and with follow-up into adolescence an association between early language delays and later antisocial behavior might be found for at least a subgroup of previously language disabled children.

MECHANISMS LINKING LANGUAGE DISABILITY AND BEHAVIOR DISORDERS

The evidence considered so far has concerned the strength and the specificity of the association between language impairment and behavior problems. We will now review the evidence about the nature of the mechanisms that might be responsible for this association.

Rutter and Lord framework for analysing comorbidity

The types of pattern of association between language impairment and behavior have been reviewed by Rutter and Lord (1987). They differentiated between the possibilities that (a) psychiatric disorder and language problems are integral parts of a common condition (e.g. autism), (b) psychiatric disorder and language sharing a common cause (e.g. mental handicap), (c) there are separate but correlated causes of the two disorders (e.g. aspects of environmental deprivation), (d) language problems arise as a consequence of a psychiatric disorder (e.g. elective mutism), and (e) psychiatric disorders arise as a consequence of language disorders (e.g. socioemotional problems secondary to specific language delays).

Single syndrome

Behavioral difficulties and language disorders may co-occur because they are both components of a single syndrome. A clear example of this is autism where deficiencies in language, social relationships and behavior can all be seen to stem from a common origin in a biological based deficit which produces a distinctive cognitive disability and which in turn produces the language and behavioral symptoms of the condition (Frith, 1989; Morton, 1989). Although there is variation in the manifestation of the symptoms in autistic children, the single syndrome formulation is different from the next category (common aetiology) in that the biological deficits if present produces the combined language and behavioral symptoms. In contrast, where a common aetiology is acting it may produce comorbidity or may produce either the language or the behavioral disturbances alone.

Common etiology

There are a wide range of factors that could act as shared causes of both language disability and behavior disorders. In the preschool child both are associated with social disadvantage and with a lack of warmth in parenting (Richman, Stevenson, & Graham, 1982). Baker & Cantwell (1987b) also reported that psychiatric diagnoses were associated with psychosocial stresses within their sample. This suggests that the high rate of disturbance in the language delayed group might be a reflection of higher levels of psychosocial stress or that language delayed children are particularly vulnerable to such stresses.

The absence of a normal control group in the Baker and Cantwell (1987b) study does not allow these two alternatives to be evaluated. There is evidence from other studies (e.g. Richman & Stevenson, 1977) that language delay is associated with high levels of social stress. However, there is also evidence from Cantwell & Baker (1987b) that the elevated rates of psychiatric disorder in language delayed children are probably not due simply to the increased exposure to psychosocial stress. They found that children with language delay were more likely to show inappropriate affect, bizarre behavior and stereotypies than matched controls referred for behavior disorders. These differences in symptomatology are consistent with distinct specific influences on the disorders shown by language delayed children. However, most studies have concentrated on within child factors as a common cause.

Mental handicap

There are two well-established findings that as samples are identified with decreasing IQ levels their relative handicap in language becomes more marked and the frequency of behavior problems increases (Scott, 1993). For some cases of language delay, both the delay itself and the associated behavior problems may be a product of a general pattern of low intellectual functioning.

Neurodevelopmental precursor

Beitchman et al. (1989) suggest that psychiatric disorder, especially attention deficit hyperactivity disorder, is associated with general linguistic impairment rather than with specific disabilities such as auditory comprehension or articulation. They considered this association as being due to a common neurodevelopmental immaturity underlying both linguistic impairment and psychiatric disorder.

A similar conclusion is reached by Tallal, Dukette, & Curtiss (1989) who go further to suggest that if neurodevelopmental items are deleted from indices of behavioral and emotional status that there are few, if any, residual behavior deficits in language impaired children. There are a number of problems with the results presented in this study. Most importantly, the distinction between neurodevelopmental items and other indices of behavior problems is not clearly justified (e.g. why is "slow moving" neurodevelopmental but not "much sleep," why "stares blankly" but not "daydreams," and so on). The actual results indicate that even after taking out the "neurodevelopmental" items that discriminate most clearly between the groups, there was still a significantly higher Total Behavior Score on the CBCL for the language impaired boys (27) than for the normal boys (19) (p < 0.05). As an index of size of effect the between group difference here is of the order of 0.75 of a standard deviation – not a trivial difference.

There is an important difference in the explanations of Beitchman et al. (1989) and of Tallal and her colleagues. Beitchman et al. (1989) found that the risk of behavior problems increased with the degree of language impairment. Benasich, Curtiss, & Tallal (1993) found in their sample that when nonverbal IQ was controlled this association disappeared. They suggest that both language impairment and behavior problems might be a consequence of a neurodevelopmental deficit. They postulate that this deficit centers on a deficiency in processing rapidly changing stimuli across modalities (Tallal, Sainburg, & Jernigan, 1991).

It must be accepted that if neurodevelopmental status is controlled there is a reduction in the level of the behavior problems shown by language impaired children (Stevenson & Richman, 1978). However, it is also clear that differences in behavior remain after such control in cross-sectional studies. Longitudinal studies also indicate that there are residual risks of disturbance once the language has improved; an issue which will be discussed in the next section.

There is an instance of language and behavior showing shared genetic aetiology which does not seem to be mediated via common neurodevelopmental precursor. For example, Stevenson et al. (1993) developed a bivariate extension of the DeFries and Fulker (1985) multiple regression analysis to detect shared genetic influences on spelling disability and attention deficit hyperactivity disorder (ADHD). Previous studies have shown that both spelling disability (DeFries et al., 1991; Stevenson, 1991) and hyperactivity (Stevenson, 1992; Gillis et al., 1992) are substantially heritable. Stevenson et al. (1993) found that to the modest extent that these disabilities tend to co-occur they do so largely for genetic reasons. This finding might arise as a result of a pleiotropic genetic effect whereby the same gene or genes produces hyperactivity and spelling disability; the common neurodevelopmental precursor explanation. Alternatively, one condition could be largely genetically determined and this condition leads to the development of the other as a secondary consequence. This latter mechanism may well apply to the shared genetic aetiology of spelling disability and hyperactivity. The phenocopy hypothesis, discussed below, put forward by Pennington, Grossier, & Welsh (1993) in their study of the comorbidity of reading disability and ADHD provides one such mechanism.

Separate but correlated causes

The possibility of separate but correlated causes has not been extensively investigated. One plausible candidate is the association between language delay and inattention. It has been found that mothers who are depressed are likely to engender a style of rapid attentional switching in the preschool children (Breznitz & Friedman, 1988). This arises from their interactional style of rapid changes of topic when playing with their children. Language delay is also associated with maternal depression (Richman & Stevenson, 1977). However, in this case the association is likely to arise through lack of appropriate and sensitive responding to the child (Davis, Stroud, & Green, 1988; Whitehurst et al., 1988). Here we have behavior and language adversely affected by different aspects of maternal care. However, these features of the mother–child relationship are correlated since they are both likely to arise in mothers who are depressed: an example of separate but correlated causes.

Language disability leads to behavior disorder

The mechanisms considered so far are based upon an association arising from the action of prior causes. The possibility that one condition leads to the other needs to be considered next. Taking this perspective, there has been much more emphasis on language disability leading to behavior problems than upon effects in the opposite direction.

Frustration stemming from communication failure

There is now a substantial body of evidence to indicate that children with language impairments have significant handicaps in the use of language skills. Lapadat (1991) undertook a meta-analysis of the results of 33 studies of the pragmatic language skills of 3 to 12-year-old children with language impairments (usually based on speech-language pathologist diagnosis following clinical assessment with a battery of tests) with and without learning disabilities (as defined by local, state or national guidelines, that is using administrative definitions). She estimated the mean effect size was −0.52 (s.e. = 0.06), that is the mean of the language impaired children was about half a standard deviation below that of controls. The effect was equally marked for language impaired children above and below 8 years of age. There are indications from this review that the pragmatic deficits were attributable to language disabilities *per se* since the effect size was more marked ($-$o.77) for children labeled language disordered than for children with a general learning disability. Clearly these pragmatic deficiencies in aspects of language use such as topic selection, turn taking, appropriate word choice and parody will interfere with effective communication. It had been proposed previously by Donahue (1983) that such pragmatic deficits would lead the language impaired child to experience communication failure and this would lead to subsequent frustration and either anxiety and social withdrawal or possibly more externalizing behavior problems.

There have been few direct tests of this frustration hypothesis. Some support for it has come from the work of Caulfield (1989). Children with expressive language delay and controls were studied in contexts where communication demands were low (a nonverbal pointing task), where communicative demands were high (a reading task) and where the task demands were particularly difficult for the language delay group (a naming task). The rates of misbehavior were same in the two groups for the first two tasks but were only elevated in the language delay group for the third task. This evidence suggests that in part some of the difficult behavior of language delayed children is a consequence of the frustration they experience in being unable to communicate effectively in certain contexts.

Phenocopy hypothesis for attention deficits and reading disability

There is one example where the mechanism has been clearly articulated which leads from language disorders to behavior. Pennington, Grossier, & Welsh (1993) found that reading disabled children showed phonological processing deficits and children with ADHD alone showed primarily deficits in executive functions. However, the children comorbid for reading disability and ADHD showed deficits in phonological processing only. They argue that the symptoms of ADHD can arise as a secondary consequence of reading disability, that is as a phenocopy. Further studies are needed to both identify the mechanisms involved and which reading disabled children are at risk of following this developmental path.

Low self-esteem

It has been suggested by McGee et al. (1986) that reading disability and antisocial behavior are linked via lowered self-esteem. Continuing experience of educational failure leads to a lowering of self-esteem which in turn predisposes the child towards antisocial behavior in early adolescence. There is evidence that children with learning disabilities such as reading disability do show lower academic self-esteem (e.g. Margalit & Zak, 1984). However, in reviewing this literature Rourke and Fuerst (1991) suggest that there is little consistent evidence that such academic self-esteem generalizes to other aspects of the child's self-evaluation or that it leads to problem behavior even in the school setting.

Language, cognition, and the regulation of behavior

The implication of language disability for the child's problem solving in general and the regulation of behavior in social settings in particular has not been extensively examined (Montgomery, 1992). If the child with language delay is deficient in developing and understanding of social situations or in using language to regulate their own behavior or social interactions, then the basis would be in place for language delay to lead to behavior disorders. There is some limited evidence that the peer interactions of children with language delay are impaired either through communication difficulties or possibly a specific deficit in social cognition (Siegel et al., 1985).

There is some evidence that language may have a role to play in the association between emotional understanding and behavior problems. Cook, Greenberg, & Kusché (1994) found that children with behavior problems (as identified by the Child Behavior Checklist) showed deficits in emotional understanding compared to nonproblems controls. Within the sample vocabulary scores were highly related to both to behavior problems and to emotional understanding. When vocabulary was controlled as a covariate the differences between the behavior problems groups in emotional understanding were still significant though attenuated. This suggests that language deficits are in part contributing to the problems in emotional understanding experienced by children with behavior problems.

There is also experimental evidence that children with language disabilities are less competent in using information they have to solve problems and to communicate effectively (e.g. Johnson & Smith, 1989). However, as Bishop and Adams (1991) have shown the extent of the language impaired child's handicap in conversation only becomes apparent in more naturalistic settings. There is scope for studies that look at the extent to which deficits in social cognition and pragmatic language skills are related to the risk of behavior disturbances within the population of language delayed children. The methods adopted by Buitelaar et al. (1994) have been shown to be sensitive to the social cognitive deficits of children with hyperactivity and could be readily applied to samples of children with language delay.

Behavior disorder leads to language disability

Most research on the association between language impairment and behavior disorder has been interpreted in terms of the impact of language deficits on behavior. There are circumstances where it is more appropriate to postulate a pattern of reciprocal effects between the two or indeed where the impact of behavior disorders on language development may be the more salient.

Inattention and language development

As has been discussed above there is repeated finding linking language impairment and components of attention deficit hyperactivity disorder. For example Cohen et al. (1993) showed these behavioral dimensions to be the most distinctive in separating psychiatrically disturbed children with and without language impairments on both parent and teacher rating. They observe that there is a need for additional investigations to ascertain whether attention deficits lead to language delays or vice versa or indeed whether there are bi-directional effects. It is certainly plausible that inattentive, impulsive, and distractible preschoolers are less likely to gain from social interaction that fosters language development. What is needed are longitudinal studies of children showing just one of these deficits, i.e. pure language delay and pure hyperactive groups. The question of interest would then be which of these two pure groups is more likely to become comorbid. Until we have data of this kind it will not be possible to decide either way on the plausibility that language development is adversely influenced by symptoms of ADHD.

The impact of child's behavior on the caretaker

There is a substantial body of evidence that the quality of early social interactions between child and caretaker is a major influence on language development (e.g. Olson, Bates, & Bayles, 1984). It has been found that behavior problems in young children are associated with a high level of parental criticism and a lack of warmth towards the child (Richman, Stevenson, & Graham, 1982). It may be that behavioral difficulties in the child feed back into the parent–child relationship to change the emotional tone and possibly the sensitivity with which parents respond and interact with their children. This in turn would act to have an adverse impact on the child's language development.

A DEVELOPMENTAL MODEL OF THE MECHANISMS LINKING LANGUAGE DEVELOPMENT AND BEHAVIOR

The account given above suggests that there is a large number of plausible mechanisms that could be acting to produce the association between language disability and behavior problems. The explanations are of course not mutually exclusive and indeed a number of mechanisms may be acting in concert. However, given the change in the type of behavior associated with language impairment with age it is likely that the salience of these mechanisms also changes with age. A possible outline of such a developmental pattern is presented in Figure 5.1.

In the preschool years the most salient feature of the behavior of children showing language delay is immaturity and overactivity. Moving into the early school years children with previous or continuing language delays are more likely to show internalizing disorders. Then towards the early adolescence there are mechanisms that would produce an association between early language delays and antisocial behavior but perhaps only in those children with language delay that go on to develop reading disability.

The model is an attempt to identify the mechanisms linking language/reading disability and behavior disorders. It does not attempt to provide a complete picture of the influence on these forms of behavior or emotional disorders. For example, low self-esteem is shown as a mediator of the association between reading disability and externalizing behavior (see Hinshaw, 1992 for evidence in support of this link). However, low self-esteem is also a vulnerability factor for the onset of internalizing disorders in response to life events. This relationship has not been incorporated since it is not postulated to be involved in the association between language/reading disorders and behavior. Similarly, it is not proposed that internalizing disorders are only produced by social cognition deficits; it is simply that these are postulated to be significant in the language/behavior context.

Late onset of language development is given as distinct from language delay since this provides one means whereby experiential factors may feed into the mechanisms linking language and behavior. Specifically, parents whose children are late in starting to develop language may acquire low expectations of the child's developmental potential and, especially if this is reinforced by behavioral immaturity and overactivity, may not provide optimal stimulation of the subsequent language development of the child. By this means social factors may feed into the development of language delay in children who are not otherwise at risk for biological reasons.

There are additional paths that could be added to the figure. For example, there may be genetic influences on phonological ability that are not mediated via language delay; this seems likely given the strong genetic effects found on phonological processing during reading and the fact that many children with reading disability do not show early delays in language development. For example, Richman, Stevenson, & Graham (1982) used a variety of definitions of reading disability at two levels of severity. The percentage of these children with reading disability who showed one of a number of types of language delay at 3 or 4 years of age was never more than 71%. Therefore nearly a third of children with reading disability at 8 years of age do not show language impairments during the preschool period.

Paths could be added indicating direct genetic influences on internalizing disorders. Again this is plausible since the genetic effects on internalizing disorders are moderately strong (Rende et al., 1993) and the majority of

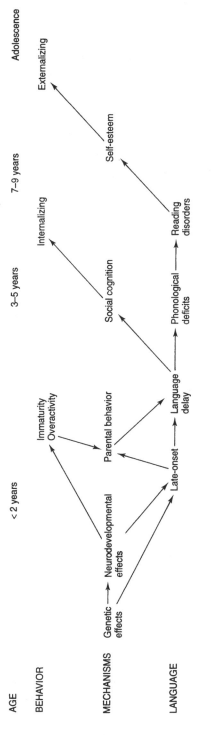

Figure 5.1. Mechanisms linking language impairment and behavior at different ages.

children with internalizing disorders do not have a history of delayed language development. For example, McConaughty, Achenbach, & Gent (1988) found that internalizing problems were associated with higher IQ and better than average performance on tests of cognitive ability. The same is true but to a lesser extent for externalizing disorders (Hinshaw, 1992).

Figure 5.1 also ignores the complexities that arise when the effects of behavior disorders on each other are considered (e.g. Fergusson & Horwood, 1992). In particular, the risk of internalizing and externalizing disorders in children showing ADHD are put to one side. Equally the full range of influences on each of the mechanisms is not reflected in the figure. For example parental behavior will be influenced by a wide range of characteristics in addition to the child's behavior and language. Social stresses, the parents own experiences in their families of origin, education, and income are just some of the additional influences on parenting behavior (Belsky, 1984). This simplification is made on the grounds that there is no evidence that these factors affect the main links between language development and behavior.

There are a number of features of this formulation that require empirical confirmation. First, the influence of genetic factors on delayed language development has been established (e.g. Bishop et al., 1995). However, it is as yet unknown to what extent the genetic effects on phonological processing of the written word are also acting on early language development and therefore to what extent there are genetic influences in common between language delay, behavioral, and reading disability.

Second, the putative effect of delayed language on internalizing problems through an influence on an impairment in social cognition needs to be investigated more fully. An impoverished early language experience and the reduced experience of language use that the language delayed child experiences have been shown to be potent factors reducing social cognitive competence. It is hypothesized that deficits in social cognitive ability will act to reduce the child's willingness to engage socially because they will be aware of their inability to understand nuances of social interaction and exchange.

Finally, we have too few studies addressing the question of the mechanisms linking language related competencies and behavior. In particular, longitudinal studies of children showing language impairments only and behavior problems only are likely to provide insight into the direction and strength of such effects. Such data is essential if the complexities and developmental shifts in mechanisms incorporated into this hypothetical framework are to be adequately tested.

REFERENCES

Achenbach, T.M. (1991). *Manual for the Child Behavior Checklist/4–18 and 1991 Profile.* Burlington, VT: University of Vermont, Department of Psychiatry.

Baker, L. & Cantwell, D.P. (1987a). Factors associated with the development of psychiatric illness in children with early speech/language problems. *Journal of Autism and Developmental Disorders*, **17**, 499–510.

Baker, L. & Cantwell, D.P. (1987b). A prospective psychiatric follow-up of children with speech and language disorders. *Journal of the American Academy of Child and Adolescent Psychiatry*, **26**, 546–553.

Beitchman, J.H. (1985). Therapeutic considerations with language impaired preschool child. *Canadian Journal of Psychiatry*, **30**, 609–613.

Beitchman, J.H., Hood, J., & Inglis, A. (1990). Psychiatric risk in children with speech and language disorders. *Journal of Abnormal Child Psychology*, **18**, 283–296.

Beitchman, J.H., Hood, J., Rochon, J., & Peterson, M. (1989). Empirical classification of speech/language impairment in children. II: Behavioral characteristics. *Journal of the American Academy of Child and Adolescent Psychiatry*, **28**, 118–123.

Beitchman, J.H., Peterson, M., & Clegg, M. (1988). Speech and language impairment and psychiatric disorder: the relevance of family demographic variables. *Child Psychiatry and Human Development*, **18**, 191–207.

Beitchman, J., Tucket, M., & Batth, S. (1987). Language delay and hyperactivity in preschoolers: evidence for a distinct sub-group of hyperactives. *Canadian Journal of Psychiatry*, **32**, 683–687.

Belsky, J. (1984). The determinants of parenting: A process model. *Child Development*, **55**, 83–96.

Benasich, A.A., Curtiss, S., & Tallal, P. (1993). Language, learning and behavior disturbances in childhood: a longitudinal perspective. *Journal of the American Academy of Child and Adolescent Psychiatry*, **32**, 585–594.

Bishop, D.V.M. & Adams, C. (1990). A prospective study of the relationship between specific language impairment, phonological disorders and reading retardation. *Journal of Child Psychology and Psychiatry*, **31**, 1027–1050.

Bishop, D.V.M. & Adams, C. (1991). What do referential communication tasks measure? A study of children with language impairment. *Applied Psycholinguistics*, **12**, 199–215.

Bishop, D.V.M., North, T., & Donlan, C. (1995). Genetic basis of specific language impairment: evidence from a twin study. *Developmental Medicine and Child Neurology*, **37**, 56–71.

Breznitz, Z. & Friedman, S.L. (1988). Toddlers concentration: does maternal depression make a difference. *Journal of Child Psychology and Psychiatry*, **29**, 267–280.

Buitelaar, J.K., Swinkles, S.H., de Vries, H., Jan van der Gaag, R., & van Hooff, J.A.R.A.M. (1994). An ethological study on behavioral differences between hyper-active, aggressive, combined hyperactive/aggressive and control children. *Journal of Child Psychology and Psychiatry*, **35**, 1437–1446.

Camarata, S.M., Hughes, C.A., & Ruhl, K.L. (1988). Mild/moderate behaviorally disordered students: a population at risk for language disorders. *Language and Hearing Services in Schools*, **19**, 191–200.

Cantwell, D.P. & Baker, L. (1987a). Prevalence and types of psychiatric disorders in three speech and language groups. *Journal of Communication Disorders*, **20**, 151–160.

Cantwell, D.P. & Baker, L. (1987b). Psychiatric symptomatology in language impaired children. *Journal of Child Neurology*, **2**, 128–133.

Cantwell, D.P. & Baker, L. (1987c). The prevalence of anxiety in children with communication disorders. *Journal of Anxiety Disorders*, **1**, 239–248.

Caulfield, M.B. (1989). Communication difficulty: A model of the relation of language delay and behavior problems. *Society for Research in Child Development Abstracts*, **7**, 212.

Caulfield, M.B., Fischel, J.E., DeBaryshe, B.D., & Whitehurst, G.J. (1989). Behavioral correlates of developmental expressive language disorder. *Journal of Abnormal Child Psychology*, **17**, 187–201.

Cohen, N.J., Davine, M., Horodezky, N., Lipsett, L., & Isaacson, L. (1993). Unsuspected language impairment in psychiatrically disturbed children: Prevalence and language and behavioral characteristics. *Journal of the American Academy of Child and Adolescent Psychiatry*, **32**, 595–603.

Cohen, N.J., Davine, M., & Meloche-Kelly, M. (1989). Prevalence of unsuspected language disorders in a child psychiatric population. *Journal of the American Academy of Child and Adolescent Psychiatry*, **28**, 107–111.

Cook, E.T., Greenberg, M.T., & Kusché, C.A. (1994). The relationships between emotional understanding, intellectual functioning and disruptive behavior in elementary school-aged children. *Journal of Abnormal Child Psychology*, **22**, 205–220.

Davis, H., Stroud, A., & Green, L. (1988). The maternal language environment of children with language delay. *British Journal of Disorders of Communication*, **23**, 252–266.

DeFries, J.C. & Fulker, D.W. (1985). Multiple regression of analysis of twin data. *Behavior Genetics*, **15**, 467–473.

DeFries, J.C., Stevenson, J., Gillis, J.J., & Wadsworth, S.J. (1991). Genetic etiology of spelling deficits in the Colorado and London twin studies of reading disability. *Reading and Writing*, **3**, 271–283.

Donahue, M. (1983). Learning disabled children as conversational partners. *Topics in Learning Disorders*, **4**, 15–27.

Fergusson, D.M. & Horwood, L.J. (1992). Attention deficit and reading achievement. *Journal of Child Psychology and Psychiatry*, **33**, 375–386.

Fuerst, D.R., Fisk, J.L., & Rourke, B.P. (1990). Psychosocial functioning of learning-disabled children: relations between WISC Verbal IQ-Performance IQ discrepancies and personality sub-types. *Journal of Consulting and Clinical Psychology*, **58**, 657–660.

Fundudis, T., Kolvin, I., & Garside, R. (eds) (1979). *Speech Retarded and Deaf Children: Their Psychological Development*. London: Academic Press.

Frith, U. (1989). *Autism: Explaining the Enigma*. Oxford: Basil Blackwell.

Gillis, J.J., Gilger, J.W., Pennington, B.F., & DeFries, J.C. (1992). Attentional deficit disorder in reading-disabled twins: evidence for a genetic etiology. *Journal of Abnormal Child Psychology*, **20**, 303–315.

Haynes, C. & Naidoo, S. (1991). *Children with Specific Speech and Language Impairment*. Clinics in Developmental Medicine No. 119. Oxford: MacKeith Press/Blackwells Scientific.

Hinshaw, S.P. (1992). Externalizing behavior problems and academic underachievement in childhood and adolescence: causal relationships and underlying mechanisms. *Psychological Bulletin*, **111**, 127–155.

Johnson, J. & Smith, L. (1989). Dimensional thinking in language impaired children. *Journal of Hearing and Speech Research*, **32**, 33–40.

Jorm, A.F., Share, D.L., Matthews, R., & Maclean, R. (1986). Behavior problems in specific reading retarded and general reading backward children: a longitudinal study. *Journal of Child Psychology and Psychiatry*, **27**, 33–43.

Kotsopoulos, A. & Boodoosingh, L. (1987). Language and speech disorders in children attending a day psychiatric programme. *British Journal of Disorders of Communication*, **22**, 227–236.

Lapadat, J.C. (1991). Pragmatic language skills of students with language and/or learning disabilities: a quantitative synthesis. *Journal of Learning Disabilities*, **24**, 147–158.

Leonard, L.B., Sabbandini, L., Leonard, J.S., & Volterra, V. (1987). Specific language impairment in children. *Brain and Language*, **32**, 233–252.

Love, A.J. & Thompson, M.G.G. (1988). Language disorders and attention deficit disorders in young children referred for psychiatric services: analysis of prevalence and a conceptual synthesis. *Journal of Orthopsychiatry*, **58**, 52–64.

Mann, V.A. & Brady, S. (1988). Reading disability: the role of language deficiencies. *Journal of Consulting and Clinical Psychology*, **56**, 811–816.

Margalit, M. & Zak, I. (1984). Anxiety and self-concept of learning disabled children. *Journal of Learning Disabilities*, **22**, 41–45.

Maughan, B., Gray, G., & Rutter, M. (1985). Reading retardation and antisocial behaviour: a follow-up into employment. *Journal of Child Psychology and Psychiatry*, **26**, 741–758.

McConaughty, S.H., Achenbach, T.M., & Gent, C.L. (1988). Multi-axial empirically based assessment: parent, teacher, observational, cognitive and personality correlates of child behavior profiles for 6–11-year-old boys. *Journal of Abnormal Child Psychology*, **16**, 485–509.

McGee, R. & Share, D.L. (1988). Attention deficit disorder-hyperactivity and academic failure: which comes first and which should be treated? *Journal of the American Academy of Child and Adolescent Psychiatry*, **27**, 318–325.

McGee, R., Williams, S., Share, D.I., Anderson, J., & Silva, P. (1986). The relationship between specific reading retardation, general reading backwardness and behavioral problems in a large sample of Dunedin boys: a longitudinal study from five to eleven years. *Journal of Child Psychology and Psychiatry*, **27**, 597–610.

Montgomery, J.W. (1992). Easily overlooked language disabilities during childhood and adolescence: A cognitive-linguistic perspective. *Pediatric Clinics of North America*, **39**, 513–524.

Morton, J. (1989). The origins of autism. *New Scientist*, 9 December, 44–47.

Olson, S.L., Bates, J.E., & Bayles, K. (1984). Mother–infant interaction and the development of individual differences in children's cognitive competence. *Developmental Psychology*, **20**, 166–179.

Pennington, B.F., Grossier, D., & Welsh, M.C. (1993). Contrasting neuropsychological deficits in attention deficit hyperactivity disorder versus reading disability. *Developmental Psychology*, **29**, 511–523.

Rende, R.D., Plomin, R., Reiss, D., & Hetherington, E.M. (1993). Genetic and environmental influences on depressive symptomatology in adolescence: Individual differences and extreme scores. *Journal of Child Psychology and Psychiatry*, **34**, 1387–1398.

Reynell, J. (1969). Reynell Developmental Language Scales. Experimental Edition. Windsor: NFER.

Richman, N. & Graham, P. (1971). A behavior screening questionnaire for use with three-year-old children. *Journal of Child Psychology and Psychiatry*, **12**, 5–33.

Richman, N. & Stevenson, J. (1977). Language delay in 3-year-olds: family and social factors. *Acta Paediatrica Belgica*, **30**, 213–219.

Richman, N., Stevenson, J., & Graham, P. (1982). *Preschool to School*. London: Academic Press.

Rourke, B.P. & Fuerst, D.R. (1991). *Learning Disabilities and Psychosocial Functioning: A Neuropsychological Perspective*. New York: Guilford Press.

Rutter, M. (1967). A children's behaviour questionnaire for completion by teachers. *Journal of Child Psychology and Psychiatry*, **8**, 1–11.

Rutter, M. & Lord, C. (1987). Language disorders associated with psychiatric disturbance. In W. Yule and M. Rutter (eds) *Language Development and Disorders*. Oxford: MacKeith Press, pp. 206–233.

Rutter, M. & Mawhood, L. (1991). The long term sequelae of specific development disorders of speech and language. In M. Rutter & P. Casaer (eds) *Biological Risk Factors in Childhood and Psychopathology*. Cambridge: Cambridge University Press.

Rutter, M. & Yule, W. (1975). The concept of specific reading retardation. *Journal of Child Psychology and Psychiatry*, **16**, 181–197.

Scott, S. (1993). Mental handicap. In M. Rutter, E. Taylor, & L. Hersov (eds) *Child and Adolescent Psychiatry*, 3rd edn. Oxford: Blackwells.

Siegel, L., Cunningham, C., & van der Spuy, H. (1985). Interactions of language-delayed and normal preschool boys with their peers. *Journal of Child Psychology and Psychiatry*, **26**, 77–83.

Silva, P.A., Justin, C., McGee, R., & Williams, S. (1984). Some developmental and behavioural characteristics of seven-year-old children with delayed speech development. *British Journal of Disorders of Communication*, **19**, 107–154.

Silva, P.A., Williams, S., & McGee, R. (1987). A longitudinal study of children with developmental language delay at three years: later intelligence, reading and behaviour problems. *Developmental Medicine and Child Neurology*, **29**, 630–640.

Stevenson, J. (1991). Which aspects of processing text mediate genetic effects? *Reading and Writing*, **3**, 249–269.

Stevenson, J. (1992). Evidence for genetic aetiology in hyperactivity in children. *Behavior Genetics*, **22**, 337–344.

Stevenson, J., Pennington, B.F., Gilger, J.W., DeFries, J.C., & Gillis, J.J. (1993). ADHD and spelling disability: testing for shared genetic aetiology. *Journal of Child Psychology and Psychiatry*, **34**, 1137–1152.

Stevenson, J. & Richman, N. (1978). Behavior, language and development in three-year-old children. *Journal of Autism and Childhood Schizophrenia*, **8**, 299–313.

Stevenson, J., Richman, N., & Graham, P. (1985). Behavior problems and language abilities at three years and behavioral deviance at eight years. *Journal of Child Psychology and Psychiatry*, **26**, 215–230.

Tallal, P., Dukette, D., & Curtiss, S. (1989). Behavioral/emotional profiles of preschool language-impaired children. *Development and Psychopathology*, **1**, 51–67.

Tallal, P., Sainburg, R., & Jernigan, T. (1991). Neuropathology of developmental dysphasia. *Reading and Writing*, **4**, 65–79.

Whitehurst, G.J., Fischel, J.E., Lonigan, C.J. Valdez-Menchaca, M.C., DeBaryshe, B.D., & Caulfield, M.B. (1988). Verbal interactions in families of normal and expressive-language-delayed children. *Developmental Psychology*, **24**, 690–699.

Williams, S. & McGee, R. (1994). Reading attainment and juvenile delinquency. *Journal of Child Psychology and Psychiatry*, **35**, 441–459.

Wirt, R.D., Lachar, D., Klinedinst, J.K., & Seat, P.D. (1984). *Multidimensional Descriptions of Child Personality: A Manual for the Personality Inventory for Children – Revised 1984*. Los Angeles, CA: Western Psychological Services.

PART II

LANGUAGE IMPAIRMENT AND PSYCHIATRIC DISORDER

Introduction

ROSEMARY TANNOCK

A relationship between communication disorders and psychiatric disorders has been described clinically and established in epidemiological studies (e.g., Beitchman et al., 1986; Cantwell & Baker, 1991; Stevenson & Richman, 1978). The next four chapters extend this literature by considering: (1) the nature of the communication impairments; (2) possible explanations for the comorbidity between communication problems and various psychiatric disorders; and (3) the implications of the association for assessment and treatment.

The chapters cover a broad spectrum of disorders diagnosed in childhood (e.g., attention deficit disorder, childhood schizophrenia, and autistic disorder), but common issues are clearly evident, including the need for a broader conceptualization of language and a developmental perspective if we are to understand the nature of the links between variation in language, learning, and behavior. Also, all of the authors conclude that the relationship between communication disorders and psychiatric disorders are complex, multidimensional and transactional.

In the first chapter in this section, Chapter 6, Cohen comments on the high rates of language impairment among children referred for psychiatric assessment and the implications for assessment, diagnosis, and treatment. She describes her program of research that has shown that many children referred for psychiatric assessment and treatment have language impairments that have not been recognized previously and may continue to be overlooked unless a systematic language assessment is done. Through the use of case examples of children during different developmental periods, Cohen illustrates how even a clinically mild language impairment can have profound effects on multiple domains of child development and family dynamics. Failure to recognize language impairments often results in misperceptions and incorrect attributions regarding the "cause" of the child's socioemotional behavior problems. She comments that an examination of the interrelation and integration of a range of associated developmental processes in children at all ages presenting for psychiatric services is important because the ability to communicate and understand language influences their experiences not only in the family and at school, but also in the context of clinical interventions. Moreover, improved communication is one goal of mental health interventions and therefore understanding language and communicative development is essential for clinical practice.

In Chapter 7, Tannock and Schachar attempt to elucidate the complex relationships between attention deficit hyperactivity disorder (ADHD), communication disorders, and learning disorders. The thesis of the chapter is that the core behavioral symptoms of ADHD (i.e., inattention, impulsiveness, and overactivity) and the pragmatic difficulties these children exhibit (e.g., poor topic maintenance, interrupting conversations, excessive talkativeness) are related to deficits in higher-order cognitive processes, known as executive function, which are believed to be central to ADHD. The authors point out that pragmatic deficits are evident even in those ADHD children with intact receptive and expressive language abilities. By contrast, they argue that deficits observed in these children's articulation, phonological processing, receptive and expressive syntax, and semantics are associated with the frequently comorbid condition of dyslexia and not ADHD *per se*.

Chapter 8 by Caplan further expands the preceding discussion of pragmatics by demonstrating how the study of language use in context contributes to our understanding of the impaired communication skills in childhood schizophrenia and their linguistic, cognitive, and clinical correlates. The results from her studies highlight the importance of analyzing the communicative process at both the macrostructural level (e.g., topic organization and maintenance) and microstructural level (e.g., linguistic devices used to build a cohesive and coherent text). These studies identify deficits at both levels in children with schizophrenia, which make it difficult for a conversational partner to follow the ideas of children with schizophrenia and to understand who and what these children are talking about, or how their talk is related to the ongoing topic of conversation. Caplan points out that communication deficits at the macro- and microstructural level are largely independent, but that the few points of convergence are particularly informative because they suggest that some deficits at the microstructural level may be related to different macrostructural deficits and cognitive/attentional impairments.

In Chapter 9, Konstantareas and Beitchman review evidence for the overlap and independence of Autistic Disorder (AD) and Developmental Language Disorder (DD). They consider various explanations for the comorbidity between AD and DD and discuss etiological factors, including genetic factors, infections during the prenatal, perinatal and neonatal periods, and neuro-anatomical or neurofunctional abnormalities. On the basis of the limited evidence available on key dimensions of language and communication, including semantic and pragmatic development in AD and DD, the authors conclude that AD and DD can be distinguished, but that their co-occurrence may be largely attributable to overlapping diagnostic criteria. Konstantareas and Beitchman propose that the key to understanding these two disorders lies in clarifying the relationship between language development, cognitive understanding, and the development of social understanding.

REFERENCES

Beitchman, J.H., Nair, R., Clegg, M., Ferguson, B., & Patel, P.G. (1986). Prevalence of psychiatric disorders in children with speech and language disorders. *Journal of the American Academy of Child Psychiatry*, **25**, 528–535.

Cantwell, D.P. & Baker, L. (1991). *Psychiatric and Developmental Disorders in Children with Communication Disorder*. Washington, DC: American Psychiatric Press.

Stevenson, J. & Richman, N. (1978). Behaviour, language and development in three-year-old children. *Journal of Autism and Childhood Schizophrenia*, **8**, 299–313.

6 Unsuspected language impairments in psychiatrically disturbed children: developmental issues and associated conditions

NANCY J. COHEN

Many children referred for psychiatric assessment and treatment have a language impairment and for some of them it remains unsuspected unless a routine systematic assessment is done. This chapter examines the association between language impairment and social-emotional disturbance as it pertains to children referred for psychiatric assessment and treatment during the period from preschool to early adolescence. Findings and case examples from this author's research program will highlight the consequences for clinical practice of overlooking even a clinically mild language impairment during different developmental periods. This chapter also will show how application of a narrow definition of language in most studies of the interface between language impairment and social-emotional disturbance sets limits on the understanding of the relation between these disorders. As well, it will illustrate the importance of examining the interrelation and integration of a range of associated developmental processes throughout childhood. The focus will be on children with at least normal nonverbal intelligence so as not to confound language impairment with more general developmental delay.

During the past decade an increased awareness of the association of language impairment and psychiatric disorder has arisen from a number of directions. First, examination of language development in samples of psychiatrically disturbed children has become part of the sustained endeavor to describe the correlates and discover the causes of childhood psychiatric disturbance. For instance, current research is examining language and other neuropsychological correlates of specific types of psychiatric symptoms and disorders (Hinshaw, 1992; Cole, Usher, & Cargo, 1993; Kuschė, Cook, & Greenberg, 1993; McBurnett et al., 1993; Moffitt, 1993) and the association of early insecure attachment relationships with language and cognitive development (Gersten et al., 1986; Morisset et al., 1990). In this context, language has been implicated as a potential mediating factor for both psychopathology and low achievement (Hinshaw, 1992; Moffitt, 1993). Second, there is an increasing awareness of the need to study comorbid conditions generally (Caron & Rutter, 1988). It is only relatively recently that the magnitude of the prevalence of language impairments in children referred for psychiatric assessment and treatment has been acknowledged with estimates running as high as 71% (Kotsopoulos & Boodoosingh, 1987; Camarata, Hughes, & Ruhl, 1988). Finally, because the ability of children to communicate and understand language colors their experiences in the family, in school, and in therapy, and because improved communication is a goal of mental health intervention, understanding language and communicative development is essential for clinical practice.

ASSOCIATION BETWEEN LANGUAGE IMPAIRMENT AND SOCIAL-EMOTIONAL DISTURBANCE

An association between language impairment and social-emotional disturbance has been observed in children presenting to speech/language clinics (Cantwell & Baker, 1977) and in children identified in community epidemiological surveys (Richman, Stevenson, & Graham, 1982; Silva et al., 1984; Beitchman et al., 1986) where approximately 50% of children consistently have been shown to have a diagnosable psychiatric disorder (Cantwell & Baker, 1977). Considerable evidence points to the persistence of language impairments over time. Children who have difficulties in multiple specific language areas and whose language problems continue beyond the age of 5 years are at the greatest disadvantage (e.g., Bashir, Wiig, & Abrams, 1987; Tallal, Curtiss, & Kaplan, 1988; Beitchman et al., 1994, in press; Whitehurst & Fischel, 1994). Moreover, children with language impairments that involve language comprehension have higher rates of learning and social-emotional problems than do children with specific expressive language delays (Bishop & Edmundson, 1987; Silva, Williams, & McGee, 1987; Cantwell & Baker, 1991; Whitehurst & Fischel, 1994). Language impairments are presumed to have a neurological basis given their predominance in males, evidence of heritability, and association with other neuropsychological attributes (Plomin, DeFries, & Fulker, 1985).

Systematic examination of the language functioning of psychiatric samples has emerged relatively recently (Grinnell, Scott-Harnett, & Glasier, 1983; Gualtieri et al., 1983; Kotsopoulos & Boodoosingh, 1987; Camarata et al., 1988; Love & Thompson, 1988; Cohen, Davine, & Meloche-Kelly, 1989; Mack & Warr-Leeper, 1989; Baltaxe & Simmons, 1990; Cohen & Lipsett, 1992; Cohen et al., 1993). However, it is now apparent that language impairment is common among children presenting for psychiatric assessment and treatment with estimates running as high as 97% (Camarata et al., 1988).

Many of the investigators studying psychiatric samples observed that some children's language impairments went unnoticed until the routine systematic research assessment was done. To determine whether these children are distinctive in a clinically meaningful way, however, they had to be compared to psychiatrically disturbed children whose language impairments had already been identified and to psychiatrically disturbed children with normally developing language. Using this group comparison design, we undertook a research program that involved systematically screening consecutive referrals of 399 4 to 12-year-old child psychiatric outpatients, excluding children who were developmentally handicapped, autistic, had frank signs of neurological damage, were hearing impaired, and who came from non-English speaking homes (Cohen et al., 1993). The methodology involved administering a comprehensive battery of standardized measures of language structure to assess the receptive and expressive components of semantics, syntax, phonology, and auditory verbal memory. As a crude index of the social communicative aspect of language, speech/language pathologists completed a checklist of pragmatic skills and administered a test of narrative discourse. Standardized behavioral rating scales assessed the parents' and teachers' perceptions of the children's behavior using the Child Behavior Checklist (CBCL: Achenbach & Edelbrock, 1983) and the Teacher Report Form (TRF: Achenbach & Edelbrock, 1986). Comparisons were then made between three subgroups: children with previously identified language impairment (PILI), children whose language impairments were not suspected until the routine systematic assessment was done ("unsuspected" language impairment, USLI), and children with normally developing language. Designation as a PILI was based on typical system indicators such as whether a child was diagnosed by a speech/language pathologist, had a special class placement, or was receiving help. Designation as an USLI was made using the standardized measures (for details see Cohen et al., 1993). To ensure that children would not be diagnosed as having an USLI based solely on what might be an attentional problem, the criteria also required that a child not be diagnosed as language impaired because of auditory verbal memory deficits alone. This systematic screening revealed that 27.8% of the clinically referred children had a PILI (see Figure 6.1). Among the remaining children, who were referred solely for psychiatric assessment and treatment, 34.4% had an USLI.

A possible reason why some children's language impairments were overlooked emerged when the patterns of language functioning and social-emotional disturbance were examined. Although children with PILI and USLI were similar in the severity of their receptive language problems, children with PILI had more severe expressive language impairments (Cohen et al., 1993). As well, although pragmatic and narrative skills were poorer in both groups of language impaired children than in children with normally developing language, children with PILI performed the poorest (Cohen, 1992a). Thus, children with PILI were more likely than those with USLI to have problems with expressive language and social communication. It is reasonable to assume that these attracted adults' attention more than the subtle receptive language problems.

When social-emotional characteristics were examined, the results were similar to other studies in that children who had language impairments exhibited a heterogeneous pattern of the psychopathology with symptoms

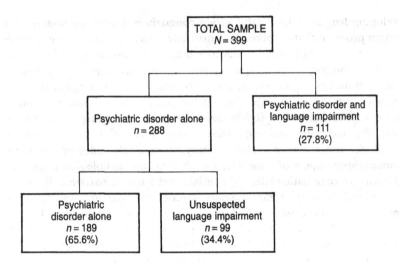

Figure 6.1. Reason for referral and outcome of language assessment.

associated with attention deficit hyperactivity disorder (ADHD) being the most common (e.g., Beitchman et al., 1986; Love & Thompson, 1988; Cantwell & Baker, 1991). However, a different pattern emerged when children with PILI and USLI were compared. Children with USLI were rated as the most delinquent and depressed by parents, and as most aggressive by teachers whereas children with PILI were rated as more socially withdrawn and anxious. Although rating scale rather than diagnostic information was used, it is notable that elsewhere in the literature it has been shown that children who are comorbid for ADHD and Conduct Disorders have a more negative outcome than children who are diagnosed only as ADHD (Moffitt, 1993).

Language and learning problems have been called "marginal" or "invisible" handicaps (Willmer & Crane, 1979; Lipsky, 1985). Thus, problems in producing or understanding language may appear to adults as noncompliance, inattentiveness, or social withdrawal (Howlin & Rutter, 1987). Consequently, parent–child interactions may be based on inappropriate expectations of the child and attributions for their behavior. For instance, language impaired children have been shown to be perceived by their mothers as more difficult than children with more severe but visible disabilities such as Down syndrome (Wulbert et al., 1975). Because children with USLI were less likely to have problems with language expression than children with PILI, their problems may be even more difficult to discern, magnifying the misperceptions and miscommunications regarding the intentionality of their misbehavior. In line with this, Barwick, Im, & Cohen (1995) found that parents and teachers of children with PILI were more likely to attribute problematic behavior to learning problems than parents of children with USLI.

The serious consequences of overlooking receptive language impairments are highlighted further by the finding that adults overestimate children's receptive language skills (e.g., Sattler, Feldman, & Bohanan, 1985). Additionally, it has been observed that toddlers' verbal comprehension skills are associated with compliance with adults (Kaler & Kopp, 1990). This is interesting in light of the large number of studies examining children's compliance with adults that typically do not measure language comprehension. As the research described above has shown, children's receptive language skills also are rarely examined when a noncompliant child is presented for psychiatric assessment and treatment.

We also found that both children with PILI and USLI experienced greater psychosocial disadvantage than children with normally developing language. They came from homes of lower socioeconomic status and their mothers had less education, a finding consistent with other studies of language impaired children (Cantwell & Baker, 1991). Furthermore, children with USLI were more likely to come from single-parent households. These stresses may contribute directly to the development of social-emotional problems as it has been shown repeatedly that environmental adversity contributes to a negative outcome (Werner, 1989). They also may be associated with circumstances that can make families less attentive to their children's language and learning development and problems. Moreover, because many language and cognitive problems have a genetic component (Plomin et al., 1985), language and cognitive deficits in parents may limit the direct help they can provide to their children.

DEVELOPMENTAL DIFFERENCES IN LANGUAGE AND SOCIAL-EMOTIONAL DISTURBANCE

The prevalence of language impairment in the population varies as a function of age. In a recent review, Whitehurst & Fischel (1994) concluded that language impairments are most prevalent in 2-year-olds (9–17%). In 3-year-olds the prevalence drops to between 3% and 8%, and in 5-year-olds to between 1% and 3%. There are fewer data concerning the prevalence of language impairments in school-aged samples but the most common estimate is 3% (Richardson, 1989).

Language and social-emotional problems overlap in the toddler period (Caulfield et al., 1990) and possibly as early as infancy (Prizant & Wetherby, 1990). However, it is during the preschool period that most speech and language impairments are identified. The early academic grades afford another identification point when language-related reading problems begin to surface. With age, language impaired children become increasingly more adept at giving the appearance of language competence and in eliciting the unwitting assistance of adults in their communicative efforts. Consequently, it might be expected that the largest proportion of children with USLI would be observed in older age groups. To examine this speculation, our sample of 4 to 12-year-olds was divided into age groups, representing three developmental periods, a kindergarten/beginning school period (4 to 6–11-year-olds), an early school period (7 to 9–11-year-olds), and a preadolescent period (10 to 12–11-year-olds).

The results indicated that the prevalence of both PILI and USLI was similar across age levels, with approximately one-third of children having an USLI (Cohen, 1992a). In our new ongoing study of 7 to 14-year-olds, preliminary findings indicate a similar prevalence in 13 and 14-year-olds. Although contrary to our expectation, these findings indicated that whereas in the general population the prevalence of language impairments declines from the preschool years onwards, in a psychiatric sample the prevalence of language impairment remains consistent into early adolesence.

Although the prevalence of language impairment remains constant, when behavioral differences between the age groups were examined, 4 to 6-year-olds with PILI were rated as having the least severe psychopathology compared to children with USLI and to older children with PILI. Thus, there may be a window of opportunity for young children with an identified handicap when caregivers have a more generous view of their child.

INTEGRATION OF LANGUAGE, COGNITIVE PROCESSES, AND SOCIAL-EMOTIONAL FUNCTIONING: DEVELOPMENTAL TRANSITIONS

The research described above has elucidated the high prevalence of language impairment in psychiatric clinic populations. To consider how language impairment and social-emotional disorder may be linked, these studies have focused primarily on language structure. In recent years, speech/language pathologists have emphasized the critical importance of examining the social communicative aspect of language. This includes the complex integration of specific language structures with other cognitive processes that mediate the relation between language and social-emotional disturbance and are represented in social discourse, pragmatic skills, and social cognitive competence (Prutting, 1982; Johnston et al., 1993; Liles, 1993; Westby & Cutler, 1994). Thus, children have to construct grammatically correct sentences and acquire an adequate vocabulary. They also must learn to link sentences to form cohesive communicative messages in order to recount experiences and give instructions, wait their conversational turn, and know the limits of body space and movement in different situations, for example, how close or distant to stand, when to touch and make eye contact. They also must be able to recognize miscommunications and repair them. Vallance (1994) found that social discourse and pragmatic skills, as opposed to structural language deficits, were related to social competence in language learning disabled children who also exhibited symptoms of social-emotional disturbance.

Only recently have the social communicative aspects of language been considered in children referred for social-emotional problems (Martin et al., 1992; Cohen et al., 1993; Tannock, Purvis, & Schachar, 1993). The most clearcut findings have been reported for children diagnosed as ADHD. Interestingly, the DSM-IV (American Psychiatric Association, 1994) criteria for ADHD include characteristics that could be considered as evidence of pragmatic dysfunction (e.g., difficulty waiting turns, interrupting others, blurting out answers to uncompleted questions).

To communicate effectively, children also must be aware of the feelings, intentions, and attributions of others. Thus, it has been suggested that social cognitive variables including processing of social cues, attributions, social problem solving, affect labeling, outcome expectations, and self-concept are important facets to examine in clinical populations (Kusché et al., 1993; Lochman & Dodge, 1994).

At this time the conclusions of studies of language impairment and social communicative skills, and social-emotional disturbance are limited by the narrow range of developmental domains that have been examined as well as the narrow definition of language and communicative development that have been applied. In light of problems in social relationships and emotional expression that bring children to clinical attention, a range of variables including language structure, social communicative skills, social communicative self-awareness, and social cognitive skills must be examined simultaneously.

In our current research we have expanded the focus to examine the interrelation and interdependence of these skills cited above and environmental events and influences. To illustrate the intricacy of the interrelationships of these skills and environmental events during different developmental periods, case examples will be drawn from our ongoing study of 7 to 14-year-old children who are in middle childhood and early adolescence.

Case example: middle childhood

Kevin, aged 7 years 10 months, was referred because of his destructive, angry, inattentive, and disruptive behaviors. He was physically violent and verbally abusive to peers, and had few friends. Kevin's parents had been separated for five years and he rarely saw his father. Kevin's mother described him as a difficult baby who cried a lot and was irritable and overactive, but reported no developmental delays. She attributed his problems to not listening and to her own inconsistency in discipline. She felt that Kevin did not have friends because he had a "bad attitude." Kevin's teacher reported that he was performing at grade level with the exception of spelling. She attributed Kevin's problems to family dysfunction, emotional problems, and social problems with other children.

Kevin received psychiatric diagnoses of ADHD and Oppositional Defiant Disorder based on maternal report on the Child Assessment Schedule structured psychiatric interview (Hodges, 1990). His mother rated Kevin in the clinically significant range on the Withdrawn, Anxious/Depressed, Social Problems, Attention Problems, Delinquent Behavior, and Aggressive Behavior scales of the CBCL. His teacher rated him in the clinical range on the Social Problems, Attention Problems, Aggressive, and Withdrawn Scales of the TRF.

Testing indicated average intelligence (Full Scale IQ = 104). On the language assessment Kevin scored below the normative mean on tests of expressive grammar and auditory verbal memory for recalling sentences and paragraphs. Problems in pragmatic skills and social discourse were evident. His narrative lacked coherence and answers often were off topic. Not only was it difficult for the examiner to understand him but Kevin himself said that he was lost in his narrative.

On academic achievement tests, Kevin performed poorly on reading decoding, word attack, reading comprehension, and mathematical computation. He also exhibited problems on orthographic and phonological reading tasks and displayed deficiencies in both verbal and nonverbal working memory.

On an emotion decoding task, Kevin made many errors. He needed a considerable amount of time to label the emotions in pictures of faces and to identify the picture expressing an emotion associated with a brief story read aloud to him. The difficulties he had were reflected in the way he examined the pictures. He looked at the cheeks and teeth in the picture, then copied them with his own facial expression, and only then gave a response. On a measure of social cognition, the Interpersonal Negotiating Strategies Task (Schultz, Yeates, & Selman, 1989), Kevin had difficulties identifying the problem to be solved, labeling the feelings of the participants in the social problem solving situation, and knowing when the problem was solved. When asked about his own worries and how he handled them, Kevin mentioned worries about his mother and his relationships with peers and acknowledged feeling sad about both. His solution was to isolate himself rather than take positive action. Kevin's responses to a self-esteem questionnaire indicated low esteem related to popularity and to feelings of happiness and satisfaction.

It was concluded that language processing problems, both expressive and receptive, had been overlooked and were a source of frustration to Kevin. Language impairments and associated social cognitive deficits interfered with both achievement and social information processing necessary for effective social interactions. When this feedback was given, Kevin's teacher questioned the results and continued to attribute Kevin's problems to emotional factors. Ultimately, however, he was placed in a class for children with specific learning disabilities. Kevin's mother was relieved that Kevin's problems were not totally her fault or the result of his living in a single parent home, and that she could implement suggestions to provide more structure for Kevin. Although clearly there were family problems that required attention, having the feedback allowed Kevin's mother and the clinician to distinguish problems that were related to the family and those that were not. This led to greater differentiation and specificity in the treatment plan and in school placement.

Developmental transitions of middle childhood

The problems that Kevin displayed can be seen in the context of important developmental transitions that characterize the early school years. A major developmental transition occurs at around 6 to 7 years when most cultures begin formal schooling. Although it is an exciting milestone for most children, it is also a time when learning and social-emotional difficulties emerge.

Learning to read and write are among the most important tasks of this period. Considerable research has shown that language impairments underlie most reading problems. By 8 to 9 years, basic language structures should be mature. For instance, children normally have all of the grammatical rules in their repertoire and can use them for language comprehension and expression. Moreover, there is a reciprocal relation between language and reading such that vocabulary and syntax knowledge decline from 3 to 11 years of age in children with reading disabilities (Share & Silva, 1987; Stanovich, 1988).

Language development is also intertwined with metacognitive or executive control skills. In particular, sufficient receptive and expressive language skills are essential to understand and later to retrieve, organize, and verbalize rules. Furthermore, the internalization of rule-governed language is associated with the development of self-control (Luria, 1961; Vygotsky, 1962). Self-regulation skills also contribute to pragmatic or communicative competence, for instance, in helping children to organize coherent conversations and to inhibit responding prematurely (Tannock et al., 1993).

Formation and maintenance of social relationships are related to language and social cognitive development, in particular, the ability to use emotion labels to reflect upon and talk about feelings, to articulate empathic feelings, and to see the consequences of actions. In the early school years the first signs of reciprocal friendships emerge concurrently with development of language and social cognitive skills. Poor social cognitive skills may contribute to misinterpreting the intentions and motives of other children as harmful, leading some language impaired children to initiate and to elicit negative interactions (Dodge & Frame, 1986). During this age period, children also become capable of masking their true feelings, and language impaired children may give a false impression of not caring, may become loners, or get into fights. Consequently, they are often both more aggressive and more rejected by peers. Moreover, it has been shown that children who are both aggressive and depressed exhibit a wider range of social cognitive deficits than children with either type of problem alone (Quiggle et al., 1992). From the preschool years onward children develop an increasingly coherent sense of self. Children with language impairments may have difficulty with this both because of their problems representing experiences symbolically and the frequent negative feedback from the environment regarding achievement and social relationships.

Developmental transitions of early adolescence

Early adolescence gives rise to further shifts in cognitive development with increasing capacity for systematic problem solving. Language continues to be a means of self-control through the use of internal language, and verbal abstract reasoning is facilitated through symbolic representation. During this period, language skills gain primarily in sophistication. For example, discourse skills become more refined and vocabulary increases. The requirements for complex structures in written work and for reading and interpreting abstract material also increase. For many children with language impairments this is a difficult time because academic demands for inferential thinking and independent learning increase. Socially, early adolescence is a time when friendships become more intense and demanding, which is related to increased capacity to appreciate fully the reciprocal nature of relationships. Adolescents have a clearer identity and understanding of themselves and see their personal characteristics as enduring qualities. The risk for social-emotional problems emerging or intensifying is considerable for children who have had a history of poor achievement and inadequate capacity for engaging in reciprocal relations with peers.

The following examples demonstrate how multiple problems in learning and achievement can be masked by extreme familial, social, and relational problems that are evident from early childhood. As is often the case, family and behavioral problems are seen as the primary focus for assessment and intervention.

Case examples: early adolescence

Michael, aged 14 years 11 months, had a history of delinquency with 18 robberies on his conviction record. As a young child he was sexually abused. He was a loner and had no positive peer relationships. Michael had been in eight different schools since Grade 1 and had missed many days of school because of truancy, suspensions, and involvement with the legal system. His parents were separated and Michael was living with his mother who worried about his angry outbursts escalating. She attributed Michael's problems to family difficulties and low self-esteem resulting from his father's verbal abuse. His mother noted that Michael had problems with math, reading, and writing. Teachers attributed Michael's learning and behavioral problems to poor attendance, lack of motivation, and being rewarded for aggressive behavior in the past.

Several comorbid psychiatric disorders were diagnosed using the Child Assessment Schedule including Conduct Disorder, ADHD, Separation

Anxiety, Dysthymia, and Overanxious Disorder. On the CBCL, particularly high scores were observed on the Withdrawn, Anxious/Depressed, Attention Problems, Delinquent, and Aggressive Behavior scales. Michael was relatively new to his school and his teacher did not want to complete the TRF.

Michael had average intelligence (Full Scale IQ = 93). Many problems were noted on standardized achievement tests with respect to word attack skills, reading comprehension, spelling, and math. On the language tests, problems were observed in expressive vocabulary, receptive syntax, auditory verbal memory for sentences and paragraphs, following directions, and narrative discourse. Michael also showed hyperacuity to sound during the audiometric screening. This sensitivity to sound might have intensified his confusion with incoming auditory stimuli. In terms of pragmatic and social discourse skills, Michael was uncomfortable expressing himself verbally and was slow to respond, giving many "I don't know" answers. However, when asked whether he did not know the answer or whether he needed more time to think, Michael replied that he needed more time. If offered this option, he often gave an acceptable answer.

Michael was able to identify emotions accurately although, here too, he needed time to process the information. He was consistently inaccurate in his perception of anger and his solutions to social problems were always aggressive. When asked about his worries, Michael stated that he was worried about what he was going to do to some people for being rude to his sister. His strategy for dealing with his feelings was to think about killing them and then isolate himself. He reported low self-esteem with respect to academic and school status. When given feedback, Michael's mother was angry with the school for failing to identify his language and learning problems earlier. Michael had difficulty accepting the feedback as he was convinced that he was "stupid." While Michael was not hopeful, the school was mobilized to help him to develop strategies for dealing with some of his academic and language and cognitive processing problems. Additionally, feedback to the clinician alerted him to potential reasons for lapses in communication as well as strategies for averting such difficulties.

Although Michael's difficult behavior seemed to be a product of a long history of failures in multiple domains, for other children problems do not emerge until the academic and social demands at higher grade levels tax their capacities. The following case example illustrates this point.

Paula, aged 12 years 1 month, was referred because she was unhappy, had irrational outbursts over minor issues and always wanted her own way. She did not complete her homework, could not take notes, had difficulty organizing her ideas and preparing written work, and interfered with classroom procedures. Difficulties were beginning to emerge in her social relationships with peers and adults. Paula's teacher attributed the problems to Paula's preoccupation with her social life, poor attitude, and low motivation.

Her mother attributed Paula's behavior to motivational and attitudinal problems, and to her parents' separation.

The structured psychiatric interview yielded no psychiatric diagnosis. On the CBCL most scores were in the nonclinical range except for the Aggressive Behavior scale score. None of the teacher's ratings were in the clinical range.

Paula had average intelligence (Full Scale IQ = 101). On the language tests, she scored one standard deviation below the mean on tests of expressive grammar. One of these, which required her to recall sentences read aloud to her, also had an auditory verbal memory component. During testing, Paula exhibited word finding difficulties and her narrative discourse lacked coherence, fluency, and specificity. Standardized test results indicated that Paula was performing at grade level with respect to word attack skill, reading decoding and comprehension, and arithmetic. The only problem she exhibited was in spelling.

On social cognitive tasks, Paula had difficulty correctly identifying emotions and took a long time to respond. She was able to generate alternative social problem solving strategies but saw the primary means of resolving problems as changing the social partner's position rather than arriving at a compromise. When asked about her worries, Paula expressed concerns about her friends being mad at her and about the possibility of her father and grandmother dying. Her way of dealing with these worries was by avoiding rather than actively coping with them. Although her score on a self-esteem scale was within normal limits, Paula reported suspiciously high self-esteem on the popularity subscale.

Since Paula had not experienced learning or social problems previously, and because there were no apparent current life changes, it was concluded that Paula's mild subtle expressive and receptive language problems were just beginning to interfere with learning and performance. Her problems were not associated with reading but with general organizational and processing skills. In Grade 7 there is typically a shift in academic demands toward greater independent learning, such as preparation of essays. The higher demands for independence and organization posed obstacles for Paula and they would be likely to intensify further when she entered high school.

Although family therapy continued, feedback helped Paula's teachers and mother to reconceptualize Paula's problems as language and social information processing problems rather than attitudinal ones. In the feedback interview, Paula's teacher recalled Paula's difficulties expressing herself and that this irritated her mother and peers, who would often say in an exasperated tone, "Just come to the point." Subsequently, Paula's teacher began to use more repetition in teaching, checked to make sure that she understood the material, and helped Paula to use a daytimer and organizer. Paula's mother helped her to structure activities at home. The feedback was a relief to Paula, as she realized that she was not stupid. By gaining the support of her teacher and mother, as well as being able to redefine her own problems, the prognosis for improvements in academic functioning, social relations, and self-esteem was felt to be good. At the time of referral, Paula's problems with aggression and peer relationships were just emerging and it is likely that without intervention these problems would have escalated and become more serious and entrenched.

CLINICAL IMPLICATIONS

The data and case examples presented in the preceding pages indicate that leaving impairments of language and communication and associated cognitive processing problems undiagnosed can lead to incorrect or incomplete diagnosis and treatment of children with social-emotional problems. In particular, parents, teachers, and clinicians may misattribute a child's difficulties in comprehending and processing information to opposition, inattention, or noncompliance. By definition, none of the children with USLI in our sample were in special classes where their language-related problems could be addressed. However, some of these children were in classes for behaviorally and emotionally disturbed children, where the chances of getting appropriate remedial help might actually be diminished.

Even when children have an identified language impairment, the impact of their specific deficits is often not taken into account in formulation and treatment planning around their social-emotional problems. Most typically when a child is enrolled in a special class for children with learning disabilities this aspect of development is viewed as somehow "being taken care of" and therefore separable from social-emotional interventions. Moreover, sometimes children are not accepted into special classes or given remedial attention until their behavior problems have been treated, reflecting a belief that behavior and learning problems are linearly rather than reciprocally related.

Recent literature on learning disabled children has been promoting the integration of family therapy into educational planning (e.g., Ziegler & Holden, 1988; Green, 1989), but little has been written about how language and learning impairments may influence mental health interventions (e.g., Silver, 1989; Cohen & Lipsett, 1992). Yet, the ability of a child to communicate and understand language clearly are factors that influence experiences in their family and in therapy. Since assessment and treatment techniques used with children and families rely almost exclusively on verbal communication, additional stresses may be imposed on children with language impairments when situations involve communications that are not only emotionally loaded but also structurally and semantically complex.

The results of research on children with an USLI suggest that routine assessment of language in psychiatric clinics is important. Although research has focused primarily on externalizing problems, language deficits also have been shown in children with internalizing problems (Kusché et al., 1993; Naylor et al., 1994). In these children, both language problems and social-emotional disturbance may be overlooked because of the children's compliant behavior. Therapists need to work collaboratively with speech/language pathologists to help parents, teachers, and children to understand how language structure, processing, pragmatic, and social discourse problems impact on children's learning and social functioning. Such information is also useful in the course of individual and family therapy in focusing attention on whether the child is comprehending what is said and communicating what is intended.

Obviously language impairment is not the only problem for children with a social-emotional disorder and their families. Nevertheless, therapists and speech/language pathologists can help children and their families to discriminate the consequences of language impairment from what may be a reflection of the children's and families' personality and functioning. In this way, sometimes what may have been labeled as inattention, lack of motivation, or noncompliance may be relabeled and correctly attributed, and what is a secondary reaction to failure can be addressed to reduce frustration and increase self-esteem. We have observed that shifting parents' attributions for their children's misbehavior to disorders in processing and sequencing information often has a noticeable immediate salutary effect for both the parents and the children. This was illustrated in the case examples described earlier. Similarly, a number of investigators have reported the positive effects of diagnostic labeling both on children's self-esteem (Ribner, 1978) and on parent stress (Marcovitch et al., 1987).

Feedback also can provide relief because it gives families something tangible to do. This might include collaborating with schools to obtain appropriate special services and the families utilizing what they have learned about their children's specific disabilities to structure home life in a way that is consistent with developmental requirements. As well, we have observed that nonreferred younger siblings of language impaired children are more likely to have a previously identified or an unsuspected language impairment than siblings of children with normally developing language (Cohen et al., in press). Thus, developmental guidelines also can be provided to alert parents to the first sign of problems with siblings so that early identification and intervention can occur and dysfunctional relational outcomes be minimized.

Given the subtle language problems of children with USLI, a future challenge is to identify children in the preschool years so as to forestall or minimize negative sequelae. Generally, early childhood has been considered a period that is particularly amenable to shifting the family influence in a direction that is more consistent with an adaptive outcome (Rutter, 1990). Furthermore, it has been suggested that interventions may have a greater influence in early childhood than either in infancy or later in childhood because competencies become less canalized at a time when children have not yet begun to choose their own environments (McCall, 1981). The notion of providing developmental check-ups, much like regular medical examinations, has been suggested by Landy and her colleagues on the basis of the results of a community screening, tracking, and intervention study (Landy et al., 1993). Wide distribution of guidelines to a range of professionals for identifying children who may have language impairments and associated developmental conditions is also essential. Young children are less likely to be identified by speech/language pathologists than by daycare workers, pediatricians, and family physicians. In deciding whether referral to a specialist is required these latter professionals may rely solely on obvious speech problems or expressive language disabilities. With more children attending day care the number of young children who could be identified early will escalate. Although surveys of developmental and social-emotional problems in daycare settings have tended to be relatively informal, here too, it has been noted that language impairments are often overlooked (see review by Cohen, 1992b).

IMPLICATIONS FOR RESEARCH AND TREATMENT

It is clear that a broader definition of language must be adopted in studies of children who have a social-emotional disorder. This definition must include a range of skills necessary for social communication. Additionally, the multiple mechanisms that mediate language and social-emotional problems must be delineated, including pragmatic, narrative discourse, and social cognitive skills. While this information is essential to inform intervention strategies it is not yet available in the existing literature. For instance, although language functioning plays a central role in achievement and social-emotional functioning (Hinshaw, 1992; Moffitt, 1993), there is no research on social cognitive characteristics of children who are language impaired and have a social-emotional disturbance. A handful of studies have incorporated social cognitive components, such as social problem solving, into therapy with clinical samples but no data are available on the language functioning of these children (Selman & Demorest, 1984). Furthermore, whereas there is some research on social cognitive characteristics of children with learning disabilities, it has not distinguished between language-based and nonverbal learning disabilities. Recently, researchers have begun to examine the relations between pathological symptoms and the range of language, cognitive, and social cognitive processing deficits in clinical (Cohen, Vallance, & Menna, 1996) and in nonclinical samples (Pellegrini et al., 1987; Kusché et al., 1993).

There are a number of developmental pathways by which an association between language impairment and social-emotional disturbance may come about (Rutter & Lord, 1987). The preponderant view currently is that many social-emotional problems evolve from a complex ongoing transaction between the psychosocial environment and language, cognitive, social, and emotional deficits (e.g., Prizant et al., 1990; Moffitt, 1993). Increasingly, researchers have been applying a developmental organizational conceptual framework to understand the dynamic process of interrelations and transactions of multiple domains of functioning in both normal and abnormal development (Cicchetti, 1993; Cicchetti & Richters, 1993). This has shown that in normal development, domains of functioning are interrelated and integrated in such a way as to facilitate adaptation whereas in pathological development this integration has not occurred. In this way, as a result of variations in levels of functioning across domains, children experience the same events differently (Cicchetti, 1993). For instance, Moffitt (1993) has suggested that language impairments and executive control deficits place children at the risk of setting into motion negative interactions first with parents, and later with peers and teachers. She further suggests that in this context, parents and teachers tend to reduce their efforts to guide children's learning and behavior. Data from our ongoing research on a large group of children referred for psychiatric assessment and treatment will provide needed information relevant both to the broader definition of language functioning discussed above and to the understanding of the interrelation between a range of developmental domains during different age periods. The most useful information for clinical practice, will derive from concurrent study of clinical and nonclinical samples.

If language and communicative deficits and associated cognitive processing problems have a central role to play in the evolution and/or maintenance of social-emotional problems, an obvious question is whether changes in language functioning will influence other aspects of development and social-emotional disorder. There have been no controlled studies that make all of the necessary comparisons of individual and combined treatment modalities to provide an empirical answer to this question. Some headway has been made in interventions for children with language and language-related learning disabilities, especially with respect to teaching phonological skills which underlie most reading problems (Stevenson, 1989; Lovett, 1991). However, these studies have not included children with social-emotional disorders or measures of social-emotional functioning.

There also has been little by way of systematic study of language interventions in psychiatric disordered samples. Follow-up studies of language impaired children, some of whom received remedial help, generally have been discouraging, showing that language problems persist and that psychiatric disorders often increase over time (Baker & Cantwell, 1987; Benasich, Curtiss, & Tallal, 1993; Beitchman et al., 1994a). In an evaluation of a preschool day treatment program, Cohen, Kolers, & Bradley (1987) found that children with normal intelligence who had dual language and social-emotional disorders made greater gains than either developmentally handicapped children or children presenting for only social-emotional problems with respect to both language and social-emotional characteristics. The greatest benefits accrued to children who remained in the program for more than one year and whose parents were involved in the treatment process (Cohen, Bradley, & Kolers, 1987). Although not directed at language impaired samples *per se*, there is also evidence that interventions that incorporated academic tutoring led to gains in a broader range of changes on achievement, behavior, and peer status measures than did social and behavioral interventions alone (Ayllon, Layman, & Kandel, 1975; Bachara & Zaba, 1978; Coie & Krehbiel, 1984).

There is evidence that psychotherapy may have a beneficial effect on language, at least for some disturbed children. Russell, Greenwald, & Shirk (1991) did a metanalysis of studies of child psychotherapy that included language measures and showed that children presenting with problems of peer rejection, low self-esteem, or underachievement exhibited language gains. In certain respects psychotherapy is similar to speech/language therapy in that both involve modeling, practice under conditions of reduced anxiety about performance, and emphasis on clarification of verbal expression. Although the impact on children with more entrenched overcontrolled and undercontrolled symptoms was less striking, the point remains that from a clinical perspective, interventions for social-emotional development and language/communication disorders overlap considerably.

Controlled studies of single variables or single interventions are unlikely to provide the best test of intervention outcomes. The children described in this chapter need help to compensate for a range of language, communicative, and social cognitive deficits that pose obstacles to their development. It is reasonable to assume that multimodal interventions such as the PATHS program developed by Greenberg and his colleagues (Greenberg et al., 1995) that deals with social cognition, emotion decoding, and behavior regulation will be required. A preventive intervention model for conduct problems has recently been suggested that combines the PATHS program with remedial work for specific linguistic and communicative deficits (Conduct Problems Prevention Research Group, 1992). Family interventions that facilitate communicative capacities will be an important adjunct to such programs. Research findings grounded within a developmental organizational perspective will be essential in guiding the design and implementation of intervention and prevention strategies because of its focus on understanding both the interrelation and timing of developmental processes. The specific challenge for helping the children with language impairments and social-emotional disorders under consideration here is to gain this understanding in relation to a range of processing difficulties and environmental influences and to monitor improvements in multiple areas of functioning in sequence and in relation to one another over time.

ACKNOWLEDGMENTS

Research described in this chapter was supported by grants from Health Canada, National Health Research and Development Program (Nos. 6606-3502 and 6606-4835). The comments of Melanie Barwick, Rosanne Menna, Denise Vallance, and Naomi Berney Horodezky on an earlier version of this chapter were greatly appreciated.

REFERENCES

Achenbach, T.M. & Edelbrock, C. (1983). *Manual for the Child Behavior Checklist*. Burlington, VT: University of Vermont Press.

Achenbach, T.M. & Edelbrock, C. (1986). *Manual for the Teacher's Report Form*. Burlington, VT: University of Vermont, Department of Psychiatry.

American Psychiatric Association (1994). *Diagnostic and Statistical Manual of Mental Disorders* (4th edn.). Washington, DC: Author.

Ayllon, T., Layman, D., & Kandel, H.J. (1975). A behavioral alternative to drug control of hyperactive children. *Journal of Applied Behavior Analysis*, **8**, 137–146.

Bachara, G.H. & Zaba, J.N. (1978). Learning disabilities and juvenile delinquency. *Journal of Learning Disabilities*, **11**, 258–262.

Baker, L. & Cantwell, D.P. (1987). A prospective psychiatric follow-up of children with speech/language disorders. *Journal of the American Academy of Child and Adolescent Psychiatry*, **26**, 546–553.

Baltaxe, C. & Simmons, J.Q. III (1990). The differential diagnosis of communication disorders in child and adolescent psychopathology. *Topics in Language Disorders*, **10**, 17–31.

Barwick, M.A., Im, N., & Cohen, N.J. (1995). Parent and teacher attributions underlying psychiatric referral for children with unsuspected language and learning impairments. Poster session presented at the Biennial Meeting of the Society for Research in Child Development, Indianapolis (March).

Bashir, A.S., Wiig, E.H., & Abrams, J.C. (1987). Language disorders in childhood and adolescence: implications for learning and socialization. *Pediatric Annals*, **16**, 145–156.

Beitchman, J.H., Brownlee, E.B., Inglis, A., Wild, J., Mathews, R., Schachter, O., Kroll, R., Martin, S., Ferguson, B., & Lancee, W. (1994). A seven year follow-up of speech/language impaired and control children: Part I. Speech/language stability and outcome. *Journal of the American Academy of Child and Adolescent Psychiatry*, **33**, 1322–1330.

Beitchman, J.H., Brownlee, E.B., Inglis, A., Wild, J., Ferguson, B., Schachter, D., Lancee, W., Wilson, B., & Mathews, R. (in press). A seven year follow-up of speech/language impaired and control children: Part II. Psychiatric outcome. *Journal of Child Psychology and Psychiatry*.

Beitchman, J.H., Nair, R., Clegg, M., Ferguson, B., & Patel, P.G. (1986). Prevalence of psychiatric disorders in children with speech and language disorders. *Journal of the American Academy of Child Psychiatry*, **25**, 528–535.

Benasich, A.A., Curtiss, S., & Tallal, P. (1993). Language, learning, and behavioral disturbances in childhood: a longitudinal perspective. *Journal of the American Academy of Child and Adolescent Psychiatry*, **12**, 585–594.

Bishop, D.V.M. & Edmundson, A. (1987). Language impaired 4 year olds: Distinguishing transient from persistent impairment. *Journal of Speech and Hearing Disorders*, **52**, 156–173.

Blechman, E.A., Tinsley, B., Carella, E.T., & McEnroe, M.J. (1985). Childhood competence and behavior problems. *Journal of Abnormal Psychology*, **94**, 70–77.

Camarata, S.M., Hughes, C.A., & Ruhl, K.L. (1988). Mild/moderate behaviorally disordered students: a population at risk for language disorders. *Language, Speech, and Hearing Services in the Schools*, **19**, 191–200.

Cantwell, D.P. & Baker, L. (1987). Clinical significance of children with communication disorders: perspectives from a longitudinal study. *Journal of Child Neurology*, **2**, 257–264.

Cantwell, D.P. & Baker, L. (1977). Psychiatric disorder in children with speech and language retardation: a critical review. *Archives of General Psychiatry*, **34**, 583–591.

Cantwell, D.P. & Baker, L. (1991). *Psychiatric and Developmental Disorders in Children with Communication Disorder*. Washington, DC: American Psychiatric Press.

Caron, C. & Rutter, M. (1988). Comorbidity in child psychopathology: Concepts, issues, and research strategies. *Journal of Child Psychology and Psychiatry*, **32**, 1063–1080.

Caulfield, M.B., Fischel, J.E., DeBaryshe, B.D., & Whitehurst, G.J. (1990). Behavioral correlates of developmental expressive language disorder. *Journal of Abnormal Child Psychology*, **17**, 187–201.

Cicchetti, D. (1993). Developmental psychopathology: reactions, reflections, projections. *Developmental Review*, **13**, 471–502.

Cicchetti, D. & Richters, J. (1993). Developmental considerations in the investigation of conduct disorder. *Development and Psychopathology*, **5**, 331–344.

Cohen, N.J. (1992a). Psychiatrically disturbed children with unsuspected language impairments: developmental differences in language and behavioural characteristics. Paper presented at the conference Integrating Language, Learning and Behaviour: Theory and applications. Toronto, Ontario (May).

Cohen, N.J. (1992b). Models and strategies for providing mental health promotion services in community day care centres. Literature review prepared for Health and Welfare (Canada). Health Services and Promotion Branch (No. 6606-4437).

Cohen, N.J., Barwick, M.A., Horodezky, N.B., & Isaacson, L. (in press). Comorbidity of language and social-emotional disturbance: Comparison of psychiatric outpatients and their siblings. *Journal of Clinical Child Psychology*.

Cohen, N.J., Bradley, S., & Kolers, N. (1987). Outcome evaluation of a therapeutic day treatment program for delayed and distributed preschoolers. *Journal of the American Academy of Child and Adolescent Psychiatry*, **26**, 687–693.

Cohen, N.J., Davine, M., Horodezky, N., Lipsett, L., & Isaacson, L. (1993). Unsuspected language impairment in psychiatrically disturbed children: prevalence and language and behavioral characteristics. *Journal of the American Academy of Child and Adolescent Psychiatry*, **32**, 595–603.

Cohen, N.J., Davine, M., & Meloche-Kelly, M. (1989). Prevalence of unsuspected language disorders in a child psychiatric population. *Journal of the American Academy of Child and Adolescent Psychiatry*, **28**, 107–111.

Cohen, N.J., Kolers, N., & Bradley, S. (1987). Predictors of the outcome of treatment in a therapeutic preschool. *Journal of the American Academy of Child Psychiatry*, **26**, 829–833.

Cohen, N.J. & Lipsett, L. (1992). Recognized and unrecognized language impairment in psychologically disturbed children: child symptomatology, maternal depression, and family dysfunction: Preliminary report. *Canadian Journal of Behavioural Science*, **23**, 376–389.

Cohen, N.J., Vallance, D., & Menna, R. (1996). Language, cognitive, and social-cognitive processing of psychiatrically referred children. Poster session presented at the Annual Meeting of the Society for Research in Child and Adolescent Psychopathology, Santa Monica, CA (January).

Coie, J.D. & Krehbiel, G. (1984). Effects of academic tutoring on the social status of low-achieving, socially rejected children. *Child Development*, **55**, 1465–1478.

Cole, P.M., Usher, B.A., & Cargo, A.P. (1993). Cognitive risk and its association with risk for disruptive behavior disorder in preschoolers. *Journal of Clinical Child Psychology*, **22**, 1154–1164.

Conduct Problems Prevention Research Group (1992). A developmental and clinical model for the prevention of conduct disorder: the FAST Track Program. *Development and Psychopathology*, **4**, 509–520.

Dodge, K.A. & Frame, C.L. (1986). Social cognitive biases and deficits in aggressive boys. *Child Development*, **53**, 620–635.

Gersten, M., Coster, W., Schneider-Rosen, K., Carlson, V., & Cicchetti, D. (1986). The socio-emotional bases of communicative functioning: Quality of attachment, language development, and early maltreatment. In M.E. Lamb, A.L. Brown, & B. Rogoff (eds) *Advances in Developmental Psychology, Vol. 4*. Hillsdale, NJ: Erlbaum (pp. 105–151).

Green, R. (1989). "Learning to learn" and the family system: new perspectives on underachievement and learning disorders. *Journal of Marital and Family Therapy*, **15**, 187–203.

Greenberg, M.T., Kusché, C.A., Cook, E.A., & Quamma, J. (1995). Promoting emotional competence in school-aged children: the effects of the PATHS Curriculum. *Development and Psychopathology*, **7**, 117–136.

Grinnell, S., Scott-Harnett, D., & Glasier, J. (1983). Letter to the editor. *Journal of the American Academy of Child and Adolescent Psychiatry*, **22**, 580–581.

Gualtieri, T., Koriath, U., Van Bourgondien, M., & Saleeby, N. (1983). Language disorders in children referred for psychiatric services. *Journal of the American Academy of Child and Adolescent Psychiatry*, **22**, 165–171.

Hinshaw, S. (1992). Externalizing behavior problems and academic underachievement in childhood and adolescence: causal relationships and underlying mechanisms. *Psychological Bulletin*, **111**, 127–135.

Hodges, K. (1990). Child Assessment Schedule (CAS) Parent Form. Military version. Michigan State University, Lansing, MI.

Howlin, P. & Rutter, M. (1987). The consequences of language delay for other aspects of development. In W. Yule & M. Rutter (eds) *Language Development and Disorders*. Oxford: Blackwell Publications (pp. 271–294).

Johnston, J.R., Miller, J.F., Curtiss, S., & Tallal, P. (1993). Conversations with children who are language impaired: asking questions. *Journal of Speech and Hearing Research*, **36**, 973–978.

Kaler, S.R. & Kopp, C. (1990). Compliance and comprehension in very young toddlers. *Child Development*, **61**, 1997–2003.

Kotsopoulos, A. & Boodoosingh, L. (1987). Language and speech disorders in children attending a day psychiatric programme. *British Journal of Disorders in Communication*, **22**, 227–236.

Kusché, C.A., Cook, E.T., & Greenberg, M.T. (1993). Neuropsychological and cognitive functioning in children with anxiety, externalizing and comorbid psychopathology. *Journal of Clinical Child Psychology*, **22**, 172–195.

Landy, S., DeV. Peters, R., Allen, A.B., Brooks, F., & Jewell, S. (1993). "Staying on track": An early identification, tracking, intervention and referral system for infants, young children and their families. Final Report to the Premier's Council on Health, Well Being and Social Justice. Toronto, Ontario.

Liles, B.Z. (1993). Narrative discourse in children with language disorders and children with normal language: a critical review of the literature. *Journal of Speech and Hearing Disorders*, **36**, 868–882.

Lipsky, D.K. (1985). A parental perspective on stress and coping. *American Journal of Orthopsychiatry*, **55**, 614–617.

Lochman, J.E. & Dodge, K.A. (1994). Social-cognitive processes of severely violent, moderately aggressive, and nonaggressive boys. *Journal of Consulting and Clinical Psychology*, **62**, 366–374.

Love, A. & Thompson, M. (1988). Language disorders and attention deficit disorders in young children referred for psychiatric services: analysis of prevalence and a conceptual synthesis. *American Journal of Orthopsychiatry*, **58**, 57–64.

Lovett, M.W. (1991). Developmental dyslexia. In S.J. Segalowitz and I. Rapin (eds) *Handbook of Neuropsychology. Vol. 7*. Amsterdam: Elsevier Science Publishers (pp. 163–185).

Luria, A.R. (1961). *The Role of Speech in the Regulation of Normal and Abnormal Behavior*. New York: Basic Books.

Mack, A.E. & Warr-Leeper, G.A. (1989). Language abilities in boys with chronic behavior disorders. *Language, Speech, and Hearing Services in the Schools*, **23**, 214–223.

Marcovitch, S., Goldberg, S., Lojkasek, M., & MacGregor, D. (1987). Concept of difficult temperament in developmentally delayed preschoolers. *Journal of Applied Developmental Psychology*, **8**, 151–164.

Martin, S., Kroll, R., Beebakhee, J., & Beitchman, J. (1992). Differential pragmatic abilities among communicatively impaired children. Poster presented at the conference Integrating Language, Learning, and Behavior: Theory and Applications. Toronto, Ontario (May).

McBurnett, K., Harris, S.M., Swanson, J.M., Pfiffner, L.J., Tamm, L., & Freeland, D. (1993). Neuropsychological and psychophysiological differentiation of inattention/overactivity and aggression/defiance symptom groups. *Journal of Clinical Child Psychology*, **22**, 165–171.

McCall, R.B. (1981). Nature-nurture and the two realms of development: A proposal for integration with respect to mental development. *Child Development*, **52**, 1–12.

Moffitt, T.E. (1993). Neuropsychology of conduct disorders. *Development and Psychopathology*, **5**, 135–151.

Morisset, C.E., Barnard, K.E., Greenberg, M.T., Booth, C.L., & Spieker, S.J. (1990). Environmental influences on early language development: the context of social risk. *Development and Psychopathology*, **2**, 127–149.

Naylor, M.W., Staskowski, M., Kenney, M.C., & King, C.A. (1994). Language disorders and learning disabilities in school-refusing adolescents. *Journal of the American Academy of Child and Adolescent Psychiatry*, **33**, 1331–1337.

Pellegrini, D.S., Masten, A.S., Garmezy, N., & Ferrarese, M.J. (1987). Correlates of social and academic competence in middle childhood. *Journal of Child Psychology and Psychiatry*, **28**, 699–714.

Plomin, R., DeFries, J.C., & Fulker, D.W. (1985). *Nature and Nurture During Infancy and Childhood*. New York: Cambridge University Press.

Prizant, B.M., Audet, L.R., Burkes, G.M., Hummel, L.J., Manor, S.R., & Theodore, G. (1990). Communication disorders and emotional/behavioral disorders in children and adolescents. *Journal of Speech and Hearing Disorders*, **55**, 179–192.

Prizant, B. & Wetherby, A. (1990). Toward an integrated view of early language and communication development and socioemotional development. *Topics in Language Disorders*, **10**, 1–16.

Prutting, C.A. (1982). Pragmatics as social competence. *Journal of Speech & Hearing Disorders*, **47**, 123–133.

Quiggle, N.L., Garber, J., Panak, W.F., & Dodge, K.A. (1992). Social information processing in aggressive and depressed children. *Child Development*, **63**, 1305–1320.

Ribner, S. (1978). The effects of special class placement on the self-concept of exceptional children. *Journal of Learning Disabilities*, **11**, 319–323.

Richardson, S. (1989). Developmental language disorders. In H.I. Kaplan & B.J. Sadcock (eds) *Comprehensive Textbook of Psychiatry*. Baltimore, MD: Williams & Wilkins (pp. 1812–1817).

Richman, N., Stevenson, J., & Graham, P. (1982). *Pre-school to School: A Behavioural Study*. New York: Academic Press.

Russell, R.L., Greenwald, S., & Shirk, S.R. (1991). Language change in child psychotherapy: a meta-analytic review. *Journal of Consulting and Clinical Psychology*, **59**, 916–919.

Rutter, M. (1990). Psychosocial resilience and protective mechanisms. In J. Rolf, A.S. Masten, D. Cicchetti, K.H. Nuechterlein, & S. Weintraub (eds) *Risk and Protective Factors in the Development of Psychopathology*. New York: Cambridge University Press (pp. 181–214).

Rutter, M. & Lord, C. (1987). Language disorders associated with psychiatric disturbance. In W. Yule & M. Rutter (eds) *Language Development and Disorders*. London: MacKeith Press (pp. 206–233).

Sattler, J.M., Feldman, J., & Bohanan, A.L. (1985). Parental estimates of children's receptive vocabulary. *Psychology in the Schools*, **22**, 303–307.

Schultz, L.H., Yeates, K.O., & Selman, R.L. (1989). *The Interpersonal Negotiation Strategies (INS) Interview: A Scoring Manual*. Cambridge, MA: Harvard Graduate School of Education.

Selman, R.L. & Demorest, A. (1984). Observing troubled children's interpersonal negotiating strategies: implications of and for a developmental model. *Child Development*, **55**, 288–304.

Share, D.L. & Silva, P.A. (1987). Language deficits and reading retardation: cause or effect? *British Journal of Disorders of Communication*, **22**, 219–226.

Silva, P.A., Justin, C., McGee, R., & Williams, S.M. (1984). Some developmental and behavioural characteristics of seven-year-old children with delayed speech development. *British Journal of Disorders of Communication*, **19**, 147–154.

Silva, P.A., Williams, S.M., & McGee, R. (1987). A longitudinal study of children with developmental language delay at age three: later intelligence, reading, and behavior problems. *Developmental Medicine and Child Neurology*, **25**, 783–793.

Silver, L.B. (1989). Psychological and family problems associated with learning disabilities: assessment and intervention. *Journal of the American Academy of Child and Adolescent Psychiatry*, **28**, 319–325.

Stanovich, K.E. (1988). The right and wrong places to look for the cognitive locus of reading disability. *Annals of Dyslexia*, **38**, 154–177.

Stevenson, J. (1989). Language development and delays and predictors of later reading failure. In M. Bambring, F. Losel, & H. Skowrorek (eds) *Children at Risk:*

Assessment, Longitudinal Research, and Intervention. New York: Walter de Gruyter (pp. 295–309).

Tallal, P., Curtiss, S., & Kaplan, R. (1988). The San Diego longitudinal study: Evaluating the outcome of preschool impairment in language development. In S. Gerber & G. Menecher (eds) *International Perspectives in Communication Disorders.* Washington, DC: Gallaudet University Press (pp. 86–126).

Tannock, R., Purvis, K.L., & Schachar, R.J. (1993). Narrative abilities in children with Attention Deficit Hyperactivity Disorder and normal peers. *Journal of Abnormal Child Psychology*, **21**, 103–117.

Vallance, D. (1994). Factors mediating the relation between language skills and social competence in language learning disabled children: A developmental-organizational perspective. Unpublished doctoral dissertation, York University, Toronto, Ontario.

Vygotsky, L.S. (1962). *Thought and Language.* New York: Wiley.

Werner, E. (1989). High-risk children in young adulthood: A longitudinal study from birth to 32 years. *American Journal of Orthopsychiatry*, **59**, 72–81.

Westby, C.E. & Cutler, S.K. (1994). Language and ADHD: understanding the bases and treatment of self-regulatory deficits. *Topics in Language Disorders*, **14**, 58–76.

Whitehurst, G.J. & Fischel, J.E. (1994). Practitioner review: early developmental language delay: what, if anything, should the clinician do about it? *Journal of Child Psychology and Psychiatry*, **35**, 613–648.

Willmer, S.K. & Crane, R. (1979). A parental dilemma: the child with a marginal handicap. *Social Casework*, **60**, 30–35.

Wulbert, M., Inglis, S., Kriegsman, E., & Mills, B. (1975). Language delay associated with mother–child interactions. *Developmental Psychology*, **11**, 61–71.

Ziegler, R. & Holden, L. (1988). Family therapy for learning disabled and attention-deficit disordered children. *American Journal of Orthopsychiatry*, **58**, 196–210.

7 Executive dysfunction as an underlying mechanism of behavior and language problems in attention deficit hyperactivity disorder

ROSEMARY TANNOCK AND RUSSELL SCHACHAR

INTRODUCTION

Attention deficit hyperactivity disorder (ADHD) is the most common psychiatric disorder diagnosed in childhood: it is conservatively estimated to occur in 3% to 6% of children from diverse cultures and geographical regions (e.g., Anderson et al., 1987; Bird et al., 1988; Szatmari, Offord, & Boyle, 1989a). This common disorder encompasses the lifespan, affecting children from preschool to school-age and continuing through adolescence into adulthood (e.g., Manuzza et al., 1993; Weiss & Hechtman, 1993). It is characterized by persistent and developmentally inappropriate levels of inattention, impulsiveness, and hyperactivity that can occur in various combinations across school, home, and social settings (American Psychiatric Association, 1994). These problematic behavioral symptoms are first evident in early childhood (i.e., prior to age 7); they are unexpected and cannot be explained by developmental or mental level, or by other disorders (e.g., psychosis, affective disorder); and they cause significant impairment in social, academic, or occupational functioning (American Psychiatric Association, 1994). ADHD is a heterogeneous disorder and exhibits marked overlap with other disorders, including oppositional defiant disorder, conduct disorder, anxiety disorders, communication disorders, and learning disorders (reviewed by Biederman, Newcorn, & Sprich, 1991). This chapter focuses on the specific link that has been proposed between ADHD and communication disorders (e.g., Beitchman, Tuckett, & Batth, 1987; Love & Thompson, 1988; Cantwell & Baker, 1991). Communication disorder is an umbrella term that refers to a delay or deviance in the acquisition of speech or language, or both.[1] Since deficits in a specific subsystem of language (phonological) are believed to underlie developmental reading disorder (RD) which frequently co-occurs with ADHD, we also address the complex interrelations between communication disorders, RD, and ADHD.

---

[1] The *Diagnostic and Statistical Manual of Mental Disorders,* 4th edition (DSM-IV; American Psychiatric Association, 1994) differentiates five types of Communication Disorders: expressive language disorder, receptive-expressive language disorder, phonological disorder, stuttering, and communication disorder not otherwise specified.

Despite the high rate of association between ADHD and communication disorders, neither the precise nature of the communication problems in children with ADHD nor the causal mechanisms for their overlap with ADHD are well understood. The comorbidity of ADHD and communication disorder presents clinicians with major challenges related to accurate diagnosis and appropriate treatment. Are the behavioral problems secondary to specific deficits in receptive and/or expressive language? Do the communication problems result from a subtle neuropsychological dysfunction underlying ADHD? Do the child's problems reflect two disorders each with its distinct etiology, course, and treatment response, or reflect a previously unrecognized and unclassified disorder with an etiology, course, and treatment response that is distinct from both ADHD and communication disorder? Clearly, an understanding of the etiology of this comorbidity will influence clinical practice as well as contribute to theories of developmental psychopathology. For example, if communication disorders give rise to ADHD, then remediation of the speech/language problems may alleviate the symptoms of ADHD as well. Alternatively, if the two disorders coexist, but with no causal relation, then both disorders must be treated.

In this chapter, we consider possible mechanisms mediating the association between ADHD and communication disorders. To do so, we first consider the nature of the fundamental deficits in ADHD. Next, we review the nature of the speech and language problems associated with ADHD. In the final section, we review various explanations for comorbidity and consider the possibility of a third underlying factor causing both ADHD and communication disorders.

FUNDAMENTAL DEFICITS IN ADHD: CURRENT CONCEPTUALIZATION

ADHD is defined by a persistent pattern of behavioral symptoms of inattention, impulsivity, and hyperactivity that may occur in various combinations (American Psychiatric Association, 1987, 1994). There is growing consensus, however, that the fundamental problems are in self-regulation and that ADHD is better conceptualized as an impairment of higher-order cognitive processing known as "executive function" (Mattes, 1980; Douglas, 1988; Benson, 1991; Shue & Douglas, 1992; Pennington, Groisser & Welsh, 1993; Schachar, Tannock, & Logan, 1993; Barkley, 1994). Executive function is required for planning, organizing, monitoring, and evaluating behavior (Luria, 1966; Goldman-Rakic, 1987). It is concerned with information utilization (i.e., how we use what we know) rather than with the processing, perception, and storage of information (i.e., what we know).

Executive function encompasses a range of abilities including the ability to inhibit a prepotent response or to defer it to a later more appropriate time, strategic planning, organizing, and monitoring action sequences (Luria, 1966;

Shallice, 1982; Duncan, 1986; Stuss & Benson, 1986; Goldman-Rakic, 1987). These abilities, which all share the requirement to disengage from the immediate external context and guide action instead by mental models or internal representations (Dennis, 1991), emerge in the first year of life and continue to develop through adolescence (e.g., Passler, Isaac, & Hynd, 1985; Grattan & Eslinger, 1991; Welsh, Pennington, & Groisser, 1991; Weyandt & Willis, 1994). Although there is general consensus that executive function is mediated by the prefrontal regions of the cortex (i.e., frontal lobes) and their interconnecting pathways or structures and that dysfunction in these areas disrupts the organization and control of behavior, the precise neural substrates have not yet been identified (Shallice, 1982; Fuster, 1985; Stuss & Benson, 1986; Goldman-Rakic, 1987; Perecman, 1987). Also, it is unclear how the various prefrontal areas that are anatomically and functionally distinct, contribute to performance on various measures of executive function (Benton, 1991; Grattan & Eslinger, 1991).

Evidence of frontal executive dysfunction in ADHD

Converging evidence from clinical, neurobiological and neuropsychological studies suggests that the surface behavioral manifestations in ADHD reflect an underlying problem in executive function. First, clinical assessments of ADHD yield a characterization that closely resembles classic descriptions of frontal executive dysfunction observed in adult patients with frontal lobe lesions (e.g., Pibram et al., 1964; Luria, 1966). For example, Douglas (1983, 1988) proposed that ADHD is best characterized as a generalized deficit in self-regulation and that this fundamental deficit arises from deficiencies in: "(1) the investment, organization and maintenance of attention and effort; (2) the inhibition of impulsive responding; (3) the modulation of arousal levels to meet situational demands; and (4) an unusually strong inclination to seek immediate reinforcement" (p. 280). These are precisely the characteristics of individuals with frontal lobe damage who typically show preservation of basic processes (memory, language, visual, etc.) but are impaired in their application and organization (Mattes, 1980).

Second, neuropsychological studies demonstrate that children with ADHD typically (but not invariably) perform more poorly than age-matched normal controls on a range of executive function measures that have been found to discriminate adult patients with circumscribed frontal lobe lesions from those with other lesions (reviewed by Barkley, Grodinsky, & DuPaul, 1992; see also the studies published subsequently to that review: Matazow & Hynd, 1992; Shue & Douglas, 1992; Kemp & Kirk, 1993; Pennington, Groisser, & Welsh, 1993; Weyandt & Willis, 1994; Reader et al., 1995). Evidence that the performance of ADHD children on frontal lobe/executive function tests often resembles that of younger normal children (Shue & Douglas, 1992; Reader et al., 1995), suggests that delayed frontal lobe maturation and development of executive function may be operative in ADHD. The deficits in ADHD appear to be relatively specific to executive function rather than reflecting generalized cognitive impairment, because executive dysfunction is evident in ADHD children with above-average IQ and deficient performance is observed on frontal-lobe tasks but not on measures of temporal-lobe functioning (Shue & Douglas, 1992) or on "nonexecutive tasks" (Weyandt & Willis, 1994; Reader et al., 1995). Also, it is important to note that executive function is a multidimensional construct and there is strong evidence that ADHD may be uniquely associated with deficits in specific components. For example, deficits in one aspect – *response inhibition* (the ability to inhibit a planned action) – differentiate children with ADHD from those with other psychopathology (e.g., conduct disorder, anxiety disorders) as well as from normally developing children (Schachar & Logan, 1990; Pliszka & Borcherding, 1992; Schachar & Tannock, 1995; Schachar et al., 1995; Oosterlaan & Sergeant, 1996). Response inhibition correlates significantly with externalizing symptomatology but not with internalizing symptoms (Oosterlaan & Sergeant, 1996). Moreover, "pure" ADHD (i.e., no learning disability) may be associated with deficits on measures of frontal executive function loading on an attention/maintenance factor (e.g., supraspan memory, accuracy of speeded addition, shift/maintenance of set), but with success on those executive function measures loading on an automaticity/language factor (e.g., solving word problems, rate of speeded math, linguistic fluency, confrontation naming) (Kemp & Kirk, 1993).

Third, results of neuroimaging and neurophysiological studies identify structural and functional aberrations of the frontal regions in individuals with ADHD that may differentiate ADHD from dyslexia (e.g., Zametkin et al., 1990; Semrud-Clikeman, et al., 1991; Hynd et al., 1993; Lou et al., 1984). Although these findings generally corroborate the neuropsychological evidence of frontal executive dysfunction, it is important to note that the findings are not always consistent, structure and function are not always well correlated, and that there may be important age- and gender-related differences (e.g., Zametkin et al., 1990; Ernst et al., 1994; also, see Logan, Chapter 14).

Impact of comorbidity

The presence of concurrent disorders may alter executive function in ADHD. For example, preliminary evidence suggests that concurrent anxiety disorder attenuates the deficit in response inhibition (Pliszka & Borcherding, 1992). By contrast, the presence of comorbid conduct disorder or aggression in ADHD does not (Schachar & Tannock, 1995; Oosterlaan & Sergeant, 1996). To our knowledge, no study to date has examined the impact of concurrent communication disorder on executive function in ADHD, but several have investigated executive function in young people with ADHD and comorbid RD (ADHD + RD). The findings are inconsistent. For example, Kemp and

Kirk (1993) reported that children with ADHD + RD exhibited deficits on an automaticity/language factor of executive function but not on an attention/ maintenance factor. By contrast (as noted previously), the ADHD-only group were impaired on the attention/maintenance factor but not on the auto-maticity/language factor (Kemp & Kirk, 1993). A dissociation between ADHD and ADHD + RD was also demonstrated by Pennington and his colleagues (1993), but in this case, only the "pure" ADHD group exhibited executive dysfunction; the ADHD + RD and RD-only groups both exhibited a language-based deficit in phonological processing, but intact executive function. Other studies failed to discriminate ADHD and ADHD + RD on measures on executive function (e.g., Reader et al., 1995). Thus, Pennington's (Pennington et al., 1993) interpretation of his data as evidence that ADHD is secondary to RD in the comorbid condition, may be premature.

Summary

There is converging evidence that frontal executive dysfunction is fundamental to ADHD. Deficits in these higher-order cognitive processes give rise to problems in the planning, organization, monitoring, and regulation of behavior, which in turn are the basis of the surface behavioral symptoms of inattention, impulsiveness and hyperactivity. Moreover, some aspects of executive function, such as response inhibition, may be specific to ADHD. This evidence has spawned a recent theory of ADHD that assumes the fundamental deficit to be an inability to inhibit and delay dominant or prepotent responses to an event, which in turn disrupts other executive functions that are critical to developing self-control and directing behavior towards the future, including the use of internalized, self-directed speech for self-regulation (Barkley, 1994; Shelton & Barkley, 1994).

COMMUNICATION DISORDERS ASSOCIATED WITH ADHD

We now shift perspective to review the prevalence and nature of com-munication disorders associated with ADHD, before considering possible mechanisms underlying the comorbidity between the two disorders. We examine the following issues: (1) the strength of the association between ADHD and communication disorder; (2) the specificity of the association; (3) the impact of comorbidity; (4) the impact of otitis media; and (5) develop-mental changes in the association.

Strength of the association

Epidemiological and clinical studies not only indicate a high degree of overlap between psychiatric disorders and moderate to severe speech/language impairments (S/LI), but also suggest a specific link between ADHD and S/LI (reviewed by Prizant et al., 1990; Cantwell & Baker, 1991; Baker & Cantwell, 1992). As shown in Table 7.1, numerous studies indicate elevated rates of S/LI in children with ADHD (or symptoms associated with ADHD) and conversely, elevated rates of ADHD (or symptoms associated with ADHD) in children with S/LI. Estimates of the overlap varies widely from a low of 8% to a high of 90%, depending on the precise definitions of S/LI, the nature of the S/LI, and the type of the methods used to diagnose ADHD. It is important to note that the data are derived almost exclusively from clinic-referred psychiatric samples in which inflated rates of comorbidity are inherent (Caron & Rutter, 1991). On the other hand, the one epidemiological study reports that a substantial proportion (30%) of the children with S/LI also had attention deficit disorder (ADD), compared to only 4% of the non-language-impaired control children (Beitchman et al., 1989). The overlap appears to be asymmetrical: children with ADHD are more likely to have S/LI (average 50%) than vice versa (average 20%), but the comorbidity patterns may reflect a sampling bias.

The association between ADHD and S/LI is greater than would be expected by chance alone, given the base rates of each disorder in the community. For example, according to epidemiological studies, the base rate ADHD ranges from 3% to 10% (e.g., Anderson et al., 1987; Szatmari et al., 1989a) and that for S/LI ranges from 1% to 17% (with most estimates in the 3% to 7% range), depending upon the methods of ascertainment, professional background of the diagnostician, and the precision in definition and diagnosis (see Cantwell & Baker, 1991, for a review of prevalence estimates of S/LI). Assuming an upper bound estimate of 10% for ADHD and 7% for S/LI, the expected association between ADHD and S/LI would be 1.7% (i.e., the product of the probability levels for each disorder alone), which is substantially lower than the observed association of 30% in the epidemiological study by Beitchman et al. (1989).

Specificity of the association

Communication disorders may be manifested by a wide range of signs that can occur singly or in different combinations. Traditionally, distinctions have been made between two broad categories; disorders of speech (i.e, the motor production of the sounds of a particular language); disorders of language (problems in the comprehension and/or production of the arbitrary system of symbols and rules used to convey meanings). However, as noted by Chaban (Chapter 2), there is a growing awareness of language related problems that may not reflect deficits in the basic subsystems of language (i.e., phonology, semantics, syntax) but rather concern problems in the appropriate use of language within social, situational, and communicative contexts. These problems are known as pragmatic deficits. Our aim here is

Table 7.1. *Studies of the association between ADHD and speech/language impairments*

Study	Sample: size, source comparison group	Age range (yrs)	Findings
Beitchman et al. (1989)	Epidemiological sample (one-in-three; *n* = 1655), from schools, Canada	Kindergarten (5-yr-olds)	30% of SLI had ADD; 13% of SLI had emotional disorders
Benasich et al. (1993)	56 children with LI & 43 NC followed longitudinally from age 4 to age 8, USA	8-yr-olds	18% of children with LI versus 0% of controls scored in the clinical range on CBCL-hyperactivity subscale
Berry et al. (1985)	134 ADD from learning disorders and pediatric clinics; 94 NC from public schools, USA	6–13	26% of ADD had expressive language problems; 8% had receptive language problems
Cantwell & Baker (1991)	600 children from community speech-hearing clinic, USA	3–16	19% of SLI had ADD; 10% of SLI had anxiety
Chess & Rosenberg (1974)	563 preschoolers from psychiatric outpatient clinic	preschool	24% had SLI, most of whom had ADD symptoms
Cohen et al. (1993)	399 consecutive referrals to psychiatric outpatient clinic, Canada	4–12	Children with SLI more likely to have ADD symptoms
Gualtieri et al. (1983)	26 consecutive admissions to psychiatry inpatient unit with completed evaluations, USA	5–13	90% of those with ADD (with or without CD) had SLI
Humphries et al. (1994)	30 boys with attention problems and 33 with learning disorder referred to a hospital child development clinic, Canada	6–14	42% of boys with attention problems had SLI according to teacher ratings
Love & Thompson (1988)	116 referrals to child psychiatric outpatient clinic, Canada	preschool	66% of ADD had SLI
Tannock et al. (1995)	20 ADHD referred for medication trial, Canada	7–11	60% ADHD had SLI, previously undiagnosed in all but one case

Table 7.1 *(cont.)*

Study	Sample: size, source comparison group	Age range (yrs)	Findings
Thorley (1984)	73 hyperkinetic syndrome 73 conduct disorder from mental health clinics, England		30% hyperkinetic syndrome with 10 > 70 had articulation disorder vs. 6% of those with conduct disorder
Trautman et al. (1990)	67 severe emotional/behavioral disordered youngsters in a special school/day treatment program, USA	6–13	69% of ADD had SLI
Warr-Leeper et al. (1994)	20 boys in residential treatment program for antisocial behavior, USA	10–14	80% with comorbid ADHD of whom most had previously undiagnosed SLI

Notes: ADD, attention deficit disorder; ADHD, attention deficit hyperactivity disorder; SLI, speech/language impairments; LI, language impairment; CBCL, Child Behavior Check List (Achenbach & Edelbrock, 1983); NC, normally developing children; CD, conduct disorder.

to determine whether there is a specific type (or types) of communication disorder associated closely with ADHD.

Speech disorders in ADHD

Problems in the motor production of the sounds of a particular language (i.e., speech disorders), include problems in articulation (frequent and recurring mispronunciations of one or more speech sounds), fluency (difficulty stringing the sounds together in a smooth rhythm), voice quality (abnormal pitch, loudness, nasality or hoarseness), and rate of speech (so rapid or slow that it is unintelligible).[2]

Speech problems (primarily articulation, fluency) may be more common in ADHD children compared to normal controls, although findings are incon-

---

[2] The DSM-IV classification system uses a different breakdown of speech disorders; phonological disorder includes problems in production (i.e., articulation) and in linguistic categorization (i.e., phonological processing) of the sounds of one's language; stuttering (a disturbance in the normal fluency and time patterning of speech), and voice disorder (i.e., an abnormality of vocal pitch, loudness, quality, tone, or resonance). The latter is classified under Communication Disorder Not Otherwise Specified (American Psychiatric Association, 1994).

sistent (cf. Humphries et al., 1994; Szatmari et al., 1989b). However, they are less strongly related to ADHD than are language problems, and typically co-exist with language problems (see Tables 7.2 and 7.3). Speech disorders *per se* are more strongly associated with emotional problems (e.g., anxiety and affective disorders) than with ADHD (see Table 7.2).

Speech problems in children with ADHD decline with age (Baker & Cantwell, 1992). Also, they may be gender related, although it is unclear in what way. According to one study, articulation problems are more common in boys than girls (84% vs. 44%; Baker & Cantwell, 1992). On the other hand, another study found that girls with ADHD were more likely to be referred for speech problems than were ADHD boys (Berry et al., 1985). The ADHD girls were also noted to be younger at age of referral and to exhibit more severe language impairments than boys, factors which are also related to speech problems.

Language disorders

Language disorders include problems in comprehending the meaning of words or grammatical and sentence structures (receptive language disorder) and problems in choosing and developing ideas, selecting appropriate words to represent the ideas, and/or in ordering the words grammatically to convey a meaningful message (expressive language disorders).[3]

Children with ADHD are more likely to be delayed in the onset of language (as assessed by the appearance of first words and short sentences) relative to normal children: delayed onset is observed in 6% to 35% of children with ADHD compared with 2% to 6% of non-ADHD children (Hartsough & Lambert, 1985; Szatmari, Offord, & Boyle, 1989b; Gross-Tsur, Shalev, & Amir, 1991; Ornoy, Uriel, & Tennenbaum, 1993). However, findings are not always consistent (e.g., Barkley, DuPaul, & McMurray, 1990).

Systematic assessment of current language abilities (using standardized tests) indicate that a substantial proportion of children with ADHD (15% to 76%) exhibit language impairments and conversely a substantial proportion of children with language impairments (20% to 60%) exhibit ADHD or symptoms associated with ADHD (see Tables 7.2 and 7.3). The variation in estimates is attributable in part to differences in how language impairment was defined in the studies. Although problems in both receptive and expressive language have been reported in children with ADHD, expressive language appears to be particularly impaired (Beitchman et al., 1987; Berry et al., 1985; Baker & Cantwell, 1992; Tannock, Ickowicz, Oram, & Fine, 1995).

---

[3] DSM-IV (American Psychiatric Association, 1994) distinguishes two types of language disorder – Expressive Language Disorder, Mixed Receptive-Expressive Language Disorder – in recognition of the fact that receptive language problems rarely occur in isolation without accompanying expressive problems.

Table 7.2. *Rates of psychiatric disorder in children with various categories of speech/language impairments*

Study	Psychiatric diagnosis	Types of speech/language impairment*		
		Speech only	Language only	Speech/language
Beitchman et al.	ADD	5%	38%	59%
(1989)	CD	9%	0%	4%
	ED	19%	0%	14%
Cantwell &	ADD	10%	33%	23%
Baker (1991)	ODD	3%	4%	6%
	CD	1%	9%	1%
	ED	15%	31%	20%
Trautman et al.	ADD	50%	38%	63%
(1990)	CDD	0%	6%	0%
	CD	17%	17%	14%
	ED	17%	0%	7%

Notes: ADD, attention deficit disorder (generic term); ODD, oppositional defiant disorder (generic term); CD, conduct disorder; ED, emotional disorder, primarily anxiety disorders; Speech-only disorders include articulation, voice and fluency problems in studies by Cantwell & Baker (1991) and Trautman et al. (1990), but only articulation problems in Beitchman et al., 1989.

* Figures indicate the percentage of children with a specific type of speech/language impairment with psychiatric disorder (e.g. 5% of children with speech only impairments have ADD).

Of concern, is the evidence that many children referred solely for disruptive behavior disorders may have coexisting S/LI that remain unrecognized and identified only upon systematic assessment (Cohen et al., 1989, 1993; Warr-Leeper, Wright, & Mack, 1994). Similar findings are emerging in our current sample of children with ADHD referred solely for an evaluation of medication treatment for their behavioral problems: 12 of the 20 (60%) children assessed to date, have been found to have moderate receptive and/or expressive language impairments which were previously undiagnosed in all but one case (Tannock, Ickowicz, Oram, & Fine, 1995). Perhaps parents and clinicians focus on the more salient disruptive behavior symptoms and fail to notice poor language skills (Cohen, 1989, 1993). In this situation, there is a risk that the child's failure to follow instructions may be attributed incorrectly to inattentiveness and/or oppositional behavior and not recognized as an impairment in decoding skills responsible for the assignment of meaning to speech (Cohen et al., 1993).

Table 7.3. *Rates and type of speech/language impairments in children with ADD*

Study	Samples	Number of ADD subjects in sample	Percentage of ADD sample with problems in:		
			Speech-only	Language-only	Speech/language
Baker & Cantwell (1992)	Clinical sample of speech/language impaired children (3–16 yr)	65	17%	22%	62%
Beitchman et al. (1989)	Epidemiological sample of kindergarten children	17	6%	18%	76%
Trautman et al. (1990)	Clinical sample; day treatment program for behavioral emotional disorders	22	14%	27%	27%

Note: ADD, attention deficit disorder.

Pragmatic disorder

Pragmatic disorder is broadly defined as difficulties in using language appropriately within a social, situational, and communicative context. Pragmatic language skills are complex and implicate executive function; they include recognition of the social and informational demands of the situation, knowledge of language to be able to select appropriate linguistic forms and meanings to meet those demands, the ability to organize and express thoughts and ideas through several channels simultaneously (vocabulary, sentence structure, pronunciation, facial expression, gesture, tone of voice), and the ability to make rapid, "on-line" changes according to moment-by-moment changes in the communicative context (Spekman, 1984; Prutting & Kirchner, 1987; see also Chaban, Chapter 2). Thus dysfunction in any of these components, alone or in combination may result in pragmatic deficits.

As shown in Table 7.4, a wide range of pragmatic deficits have been demonstrated in children with ADHD. These studies indicate that compared to normal children, those with ADHD exhibit: (1) excessive verbal output during spontaneous conversations, task transitions, and in play settings (Barkley, Cunningham, & Karlsson, 1983; Zentall, 1988); (2) decreased verbal output and more dysfluencies when confronted with tasks which require planning and organization of verbal responses, as in story retelling and giving directions (Hamlett, Pellegrini, & Connors, 1987; Zentall, 1988; Tannock, Purvis, & Schachar, 1993); (3) difficulties in introducing, maintaining, and changing topics appropriately and in negotiating smooth interchanges or turn taking during conversation (Humphries et al., 1994; Ludlow et al., 1978; Zentall et al., 1983); (4) problems in being specific, accurate and concise in the selection and use of words to convey information in an unambiguous manner (Tannock et al., 1993); and (5) difficulties in adjusting language to the listener and specific contexts (Whalen et al., 1979; Landau & Milich, 1988; Zentall, 1988).

In addition to the preceding deficits in the use of language in social and communicative contexts, ADHD is also associated with deficits in the use of language for problem solving. For example they exhibit deficits in verbal and semantic organizational strategies (Tant & Douglas, 1982; Ackerman et al., 1986; August, 1987; Felton et al., 1987) and in self-talk (Copeland, 1979; Berk & Potts, 1991). Self-talk or private-speech, which is defined as speech uttered aloud that is addressed to the self or to no particular listener, is "thought spoken out loud" for the purpose of self-guidance and self-regulation (Vygotsky, 1934/1987). Cross-sectional and longitudinal data demonstrate that private speech consistently follows a developmental sequence from audible, externalized speech to more internalized, less audible forms (e.g., Berk, 1986, 1992). Moreover, the movement towards internalized forms of private speech is positively associated with concurrent task behavior, such as focused attention and motor quiescence (Berk, 1986; Berk & Potts, 1991). Children with ADHD are delayed in the development of private speech. These children engage in more externalized, self-guiding task and less inaudible, internalized speech than normal controls. Moreover, they are less able to use private speech as a self-regulatory mediational strategy to ameliorate behavioral and at-tentional problems (Berk & Potts, 1991). Also, deficits in private speech are much greater in children with comorbid ADHD and LD, compared to those with LD only (Berk & Landau, 1993).

Pragmatic deficits are evident in the majority of ADHD children, even in those with adequate phonological, morphological, syntactic, and semantic abilities (Ludlow et al., 1978; Humphries et al., 1994; Tannock et al., 1991, 1993). Moreover, although pragmatic disorders are also evident in children with learning disabilities (e.g., Lapadat, 1991), they appear to be more strongly associated with ADHD. For example, Humphries and his colleagues (1994) found that 60% of boys with attention problems exhibited pragmatic deficits, compared to 15% of those with learning disabilities and 7% of normally developing children.

Impact of comorbid RD

One limitation of many of the survey studies is that they did not distinguish between children with ADHD only and those with comorbid disorders and

Table 7.4. *Pragmatic deficits in children with attention deficit disorder*

Study	Sample	Method	Findings
Berk & Landau (1993)	9 LD/AD 47 LD 47 NC	Self-talk, motor activity and attention during academic seatwork, at school and in the lab	LD/AD group used more task-relevant, externalized and less internalized self-talk than LD and NC groups (analysis based on matched groups of 9)
Berk & Potts (1991)	19 ADHD 19 NC	Self-talk and its relationship to self-controlled behavior during academic seatwork	ADHD group used more externalized and less internalized self-talk than NC. Self-talk of ADHD children less effective in controlling task-related behavior
Hamlett et al. (1987)	16 ADDH 16 NC	Social communication task; procedural narrative	ADDH group were less informative, less easy to follow, and more dysfluent
Humphries et al. (1994)	30 AP 32 LD 32 NC	Teacher ratings of language functioning	Pragmatic problems rated as the most problematic in AP boys and more common than in LD or NC boys
Landau & Millich (1988)	17 ADD 18 NC	Peer interaction during a role playing task	ADD boys less able to modulate communication when role requirements changed
Ludlow et al. (1978)	12 hyperactive 12 NC	Communication tasks: picture description, story telling, referential communication	Hyperactive boys produced more disruptive and child-initiated speech and fewer instructions, but did not differ in speech fluency or syntactic complexity, compared to NC, matched on verbal ability and language development

Table 7.4 *(cont.)*

Study	Sample	Method	Findings
Tannock et al. (1993)	30 ADHD 30 NC	Comprehension and production of story narratives	ADHD boys provided less information and their stories were more poorly organized, less cohesive and more inaccurate, but they did not differ in comprehension
Whalen et al. (1979)	23 hyperactive 39 NC	Peer communication during a dyadic referential communication task	Hyperactive boys less able to adjust their communication as required when shifting role from message sender to message recipient
Zentall (1988)	23 ADDH 22 NC	Spontaneous language during elicited (four narrative tasks) and nonelicited conditions (transitions non-verbal task)	ADDH group more talkative during nonelicited condition, but less talkative during elicited conditions, particularly during tasks requiring organization and planning
Zentall et al. (1983)	13 hyperactive 13 NC	Language and behavior during transitions and a referential communication task	Hyperactive preschoolers were more verbally and motorically active; produced more impulsive verbalization during transitions and tasks; and were more dysfluent and used less commentary during referential tasks

Notes: ADD, attention deficit disorder; ADDH, attention deficit with hyperactivity; ADHD, attention deficit hyperactivity disorder; AP, attention problems; LD, learning disorders; LD/AD, learning disorders with concurrent attention deficit hyperactivity disorders; NC, normal comparison group.

so one cannot determine whether the language impairments are more a function of the comorbid disorder than of ADHD. Findings from our recent studies demonstrate that receptive and expressive impairments in the basic language systems (phonology, semantics, syntax) are more closely linked with developmental reading disorders than with ADHD (Tannock, Purvis, & Schachar, 1991; Tannock et al., 1994). For example, we found that children (aged 7 to 11 years) with "pure" RD ($n = 10$) and those with ADHD + RD ($n = 21$) scored significantly lower than children with "pure" ADHD ($n = 28$) and normal controls ($n = 15$) on standardized measures of receptive and expressive abilities in semantic aspects of language (The Word Test: Jorgeson et al., 1981; Language Processing Test: Richard & Hanner, 1985). RD was defined by a combined achievement-discrepancy formula (a reading achievement score at least 1.5 standard deviations below the mean for age, and 1 standard deviation (SD) below IQ). Moreover, a substantially higher proportion of children in the ADHD + RD and RD groups were classified as "language impaired" (defined as a score of at least 1.0 SD below the mean for age on one or both tests): 7% of ADHD, 24% of ADHD + RD, 60% of RD and none of the NC group. By contrast, all three clinical groups exhibited impairments in a story narrative task, which requires pragmatic skills: their story narratives were less informative and cohesive, poorly organized, and more difficult to understand compared to those produced by normal peers (Purvis & Tannock, 1995).

In another study (Tannock et al., 1994), we assessed phonological processing in a large clinical sample of children with a diagnosis of ADHD ($n = 75$) confirmed by clinical diagnostic interviews and behavior rating scales. Phonological processing refers to the use of the sounds of one's language to process written and oral language (see Vandervelden & Siegel, Chapter 11 for a detailed exposition). The sample was dichotomized into "adequate readers" and "poor readers"; poor readers had scores of at least 1.5 SD below the mean for age on a standardized word identification test (Wide Range Achievement Test-Revised; Jastak & Wilkinson, 1984). These two subgroups did not differ in age, nonverbal IQ, or severity of ADHD. The results indicated that only the ADHD/poor readers exhibited marked deficits on all of the standardized measures of phonological processing, which included a measure of nonword reading (Woodcock Reading Mastery Test-Revised, Word Attack Subtest), phoneme deletion and blending (Rosner Auditory Analysis Test) and speed of naming (Rapid Automatized Naming: letters, numbers, colors). Moreover, the deficits were not attenuated with increasing age. By contrast, there was no evidence of phonological deficits in the ADHD group with adequate achievement in reading.

Collectively, these findings suggest that receptive and expressive deficits in the basic language systems of phonology, syntax, and semantics are more closely linked with RD than ADHD. Furthermore, the results suggest that poor reading abilities in children with ADHD children are related to deficient phonological abilities and not ADHD symptomatology *per se* (e.g., inattentiveness, impulsiveness). Stronger evidence for the independence of attentional impairments and phonological impairments is provided by the findings from a series of longitudinal studies by Wood and Felton (1994). More specifically, Wood & Felton (1994) demonstrated that phonological processing abilities in childhood are powerful predictors of reading ability, whereas childhood ADD has no measurable impact on reading ability in either childhood or in adulthood.

Impact of otitis media

Otitis media with effusion (fluid in the ear following inflammation of the middle ear), which is a prevalent condition in early childhood, is often associated with transient conductive hearing loss (Paradise, 1980; Bluestone, 1983). High rates of otitis media (with effusion) in preschool children have been associated with later language deficits and problems in attention and hyperactivity (e.g., Teale et al., 1984; Feagans et al., 1987; Hagerman & Falkenstein, 1987; Roberts et al., 1989). Also, school-aged children with ADHD have been found to experience more middle ear problems (and more upper respiratory infections) in the past year, compared to children with learning disabilities (Adesman et al., 1990). The precise role of middle ear disease in communication disorders or other learning disabilities associated with ADHD is unknown. Nevertheless, these data indicate the need to screen for middle ear disease and current audiological status, particularly in children presenting with both ADHD and communication impairments.

Developmental changes in the association between ADHD and S/LI

The co-occurrence of receptive/expressive language impairments and ADHD emerges in the preschool years and continues throughout the elementary school years into adolescence (e.g., Beitchman et al., 1987; Benasich et al., 1993; Cantwell & Baker, 1991; McGee et al., 1991). Longitudinal studies suggest that hyperactive preschoolers with language impairments are at high risk for the development of comorbid learning disabilities, particularly reading disorder which persists through adolescence (McGee et al., 1991; Ornoy et al., 1993). For example, Ornoy et al. (1993) found that 80% of preschoolers who exhibited the triad of language impairments, inattentiveness/hyperactivity and "soft" neurological signs at age 3, met the diagnosis for ADHD in middle childhood and most had comorbid learning disabilities. Similarly, McGee et al. (1991) found in his 12-year follow-up of a group of pervasively hyperactive 3-year-olds with receptive and expressive language impairments, that 35% of the hyperactive-language impaired group had reading disabilities at age 15, compared to 17% of children who had been classified as "difficult to manage" (but not ADHD) at age 3, 10% of the language impaired only group, and 10% of the normal comparison group. The findings of high rates of reading disorders among the children with early language impairments are consistent with those from longitudinal studies of specifically language impaired children (e.g., Aram, Ekelman, & Nation, 1984; Silva et al., 1987; Bishop & Adams, 1990; Benasich et al., 1993).

Summary

To summarize the evidence reviewed so far for the relationships between ADHD and communication disorders, the strongest association is between ADHD and expressive language deficits, particularly deficits in the pragmatic domain. These deficits are evident in both interpersonal and personal domains (i.e., in language used for social, communication and in that used for self-regulation). Many (but not all) preschoolers with symptoms consistent with both ADHD and speech/language impairments present in middle school years as youngsters with ADHD and comorbid RD. Some types of communication disorders (pragmatic disorders) appear to be more specifically linked with ADHD, whereas others (phonological disorders, receptive and expressive semantic and syntactic disorders) appear to be linked with RD rather than ADHD. Factors other than ADHD, such as age, gender, and comorbidity with other disorders, must be taken into account when considering the relationship between ADHD and communication disorders.

MECHANISMS UNDERLYING COMORBIDITY

There are several possible explanations for the comorbidity of ADHD and S/LI (e.g., Rutter & Lord 1987; Prizant et al., 1990; Caron & Rutter, 1991). Some can be excluded on the basis of existing evidence. First, the comorbid condition of ADHD + S/LI cannot be attributed to the chance occurrence of two unrelated disorders. As noted previously, the high degree of overlap of these two disorders is well above the rates expected by chance alone. Nor is the degree of overlap so great that ADHD and S/LI can be assumed to be a single disorder: Each disorder alone can be identified in both community and clinical samples (e.g., Berry et al., 1985; Beitchman et al., 1989; McGee et al., 1991). Second, the evidence that ADHD + S/LI is common in both clinic and community samples indicates that this comorbidity is not an artefact of referral bias (e.g., Love and Thompson, 1988; Beitchman et al., 1989; McGee et al., 1991; Cohen et al., 1993). Third, the high rate of ADHD + S/LI is not simply an artefact of measurement problems, because high rates of comorbidity are found with a range of diagnostic methods, including symptom checklists and rating scales, diagnostic interviews, and discriminatory measures of speech/language abilities. Fourth, it is unlikely that the comorbidity of ADHD and S/LI is the artefactual result of overlapping diagnostic criteria, although many of the symptoms of ADHD described in the DSM-IV list are also characteristic of pragmatic dysfunction (e.g., talking excessively, blurting out answers before questions have been completed, interrupting others by butting into conversations). Eliminating overlapping symptoms, such as talking excessively/interrupting conversations, would not be expected to result in a significant decrease in the rate of comorbid ADHD and S/LI.

Common etiology

Other explanations for the common overlap between ADHD and S/LI have yet to be evaluated. One explanation is that one disorder may give rise to the other (e.g., speech/language problems lead to ADHD or vice versa). A variant of this hypothesis is that one disorder is primary and produces a symptomatic phenocopy of the other disorder, but without its core or primary characteristics (Pennington et al., 1993). A second possible explanation is that a common underlying factor may produce the comorbid condition of ADHD + S/LI or give rise to ADHD or S/LI alone.

The fact that the overlap between ADHD and S/LI appears early in development (i.e., in preschool years) suggests that common underlying causal factors might be operative in shaping eventual comorbidity (Hinshaw, 1992). Several factors have been proposed, including psychosocial factors (e.g., low socioeconomic status, single parent, parental psychopathology, stress, or style of caregiving/behavior management), specific cognitive factors, and neuro-developmental immaturity (Beitchman et al., 1987, 1989; Tallal, Dukette & Curtiss, 1989). Stevenson (Chapter 5) provides a thoughtful discussion of psychosocial factors (as well as other explanations for comorbidity) and so we will not reiterate the exposition here. Rather, we address the hypothesis that shared cognitive factors and/or neurodevelopmental immaturity might account for the observed comorbidity between ADHD and communication disorders.

Executive dysfunction as a shared risk factor

We propose that frontal executive dysfunction may account for both the core behavioral problems and the pragmatic disorders commonly observed in ADHD. By contrast, we argue that deficits in the basic systems of language (phonology, syntax, semantics) that have been attributed previously to ADHD are more related to RD. ADHD and RD are distinct clinical entities, that frequently co-occur (e.g., Pennington et al., 1993; Wood & Felton, 1994).

A number of factors have led us to the formulation of executive dysfunction as a common factor underlying both the behavioral and communication problems observed in ADHD. First, we concluded from the preceding literature review that deficits in higher-order cognitive processes – executive function – are fundamental to ADHD and account for the core behavioral symptoms of this disorder. Moreover, based on the evidence that ADHD children tend to perform more like younger normal children on measures of frontal lobe/executive function, we suggest that a delay in frontal lobe maturation and in the development of executive function might be operative in ADHD. Given the importance of genetic influences in ADHD (e.g., Biederman et al., 1991b; Gillis et al., 1992; Stevenson, 1992), it is possible that frontal lobe maturation has a genetic origin.

Second, we note that the prefrontal regions of the cortex are not only involved in the temporal (serial, sequential) organization of behavior and cognition, but also they are involved in the production and interpretation of language (Luria, 1966; Ingvar, 1993). For example, frontal lobe lesions disturb the regulatory function of speech, but not the phonetic, lexical, or grammatical functions (Luria, 1966, 1973). That is, adults with frontal lobe lesions can no longer control their behavior with the aid of their own speech, or that of another person. Disturbances in the verbal regulatory function have been related to disturbances of planning, organizing, and monitoring behavior (Milner, 1963; Petrides & Milner, 1982).

Third, our review of the types of communication disorders associated with ADHD revealed the strongest link to be between ADHD and problems in the expression of language, most notably in the pragmatic system that provides rules for selecting particular forms of language for use in different situations. Recall that children with ADHD exhibit problems in the development of self-regulatory speech, verbal mediation, and in the production and processing of discourse (i.e., extended stretches of language used in conversations and narratives, which place heavy demands on planning, organization, and monitoring). These are precisely the type of deficits that would be predicted to occur with frontal executive dysfunction. Also, problems in the basic language systems (phonology, semantics, syntax), which are not thought to be influenced by frontal executive function, appear to be related to RD rather than ADHD. Empirical support exists for the underlying assumption that frontal executive function and specific language processes (e.g., phonological processing) are separable, independent subcomponents of cognitive function (e.g., Kemp & Kirk, 1993; Pennington et al., 1993).

Finally, we argue that if executive dysfunction underlies both language and behavior problems, then treatment of this common factor should produce concomitant changes in both language and behavior. Specifically, the treatment should influence executive function and pragmatic components of language but not the basic language systems. There is strong evidence that stimulant medication, which is the most widely used treatment for ADHD is effective in ameliorating the overt behavioral symptoms of ADHD and enhancing performance on measures of executive function (e.g., Douglas et al., 1988; Tannock et al., 1989; Tannock, Schachar, & Logan, 1995). Moreover, the limited available evidence suggests that stimulants influence pragmatic aspects of language but not the basic language systems. For example, Berk & Potts (1991) noted that stimulant medication not only reduced off-task and restless behavior, but also it increased the developmental maturity of private speech and its association with visual attention to task and motor quiescence. In addition Ludlow and colleagues (Ludlow et al., 1978) reported that stimulant treatment was effective in reducing disruptive and non-task related talk in a group of hyperactive boys with normally developing language. By contrast, stimulants had no impact on speech fluency or task-related talk. Moreover, there is no evidence to date that stimulants have any direct impact on the phonological system of language (Richardson et al., 1988; Balthazor, Wagner, & Pelham, 1991).

Bidirectional model

Implicit in our argument so far is that the direction of influence is unidirectional: executive dysfunction gives rise to ADHD symptomatology and to problems in using language appropriately within social and situational contexts. We suspect that a bi-directional or transactional model would more accurately reflect the situation. That is, executive dysfunction impedes the development of internalized self-directed talk and self-regulation, which in turn has a negative effect on the development and use of these high-order cognitive processes.

CONCLUSIONS AND IMPLICATIONS

Complex relationships exist among ADHD, communication disorders, and learning disabilities (specifically, RD), which frequently co-occur. We theorize that the core behavioral symptoms of ADHD (inattention, hyperactivity/impulsiveness) and the pragmatic difficulties that these children exhibit (e.g., poor topic maintenance, interrupting conversation, excessive talk) are related to deficits in executive function (i.e., higher-order cognitive processes), which is believed to be central to ADHD. Pragmatic deficits are evident even in ADHD children with intact receptive and expressive abilities in the basic language systems (phonology, syntax, semantics). By contrast, deficits in the basic language systems are related to RD and not ADHD: RD is a distinct clinical entity that frequently co-occurs with ADHD. Delayed development of the basic language systems in hyperactive preschoolers is a strong risk factor for learning disabilities, particularly reading disorder, in middle childhood.

Notwithstanding the speculative nature of our formulation of the relationships, the high rate of comorbidity between communication disorders and ADHD has important implications for clinical practice. The language and communication difficulties in children with ADHD may remain undetected unless language functioning is made a formal part of the diagnostic assessment for ADHD. Clinicians responsible for the diagnosis and management of children and adolescents with ADHD need to become better informed about the nature of communication disorders in these young people and the impact on academic and social functioning. Treatment prescribed for ADHD (e.g., stimulant medication) may improve some aspects of the communication disorder (i.e., pragmatic dysfunction), but it is unlikely to have any impact on deficits in those aspects that are central to reading ability (e.g., phonological processing). Deficits in the basic language systems require specific intervention in consultation with speech/language pathologists. Conversely, speech-language pathologists need to acquire a better understanding and appreciation of the fundamental deficits and defining characteristics in ADHD as well as the nature of the communication disorders most closely linked to ADHD. Effective treatments and management techniques are available for ADHD, which may enable young people to obtain greater benefit from speech/language intervention.

ACKNOWLEDGMENTS

The research described in this chapter was supported by grants from the Medical Research Council of Canada and Health Canada, National Health Research and Development Program.

REFERENCES

Achenbach, T.M. & Edelbrock, C.S. (1983). *Manual for the Child Behavior Checklist and Revised Child Behavior Profile*. Burlington, CT: University of Vermont, Department of Psychiatry.

Ackerman, P.T., Anhalt, J., Dykman, R.A., & Holcomb, P. (1986). Effortful processing deficits in children with reading and/or attention disorders. *Brain & Cognition*, **5**, 22–40.

Adesman, A.R., Alshuler, L.A., Lipkin, P.H., & Walco, G.A. (1990). Otitis media in children with learning disabilities and in children with attention deficit disorder with hyperactivity. *Pediatrics*, **85**, 442–446.

American Psychiatric Association (1987). *Diagnostic and Statistical Manual of Mental Disorders*, 3rd edn. Washington, DC: Author.

American Psychiatric Association (1994). *Diagnostic and Statistical Manual of Mental Disorders*, 4th edn (DSM-IV). Washington, DC: American Psychiatric Association.

Anderson, J.C., Williams, S., McGee, R., & Silva, P.A. (1987). DSM-III-R disorders in preadolescent children: prevalence in a large sample from the general population. *Archives of General Psychiatry*, **44**, 69–76.

Aram, D.M., Ekelman, B., & Nation, J.E. (1984). Preschoolers with language disorders: 10 years later. *Journal of Speech and Hearing Research*, **27**, 232–244.

August, G.J. (1987). Production deficiences in free recall: a comparison of hyperactive, learning-disabled, and normal children. *Journal of Abnormal Child Psychology*, **15**, 429–440.

Baker, L. & Cantwell, D.P. (1992). Attention deficit disorder and speech/language disorders. *Comprehensive Mental Health Care*, **2**, 3–16.

Baker, L. & Cantwell, D. (1987). Comparison of well, emotionally disordered, and behaviorally disordered children with linguistic problems. *Journal of the American Academy of Child and Adolescent Psychiatry*, **26**, 193–196.

Balthazor, M.J., Wagner, R.K., & Pelham, W.E. (1991). The specificity of effects of stimulant medication on classroom learning-related measures of cognitive processing for attention deficit disorder children. *Journal of Abnormal Child Psychology*, **19**, 35–52.

Barkley, R.A. (1994). Delayed responding and attention deficit hyperactivity disorder: A unified theory. In D.K. Routh (ed.) *Disruptive Behavior Disorders in Children: Essays in Honor of Herbert Quay*. New York: Plenum (pp. 12–57).

Barkley, R.A., Cunningham, C., & Karlsson, J. (1983). The speech of hyperactive children with their mothers: comparisons with normal children and stimulant effects. *Journal of Learning Disabilities*, **16**, 105–110.

Barkley, R.A., DuPaul, G.J. & McMurray, M.B. (1990). Comprehensive evaluation of attention deficit disorder with and without hyperactivity as defined by research criteria. *Journal of Consulting and Clinical Psychology*, **58**, 775–789.

Barkley, R.A., Grodinsky, G., & DuPaul, G.J. (1992). Frontal lobe functions in attention deficit disorder with and without hyperactivity: A review and research report. *Journal of Abnormal Child Psychology*, **20**, 163–188.

Beitchman, J.H., Hood, J., & Inglis, A. (1990). Psychiatric risk in children with speech and language disorders. *Journal of Abnormal Child Psychology*, **18**, 283–296.

Beitchman, J.H., Hood, J., Rochon, J., & Peterson, M. (1989). Empirical classification of speech/language impairment in children II. Behavioral characteristics. *Journal of the American Academy of Child and Adolescent Psychiatry*, **28**, 118–123.

Beitchman, J., Tuckett, M., & Batth, S. (1987). Language delay and hyperactivity in preschoolers: evidence for a distinct group of hyperactives. *Canadian Journal of Psychiatry*, **32**, 683–687.

Benasich, A.A., Curtiss, A., & Tallal, P. (1993). Language, learning, and behavioral disturbances in childhood: a longitudinal perspective. *Journal of the American Academy of Child and Adolescent Psychiatry*, **32**, 585–594.

Benson, D.F. (1991). The role of frontal dysfunction in attention-deficit hyperactivity disorder. *Journal of Child Neurology*, **6**, 9–12.

Benton, A. (1991). Prefrontal injury and behavior in children. *Developmental Neuropsychology*, **7**, 275–282.

Berk, L. (1986). Relationship of elementary school children's private speech to behavioral accompaniment to task, attention, and task performance. *Developmental Psychology*, **22**, 671–680.

Berk, L.E. (1992). Children's private speech: An overview of theory and status of research. In Diaz, R.M. & Berk, L.E. (eds) *Private Speech: From Social Interaction to Self-Regulation*. Hillsdale, NJ: Lawrence Erlbaum (pp. 17–53).

Berk, L. & Potts, M. (1991). Development and functional significance of private speech among Attention-Deficit Hyperactivity Disordered and normal boys. *Journal of Abnormal Child Psychology*, **19**, 357–377.

Berk, L.E. & Landau, S. (1993). Private speech of learning disabled and normally achieving children in classroom academic and laboratory contexts. *Child Development*, **64**, 556–571.

Berry, C.A., Shaywitz, S.E., & Shaywitz, B.A. (1985). Girls with attention deficit disorder: a silent minority? A report on behavioral and cognitive characteristics. *Pediatrics*, **76**, 801–809.

Biederman, J., Faraone, S.V., Keenan, K., et al. (1991b). Family-genetic and psychosocial risk factors in DSM-III attention deficit disorder. *Journal of the American Academy of Child and Adolescent Psychiatry*, **29**, 526–533.

Biederman, J., Newcorn, J., & Sprich, S. (1991). Comorbidity of attention deficit hyperactivity disorder with conduct, depressive, anxiety and other disorders. *American Journal of Psychiatry*, **148**, 564–577.

Bird, H., Canino, G., Rubio-Stipec, M., et al. (1988). Estimates of the presence of childhood maladjustment in a community survey in Puerto Rico. *Archives of General Psychiatry*, **45**, 1120–1126.

Bishop, D.V.M. & Adams, C. (1990). A prospective study of the relationship between specific language impairment, phonological disorders and reading retardation. *Journal of Child Psychology and Psychiatry*, **31**, 1027–1050.

Bluestone, C.D. (1983). Workshop on effects of otitis media on the child: goals, definitions, and classification of otitis media. *Pediatrics*, **71**, 639–651.

Cantwell, D. & Baker, L. (1987). Psychiatric symptomatology in language-impaired children: a comparison. *Journal of Child Neurology*, **2**, 128–133.

Cantwell, D.P. & Baker, L. (1991). *Psychiatric and Developmental Disorders in Children with Communication Disorder*. Washington, DC: American Psychiatric Press.

Caron, C. & Rutter, M. (1991). Comorbidity in child psychopathology: concepts, issues and research strategies. *Journal of Child Psychology and Psychiatry*, **32**, 1063–1080.

Chess, S. & Rosenberg, M. (1974). Clinical differentiation among children with initial language complaints. *Journal of Autism and Childhood Schizophrenia*, **4**, 99–109.

Cohen, N., Davine, M., Horodezky, N., Lipsett, L., & Isaacson, L. (1993). Unsuspected language impairment in psychiatrically disturbed children: prevalence and language and behavioral characteristics. *Journal of the American Academy of Child and Adolescent Psychiatry*, **32**, 595–603.

Cohen, N., Davine, M., & Meloche-Kelly, M. (1989). Prevalence of unsuspected language disorder in a child psychiatric population. *Journal of the American Academy of Child and Adolescent Psychiatry*, **28**, 107–111.

Copeland, A. (1979). Types of private speech produced by hyperactive and non-hyperactive boys. *Journal of Abnormal Child Psychology*, **7**, 169–177.

Dennis, M. (1991). Frontal lobe function in childhood and adolescence: a heuristic for assessing attention regulation, executive control, and the intentional states important for social discourse. *Developmental Neuropsychology*, **7**, 327–358.

Douglas, V.I. (1983). Attentional and cognitive problems. In M. Rutter (ed.) *Developmental Neuropsychiatry*. New York: Guilford (pp. 280–329).

Douglas, V.I. (1988). Cognitive deficits in children with attention deficit disorder with hyperactivity. In L. Bloomingdale & J. Sergeant (eds) *Attention Deficit Disorder: Critique, Cognition, and Intervention*. New York: Pergamon Press (pp. 65–82).

Douglas, V.I., Barr, V.G., Amin, K., et al. (1988). Dosage effects and individual responsivity to methylphenidate in attention deficit disorder. *Journal of Child Psychology and Psychiatry*, **29**, 453–475.

Duncan, J. (1986). Disorganization of behavior after frontal lobe damage. *Cognitive Neuropsychology*, **3**, 271–290.

Ernst, M., Liebenauer, L.L., King, A.C., Fitzgerald, G.A., Cohen, R.M., & Zametkin, A.J. (1994). Reduced brain metabolism in hyperactive girls. *Journal of the American Academy of Child and Adolescent Psychiatry, 33,* 858–868.

Feagans, L., Sanyal, M., Henderson, F., Collier, A., & Appelbaum, M. (1987). Relationship of middle ear disease in early childhood to later narrative and attention skills. *Journal of Pediatric Psychology, 12,* 581–594.

Felton, F.H., Wood, F.B., Brown, I.S., Campbell, S.K., & Harter, M.R. (1987). Separate verbal memory and naming deficits in attention deficit disorder and reading disability. *Brain and Language, 31,* 171–184.

Fuster, J.M. (1985). The pre-frontal cortex, mediator of cross-temporal contingencies. *Human Neurobiology, 4,* 169–179.

Gillis, J.J., Gilger, J.W., Pennington, B.F., & DeFries, J.C. (1992). Attention deficit disorder in reading disabled twins: Evidence for a genetic etiology. *Journal of Abnormal Child Psychology, 20,* 303–315.

Goldman-Rakic, P.S. (1987). Development of cortical circuitry and cognitive function. *Child Development, 58,* 601–622.

Grattan, L.M. & Eslinger, P.J. (1991). Frontal lobe damage in children and adults: a comparative review. *Developmental Neuropsychology, 7,* 283–326.

Gross-Tsur, V., Shalev, R.S., & Amir, N. (1991). Attention deficit disorder: association with familial-genetic factors. *Pediatric Neurology, 7,* 258–261.

Gualtieri, C., Koriath, U., van Bourgondien, M., & Saleeby, N. (1983). Language disorders in children referred for psychiatric services. *Journal of the American Academy of Child Psychiatry, 22,* 165–171.

Hagerman, R.J. & Falkenstein, A.R. (1987). An association between recurrent otitis media in infancy and later hyperactivity. *Clinical Pediatrics, 26,* 253–257.

Hamlett, K.W., Pellegrini, D.S., & Connors, C.K. (1987). An investigation of executive processes in the problem solving of attention deficit disorder-hyperactive children. *Journal of Pediatric Psychology, 12,* 227–240.

Hartsough, C.S. & Lambert, N.M. (1985). Medical factors in hyperactive and normal children: Prenatal, developmental, and health history findings. *American Journal of Orthopsychiatry, 55,* 190–201.

Hinshaw, S.P. (1992). Externalizing behavior problems and academic underachievement in childhood and adolescence: causal relationships and underlying mechanisms. *Psychological Bulletin, 111,* 127–155.

Humphries, T., Koltun, H., Malone, M., & Roberts, W. (1994). Teacher-identified oral language difficulties among boys with attention problems. *Developmental and Behavioral Pediatrics, 15,* 92–98.

Hynd, G.W., Hern, K.L., Novey, E.S., Eliopulos, D., Marshall, R., Gonzalez, J.J., & Voeller, K.K. (1993). Attention deficit-hyperactivity disorder and asymmetry of the caudate nucleus. *Journal of Child Neurology, 8,* 339–347.

Ingvar, D.H. (1993). Language functions related to prefrontal cortical activity: neurolinguistic implications. *Annals of the New York Academy of Sciences, 782,* 240–247.

Jastak, S. & Wilkinson, G.S. (1984). *The Wide Range Achievement Test – Revised (WRAT-R).* Wilmington, DE: Jastak Associates.

Jorgeson, C., Barrett, M., Huisingh, R., & Zachman, L. (1981). *The Word Test: A Test of Expressive Vocabulary and Semantics.* Moline, IL: Linguisystems, Inc.

Kemp, S.L. & Kirk, U. (1993). An investigation of frontal executive dysfunction in attention deficit disorder subgroups. *Annals of the New York Academy of Sciences*, **782**, 363–365.

Landau, S. & Milich, R. (1988). Social communication patterns of attention-deficit-disordered boys. *Journal of Abnormal Child Psychology*, **16**, 69–81.

Lapadat, J.C. (1991). Pragmatic language skills of students with language and/or learning disabilities: a quantitative synthesis. *Journal of Learning Disabilities*, **24**, 147–158.

Lezak, M.D. (1983). *Neuropsychological Assessment*, 2nd edn. New York: Oxford University Press.

Lou, H.C., Henriksen, L., & Bruhn, P. (1984). Focal cerebral hypoperfusion in children with dysphasia and/or attention deficit disorder. *Archives of Neurology*, **41**, 825–829.

Love, A.J. & Thompson, M.G.G. (1988). Language disorders and attention deficit disorders in young children referred for psychiatric services. *American Journal of Orthopsychiatry*, **58**, 52–63.

Ludlow, C., Rapoport, J., Basich, C., & Mikkelsen, E. (1978). Differential effects of dextroamphetamine on language performance in hyperactive and normal boys. In R. Knights & D. Bakker (eds) *Treatment of Hyperactive and Learning Disordered Children*. Baltimore, MD: University Park Press (pp. 185–205).

Luria, A.R. (1966). *Higher Cortical Function in Man*. New York: Basic Books.

Luria, A.R. (1973). The frontal lobes and the regulation of behavior. In K.H. Pibram & A.R. Luria (eds) *Psychophysiology of the Frontal Lobes*. New York: Academic Press (pp. 3–26).

Manuzza, S., Klein, R.G., Bessler, A., Malloy, O. & LaPadula, M. (1993). Adult outcome of hyperactive boys: educational achievement, occupational rank, and psychiatric status. *Archives of General Psychiatry*, **50**, 565–576.

Matazow, G.S. & Hynd, G.W. (1992, February). Analysis of the anterior posterior gradient hypothesis as applied to attention deficit disorder children. Paper presented at the 20th annual convention of the International Neuropsychological Society, San Diego, CA.

Mattes, J.A. (1980). The role of frontal lobe dysfunction in childhood hyperkinesis. *Comprehensive Psychiatry*, **21**, 358–369.

Maxwell, S.E. & Wallach, G.P. (1984). The language-learning disabilities connection: Symptoms of early language disability over time. In G. Wallach & K. Butler (eds) *Language Learning Disabilities in School Age Children*. Baltimore, MD: Williams and Wilkins (pp. 15–34).

McGee, R., Partridge, F., Williams, S., & Silva, P.A. (1991). A twelve year follow-up of preschool hyperactive children. *Journal of the American Academy of Child and Adolescent Psychiatry*, **30**, 224–232.

Milner, B. (1963). Effects of different brain lesions on card sorting. *Archives of Neurology*, **9**, 90–100.

Oosterlaan, J. & Sergeant, J.A. (1996). Inhibition in ADHD, aggressive and anxious children: A biologically based model of child psychopathology. *Journal of Abnormal Child Psychology* (in press).

Ornoy, A., Uriel, L., & Tennenbaum, A. (1993). Inattention, hyperactivity and speech delay at 2–4 years of age as a predictor for ADD-ADHD syndrome. *Israel Journal of Psychiatry & Related Sciences*, **30**, 155–163.

Paradise, J.L. (1980). Otitis media in infants and children. *Pediatrics*, **65**, 917–943.

Passler, M.A., Isaac, W., & Hynd, G.W. (1985). Neuropsychological development of behavior attributed to frontal lobe functioning in children. *Developmental Neuropsychology*, **1**, 349–370.

Pennington, B.F., Groisser, D., & Welsh, M.C. (1993). Contrasting cognitive deficits in attention deficit hyperactivity disorder versus reading disability. *Developmental Psychology*, **29**, 511–523.

Perecman, E. (1987). *The Frontal Lobes Revisited*. New York: IRBN Press.

Petrides, M. & Milner, B. (1982). Deficits on subject-ordered tasks after frontal and temporal lobe lesions in man. *Neuropsychologia*, **20**, 249–262.

Pibram, K.H., Ahumada, A., Hartog, J., & Roos, L. (1964). A progress report on the neurological processes disturbed by frontal lesions in primates. In J.M. Warren & K. Akert (eds) *The Frontal Granular Cortex and Behavior*. New York: McGraw-Hill (pp. 28–55).

Pliszka, S.R. & Borcherding, S.H. (1992). Measurement of impulsivity in attention deficit hyperactivity disorder (ADHD) and controls (abstract). *Scientific Proceedings of the Annual Meeting of the American Academy of Child and Adolescent Psychiatry*. San Antonio, Texas, October 1993 (p. 41).

Prizant, B.M., Audet, L.R., Burke, G.M., Hummel, L.J., Maher, S.R., & Theadore, G. (1990). Communication disorders and emotional/behavioral disorders in children and adolescents. *Journal of Speech and Hearing Disorders*, **55**, 179–192.

Prutting, C.A. & Kirchner, D.M. (1987). A clinical appraisal of the pragmatic aspects of language. *Journal of Speech and Hearing Disorders*, **52**, 105–119.

Purvis, K.L. & Tannock, R. (1995). Language abilities in children with Attention Deficit Hyperactivity Disorder, reading disabilities, and normal controls. Submitted for publication.

Reader, M.J., Harris, E.L., Schuerholz, L.J., & Denckla, M.B. (1995). Attention deficit hyperactivity disorder and executive dysfunction. *Developmental Neuropsychology*, **10**, 493–512.

Richard, G. & Hanner, M. (1985). *Language Processing Test*. Moline, IL: Linguisystems, Inc.

Richardson, E., Kupietz, S.S., Winsberg, B.G., et al. (1988). Effects of methylphenidate dosage in hyperactive reading-disabled children: II. Reading achievement. *Journal of the American Academy of Child and Adolescent Psychiatry*, **27**, 78–87.

Roberts, J.E., Burchinal, M.R., Collier, A.M., et al. (1989). Otitis media in early childhood and cognitive, academic, and classroom performance of the school-aged child. *Pediatrics*, **83**, 477–485.

Rutter, M. & Lord, C. (1987). Language disorders associated with psychiatric disturbance. In W. Yule & M. Rutter (eds) *Language Development and Disorders*. Oxford: MacKeith Press (pp. 206–233).

Schachar, R. & Logan, G. (1990). Impulsivity and inhibitory control in normal development and childhood psychopathology. *Developmental Psychology*, **26**, 710–720.

Schachar, R. & Tannock, R. (1995). Test of four hypotheses for the comorbidity of attention-deficit hyperactivity disorder and conduct disorder. *Journal of the American Academy of Child and Adolescent Psychiatry*, **34**, 639–648.

Schachar, R., Tannock., R., & Logan, G. (1993). Inhibitory control, impulsiveness, and Attention Deficit Hyperactivity Disorder. *Clinical Psychology Review*, **13**, 721–739.

Schachar, R., Tannock, R., Marriott, M., & Logan, G. (1995). Deficient inhibitory control in Attention Deficit Hyperactivity Disorder. *Journal of Abnormal Child Psychology* **23**, 411–437.

Semel, E., Wiig, E.H., & Secord, W. (1987). *Clinical Evaluation of Language Fundamental – Revised*. New York: The Psychological Corporation, Harcourt Brace Jovanovitch Inc.

Semrud-Clikeman, M., Hynd, G.W., Novey, E.S., & Eliopulos, D. (1991). Dyslexia and brain morphology: relationship between neuroanatomical variation and neuro-linguistic tasks. *Learning and Individual Differences*, **3**, 225–242.

Shallice, T. (1982). Specific impairments in planning. *Royal Society of London*, **B298**, 199–209.

Shelton, T.L. & Barkley, R.A. (1994). Critical issues in the assessment of attention deficit disorders in children. *Topics in Language Disorders*, **14**, 26–41.

Shue, K.L. & Douglas, V.I. (1992). Attention deficit hyperactivity disorder and the frontal lobe syndrome. *Brain & Cognition*, **20**, 104–124.

Silva, P.A., Williams, S., & McGee, R. (1987). A longitudinal study of children with developmental language delay at three years: later intelligence, reading and behaviour problems. *Developmental Medicine and Child Neurology*, **29**, 630–640.

Spekman, N.J. (1984). Learning-disabled students and language use: discourse and narrative skills. *Learning Disabilities*, **3**, 103–115.

Stevenson, J. (1992). Evidence for a genetic aetiology in hyperactivity in children. *Behavior Genetics*, **22**, 337–344.

Stuss, D.T. & Benson, D.F. (1986). *The Frontal Lobes*. New York: Raven.

Szatmari, P., Offord, D.R., & Boyle, M.H. (1989a). Ontario Child Health Study: prevalence of attention deficit disorder with hyperactivity. *Journal of Child Psychology and Psychiatry*, **30**, 219–230.

Szatmari, P., Offord, D.R., & Boyle, M.H. (1989b). Correlates, associated impairments and patterns of service utilization of children with attention deficit disorder: findings from the Ontario Child Health Study. *Journal of Child Psychology and Psychiatry*, **30**, 205–217.

Tallal, P., Dukette, D., & Curtiss, S. (1989). Behavioral/emotional profiles of preschool language-impaired children. *Development and Psychopathology*, **1**, 51–67.

Tannock, R., Corkum, P., Schachar, R., & Purvis, K. (1994). Phonological processing in children with attention deficit hyperactivity disorder. Poster presentation at the Annual Child Psychiatry Day, The Hospital for Sick Children, Toronto, Canada.

Tannock, R., Ickowicz, A., Oram, J., & Fine, J. (1995). Language impairment and audiological status in ADHD: Preliminary results. Poster presentation at the Annual Child Psychiatry Day, The Hospital for Sick Children, Toronto, Canada.

Tannock, R., Purvis, K., & Schachar, R. (1991). Language processing abilities in children with attention deficit hyperactivity disorder. Paper presented at the 38th Annual Meeting of the American Academy of Child and Adolescent Psychiatry, San Francisco (October 16–20).

Tannock, R., Purvis, K., & Schachar, R. (1993). Narrative abilities in children with Attention Deficit Hyperactivity Disorder and normal peers. *Journal of Abnormal Child Psychology*, **21**, 103–117.

Tannock, R., Schachar, R., Carr, R., Chajczyk, D., & Logan, G. (1989). Effects of methylphenidate on inhibitory control in hyperactive children. *Journal of Abnormal Child Psychology*, **17**, 473–491.

Tannock, R., Schachar, R., & Logan, G. (1995). Methylphenidate and cognitive flexibility: Dissociated dose effects in hyperactive children. *Journal of Abnormal Child Psychology*, **23**, 235–266.

Tant, J.L. & Douglas, V.I. (1982). Problem solving in hyperactive, normal, and reading disabled boys. *Journal of Abnormal Child Psychology*, **10**, 285–306.

Teale, D.W., Klein, J.O., & Rosner, B.A. (1984). Otitis media with effusion during the first three years of life and development of speech and language. *Pediatrics*, **74**, 282–287.

Thorley, G. (1984). Hyperkinetic syndrome of childhood: clinical characteristics. *British Journal of Psychiatry*, **144**, 16–24.

Trautman, R.C., Giddan, J.J., & Jurs, S.G. (1990). Language risk factor in emotionally disturbed children within a school and day treatment program. *Journal of Childhood Communication Disorders*, **13**, 123–133.

Vygotsky, L. (1978). *Mind in Society*. Cambridge, MA: Harvard University Press (original works published 1930, 1933, 1935).

Vygotsky, L. (1934/1987). Thinking and speech. In *The Collected Works of L.S. Vygotsky: Vol. 1. Problems of General Psychology*, trans. N. Minick. New York: Plenum Press (original work published 1934).

Warr-Leeper, G., Wright, N.A., & Mack, A. (1994). Language disabilities of antisocial boys in residential treatment. *Behavioral Disorders*, **19**, 159–169.

Weiss, G. & Hechtman, L.T. (1993). *Hyperactive Children Grown Up: ADHD in Children, Adolescents, and Adults*, 2nd edn. New York: Guilford Press.

Welsh, M.C. & Pennington, B.F. (1988). Assessing frontal lobe functioning in children: views from developmental psychology. *Developmental Neuropsychology*, **4**, 199–230.

Welsh, M.C., Pennington, B.F., & Groisser, B.B. (1991). A normative-developmental study of executive function: A window on prefrontal function in children. *Developmental Neuropsychology*, **7**, 131–149.

Weyandt, L.L. & Willis, W.G. (1994). Executive functions in school-aged children: potential efficacy of tasks in discriminating clinical groups. *Developmental Neuropsychology*, **10**, 27–38.

Whalen, C.K., Henker, B., Collins, B.E., McAuliffe, S., & Vaux, A. (1979). Peer interaction in a structured communication task: comparisons of normal and hyperactive boys and of methylphenidate (Ritalin) and placebo effects. *Child Development*, **50**, 388–401.

Wood, F.B. & Felton, R.H. (1994). Separate linguistic and attentional factors in the development of reading. *Topics in Language Disorders*, **14**, 42–57.

Zametkin, A.J., Nordhal, T.E., Gross, M., et al. (1990). Cerebral glucose metabolism in adults with hyperactivity of childhood onset. *New England Journal of Medicine*, **323**, 1361–1366.

Zentall, S.S. (1988). Production deficiencies in elicited language but not in the spontaneous verbalizations of hyperactive children. *Journal of Abnormal Child Psychology*, **16**, 657–673.

Zentall, S.S., Gohs, D.E., & Culatta, B. (1983). Language and activity of hyperactive and comparison children during listening tasks. *Exceptional Children*, **50**, 255–266.

8 Discourse deficits in childhood schizophrenia

ROCHELLE CAPLAN

INTRODUCTION

Discourse refers to the communicative process whereby the speaker presents the listener with a clear and coherent message. The impaired communication skills of patients with schizophrenia has been regarded as one of the hallmarks of this disorder since Kraepelin first described dementia praecox (Kraepelin, 1896). The difficulties schizophrenic adults have presenting the listener with a clear and coherent message have been described by clinical terms, such as formal thought disorder (Andreasen, 1979; Andreasen & Grove, 1986) and by linguistic terms, such as aphasia (Chaika, 1982; Lecours, 1982) and discourse deficits (Rochester & Martin, 1979).

These different approaches in the past led to a debate on whether the communication impairments of schizophrenic adults reflected a thought disorder or a language disorder (see Schwartz, 1982 for review). Numerous clinical (Andreasen & Grove, 1986; Harrow and Marengo, 1986; Holzman, Shenton, & Solovay, 1986), cognitive/information processing (Nuechterlein et al., 1986; Cornblatt, Lenzenweger, & Erlenmeyer-Kimling, 1989; Asarnow, Granholm, & Sherman, 1991), and linguistic studies (Gerver, 1967; Fromkin, 1975; Rochester & Martin, 1979) over the past four decades have demonstrated, however, that schizophrenic adults have a thought disorder rather than a language disorder (Schwartz, 1982).

Several clinical signs have been used to describe the communicative characteristics of schizophrenic adults, such as illogical thinking, incoherence, loose associations, digressive speech, circumstantiality, tangentiality, vague speech, overelaborate speech, clanging, neologisms, poverty of speech, poverty of content of speech, echolalia speech, and others (Andreasen, 1979). When present, some of these signs indicate that the patient presents his/her thoughts with inadequate reasoning (illogical thinking), unpredictable changes in the topic of conversation (loose associations), syntactical errors (incoherence), and minimal elaboration on the topic of conversation (poverty of content of speech). The discourse deficits of schizophrenic adults include impaired use of linguistic cohesive ties that link the content of one sentence to that of neighboring sentences (Rochester & Martin, 1979; Harvey, 1983; Harvey

& Brault, 1986). Thus, during a conversation schizophrenic adults appear to have difficulties processing and organizing their thoughts at the level of the paragraph, as well as at the level of the connections between sentences. Like schizophrenic adults, schizophrenic children have formal thought disorder (Arboleda & Holzman, 1965; Caplan et al., 1989, 1990a) and impaired use of cohesive devices that tie together the objects, events, and ideas across contiguous sentences (Caplan, Guthrie, & Foy, 1992).

From the functional perspective, the communicative process is complex and involves interaction between cognitive, linguistic, and social mechanisms. According to van Dijk (1972), to understand discourse as a communicative unity, one needs to analyze the contributions of the macrostructure (i.e., the overall communicative plan) and the microstructure (i.e., the words and sentences).

At the macrostructural level the speaker presents ideas, facts, and events that are logically related and either overtly or covertly explicit so that his/her message is coherent (Paty & Nespoulous, 1990). The string of facts and events that the speaker presents to the listener form a unity. Communication at the macrostructural level or the level of the paragraph involves mainly cognitive processes.

At the microstructural level (i.e., word- or sentence-level), however, there is a step-by-step construction of discourse continuity, cohesion, through relations between word-level entities across sentence boundaries (Halliday & Hasan, 1976). For example, linguistic cohesive devices tie together the objects, events, and ideas that the speaker presents within and across sentence boundaries.

In addition to the macrostructural (i.e., cognitive) and microstructural (i.e., linguistic) levels of communication, the interaction between speaker and listener is also governed by social, pragmatic principles, such as turn-taking, use of formal rather than colloquial speech as deemed necessary, or increase or decrease in the amount of speech (Paty & Nespoulous, 1990). Although linguistic mechanisms function only at the microstructural level, cognitive mechanisms play a role at all levels (Paty & Nespoulous, 1990). For example, impaired memory could handicap the formulation of ideas at the macro-structural level as well as social judgment at the pragmatic level. At the microstructural level it could also impair referential continuity across sentence boundaries, as in the relationship between the noun and subsequent pronoun in "This is the man. I like him."

As previously described, discourse breaks down in both adult onset and childhood onset schizophrenia. In the normal child the communicative process, as well as cognition, language, and emotions develop from early childhood through adolescence (Shatz, 1982). A developmental approach could have important ramifications for furthering our understanding of the discourse breakdown in childhood onset schizophrenia.

This chapter first describes the acquisition of discourse skills in normal children and focuses on microstructural measures of the linguistic (cohesive) devices that tie together who and what the child is talking about across sentences. It will also present developmental data on macrostructural measures of thought processing, such as clinical measures of formal thought disorder and their associated cognitive/information processing correlates in children. The chapter then describes the discourse deficits of schizophrenic children, and presents data on the microstructural and macrostructural deficits, as well as the relationship between these two types of discourse deficits.

DEVELOPMENT OF DISCOURSE IN CHILDHOOD

Cohesion

Definition

Halliday & Hasan (1976) described different linguistic devices that speakers use to tie together references made to people, objects, events, and ideas expressed across sentence boundaries. Several grammatical devices provide continuity between referents or between ideas presented in the conversation (Paty & Nespoulous, 1990). *Conjunction* ties together contiguous clauses (sentences) by using additive, contrastive, causal, temporal, and continuative relationships (Table 8.1). *Referential cohesion* involves use of a pronoun, demonstrative, definite article, or comparative to refer back to people or objects in the preceding spoken text (Table 8.1). Sometimes, however, the speaker makes a reference which confuses the listener (Table 8.1). In *unclear reference* this occurs because the speaker uses a pronoun, demonstrative, definite article, or comparative to refer to a person or object that has not been previously mentioned in the spoken text. Similarly, the listener becomes confused if the speaker makes an *ambiguous reference* by using a referent that can apply to more than one person or object. Under most circumstances the speaker and listener are involved in the verbal context of the ongoing conversation. If the speaker makes reference to the immediate environment during conversation, this is called *exophora*. If used in excess and the speaker breaks the flow of conversation to refer to items in the immediate environment that are unrelated to the conversational text, the listener might have difficulty following the ongoing conversation.

The following cohesive devices are semantic rather than grammatical (Table 8.2). *Lexical cohesion* provides the listener with ties between notions through word repetition, a synonym, or an antonym. *Substitution* ties the spoken text together by replacing nominal, verbal, or clausal units with a word or group of words. *Ellipsis* deletes a word, phrase, or clause whose referent is unambiguously located in the previous utterance. Ellipsis can be viewed as a form of substitution in which a nominal or verbal unit is substituted by nothing. Marked use of substitution and ellipsis, however, could also tax the

Table 8.1. *Grammatical categories of cohesion and examples*[1]

Category	Type	Examples[2]
Conjunction	Additive	*The witch gets burned* **and** that's the end of the story.
	Adversative	*I don't know how,* **but** he makes me be bad, bad.
	Causal	*I have nightmares* **because** I start to laugh.
	Temporal	*I'll go play* **when** I'm done eating.
	Continuative	I: Do you have scary dreams? S: **Well**, last night I saw this big monster in my closet.
Referential Cohesion	Pronomial	A boy called *Peter* saw a ghost. **He** was scared.
	Demonstrative	*The boy* was crying and then **this boy** called his mother.
	Comparative	I don't like *this story*. I like the **first one more**.
Impaired Reference	Unclear	Uh, I went and looked at *the guy* to see what **they** were doing.
	Ambiguous	And – and – and so when Halloween came *her* Dad made a hat and then *her mother* made a witch costume and **she** was happy.
	Exophora	I: Did you like that story? S: How does *this* tape recorder work? (Situational)
		This is a story about a witch. Once upon a time there was an old ugly witch. *I* don't like witches to come to my house (Self).

Notes: [1] Terms adapted from Halliday & Hasan (1976), Rochester & Martin (1979), and Harvey (1983).
   [2] *Referant* and **referring/presumed item**.

listener's ability because he/she needs to expend more effort retrieving previously mentioned groups of words that were substituted or deleted.

Associated skills

In addition to linguistic abilities, use of cohesive devices involves the speaker's ability to be aware of the listener's perspective as he/she speaks. From the cognitive perspective, Piaget (1955) argued that the young child is unable to take the listener's perspective into consideration because of egocentricity. He maintained that egocentricity decreases between ages 6 and 8 years. Several studies indicate, however, that children are aware of the listener's needs from the toddler period and that these skills increase through middle childhood (Shatz, 1982). In fact, the development of representation of the mind occurs in parallel with this process (Astington, Harris, & Olson, 1988). Thus, young children modify the way they speak when they need to present information to children who are younger than themselves (Keenan,

Table 8.2. *Semantic categories of cohesion and examples*[1]

Category	Type	Examples[2,3]
Lexical cohesion	Same root	The kids were *bad*. Tim was **bad**, too.
	Synonym	The kids were *mean* to Tim. They were always **nasty** to him.
	Superordinate	I don't mind *spaniels*. But really, I don't like **dogs**.
Substitution	Nominal	I: Why did you say that *was a true story*? S: Cause it's a made up **one**.
	Verbal	That boy *says "Hi"* and **so does** the other one.
	Clausal	*That's the only thing magic does*. I know it's **so**.
Ellipsis	Nominal	Ghosts have a lot of *power*. They have more ∧ than monsters.
	Verbal	I: Do you think a child *could have a dream* like this about a ghost? S: Maybe **he could** ∧.
	Clausal	I: *Have you been to Disneyland?* S: No, my brother has ∧.

Notes: [1] Terms adapted from Halliday & Hasan (1976), Rochester & Martin (1979), and Harvey (1983).
[2] *Referant* and **referring/presumed item**.
[3] ∧ Indicates ellipted word or phrase.

1974; Shatz, 1982). These findings attest to the fact that even young children are aware of the listener's needs and can modify their speech accordingly.

In terms of pragmatic skills, children's early speech is characterized by one utterance per turn (McTear, 1984). Between age 2 and 4 years children become competent at responding to the speaker consistently, initiating conversational exchanges, using turntaking, and maintaining the topic of conversation (Bloom, Rocissano, & Hood, 1976; Ervin-Tripp, 1978; McTear, 1984). From age 4 years, children not only respond to the speaker but also provide possibilities so that they or the listener can continue the conversation beyond one utterance per turn (McTear, 1984).

Development of cohesive skills

Connectives

Children begin to use connectives, such as the conjunctions *and, because,* and *but* from the toddler period (Clark, 1973; Bloom et al., 1980; French & Nelson, 1985; Sprott, 1992). Vygotsky (1962, p. 46) observed that "the child may operate with subordinate clauses, with words like *because, if, when* and *but,* long before he really grasps causal, conditional or temporal relations themselves." In support of Vygotsky's observation, several studies have found that children acquire the semantic meaning of conjunctions long after they start using conjunction or responding to utterances that include them (McTear, 1984; Gopnik, 1986; Peterson & Dodsworth, 1991; Sprott, 1992). Other investigators have reported a lag between production and comprehension of conjunctions (Amidon, 1976; Johnson & Chapman, 1980; Flores D'Arcais, 1981). Flores D'Arcais (1981) has suggested that the child makes use of the information provided by the sentence as a whole without processing the connectives.

Peterson & McCabe (1988) found that young children use the conjunction *and* primarily as a general signal of cohesion that indicates to the listener that contiguous utterances are thematically connected (Peterson & McCabe, 1988). From the pragmatic perspective, in using *and* the young child also indicates to the listener that his/her turn as speaker continues (Peterson & McCabe, 1988).

Acquisition of the semantic meaning of connectives occurs gradually through middle childhood. By age 12 years children are able to differentiate the semantic meaning of different conjunctions (Flores D'Arcais, 1981). Amidon (1976) has also shown that between age 5 to 7 years old children become more adept at retaining information expressed in subordinate clauses. These findings imply that between middle and late childhood children process the meaning of connectives and how they connect between the ideas presented in contiguous clauses.

In addition to the qualitative change involved in comprehending conjunctions, with increasing age children also use conjunctions more frequently in their utterances and utilize a wider range of conjunctions. By age 6 years, 78% of the child's sentences contain conjunctions (Gopnik, 1986). Silva (1991) has suggested that the gradual acquisition of these skills might reflect the disparate linguistic and information processing constraints associated with use of different conjunctions. For example, Silva (1991) has shown that children aged 4.1–11.11 years are competent users of *when* before *while* and of *while* before *as* during a narrative. Silva (1991) hypothesized that this phenomenon reflects the child's ability with age to appreciate the increasing specificity and constraints involved in use of these different temporal terms. In addition, the child also acquires the ability to take the listener's point of view into account and to control the type and flow of information to the listener by choice of the different conjunctions.

From the cognitive perspective, Ingram (1975) has stated that competent use of conjunctions implies the presence of reversible cognitive operations, as described by Piaget (1962). More specifically, Ingram (1975) proposed that children under age 7 years relate one sentence to another by juxtaposition. After age 7 years, however, children relate the different elements of two juxtaposed propositions to each other by use of a conjunction (Ingram, 1975). Ferreiro & Sinclair (1971) presented 130 4 years and 10-months-old children with a conservation task in which water was poured from one of two short and wide glasses to a tall and narrow glass. The children also needed to answer *when* questions about a girl doll who washed a boy doll who then went upstairs. The preoperational children who were not yet able to conserve did not use the temporal conjunctions *before* and *after* appropriately when asked "When did the boy go up? When did the girl doll wash the boy doll?" In contrast, the children who were able to perceive that no water was added or taken away despite the higher water level in the tall and narrow glass used these conjunctions well.

Unlike the previously reviewed studies, French & Nelson (1985) have demonstrated that children between the age of 2 years 11 months and 5 years 6 months use a wide range of temporal, causal, and contrastive conjunctions appropriately. According to French & Nelson (1965), this occurs if the children are asked to perform a task that reflects their everyday knowledge, such as a script of going to a restaurant. These investigators maintain that the studies that reveal a discrepancy between production and comprehension of conjunctions have used "enactment, picture selection, attributing a statement to a 'silly' or 'sensible' character, more direct grammatical judgments, and sentence completion" (p. 77) rather than more familiar tasks that children use in their daily lives.

Reference

Toddlers first use pronouns as substitutes for nouns and for pointing rather than as discourse markers that make anaphoric reference (i.e., to refer to a previously mentioned person) (Gopnik, 1986). As children acquire language they use pronouns deictically (Karmiloff-Smith, 1985) or exophorically (Gopnik, 1986) to refer to objects they see around them. Between ages 2 to 3.6 years they incorporate more pronouns into their conversation (Gopnik, 1986), use pronouns more frequently for reference (Karmiloff-Smith, 1985; Peterson & Dodsworth, 1991), and make frequent unclear and ambiguous reference (Karmiloff-Smith, 1985; Pratt & MacKenzie-Keating, 1985; Gopnik, 1986).

During narratives children often have difficulty focusing on the story and break the flow of narrative by referring to the nonverbal context using exophoric pronouns. As a result, the listener often has difficulty following who and what the young child is talking about during a conversation or a narrative. Between ages 4 and 6 years, children succeed in making the listener's task easier by using less unclear reference and ambiguous reference, as well as fewer exophoric pronouns (Gopnik, 1986; Pratt & Mackenzie-Keating, 1985). Children also learn not to use exophoric reference during story telling and that this situation implicates ignoring the shared pragmatic context and focusing on the narrative (Gopnik, 1986).

As the child's speech includes more noun phrases and becomes more complex and elaborate, he/she is faced with the cognitive task of organizing his speech into a coherent message (Bennett-Kastor, 1986). Shatz (1982) hypothesized that communication competence involves deployment of processing from a "limited capacity processor." In support of Shatz's information-processing theory, Pratt & MacKenzie-Keating (1985) have compared the communication competence of impulsive and reflective first and third graders. Using the Matching Familiar Figures Test (Kagan et al., 1964), Pratt & MacKenzie-Keating demonstrated that as task difficulty increased more impulsive children with a shorter reaction time used more inappropriate reference than reflective children with a longer reaction time.

Based on findings in 420 children, Karmiloff-Smith (1985) concluded that children achieve referential competence when retelling a narrative by age 8 to 9 years. She described three developmental stages. In the first stage, 4 to 5-year-old children use primarily noun phrases and pronouns to identify objects or people in the narrative. In the second stage, 5 to 7-year-old children use the indefinite article when they first describe the protagonist of the story. Subsequently, they use only pronouns to refer to the protagonist and always present the protagonist as the subject of the sentence. The stage 2 child always refers to subsidiary protagonists using noun phrases. In the third stage, 8 to 9-year-old children use pronouns as discourse markers for both primary and subsidiary protagonists based on the listener's need for clarity.

From the cognitive perspective, Karmiloff-Smith (1985) hypothesized that the development of these discourse skills is associated with the interplay between cognitive processing and linguistic encoding of the narrative. At level 1, the child processes the story cognitively and focuses on the individual events of the narrative. At level 2, the child linguistically encodes what is happening to the main protagonist sometimes to the exclusion of important detail. At level 3, however, the child flexibly uses both cognitive processing and linguistic encoding to determine how each event fits into the overall discourse structure.

Other cohesive devices

Regarding the development of lexical cohesion, Greenfield & Savage-Rumbaugh (1993) underscore repetition as an early pragmatic and cohesive precursor of this cohesive device. As previously described, lexical cohesion provides continuity of the topic of conversation across utterances by use of synonyms, antonyms, or superordinates. The preverbal child uses repetition to establish joint attention. Once the child acquires words, he/she repeats words as a way of maintaining attention and continuing the topic of conversation. Although the child uses less word repetition with increasing age, he/she continues to use this cohesive device in the form of lexical cohesion (Greenfield & Savage-Rumbaugh, 1993).

Whereas young children use conjunctions and reference as their main cohesive device, older children use other cohesive devices (Peterson &

Dodsworth, 1991). Of the other cohesive links described by Halliday & Hasan (1976) (Tables 9.1 and 9.2), comparative reference, nominal ellipsis, and substitution occur later as the child becomes cognitively adept to code an increasing number of components within and across utterances (Peterson & Dodsworth, 1991). For example, Peterson & Dodsworth (1991) suggest that for children to use substitution they need an "abstract counter" that will enable them to replace the substituted linguistic component.

In addition to a wider range of cohesive ties, maturation is also associated with a gradual increase in the number of cohesive ties per utterance from 1 tie per utterance in early childhood to 3 to 4 ties per utterance by adulthood (Peterson & Dodsworth, 1991). The distribution of types of cohesive devices also changes with age. Referential cohesion, conjunctions, and lexical cohesion constitute 25%, 20%, and 42%, respectively of the cohesive ties in children (Peterson & Dodsworth, 1991). In adults, however, referential cohesion, conjunctions, and lexical cohesion account for 30%, 20%, and 48%, respectively of the cohesive ties (Peterson & Dodsworth, 1991; Rochester & Martin, 1979). Peterson & Dodsworth (1991) have not found an age related increase in the proportion of conjunctions in cohesive ties from childhood to adulthood.

In summary, from the toddler period through adolescence children gradually acquire cognitive, linguistic, and pragmatic skills that enable them to use grammatical and semantic cohesive devices to link their utterances together. Conjunctions are used as pragmatic markers in the toddler period and as cohesive markers during middle childhood. Appropriate semantic usage of conjunctions, however, evolves more slowly and matures by adolescence. Children first use pronouns for exophoric reference and then for endophoric reference. As they use pronouns more for endophoric reference, they make unclear and ambiguous referential errors. By age 6 to 8 years, they make few referential errors. During middle childhood, children begin to join their more complex utterances by hierarchical means and establish ties across neighboring as well as contiguous sentence by lexical cohesion. As they acquire more abstract skills, children increase the range of cohesive devices they use to include comparative reference, nominal ellipsis, and substitution.

Method for eliciting speech samples

In considering developmental changes in the use of cohesive devices several investigators have emphasized the importance of the procedures used to elicit speech samples or narratives (Pellegrini, 1984; Wigglesworth, 1990; Clancy, 1992; Peterson & Dodsworth, 1991). For example, if children undergo an interview that involves questions and answers, there is more chance of obtaining frequent clausal ellipsis (Peterson & Dodsworth, 1991). Clancy (1992) has pointed out that the child uses different referential strategies if he/she produces a narrative based on visual (i.e., pictures) rather than on auditory stimuli (i.e., verbal instructions). She also noted that the referential strategies used by the child during narrative differ from those in a question and answer dialogue where the listener can ask questions to clarify who and what the child is talking about. Pellegrini (1984) has shown that children in kindergarten, first grade, and second grade modified their referential strategies when telling a story to a naive listener versus a listener who already knew the story. In the former case, the children used referential cohesion which enabled the listener to identify the referents. In the latter case, the children used ellipsis on the assumption that the listener knew who they were talking about.

Development of thought processing in children

Definition

Formal thought disorder represents clinical measures of the form or manner in which the patient presents his or her thoughts to the listener. The DSM-IV (American Psychiatric Association, 1994) uses the term disorganized speech (e.g., frequent derailment or incoherence) rather than formal thought disorder. The DSM-III-R (American Psychiatric Association, 1987) required the presence of loose associations or incoherence to diagnose formal thought disorder. The DSM-III (American Psychiatric Association, 1980) included four formal thought disorder signs: illogical thinking, loose associations, incoherence, and poverty of content of speech.

Two reliable and valid instruments have been used to measure formal thought disorder in children: the Thought Disorder Index (TDI; Johnston & Holzman, 1979) and the Kiddie Formal Thought Disorder Rating Scale (K-FTDS) (Caplan et al., 1989). Arboleda & Holzman (1985) were the first to use a formal psychological instrument, the TDI to measure formal thought disorder in children. The TDI codes the frequency and severity of 20 categories of verbal responses to standard Rorshach cards that have been grouped into four broad categories of thought disorder: associative, combinatory, disorganized, and unconventional verbalizations (Johnston & Holzman, 1979; Holzman et al., 1986).

The K-FTDS operationalized the four DSM-III signs of formal thought disorder so that they can be used even if children speak in short paragraphs of one to two utterances (Caplan et al., 1989) (Table 8.3). To be rated as having illogical thinking, the child's speech meets one of three criteria. First, the child uses causal utterances inappropriately. Second, the child presents the listener with unfounded and inappropriate reasoning in noncausal utterances. Third, the child contradicts him or herself within one to two utterances by simultaneously making and refuting statements.

Loose associations is rated when the child makes an utterance that is off-topic without having previously prepared the listener for the topic change.

Table 8.3. *Synopsis of the Kiddie Formal Thought Disorder Rating scale (K-FTDS)*

K-FTDS sign	Definition	Example
Illogical thinking	Inappropriate and immature use of causal utterances.	"I left my hat in her room because her name is Mary."
	Unfounded and inappropriate reasoning in noncausal utterances.	"Sometimes I'll go to bed and when I'm done laughing, I start wheezing and that's when I relax."
	Utterances in which statements are simultaneously made and refuted.	"I don't like that story, but I liked it as a story."
Loose associations	The child changes the topic of conversation to a new unrelated topic without preparing the listener for the topic change.	Interviewer: "Why do you think that's a reason not to like Tim?" Child: "And I call my mom sweetie."
Incoherence	The contents of an utterance are not understood by the listener because of scrambled syntax.	Interviewer: "What happened next in your story?" Child: "The day witches no day goes."
Poverty of content of speech	In the presence of at least two utterances, the child does not elaborate on the topic.	"I suppose – What? Maybe – Well yes, I see. I suppose that's all."

An utterance is rated as incoherence if the rater cannot comprehend its contents because of scrambled syntax. Poverty of content of speech is rated if, in the presence of at least two utterances, the child does not elaborate on the topic of conversation.

Associated skills and development of thought processing

Arboleda & Holzman (1985) demonstrated the importance of controlling for the level of cognitive development in a sample of 79 normal children. Normal children under age 10 years had higher mean global TDI scores than those above age 10 years. Arboleda & Holzman (1985) found no relationship between the TDI scores of the normal children and sex, verbal IQ, or socioeconomic status.

In a sample of 71 normal children Caplan (Caplan et al., 1989, 1990a; Caplan, 1994) found that normal children under age 7 years scored above the cut-point for pathology for illogical thinking and loose associations. There were no statistically significant differences in the illogical thinking scores of the normal children above age 7 and age 10 years. Normal children below, but not above age 7 years had loose associations. These findings were unrelated to IQ scores and ethnicity. To date, there have been no studies on the relationship between illogical thinking, loose associations, and associated cognitive skills in normal children under age 7 years.

DISCOURSE DEFICITS IN CHILDREN WITH SCHIZOPHRENIA SPECTRUM DISORDERS

Cohesion in childhood onset schizophrenia

Using Halliday and Hasan's (1976) analysis of cohesion, we examined cohesion in 31 schizophrenic children (25 male and 6 female) with a mean chronological age of 10.2 years (SD = 1.5) and mental age of 9.1 years (SD = 2.0) (Caplan et al., 1992) (Table 8.4). Each schizophrenic child was matched by sex and mental age with a normal child. The 31 normal subjects were younger children whose chronological ages were matched to the mental age of the individual patients. Trained undergraduate students with no knowledge of the children's diagnoses transcribed videotapes of the Story Game (Caplan et al., 1989). The Story Game includes two audiotaped stories, one about a ghost, the other about an ostracized boy, respectively. After each story, the child retells the tale and answers open-ended standardized questions on the story to the experimenter who sits with the child throughout the interview. The child also makes up a story chosen from several topics: the Incredible Hulk, a witch, an unhappy child, or a good or bad child.

Two blind raters coded the transcriptions independently to obtain the frequency of the cohesive devices presented in Tables 8.1 and 8.2 during the entire Story Game. To control for the variation in the number of clauses elicited from each child during the entire Story Game, they divided each frequency score by the total number of clauses the child used during the Story Game.

The interrater agreement (Pearson correlation coefficient) of the cohesion and reference pattern scores on 10 schizophrenic and 10 normal children was 0.94 for referential cohesion, 0.99 for conjunction, 0.89 for lexical cohesion, 0.70 for ellipsis, 0.67 for substitution, 0.72 for exophora, and 0.92 for unclear/ambiguous reference. We combined the ratings of ambiguous and unclear reference because of their low base rate.

Compared to normal mental age matched children, the schizophrenic children spoke less and did not provide the listener with enough links (cohesive ties) to previous utterances. They also provided the listener with fewer references (referential cohesion) to people, objects, or events mentioned in earlier utterances. In addition, the schizophrenic children broke the flow of conversation frequently by referring to people, objects, or events in their immediate surroundings and by not focusing on the ongoing conversation (exophora). The schizophrenic children with loose associations confused the listener by the unclear and ambiguous way they referred to people, objects, and events (unclear/ambiguous reference) more than the schizophrenic

Table 8.4. *Age, sex and IQ of schizophrenic and normal children*

	Schizophrenia	Normal
N	31	31
SEX		
Male	25	25
Female	6	6
AGE		
Chronological	10.3	9.1
	(SD = 3.06)	(SD = 2.10)
Mental	9.3	9.1
	(SD = 1.99)	(SD = 2.10)
IQ	90	113
	(SD = 12.37)	(SD = 13.8)

children with no loose associations. Underutilization of cohesive ties, number of words per utterance, and referential cohesion together with overutilization of exophora and unclear/ambiguous reference were also found by Harvey (1983) and by Rochester & Martin (1979) in schizophrenic adults.

The schizophrenic children also had discourse deficits which distinguished them from the adult schizophrenic patients studied by Harvey (1983) and by Rochester & Martin (1979). Compared to normal children, the schizophrenic children provided the listener with fewer connectives between contiguous clauses (conjunction) and with less repetition of words or word roots (lexical cohesion) than normal children. By using fewer conjunctions and lexical cohesion than normal children, the conversing schizophrenic child made it difficult for the listener to piece together the links in his/her speech.

Finally, in a previous study (Caplan et al., 1992) we reported that schizophrenic children omitted part of a previous clause on the presumption that the listener retained enough information from this clause (ellipsis) more frequently than normal children. This finding was related to the presence of loose associations and to distractibility. Due to revisions in our coding methodology for ellipsis, we reanalyzed our ellipsis data.[1] These analyses revealed that schizophrenic children underutilized ellipsis compared to normal children. In addition, the use of ellipsis by the schizophrenic children was unrelated to measures of formal thought disorder and distractibility.

From the developmental perspective, normal children increase the use of referential cohesion, conjunction, lexical cohesion, and ellipsis and decrease the use of exophora and unclear/ambiguous reference with age. We found no relationship between age and use of these cohesive devices in the schizophrenic

---

[1] Our earlier, but not our current, definition of ellipsis included conjunctions that were used at the beginning of a sentence.

children we studied. Irrespective of age, the schizophrenic children under-utilized referential cohesion, conjunctions, lexical cohesion, and ellipsis, but overutilized exophora and unclear/ambiguous reference. These findings have led us to hypothesize that onset of schizophrenia during middle childhood might impair the development of cohesive skills.

Formal thought disorder in childhood schizophrenia

Using the previously described sample of schizophrenic and normal children, two raters with no knowledge about the diagnosis of the children coded videotapes of the Story Game for the frequency of illogical thinking, loose associations, incoherence, and poverty of content of speech. The raters divided these frequency scores by the number of utterances per minute. The inter-rater agreement using Kappa (Fleiss, 1973) was 0.78 (SE = 0.03) and 0.66 (SE = 0.01), respectively for illogical thinking and loose associations (Caplan et al., 1989). Incoherence and poverty of content of speech occurred infrequently in the schizophrenic and normal children studied (Caplan et al., 1989; 1990a).

The schizophrenic children used significantly more illogical thinking and loose associations than the normal children. The sum of these two macro-structural measures correctly diagnosed 85% of the schizophrenic (i.e., sensitivity) and the normal (i.e., specificity) children (Caplan et al., 1990a). Illogical thinking alone had a sensitivity and specificity of 82% and 66%, respectively. Loose associations had a sensitivity of 71% and specificity of 97%.

The severity of illogical thinking and loose associations was a function of age of onset rather than of duration of illness (Caplan et al., 1990a). The younger schizophrenic children used significantly more illogical thinking and loose associations than the older children with this diagnosis. Eighty per cent (4/5) of the schizophrenic children with a mental age under 7 years had illogical thinking compared to 58% (7/12) and 36% (5/14) of the schizophrenic children above ages 7 and 9.6 years, respectively (Caplan, 1994). Loose associations was found in 90%, 75%, and 50% of the schizophrenic children with a mental age below 7 years, between 7 and 9.6 years, and above 9.6 years (Caplan, 1994).

Similar to the findings on cohesion, the formal thought disorder findings led to the hypothesis that onset of schizophrenia in middle childhood might be associated with impaired maturation of the cognitive skills associated with the development of logical thinking and topic maintenance. The infrequency of incoherence in schizophrenic children was not surprising given the low base rate of this formal thought disorder sign in adult schizophrenia (Andreasen, 1979). The absence of poverty of content, a consistent finding in adult schizophrenia (Andreasen & Grove, 1986) was surprising. Latency aged children use non-discursive and unelaborated speech. It is possible that children must be competent users of discursive speech for a reliable rating of poverty of content of speech to be made (Caplan et al., 1989).

Relationship between cohesion and formal thought disorder in schizophrenic children

To examine if impairments at the microstructural level are independent of the macrostructural discourse disturbances of schizophrenic children, a principal components analysis was computed (Caplan et al., 1994). This analysis revealed that the communication deficits of schizophrenic children included three separate principal components (Table 8.5). The first component included discourse measures other than exophora. The second factor included loose associations, the WISC-R distractibility factor score, and the WISC-R verbal comprehension factor score. The third factor consisted primarily of illogical thinking and exophora. These findings suggested that, with the exception of exophora, impaired use of cohesive devices in the schizophrenic children was not associated with clinical measures of formal thought disorder.

The association between illogical thinking and exophora can be understood in light of previous findings indicating that this macrostructural deficit was associated with the schizophrenic child's performance on the partial report span of apprehension task (Caplan et al., 1990b) and conservation of continuous and discontinuous matter (Caplan et al., 1990c) (Figure 8.1). From the information processing perspective, illogical thinking, exophora, and performance on the partial report span of apprehension and conservation of continuous and discontinuous matter tap similar information processing functions (Caplan 1994).

In support of this hypothesis, Asarnow et al. (1991) have hypothesized that the poor performance of schizophrenic children on the partial report span of apprehension represents a core deficit in recruiting and allocating information processing capacity for controlled attentional processes. Similarly, the child with illogical thinking is unable to present the listener with adequate reasoning as the demand for this arises during a conversation. Furthermore, the acquisition of conservation skills involves the ability to attend to multiple cues simultaneously (O'Bryan & Boersma, 1971; Flavell, 1985), to discriminate salient cues (O'Bryan & Boersma, 1971; Flavell, 1985), and to respond to perceptual stimuli using socially-appropriate reality-based reasoning (Mehler & Bever, 1967; Acredolo, 1982; Flavell, 1985). Thus, to conserve continuous and discontinuous matter successfully, the child needs to screen out extraneous information derived from the containers of the matter and to focus his/her attention on the matter alone (Caplan et al., 1990c). Finally, the schizophrenic child with exophora breaks the flow of conversation by not screening out extraneous stimuli from the non-conversational context.

The remaining measures of cohesion were unrelated to illogical thinking,

Table 8.5. *Principal components of the communication deficits of schizophrenic children*

Factor 1	Loading	Factor 2	Loading	Factor 3	Loading
Conjunction	0.89	WISC-RF$_3$[1]	0.86	ILL[2]	0.83
Referential c[3]	0.84	WISC-RF$_1$[1]	0.74	Exophora	−0.73
Words/clause	0.83	LA[2]	−0.69		
Lexical c[3]	0.67				
Ellipsis	−0.56				

Notes: [1] F$_3$ = Distractibility, F$_1$ = Verbal comprehension.
  [2] ILL = Illogical thinking, LA = Loose associations.
  [3] c = cohesion.

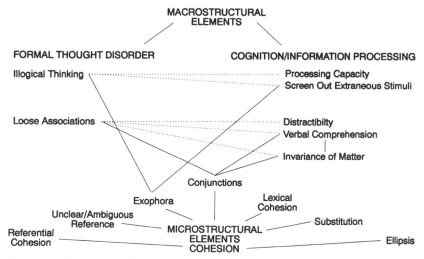

Figure 8.1. Discourse deficits of schizophrenic children.

loose associations, or the WISC-R factor scores used in the principal components analysis (Table 8.5). The partial report span of apprehension and conservation scores were not included in the principal components analysis because they were available for only 19 and 15 schizophrenic children, respectively. Within this subgroup of schizophrenic children, there was no statistically significant correlation between the span of apprehension and cohesion scores (Caplan, 1994). An examination of the relationship between conservation and measures of cohesion, however, demonstrated that schizophrenic and schizotypal children with better conservation competence used more conjunctions, were more verbally productive (words per clause), and had higher verbal comprehension WISC-R factor scores than those with poor conservation competence (Figure 8.1). An analysis of covariance adjusted for the formal thought disorder measures revealed a main effect of loose associations on the relationship of conservation competence with the scores for conjunction and verbal productivity (i.e., words per clause) (Figure 8.1).

To join the statements presented in two contiguous clauses with a conjunction, the child needs to perceive the contiguity between these two clauses. Similarly, to conserve competently, the child needs to perceive the invariance or contiguity of matter despite the change in its shape. The child with loose associations does not recognize the need to present the listener with the conversational links that maintain the topic of conversation. From an information processing perspective, therefore, similar processing impairments might underlie the schizophrenic child's difficulty using conjunctions, detecting the invariance of matter, and maintaining the topic of conversation (Figure 8.1). This hypothesis is also supported by Ferreiro and Sinclair's (1971) previously described findings on the relationship between conservation and the use of conjunctions in normal children.

Finally, in terms of the relationship between illogical thinking and loose associations, several studies have demonstrated that these two macrostructural measures represent different aspects of impaired attention/information processing in schizophrenic children (Caplan et al., 1990a, b; Caplan, 1994). Loose associations is associated with distractibility (Caplan et al., 1990b), reduced verbal comprehension (Caplan, 1994), and conservation of matter that does not involve a concomitant change in the container (Caplan et al., 1990c). As previously described, illogical thinking is not related to WISC-R scores or factor scores, but to the partial report span of apprehension and the conservation of matter within containers.

In summary, these studies demonstrate that the communication deficits of schizophrenic children reflect impairments at the microstructural and macrostructural levels. More specifically, the listener has difficulty following the communication of these children at the level of the paragraph (i.e., illogical thinking and loose associations) and at the level of the connections between sentences (i.e., impaired use of cohesion devices). Certain aspects of their microstructural discourse deficits, exophora and conjunctions, appear to be related to different macrostructural and cognitive/attentional impairments deficits. Other than these points of association, the microstructural discourse deficits of schizophrenic children appear to be independent of their macrostructural discourse deficits. The two macrostructural discourse deficits of these children, illogical thinking and loose associations, appear to reflect different aspects of impaired attention/information processing.

CONCLUSION

This chapter has highlighted how the study of discourse has enabled us to further understand the impaired communication skills of children with schizophrenia and their linguistic, cognitive, and clinical correlations. In schizophrenic children the clinical concept of "formal thought disorder" involves deficits at the macrostructural and microstructural levels. The macrostructural deficits involve poor organization of topic maintenance and inadequate reasoning. The microstructural deficits involve impaired use of linguistic devices that link the contents of contiguous and neighboring sentences. As a result of these deficits, the listener has difficulty following the ideas presented by schizophrenic children, who and what they are talking about, and how this is related to the ongoing topic of conversation and to what has been previously said.

In terms of general psychopathology, the communicative process and the child's macrostructural and microstructural discourse skills play an important part in his/her social and academic performance. Recent studies have shown that one-third of children seen in a psychiatric clinic for behavioral and learning problems have underlying language disorders (Cohen & Lipsett, 1987). Similarly, children presenting with a communication disorder are at risk of developing behavioral disturbances (Cantwell & Baker, 1987; Beitchman, Hood, & Inglis, 1990). Since discourse involves cognitive and social/emotional skills as well as linguistic skills, further study of discourse in child psychiatric disorders might have important implications for increasing our understanding of psychopathology in other child psychiatric disorders.

REFERENCES

Acredolo, C. (1982). Conservation/nonconservation: alternative explanations. In C.J. Brainerd (ed.) *Progress in Cognitive Development, Vol. 1*. New York: Springer Verlag (pp. 1–31).

American Psychiatric Association (1980). *Diagnostic and Statistical Manual of Mental Disorders*, 3rd edn. Washington, DC: American Psychiatric Association Press.

American Psychiatric Association (1987). *Diagnostic and Statistical Manual of Mental Disorders*, 3rd edn (rev.). Washington, DC: American Psychiatric Association Press.

American Psychiatric Association (1994). *Diagnostic and Statistical Manual of Mental Disorders*, 4th edn. Washington, DC: American Psychiatric Association Press.

Amidon, A. (1976). Children's understanding of sentences with contingent relations: why are temporal and conditional connective so difficult? *Journal of Experimental Child Psychology*, **22**, 423–437.

Andreasen, N.C. (1979). Thought, language, and communication disorders. I. Clinical assessment, definition of terms, and evaluation of their reliability. *Archives of General Psychiatry*, **36**, 1315–1323.

Andreasen, N.C. & Grove, W.M. (1986). Thought, language, and communication in schizophrenia: Diagnosis and prognosis. *Schizophrenia Bulletin*, **12**, 348–359.

Arboleda, C. & Holzman, P.S. (1985). Thought disorder in children at risk for psychosis. *Archives of General Psychiatry*, **42**, 1004–1013.

Asarnow, R.F., Granholm, E., & Sherman, T. (1991). Span of apprehension in schizophrenia. In H.A. Nasrallah, J. Zubin, S. Steinhauser, & J.H. Gruzelier (eds)

Handbook of Schizophrenia, Vol. 4, Experimental Psychopathology, Neuropsychology, and Psychophysiology. Amsterdam: Elsevier Science Publishers (pp. 335–370).

Astington, J.W., Harris, P.L., & Olson, D.R. (1988). *Developing Theories of Mind*. New York: Cambridge University Press.

Beitchman, J.H., Hood, J., & Inglis, A. (1990). Psychiatric risk in children with speech and language disorders. *Journal of Abnormal Child Psychology*, **18**, 283–296.

Bennett-Kastor, T.L. (1986). Cohesion and predication in child narrative. *Journal of Child Language*, **13**, 353–370.

Bloom, L., Lahey, M., Hood, L., Lifter, K., & Fiess, K. (1980). Complex sentences: acquisition of syntactic connectives and the semantic relations they encode. *Journal of Child Language*, **7**, 235–261.

Bloom, L., Rocissano, L., & Hood, L. (1976). Adult–child discourse: Developmental interaction between information processing and linguistic knowledge. *Cognitive Psychology*, **8**, 521–552.

Cantwell, D.P. & Baker, L. (1987). Clinical significance of childhood communication disorders: Perspectives from a longitudinal study. *Journal of Child Neurology*, **2**, 257–264.

Caplan, R. (1994). Communication deficits in childhood onset schizophrenia spectrum disorder. *Schizophrenia Bulletin*, **20**, 671–684.

Caplan, R., Guthrie, D., & Foy, J.G. (1992). Communication deficits and formal thought disorder in schizophrenic children. *Journal of the American Academy of Child and Adolescent Psychiatry*, **31**, 151–159.

Caplan, R., Perdue, S., Tanguay, P.E., & Fish, B. (1990a). Formal thought disorder in childhood onset schizophrenia and schizotypal personality disorder. *Journal of Child Psychology, Psychiatry and Allied Disciplines*, **31**, 1103–1114.

Caplan, R., Foy, J.G., Asarnow, R.F., & Sherman, T. (1990b). Information processing deficits of schizophrenic children with formal thought disorder. *Psychiatric Research*, **31**, 169–177.

Caplan, R., Foy, J.G., Sigman, M., & Purdue, S. (1990c). Conservation and formal thought disorder in schizophrenic and schizotypal children. *Developmental Psychopathology*, **2**, 183–190.

Caplan, R., Guthrie, D., Fish, B., Tanguay, P.E., & David-Lando, G. (1989). The Kiddie Formal Thought Disorder Rating Scale (K-FTDS). Clinical assessment, reliability, and validity. *Journal of the American Academy of Child and Adolescent Psychiatry*, **28**, 208–216.

Chaika, E. (1982). Accounting for linguistic data in schizophrenia research. *Behavioral and Brain Sciences*, **5**, 594.

Clancy, P.M. (1992). Referential strategies in the narrative of Japanese children. *Discourse Processes*, **15**, 441–467.

Clark, E.V. (1973). How children describe time and order. In C.A. Ferguson & D.I. Slobin (eds) *Studies of Child Language*. New York: Holt, Rinehart & Winston (pp. 586–606).

Cohen, N.J. & Lipsett, L. (1987). Recognized and unrecognized language impairment in psychologically disturbed children: child symptomatology, maternal depression, and family function. Preliminary report. *Canadian Journal of Behavioral Science*, **23**, 376–389.

Cornblatt, B.A., Lenzenweger, M.F., & Erlenmeyer-Kimling, L. (1989). The continuous performance test, identical pairs version: II. Contrasting attentional profiles in schizophrenic and depressed patients. *Psychiatric Research*, **29**, 65–85.

Ervin-Tripp, S. (1978). Some features of early child-adult dialogues. *Language Society*, **7**, 357–373.

Ferreiro, E., & Sinclair, H. (1971). Temporal relations in language. *Journal of Psychology*, **6**, 39–47.

Flavell, J.H. (1985). *Cognitive Development*. Englewood Cliffs, NJ: Prentice-Hall.

Fleiss, J. (1973). *Statistical Methods for Rates and Proportions*. New York: John Wiley.

Flores D'Arcais, G.B. (1981). The acquisition of meaning of the connectives. *Behavioral Development: A Series of Monographs* (pp. 265–298).

French, L.A. & Nelson, K. (1985). *Young Children's Knowledge of Relational Terms. Some Ifs, Ors and Buts*. Springer Series in Language and Communication v. New York: Springer-Verlag.

Fromkin, V.A. (1975). A linguist looks at "A linguist looks at 'schizophrenic' language." *Brain Language*, **2**, 498–503.

Gallagher, Y. (1981). Contingent query sentences with adult-child discourse. *Journal of Child Language*, **8**, 51–62.

Garvey, C. (1977). The contingent query: a dependent act in conversation. In M. Lewis & L.A. Rosenblum (eds) *Interaction, Conversation, and the Development of Language*. New York: Wiley (pp. 63–93).

Gerver, D. (1967). Linguistic rules and the perception and recall of speech by schizophrenic patients. *British Journal of Society and Clinical Psychology*, **6**, 204–211.

Gopnik, M. (1986). The development of connexity in young children. In J.J. Petrofi (ed.) *Text Connextedness for a Psychological Point of View*. Hamburg: Helmut Buske (pp. 64–95).

Greenfield, P.M. & Savage-Rumbaugh, E.S. (1993). Comparing communicative competence in child and chimp: the pragmatics of repetition. *Journal of Child Language*, **20**, 1–26.

Halliday, M.A.K. & Hasan, R. (1976). *Cohesion in Spoken and Written English*. London: Longmans.

Harrow, M. & Marengo, J.T. (1986). Schizophrenic thought disorder at followup: its persistence and prognostic significance. *Schizophrenia Bulletin*, **12**, 373–393.

Harvey, P.D. & Brault, J. (1986). Speech performance in mania and schizophrenia: The association of positive and negative thought disorders and reference failure. *Journal of Communication Disorders*, **19**, 161–174.

Harvey, P.D. (1983). Speech competence in manic and schizophrenic psychoses: the association between clinically rated thought disorder and performance. *Journal of Abnormal Psychology*, **92**, 368–377.

Holzman, P.S. (1986). Thought disorder in schizophrenia: editor's introduction. *Schizophrenia Bulletin*, **12**, 342–345.

Holzman, P.S., Shenton, M.E., & Solovay, M.R. (1986). Quality of thought disorder in differential diagnosis. *Schizophrenia Bulletin*, **12**, 360–371.

Ingram, D. (1975). If and when transformations are acquired by children. In D.P. Dato (ed.) *Developmental Psycholinguistics Theory and Applications*. Georgetown University Round Table on Languages and Linguistics. Washington, DC: Georgetown University Press (pp. 99–127).

Johnson, H.L. & Chapman, R.S. (1980). Children's judgment and recall of causal connectives: a developmental study of "because," "so," and "and." *Journal of Psycholinguistic Research*, **9**, 243–260.

Johnston, M.H. & Holzman, P.S. (1979). *Assessing Schizophrenic Thinking: A Clinical and Research Instrument for Measuring Thought Disorder.* San Francisco, CA: Jossey-Bass.

Kagan, J., Rosman, B., Day, D., Albert, J., & Phillips, W. (1964). Information processing in the child: significance of analytic and reflective attitudes. *Psychological Monographs*, No. 578.

Karmiloff-Smith, A. (1985). Language and cognitive processes from a developmental perspective. *Language and Cognitive Processes*, **1**, 61–85.

Keenan, E.O. (1974). Conversational competence in children. *Journal of Child Language*, **1**, 163–183.

Kraepelin, E. (1896). *Psychiatrie: Ein Lehrbuch für Studierende und Ärzte.* Leipzig: Barth.

Langford, D. (1981). The clarification request sequence in conversation between mothers and their children. In P. French & M. Maclure (eds) *Adult-Child Conversation.* New York: St. Martin's Press (pp. 159–184).

Lecours, A.R. (1982). Schizophasia. *The Behavioral and Brain Sciences*, **5**, 605.

MacLachlan, B.G. & Chapman, R.S. (1988). Communication breakdowns in normal and language-learning disabled children's conversation and narration. *Journal of Speech and Hearing Disorders*, **53**, 2–7.

MacWhinney, B. & Osser, H. (1977). Verbal planning functions in children's speech. *Child Development*, **48**, 978–985.

McTear, M.F. (1984). Structure and process in children's conversational development. In S. Kuczaj (ed.) *Discourse Development.* New York: Springer-Verlag (pp. 37–76).

Mehler, J. & Bever, T.G. (1967). Cognitive capacities of young children. *Science*, **158**, 141–142.

Nuechterlein, K.H., Edell, W.S., Norris, M., & Dawson, M.E. (1986). Attentional vulnerability indicators, thought disorder, and negative symptoms. *Schizophrenia Bulletin*, **12**, 408–426.

O'Bryan, K.G. & Boersma, F.J. (1971). Eye-movements, perceptual activity, and conservation development. *Journal of Experimental Child Psychology*, **12**, 157–169.

Paty, R. & Nespoulous, J.L. (1990). Discourse analysis in linguistics. In Y. Joanette & H.H. Brownell (eds) *Discourse Ability and Brain Damage. Theoretical and Empirical Perspectives.* Springer-Verlag: New York (pp. 3–27).

Pellegrini, A.D. (1984). The effect of dramatic play on children's generation of cohesive text. *Discourse Processes*, **7**, 57–67.

Peterson, C. & Dodswoth, P. (1991). A longitudinal analysis of young children's cohesion and noun specification in narratives. *Journal of Child Language*, **18**, 397–415.

Peterson, C. & McCabe, A. (1988). The connective AND as discourse glue. *First Language*, **8**, 19–28.

Piaget, J. (1955). *The Language and Thought of the Child.* New York: World Publishing (first published in 1923).

Piaget, J. (1962). *Play, Dreams, and Imitation in Childhood.* New York: Norton.

Pratt, M.W. & MacKenzie-Keating, S. (1985). Organizing stories: effect of development and task difficulty on referential cohesion in narrative. *Developmental Psychology*, **21**, 350–356.

Rochester, S.R. & Martin, J.R. (1979). *Crazy Talk: A Study of the Discourse of Schizophrenic Speakers.* New York: Plenum Press.

Roth, F. & Spekman, N. (1984). Assessing the pragmatic abilities of children: Part I. Organizational framework and assessing parameters. *Journal of Speech and Hearing Disorders*, **49**(2), 2–11.

Schwartz, S. (1982). Is there a schizophrenic language? *Behavioral and Brain Sciences*, **5**, 579–626.

Shatz, M. (1982). Communication. In P. Musson (ed.) *Carmichael's Manual of Child Psychology*. New York: John Wiley (pp. 841–889).

Shatz, M. & O'Reilly, A.W. (1990). Conversational or communicative skill? A reassessment of two-year-olds' behavior in miscommunication episodes. *Journal of Child Language*, **17**, 131–146.

Silva, M. (1991). Simultaneity in children's narratives: the case of when, while, and as. *Journal of Child Language*, **18**, 641–662.

Spilton, D. & Lee, C.L. (1977). Some determinants of effective communication in 5-year-olds. *Child Development*, **48**, 968–977.

Sprott, R.A. (1992). Children's use of discourse markers in disputes: form-function relationship and discourse in child language. *Discourse Processes*, **15**, 423–439.

van Dijk, T.A. (1972). *Some Aspects of Text Grammars*. Mouton: The Hague.

Vygotsky, L.S. (1962). *Thought and Language*. Cambridge, MA.: MIT Press.

Wigglesworth, G. (1990). Children's narrative acquisition: A study of some aspects of reference and anaphora. *First Language*, **10**, 105–125.

9 Comorbidity of autistic disorder and specific developmental language disorder: existing evidence and some promising future directions

M. MARY KONSTANTAREAS AND J.H. BEITCHMAN

It has long been recognized that high functioning individuals with autistic disorder (AD) and those with specific developmental language disorder or developmental dysphasia (DD) share a number of characteristics in common. However, the terrain of convergence is as yet very poorly understood (Shea & Mesibov, 1985; Rumsey & Hamburger, 1990). Because of this paucity of systematic comparative work, there is considerable scope for research on presenting characteristics and points of divergence and convergence, epidemiologic issues, taxonomic and classification issues, correlates, intervention strategies, and outcome.

PRESENTING CHARACTERISTICS

Language problems in children appear to persist to varying degrees well beyond the preschool period, and in some instances to worsen with time (Baker & Cantwell, 1987; Beitchman et al., 1994). Although earlier accounts of this relatively broad spectrum of difficulties have tended to be poorly focused, more recently some degree of consensus appears to have been reached regarding the importance of conceptualizing these difficulties according to more homogeneous subgroupings.

Several DD syndromes have been classified into subtypes. The most common is the "phonologic-syntactic" subtype, in which a child has selective difficulty with language form but not content, has a normal urge to communicate and says sensible things. Children who use superficially complex language with clear articulation, but whose use and understanding is defective, have been identified as presenting a "semantic-pragmatic" disorder (Rapin & Allen, 1983). Bishop and Rosenbloom (1987) believe that this subtype coexists with cognitive abnormalities of the type frequently found in children with AD. Their history is one of delayed language development. Once it appears, language may be characterized by echolalia and comprehension difficulties. The child may express fascination and enjoyment with the sound of language rather than with its use as a communication tool. He/she may fail to understand facial expression or tone of voice. Pronoun and tense distinctions give particular difficulty. Marked difficulties in understanding abstract concepts are also evident, with highly literal and concrete concepts being best understood. In contrast, imaginative play and social cognition may be poorly developed.

It is well recognized that AD constitutes the most severe variant of the pervasive developmental disorders (PDDs) (Rutter & Schopler, 1987). According to the DSM-IV, AD is defined by three clusters of abnormalities: (a) qualitative impairment in reciprocal social interaction, (b) qualitative impairment in communication and, (c) a markedly restricted repertoire of activities and interests. Communication difficulties are considered: (i) delay in or total lack of the development of spoken language, (ii) in individuals with adequate speech, marked impairment in the ability to initiate or sustain conversation with others, (iii) stereotypical use of language, and (iv) lack of varied, spontaneous, make-believe play or social play appropriate to the child's developmental level (American Psychiatric Association, 1994).

Confusion as to the nature of DD comorbid with AD has arisen because language disorders are themselves heterogeneous and the types of language disorders specific to AD have not yet been specified. Although, recently, most authors have argued that the semantic-pragmatic subtype of the DDs is most likely comorbid with AD (Bishop, 1989), others take the view that more than one subtype of the DD coexists with AD, at least occasionally (Resnick & Rapin, 1991). For ease of presentation, unless otherwise specified, the acronym DD will be used interchangeably with semantic-pragmatic disorder.

Recent interest in the relation between AD and DD has stemmed from three sources: (a) the presence of differential diagnosis which has resulted in diagnostic and methodological challenges due to a small but demanding percentage of cases; (b) follow-up work which has called into question original views on the outcome of DD that may require revision; and (c) the upsurge of interest in the concept of comorbidity which seems destined to create a minor revolution in the area of assessment, research, and modes of treatment. This chapter will attempt to critically examine the key differentiating factors between the two disorders on the basis of available research, as well as address issues of cla ,sification, assessment and etiology, in an attempt to inform future directions in clinical work and research.

Commonalities and differences: the issue of comorbidity

Until recently, classification systems such as the DSM have attempted to deal with diagnostic gray areas by using more than one axis. Recently, a more molecular approach to symptom clustering and differentiation (Achenbach, 1991) has paved the way for inductively derived, multivariate classifications. Such classification systems have permitted consideration of the relative expression of more than one formerly considered distinct disease entity in the same patient. This new strategy promises not only to revolutionize diagnostic practice, but to also improve our understanding of etiology and intervention.

Comorbidity is said to be present when two supposedly separate conditions co-occur with greater than chance frequency (Caron & Rutter, 1991). According to these authors, apparent comorbidity may arise from various nosological considerations: the use of discrete categories when dimensions might be more appropriate, overlapping diagnostic criteria, artificial sub-divisions of syndromes, one disorder representing an early manifestation of the other, and one disorder being part of the other. True comorbidity is considered to be the result of shared and overlapping risk factors, with one disorder creating an increased risk for the other.

To test the existence of true comorbidity we must ask the question: are there overlapping diagnostic criteria between AD and DD? Since language problems that constitute one of the three main symptom clusters used for arriving at a diagnosis of AD also appear in DD, by definition DD has to always be present in AD. Indeed, when Rapin and Allen (1987) allowed for both AD and DD to be independently coded in a group of children who were identified as presenting with either AD or DD, they reported that 65% of those coded as AD also showed dysphasia, including semantic-pragmatic disorder. On the other hand, since no behavioral or social parameters are specified as criteria for diagnosing DD, the presence of behavioral or social symptoms, suggestive of AD, would, by default, exclude a diagnosis of "simple" DD and lead instead to a diagnosis of AD (cf. Bishop, 1989). In this circumstance, AD cannot coexist with DD because of the way in which the latter is defined, but DD can coexist with AD. Thus the criteria overlap but only from AD to DD, not the other way around.

Could DD be an earlier manifestation of AD? If valid, such a view would be substantiated by evidence that young children with DD later develop AD. There are two reports in which aspects of this issue have been considered. Paul & Cohen (1984) noted that a group of preschoolers diagnosed with atypical developmental language delay (ADLD) appeared in adolescence to be almost indistinguishable from others who as preschoolers would have been considered AD. It is not clear whether as preschoolers the ADLD group should have been diagnosed with AD or whether the social and behavioral symptoms were not initially present but developed over time. Another report by Cantwell et al. (1989) raised similar issues. A group of DD children, when followed to adolescence, were found to show "autistic-like" social and behavioral problems. Again, it is not clear whether the so-called DD young people had, in reality, AD at first assessment but were misdiagnosed or whether some of the DD children subsequently developed autistic-like features which could warrant the diagnosis of AD. Changes in classification schemes over the last 30 years further confuse the issue. Clearly, most DD children do not go on to develop AD. What accounts for the differential outcome? Could one of the determining factors be the severity of the semantic-pragmatic disorder likely to be present in the overlap group, with the more severely affected members of that group presenting as AD at follow-up? To date, there is little evidence that bears on this question.

Is the distinction between DD and AD artificial? Because of the way AD is defined, it is not possible to have AD without having DD. Language problems alone are the necessary but not sufficient condition for AD while they are sufficient for DD. Is this differentiation artificial? We have seen that some children with DD subsequently become indistinguishable from those originally diagnosed with AD (Paul & Cohen, 1984). It may therefore be the case that there are instances of pure DD, and instances of DD and AD, but no instances of AD without DD. This exercise alerts us to the limited information we have on this issue. Further, this conceptualization fits a dimensional rather than a qualitative view of the relation between the two conditions.

The dimensions of autism and dysphasia

Turning to dimensionality, there is little doubt that both DD and AD are spectrum disorders. In the case of AD, the idea of a spectrum within the condition is not new (Coleman & Gillberg, 1993), and many workers in the field concur with the view that AD can vary considerably in severity of expression (Rutter & Schopler, 1987). Profound retardation and mutism constitute the most severe end of the continuum with Asperger's syndrome (AS) often being seen as AD's milder variant (Bishop, 1989; Schopler, 1985). Yet the DSM-IV has qualitatively differentiated the two conditions, by simply omitting language problems as a criterion for AS. Since subtle language and communication problems of a semantic-pragmatic nature are clinically evident in the high functioning AD children who will henceforth be diagnosed with AS, the issue may be far from being resolved. Bishop (1989) proposes that the use of the AS diagnosis over AD may be due to its greater acceptability among parents and professionals, who may have a stereotyped view of AD based on the clinical profile of younger AD children who tend to present with more severe symptoms. If AS were to be shown to be qualitatively different from AD, it may provide the ideal contrast group for studying socioaffective and behavioral difficulties as they may exist without the overlapping language difficulties. Hence, it would be the counterpart of "pure" DD (i.e. a language disorder without concomitant socioaffective and behavioral difficulties).

If DD, much as AD, is on a continuum (Bishop, 1989; Resnick & Rapin, 1991), then mild forms of DD may appear without the behavioral and social impairments typical of AD. Severe forms would be accompanied by the typical social and behavioral features related to AD while intermediate forms may be accompanied by some AD symptoms. Over time, if the DD improves, the AD-related social and behavioral symptoms may also improve. If it does not, social and behavioral symptoms would emerge and may become more apparent as the discrepancy between the child's chronological age and receptive language age widens. In this view, the presence of severe forms of DD without AD symptoms would be an important challenge to the notion of a dimensional concept of AD with DD as its core feature.

Research findings

Bartak, Rutter, & Cox (1975) were the first researchers to examine the relationship between AD and DD. They looked at the language and communication characteristics of high-functioning AD and "dysphasic" boys and found that language disorders were more severe and qualitatively different in boys with AD. Autistic impairment included language deviance as well as delay, and involved more severe problems in abstraction, use of spontaneous gesture, and a more extensive display of echolalia, pronoun reversal and metaphorical language use. However, there were also considerable similarities between the two, insofar as many DD boys also displayed a tendency to ignore sound, to use the third person to refer to themselves, to echo, and to reverse pronouns. Interestingly as well, approximately 20% of the cases could not be classified with certainty into either diagnosis, constituting what would now be classified as the comorbid subgroup. However, it is worth noting that the two groups differed in a critical dimension, namely receptive language ability, with the DD group having a mean receptive language age of 4.8 while the AD group's was only 3.8.

In a follow-up study contrasting higher functioning AD boys with severe receptive language DD boys, Cantwell, Baker, & Rutter (1978) revealed that the higher functioning AD boys showed major deficits in receptive language, with only one boy reaching the ceiling on the Reynell Comprehension Scale. In contrast, boys from the DD group showed much more progress. Although different from the AD group, a substantial number of the DD boys showed problems with peer relationships in middle childhood and an inability to show empathy. The presence of socioemotional difficulties has been a feature of other studies of children with developmental language disorders, particularly prevalent in those with receptive language impairments. This follow-up (Cantwell et al., 1978) leaves ambiguous the issue of the relation between receptive language difficulties and peer interactional problems, since the results suggest that within-group peer interaction differences might account for the differences in the level of receptive language, and not constitute genuine group differences, a possibility not explicitly examined. The results also hint at the chance that in a subgroup of children, AD might have begun as DD and, over time, evolved into a clinical picture akin to or identical to AD. These suppositions can only be examined prospectively, however, with careful assessment of the socioemotional development of youth, along with appropriate evaluation of their language development, with particular reference to receptive language and semantic-pragmatic abilities.

Allen, Lincoln, & Kaufman (1991) studied 20 AD and 20 developmental receptive language disordered (RLD) children, matched on age and gender. They found evidence that both groups had greater capacity for simultaneous over sequential processing, with no between-group differences, once degree of language impairment was controlled. The groups differed clearly, however, in degree and range of deficit, with the AD group having the more severe and pervasive difficulties. Similar issues have been raised in the study by Paul & Cohen (1984). They described the outcome of a group of DD children, dividing them into three subgroups: a high IQ, a low IQ, and an atypical group. When followed to adolescence, the atypical group could not be easily distinguished from adolescents diagnosed in childhood as classic AD, since they showed the verbal oddities, failure of communicative intent, language deficits and social withdrawal characteristic of AD in adolescence. The authors also noted that outcomes did not appear to vary much whether a child showed clear AD, PDD (the milder variant), or a form of the disorder too mild to be considered as either. They concluded that a conceptualization that viewed AD as a spectrum disorder, with varying degree of severity, may be more valid than the current scheme of describing AD.

In a related study, Paul, Fischer, & Cohen (1988) found that children with both AD and DD responded to a sentence comprehension task in a manner similar to that used by normal younger children at similar levels of comprehension ability. They suggested that the findings are consistent with the view that AD children show a restricted ability in semantic-pragmatic development, and concluded that the language processing deficits seen in AD children may be less unique to the syndrome than previously thought.

It appears that in the few studies in which the level of semantic-pragmatic competence of the DD subjects has been examined and compared with the level of the AD group, few differences between them have emerged. This should not be surprising. For example, Churchill (1972) proposed much earlier that there was no qualitative distinction between "developmental aphasia" and AD, with any difference being one of degree. Wing (1976) also argued that, while it is easy to recognize children with the classic Kanner syndrome and those with clear developmental receptive language disorder, the border lines between the two are not at all clear. Wing states, "If children with these problems could be arranged in an orderly series, starting from the most autistic child at one end and extending to the child who most clearly had nothing but a developmental receptive speech disorder at the other, to say where the dividing line should be drawn would need the judgement of Solomon" (Wing, 1976, p. 18).

Rutter (1978) reviewed the Bartak et al. (1975) and the Cantwell et al. (1978) studies and concluded that, while there were major differences between "developmental receptive aphasia" and "infantile autism" in severity, range, and nature of language problems and in behavioral terms, the existence of intermediate cases emphasized the difficulty of drawing a sharp boundary. He also noted that with the DD as well as the AD group, the more autistic-like the language the more autistic-like the behavior was found to be, indicating that degrees of AD can be considered in children who do not have the full syndrome.

It has been repeatedly argued that the major difference between AD and DD children is the impairment in socioaffective development and the markedly restricted repertoire of behaviors and activities characterizing the AD child. It is not certain, however, that this distinction is valid at all levels or degrees of severity of DD. As noted above, in those studies comparing the two conditions, when the language level was controlled, between-group differences disappeared. It is our view that as more research focusing on the issue of differences is carried out, the greater the impression of difficulty in recognizing the boundaries between these conditions will be. It may be that AD is a disorder without clear boundaries.

KEY DIMENSIONS OF LANGUAGE AND COMMUNICATION

Semantic development

Although there is considerable work on semantic development in normal children, dating from the classic studies of Roger Brown, there is little on the semantic development of dysfunctional children, despite the extensive clinical lore. The longitudinal study by Tager-Flusberg et al. (1990) will provide ongoing information on the AD children, but aside from its small sample size, it includes contrasting groups of Down syndrome and normal children, not those with the DD. Hermelin & O'Connor (1970) have also done some work in this area but, once again, the contrast group employed were mentally delayed children and the thrust of the research was limited to memory tasks. We need a systematic, longitudinal examination of the semantic development of AD and DD children at varying levels of severity to clarify aspects of semantic development in the two groups.

It is well documented that AD children do not communicate context-relevant information to the listener, showing evidence of a "form-context" mismatch (Swisher & Demetras, 1985). Their utterances, although grammatically correct, lack firm connections to a semantic base. They are frequently a simple recombination of words heard or "a store of phrases." An example of this dissociation was evident in a recent study by Konstantareas & Lunsky (1995) on the sexual knowledge, experience, attitudes, and interests of AD and mentally retarded adults. When asked to define sexuality-relevant terms, many AD individuals provided homophones: homosexual – having sex at home, lesbians – gaysians, diaphragm – frying pan, orgasm – playing the organ, and erection – west, east, south and north! None of the mentally retarded people who participated offered such superficial and context-irrelevant definitions. The literature is replete with other examples of this difficulty (Schuler & Prizant, 1985). Few studies exist in which these context-relevant errors have been examined in DD children but they may be more common among those with the semantic-pragmatic disorder (Bishop, 1989). Again, this raises the issue of the comparability and divergence between children with semantic-pragmatic disorder and those with AD. Related to this issue, Frith (1989) advanced the theory of mind paradigm with AD children by showing that as many as 80% of the high functioning subjects lacked "a theory of mind." That is, they could not impute motives to others as their peers typically did to guide their behavior accordingly. It would be of interest to determine: (a) the characteristics which differentiate the 20% of children who do "read minds" from the remaining 80%, and (b) the performance of children with DD on these tasks. Also, would children with AS, who are apparently free of language difficulties, possess a theory of mind? On the basis of the previous discussion, it would not be surprising to find that the performance of children with DD and AS may fall on a continuum in this regard.

Pragmatic development

Most studies on the pragmatic deficits of language impaired children have tended to deal with the AD population whose problems in this area are reported to be extensive (Baltaxe & Simmons, 1975; Curcio & Paccia, 1987). The speech of AD children has long been described as "wooded," "robot-like," and "flat," that is, lacking in pitch, intonation, and stress. Once again, there is little systematic evidence on this deficit, either in terms of spontaneous speech or in speech acquired after extensive training.

The study by Cantwell et al. (1978), quoted earlier, also examined pragmatic competencies in AD and DD children, by looking at "socialized speech," such as spontaneous remarks, directions, abnormal and egocentric speech, immediate and delayed echolalia, and nonverbal speech. Considerable differences emerged in this examination. The DD children used significantly more socialized speech, far fewer delayed echoes, and less abnormal and egocentric speech. When the two samples were compared, it was revealing to find that none of the children with DD displayed more than 1% of abnormal speech while 7 of the 12 AD children did. The remaining 5 did not do so perhaps because they also tended to show a low rate of spontaneous remarks. In view of the previously mentioned lack of equivalence in the receptive language abilities of the two groups, it is unclear whether the pragmatic differences described were true semantic ones or a function of differences in the groups' receptive language skills.

In addition to the linguistic functions originally developed by Bloom (1974) and elaborated into functional codes by McNeil & McNeil (1975), pragmatics encompasses a number of other elements not sufficiently studied in either normal or language impaired children. They are intonation, pitch, voice stress and modulation, facial expression, gesture, and body posture, to name the main ones. Considerable descriptive work on all these parameters has been carried out by communication theorists (Birdwhister, 1970). More systematic work has been reported on interactional and self-synchrony by Condon (1975). He defined impairment as a delayed body movement to linguistic or nonlinguistic sound and/or a repeated response to it upon microkinetic, sound-body videotaped analysis. Of all the dysfunctional children he examined, including the dysphasic, he found those with AD to respond with most delay and repetition. Our attempt to replicate the phenomenon with AD children yielded only a higher total body movement compared to normals (Oxman, Webster, & Konstantareas, 1978).

Pragmatics also includes elements of correspondence and tracking in the speech of two interlocutors. Feldstein et al. (1982) examined "conversational synchrony" with 12 high-functioning and verbal AD individuals over the age of 19. A stranger, the experimenter, and the individual's mother functioned as interlocutors. Although synchrony was achieved by the end of the 15-minute interval between the mother and the experimenter, none of the AD adults achieved it. A replication of this study including a group of DD individuals, ideally with semantic-pragmatic disorder, would contribute to our understanding of the association between AD and DD with respect to pragmatic development.

The features that make a conversation seem inappropriate to others have recently been examined by Bishop & Adams (1989) in the language samples of 57 language impaired children, including those with semantic-pragmatic deficit and 67 control children. The language of the semantic-pragmatic subgroup was characterized by high rates of inappropriacy. The measure of inappropriacy distinguished language impaired children from controls, with the semantic-pragmatic subgroup obtaining particularly high scores. They resembled younger normal language children in that they misunderstood the literal or implicit meaning of adult utterances and violated normal rules of exchange. Yet they differed from them in their tendency to provide the listener with too little or too much information. This study is important in showing differences in pragmatic competencies among language impaired groups. Comparisons with an AD group would represent the next logical extension of this work.

In sum, the AD children's difficulties in the area of pragmatics has been receiving increasing emphasis in recent years. Many published accounts of the language abnormalities of AD children appear to conclude that it is in pragmatics that they show qualitative differences from other language impaired groups (Frith, 1989; Swisher & Demetras, 1985; Tager-Flusberg et al., 1990). This conclusion may be premature, however, since it is based on limited systematic work. The shift in language acquisition research from transformational grammar to pragmatics (Bates, 1976) has not yet been fully realized in research with language disordered individuals. We have only a handful of studies systematically addressing the issue, and even fewer with appropriately selected or matched groups. Also, as indicated earlier, we have little evidence on semantic development which itself could be another differentiating area. In fact, only the Cantwell et al. (1978) study comes close to a well-controlled undertaking, and even here the number of children examined was certainly small. Furthermore, despite its many strengths, the study has become dated by now and in need of revision and replication. Clearly, however, progress in uncoupling AD from DD will be made in the area of semantics and pragmatics.

ASSESSMENT ISSUES

The advent of the concept of comorbidity will be likely to require that classification systems such as the DSM and the ICD adopt drastic changes to their configurations. Symptom algorithms against which a given clinical case is to be evaluated may be required. In addition, two other considerations come to mind. The first relates to the need for data from normal development to be used as benchmarks against which each symptom can be examined (Siegel, 1991). The relevant normal developmental benchmarks here are social development and the development of cognitive understanding. Social development normally proceeds through a series of stages from unoccupied and solitary activity to symbolic play to mutual play, culminating in play with rules (Freud, 1965). The particular level of play a child shows reflects, among other things, his/her cognitive development as well as his/her socioemotional growth. We would not judge a 3-year-old child who cannot engage in sophisticated cooperative play with rules as abnormal. However, we would consider this abnormal if it occurred in older children.

Among the many ingredients that contribute to the level and form of social play, such as attunement to socioaffective cues, temperamental qualities, theory of mind, and so on, the level of cognitive understanding must also be considered. The child's level of cognitive understanding may be considered an alternate expression of his/her level of semantic development. Evidence suggests that delayed or disordered semantic development results in disturbed or disordered conversational characteristics. When a child's cognitive age is not taken into consideration, the level and form of his/her social development may appear bizarre or autistic-like (Beitchman, 1975). We need to better understand how to assess the child's level of cognitive understanding and what instruments should be used for this purpose. For instance, should the level of receptive language age be considered the benchmark? What about mental age? What about nonverbal IQ? Different measures are suitable for different purposes. However, there is no consensus as to what measure should be utilized to reflect the child's expected level of social development.

If normal developmental milestones are taken as the benchmark against which assessments are compared, it will require that: (a) verbal IQ, as a measure of cognitive ability for dysfunctional populations, be replaced with nonverbal mental age or receptive language age, or some other measure of cognitive understanding, (b) normal developmental milestones be used as a basis of comparison for each atypical behavior, (c) for each diagnostic criterion, mental age cutoffs be used below which a given symptom cannot be assessed owing to the child's low mental age. Looking for echolalia in a nonverbal AD child and checking its absence as a negative for the criterion, for example, would clearly result in a lower pathology score when in fact the reverse is the case, and (d) cutoffs for degree of delay be used, such as percent of delay, to evaluate progress across time.

A second point relates to the need for quantitative information to measure the degree of overall symptomatology in order to make differential diagnoses. Checklists such as the Classification of Autism Rating Scale (Schopler, Reichler, & Renner, 1988) may be of utility. They allow for degree of symptomatology to guide diagnostic decision-making. Because checklists yield quantitative information, they can also help to determine the degree of comorbidity which would be relevant to clinical and research issues.

Assessment protocols need to include at least the following elements: (a) information on nonverbal intelligence, including sensorimotor functioning (cf. Uzgiris & Hunt, 1975), and data on object permanence and operational causality for children functioning at or below the 2-year-old level, which formal psychometric scales cannot reach; (b) broader than existing protocols to allow for the evaluation of a much more comprehensive range of psycholinguistic functions than are currently being assessed; (c) data on degree of play complexity (Wintre & Webster, 1974) and peer interaction, both at school and home; and (d) information on communicative intent, a concept central to pragmatics (Prizant & Wetherby, 1987) should also be gathered for its relevance to differential diagnosis and prognosis.

In sum, we need to develop more detailed and specific classification schemes as well as more complete assessment protocols to allow for a more precise determination of the main disorders under consideration as well as the area of overlap. As to the magnitude of the overlapping area, it can only be established with relative certainty when we sharpen our diagnostic instruments and classification models. We also need to keep in mind that the prevalence of the discrete disorders and their overlap need to be considered longitudinally since it may change with maturation. Most of the available evidence points to pragmatics as a key area to focus on for assessment and differential diagnosis.

ETIOLOGIC FACTORS

Genetics

Considerable recent evidence has alerted us to the fact that for both conditions genetic factors are responsible for an as yet undetermined percentage of affected individuals. To begin with AD, because of its low incidence in the population and the fact that affected individuals seldom procreate, it was originally not thought to be a genetic disorder. More recently, studies have pointed to probable genetic etiology. They have relied on two general strategies in delineating possible influences: (a) the behavior-brain-gene pathway and (b) the gene-brain-behavior pathway. The first pathway is used in behavioral genetics research and relies on examination of the phenotype to infer genetic contribution. The second pathway involves the identification of a known genetic disorder, and considers the possibility of linkage, that is, the cosegregation of the trait with the known gene marker (Smalley, 1991).

Relying on the first strategy, twin studies (Folstein & Rutter, 1977; Ritvo, Ritvo, & Brothers, 1982) have demonstrated higher concordance rates for MZ versus DZ twin pairs where at least one was AD. Folstein & Rutter (1977) reported concordance rates of approximately 40% for MZ twin pairs and 0% for DZ pairs while Ritvo et al. (1982) reported concordance rates as high as 96% for MZ twins and 24% for DZ. The latter study has been criticized for ascertainment bias since it relied on self-referral rather than random sampling (Paul, 1987). Thus rates are likely to be closer to those reported by Folstein and Rutter (1977), although the N of that sample was small.

As to the transmission pattern, autosomal recessive inheritance has been proposed by Ritvo et al. (1985). Smalley (1991) disputes it on the basis of the significant sex difference in frequency of expression. The increased lethality and/or reduced penetrance among the females, which has been proposed by Ritvo et al. (1985) to account for the sex difference in frequency of expression, appear of dubious relevance. Tsai, Stewart, & August (1981) have argued in favor of a multifactorial model. In such a model a large number of genes and environmental effects contribute to an underlying liability. The observed sex difference is thought to be the result of two thresholds on the liability scale, one for females and another for males. The less frequently affected sex, according to this model, is expected to have more affected relatives, because they require a greater loading of liability factors, including those of a genetic origin, to be affected. Once affected, relatives are expected to express the condition more severely. Konstantareas, Homatidis, & Busch (1989) have provided preliminary support for this model. They analyzed extensive assessment protocol data from 89 AD children, 67 males and 22 females, and found that scores on nonverbal IQ, mental age, object permanence, operational causality, receptive language, peer interaction and ability to verbalize, and overall developmental skills were higher for boys. Girls also had a higher total autism symptom score on the CARS. In not a single instance were the competence scores of AD females higher than those of males. That AD is partly genetically transmitted has also been shown in studies of its incidence among siblings of AD individuals. While the incidence is 5/10,000, the frequency of the disorder in the siblings of an AD proband is much higher,

3-5/100 (Smalley, Asarnow, & Spence, 1988). This represents a high heritability of from 80% to 90%.

The second strategy involves the identification of a known genetic disorder
and then studying the behavioral sequelae of the gene or chromosomal
abnormality related to it. Two good candidates are the fragile X condition,
present in 8% to 30% of AD males, and tuberous sclerosis present,
conservatively, in 3% of cases (Olsson, Steffenburg, & Gillberg, 1988).

Of import to our interest here, siblings of AD children were more likely
to present with cognitive deficits, particularly in the form of speech and
language disorders (August, Steward, & Tsai, 1981). A next line of action
may be: (1) to systematically examine the presenting characteristics of the DD
siblings of AD individuals and contrast them to those of the AD probands
but also to the characteristics of other language impaired children. This has
already been done to advantage with fragile-X syndrome cases (Smalley,
1991). A high incidence of avoiding eye contact, hand-flapping, hand-biting
or other stereotypies were present in 88% of 50 fragile-X males while in the
area of language 95% displayed perseverative bursts of speech, all characteristics
AD children are known to display (Hagerman, 1989). One of the possible
difficulties here is finding enough cases to allow for meaningful comparisons
to be carried out. (2) It will be useful to determine if the heritability is constant,
regardless of level of functioning of the AD proband. Studies (e.g. Lord &
Schopler, 1985) have reported that the uneven sex ratios become progressively
larger as level of cognitive functioning increases. It would be useful to also
examine whether the comorbid individuals display these highly uneven ratios.
If they do, this will speak to the validity of etiologic views that see disordered
behavior as falling along a continuum rather than consisting of a series of
discrete and discontinuous entities. Such models are likely to be more
comfortable with the notion of comorbidity since it allows for the smooth
gradation from more to less severe disorders.

Although speech and language disorders have been shown to be familial
(Bishop, 1987; Beitchman, Hood, & Inglis, 1992), the extent of their
heritability remains unknown. In part this is because syndromes appearing
clinically similar may be etiologically and genetically different. For instance,
similar clinical groups may represent phenocopies with different genotypes.
DD secondary to chromosomal abnormalities such as XXY, may appear to
be clinically similar to DD of unknown origin. In addition, the AD spectrum
has been broadened to include the heritability of language and cognitive delays
(e.g., Folstein & Rutter, 1977). This approach suggests that, from the point
of view of genetic studies, AD may be thought of as existing on a continuum
with degrees of cognitive and language delays along that continuum.
Although DD would also be on that continuum, the point of separation
between AD and DD is yet to be specified. An important next step in the
investigation of the heritability of AD and DD would be to examine the
nature of their language and cognitive delays and to identify their genetic or

other biological markers. If these markers are the same for both AD and DD, this would support the notion of a shared genetic etiology.

The examination of heritability of the two disorders is likely to shed considerable light on every aspect of relevance to our concern here, including characteristics and taxonomy, etiology and even intervention strategies and long-term outcome.

Infections during the pre-, peri- and neonatal periods

Aside from genetics, other factors have also been shown to be of etiologic relevance such as environmental risk factors during the pre-, peri- and neonatal periods. These have been reviewed for the AD (Konstantareas, 1986) and for the DD (Beitchman, Wild, & Kroll, in press) individuals. However, most studies have contrasted these groups with asymptomatic controls or mentally retarded children. To our knowledge, no systematic effort has been made to compare the backgrounds of the AD and DD groups in the same study. Viral infections and immunodeficiencies have also featured prominently in the backgrounds of both groups of children, best documented with AD children. Coleman & Gillberg (1993) have provided a comprehensive review of all biological conditions that coexist with AD, including metabolic, structural, biochemical, and neuropathological abnormalities. Although it has not been documented, it is possible that such conditions are more likely to be evident in the more severely affected AD individuals, 50% of whom are nonverbal and have IQs below 50.

Brain mechanisms and functioning

In recent years, researchers have begun to examine brain mechanisms in relation to developmental language disorders and related conditions (see Logan, Chapter 14). For the DD group, Galaburda & Kemper (1979) have reported the results of autopsies of the brains of adults with lifelong histories of language and reading disorders. They showed evidence of cytoarchitectural abnormalities all related to the left hemisphere, and specifically to the posterior parts of Heschl's gyrus and the left planum temporale. This area corresponds to the auditory association region which has long been known as Wernicke's area. More recently, magnetic resonance imaging (MRI) studies have revealed that a subgroup of DD children had an enlarged right rather than left planum temporale, which is a reversal from the brain formation of normal children (Jernigan et al., 1991).

Using MRI with AD children, Courchesne et al. (1988), reported hypoplasia of neocerebellar structures. Horowitz et al. (1988), using positron emission tomography (PET) with 14 healthy AD individuals, also reported functionally impaired interactions between frontal/parietal regions of the brain and the neostratum and thalamus, regions that subserve directed attention.

The search for anatomical specificity among children with DD and AD may however be misplaced. Recent work with aphasia in adults has led to a profound change in the conceptualization of the neural systems thought to underlie complex functions such as language and memory. These are now thought to be the result of synchronized activity in vast neuronal networks, made up of many functional regions in the cerebral cortex and subcortical nuclei. Numerous pathways are thought to interconnect these regions in a reciprocal fashion (Damasio, 1992). Any one of many interconnecting neural networks could be implicated in populations of children with DD and AD. Studies of brain function (e.g., PET or SPECT or computerized evoked potentials, see Logan, Chapter 14) are likely to hold more prospects for identifying some of the potential neuronal pathways implicated in these dysfunctional populations.

Future studies should, whenever possible, include both groups in direct comparison as well as comorbid groups to clarify possible areas of overlap between the conditions. Clearly different areas appear affected in the two. Furthermore, not all studies show evidence of abnormalities. It is possible that discrepant cases are best described as comorbid rather than "pure" disorders, with different structures perhaps being involved. Of course diagnostic precision and careful matching on key presenting characteristics and epidemiologic features, are also of relevance as Garber, Ritvo, & Chiu (1989) have argued.

Even when AD and DD can be distinguished, they share a number of broadly defined characteristics such as developmental immaturity, uneven intellectual skills, delayed and deviant language development, and inter-personal and social deficits. In an effort to more precisely clarify points of convergence and divergence, an extensive program of longitudinal research, whose goal will be to critically examine and follow through groups of carefully matched AD, dysphasic and comorbid children, is needed.

CONCLUSION

In conclusion, it is evident from the above review and comments that, on the basis of the available evidence, AD and DD can be distinguished but it may be that the distinction is less real and more of an artifact owing to the method by which these disorders are defined. These conditions are most easily separable at their extremes. The intermediate zone contains the comorbid cases where differentiation is difficult. It is likely that a better understanding of the relation between DD and AD will lead to a new conceptualization of the fundamental nature of Autism. The key to this understanding may lie in clarifying the relation between language development, cognitive understanding and the development of social relatedness.

REFERENCES

Achenbach, T.M. (1991). *Manual for the Child Behavior Checklist/4–18 and 1991 Profile.* Burlington, VT: University of Vermont Department of Psychiatry.

Allen, M.H., Lincoln, A.J., & Kaufman, A.S. (1991). Sequential and simultaneous processing abilities of high-functioning autistic and language-impaired children. *Journal of Autism and Developmental Disorders,* **21**, 483–502.

American Psychiatric Association (1994). *Diagnostic and Statistical Manual of Mental Disorders (DSM-IV),* 4th edn. Washington, DC: American Psychiatric Association.

August, G.J., Stewart, M.A., & Tsai, L. (1981). The incidence of cognitive disabilities in the siblings of autistic children. *British Journal of Psychiatry,* **138**, 416–422.

Baker, L. & Cantwell, D.P. (1987). A prospective psychiatric follow-up of children with speech/language disorders. *Journal of the American Academy of Child and Adolescent Psychiatry,* **26**, 546–553.

Baltaxe, C.A. & Simmons, J.Q. (1975). Language in childhood psychosis: a review. *Journal of Speech and Hearing Disorders,* **30**, 439–458.

Bartak, L., Rutter, M., & Cox, A. (1975). A comparative study of infantile autism and specific developmental receptive language disorder – I. The children. *British Journal of Psychiatry,* **126**, 127–145.

Bartak, L., Rutter, M., & Cox, A. (1977). A comparative study of infantile autism and specific developmental receptive language disorder – III. Discriminant function analyses. *Journal of Autism and Childhood Schizophrenia,* **7**, 383–396.

Bates, E. (1976). *Language and Context.* New York: Academic Press.

Beitchman, J.H. (1975). Therapeutic considerations with the language-impaired preschool child. *Canadian Journal of Psychiatry,* **30**, 609–613.

Beitchman, J.H., Hood, J., & Inglis, A. (1992). Familial transmission of speech and language impairment: a preliminary investigation. *The Canadian Journal of Psychiatry,* **37**, 151–156.

Beitchman, J.H., Brownlie, E.B., Inglis, A., Wild, J., Mathews, R., Schachter, D., Kroll, R., Martin, S., Ferguson, B., & Lancee, W. (1994). Seven year follow-up of speech/language impaired and control children: speech/language stability and outcome. *Journal of the American Academy of Child and Adolescent Psychiatry,* **33**, 1322–1330.

Beitchman, J.H., Wild, J., & Kroll, R. (in press). An overview of childhood speech and language disorders. In J. Noshpitz (ed.) *Basic Handbook of Child Psychiatry.*

Birdwhister, R.L. (1970). *Kinesics and Content.* Philadelphia, PA: University of Pennsylvania Press.

Bishop, D.V.M. (1989). Autism, Asperger's syndrome and semantic-pragmatic disorder: where are the boundaries? *British Journal of Disorders of Communication,* **24**, 241–263.

Bishop, D.V.M. (1987). The causes of specific developmental language disorder ("Developmental Dysphasia"). *Journal of Child Psychology and Psychiatry,* **28**, 1–8.

Bishop, D.V.M. & Adams, C. (1989). Conversational characteristics of children with semantic-pragmatic disorder: II. What features lead to a judgement of inappropriacy? *British Journal of Disorders of Communication,* **24**, 241–263.

Bishop, D.V.M. & Rosenbloom, L. (1987). Childhood language disorders: Classification and overview. In W. Yule & M. Rutter (eds) *Language Development and Disorders.* Oxford: MacKeith Press (pp. 16–41).

Bloom, L. (1974). Talking, understanding and thinking. In R.L. Schiefelbusch & L.L. Lloyd (eds) *Language Perspectives, Acquisitions, Retardation, and Intervention*. Baltimore, MD: University Park Press (pp. 285–311).

Cantwell, D.P., Baker, L., & Rutter, M. (1978). A comparative study of infantile autism and specific developmental receptive language disorder. IV. Analysis of syntax and language function. *Journal of Child Psychology and Psychiatry*, **19**, 351–362.

Cantwell, D.P., Baker, L., Rutter, M., & Mawhood, L. (1989). Infantile autism and developmental receptive dysphasia: a comparative follow-up into middle childhood. *Journal of Autism and Developmental Disorders*, **19**, 19–31.

Caron, C. & Rutter, M. (1991). Comorbidity in child psychopathology: Concepts, issues and research strategies. *Journal of Child Psychology and Psychiatry and Allied Disciplines*, **32**, 1063–1080.

Churchill, D.W. (1972). The relation of infantile autism and early childhood schizophrenia to developmental language disorders of childhood. *Journal of Autism and Childhood Schizophrenia*, **2**, 182–197.

Coleman, M. & Gillberg, C. (1993). *The Biology of the Autistic Syndromes*, 2nd edn. New York: Praeger.

Condon, W.S. (1975). Multiple response to sound in dysfunctional children. *Journal of Autism and Childhood Schizophrenia*, **5**, 37–56.

Courchesne, E., Yeung-Courchesne, R., Press, G.A., Hesselink, J.R., & Jerningan, T.L. (1988). Hypoplasia of cerebellar vermal lobules VI and VII in autism. *New England Journal of Medicine*, **318**, 1349–1354.

Curcio, F. & Paccia, J. (1987). Conversations with autistic children: contingent relationships between features of adult input and children's response adequacy. *Journal of Autism and Developmental Disorders*, **17**, 81–93.

Damasio, A.R. (1992). Aphasia. *New England Journal of Medicine*, **326**, 531–539.

Feldstein, S., Konstantareas, M.M., Oxman, J., & Webster, C.D. (1982). The chronography of interactions with autistic speakers: an initial report. *Journal of Communication Disorders*, **15**, 451–460.

Folstein, S. & Rutter, M. (1977). Genetic influences and infantile autism. *Nature*, **265**, 726–728.

Freud, A. (1965). *The Writings of Anna Freud – Volume VI: Normality and Pathology in Childhood: Assessments of Development*. New York: International Universities Press.

Frith, U. (1989). A new look at language and communication in autism. Special issue: Autism. *British Journal of Disorders of Communication*, **24**, 123–150.

Galaburda, A.M. & Kemper, T. (1979). Cytoarchitectonic abnormalities in developmental dyslexia: a case study. *Annals of Neurology*, **6**, 94–100.

Garber, H.J., Ritvo, E.R., & Chiu, L.C. (1989). A magnetic resonance imaging study of autism: Normal fourth ventricle size and absence of pathology. *American Journal of Psychiatry*, **146**, 532–534.

Hagerman, R.J. (1989). Chromosomes, genes and autism. In C. Gillberg (ed.) *Diagnosis and Treatment of Autism*. New York: Plenum (pp. 105–131).

Hermelin, B. & O'Connor, J. (1970). *Psychological Experiments with Autistic Children*. Oxford: Pergamon Press.

Horowitz, B., Rumsey, J.M., Grady, C.L., & Rapoport, S.I. (1988). The cerebral metabolic landscape in autism: Intercorrelations of regional glucose utilization. *Archives of Neurology*, **45**, 749–755.

Jernigan, T.L., Hesselink, J.R., Sowell, E., & Tallal, P.A. (1991). Cerebral structure on magnetic resonance imaging in language- and learning-impaired children. *Archives of Neurology,* **48**, 539–545.

Konstantareas, M.M., Homatidis, S., & Busch, J. (1989). Cognitive, communication, and social differences between autistic boys and girls. *Journal of Applied Developmental Psychology*, **10**, 411–424.

Konstantareas, M.M. & Lunsky, Y. (1995). Sociosexual knowledge, experience, attitudes and interests of autistic and delayed individuals. Poster presented at the Society for Research in Child Development, Indianapolis (April).

Konstantareas, M.M. (1986). Early developmental backgrounds of autistic and mentally retarded children: future research directions. *Psychiatric Clinics of North America*, **9**, 671–688.

Lord, C. & Schopler, E. (1985). Differences in sex ratios in autism as a function of measured intelligence. *Journal of Autism and Developmental Disorders*, **15**, 185–193.

McNeil, N. & McNeil, D. (1975). *Linguistic Interactions among Children and Adults.* Committee on Cognition and Communication. Chicago, IL: University of Chicago Press.

Olsson, I., Steffenburg, S., & Gillberg, C. (1988). Epilepsy in autism and autisticlike conditions. *Archives of Neurology*, **45**, 666–668.

Oxman, J., Webster, C.D., & Konstantareas, M.M. (1978). Condon's multiple response phenomenon in severely dysfunctional children: an attempt at replication. *Journal of Autism and Childhood Schizophrenia*, **8**, 395–402.

Paul, R. (1987). Communication. In D.J. Cohen & A.M. Donnellan (eds) *Handbook of Autism and Pervasive Developmental Disorders.* New York: Wiley.

Paul, R. & Cohen, D.J. (1984). Outcomes of severe disorders of language acquisition. *Journal of Autism and Developmental Disorders*, **14**, 405–421.

Paul, R., Fischer, M.L., & Cohen, D.J. (1988). Brief report: Sentence comprehension strategies in children with autism and specific language disorders. *Journal of Autism and Developmental Disorders*, **18**, 669–679.

Prizant, B.M. & Wetherby, A.M. (1987). Communicative intent: a framework for understanding social-communicative behavior in autism. *Journal of the American Academy of Child and Adolescent Psychiatry*, **26**, 472–479.

Rapin, I. & Allen, D.A. (1987). Developmental dysphasia and autism in preschool children: characteristics and subtypes. Paper presented at the First International Symposium on Specific Speech and Language Disorders (AFASIC), Reading, England.

Rapin, I. & Allen, D.A. (1983). Developmental language disorders: nosologic considerations. In U. Kirk (ed.) *Neuropsychology of Language, Reading and Spelling.* New York: Academic Press (pp. 155–184).

Resnick, T. & Rapin, I. (1991). Language disorders in childhood. *Psychiatric Annals*, **21**, 709–716.

Ritvo, E.R., Ritvo, E.C., & Brothers, A.M. (1982). Genetic and immunohematologic factors in autism. *Journal of Autism and Developmental Disorders*, **12**, 109–114.

Ritvo, E.R., Freeman, B.J., Mason-Brothers, A., Mo, A., & Ritvo, A.M. (1985). Concordance for the syndrome of autism in 40 pairs of afflicted twins. *American Journal of Psychiatry*, **142**, 74–77.

Rumsey, J.M. & Hamburger, S.D. (1990). Neuropsychological divergence of high-level autism and severe dyslexia. *Journal of Autism and Developmental Disorders*, **20**, 155–168.

Rutter, M. (1978). Language disorder and infantile autism. In M. Rutter & E. Schopler (eds) *Biology of Play*. London: Heinemann Medical Books (pp. 33–44).

Rutter, M. & Schopler, E. (1987). Autism and pervasive developmental disorders: concepts and diagnostic issues. *Journal of Autism and Developmental Disorders*, **17**, 159–186.

Schopler, E. (1985). Editorial: convergence of learning disability, higher-level autism, and Asperger's syndrome. *Journal of Autism and Developmental Disorders*, **15**, 359.

Schopler, E., Reichler, R.J., & Renner, B.R. (1988). *The Childhood Autism Rating Scale (CARS)*. Los Angeles, CA: Western Psychological.

Schuler, A.L. & Prizant, B.M. (1985). Echolalia. In E. Schopler & G. Mesibov (eds) *Communication Problems in Autism*. New York: Plenum.

Shea, V. & Mesibov, G.B. (1985). The relationship of learning disabilities and higher-level autism. *Journal of Autism and Developmental Disorders*, **15**, 425–435.

Siegel, B. (1991). Toward DSM-IV: a developmental approach to autistic disorder. *Psychiatric Clinics of North America*, **14**, 53–68.

Smalley, S.L. (1991). Genetic influences in autism. *Psychiatric Clinics of North America*, **14**, 125–139.

Smalley, S.L., Asarnow, R.F., & Spence, A. (1988). Autism and genetics. *Archives of General Psychiatry*, **45**, 953–961.

Swisher, L. & Demetras, M.J. (1985). The expressive language characteristics of autistic children compared with mentally retarded or specific language-impaired children. In E. Schopler & G. Mesibov (eds) *Communication Problems in Autism*. New York: Plenum (pp. 147–162).

Tager-Flusberg, H., Calkins, S., Nolin, T., Baumberger, T., Anderson, M., & Chadwick-Dias, A. (1990). A longitudinal study of language acquisition in autistic and Down syndrome children. *Journal of Autism and Developmental Disorders*, **20**, 1–22.

Tsai, L., Stewart, M.A., & August, G. (1981). Implications of sex differences in the familial transmission of infantile autism. *Journal of Autism and Developmental Disorders*, **11**, 165–173.

Uzgiris, I. & Hunt, J. (1975). *Assessment in Infancy: Ordinal Scales of Psychological Development*. Urbana, IL: University of Illinois Press.

Wing, L. (1976). Diagnosis, clinical description and prognosis. In L. Wing (ed.) *Early Childhood Autism: Clinical, Educational and Social Aspects, Ed. 2*. Oxford, England: Pergamon Press (pp. 15–48).

Wintre, M.G. & Webster, C.D. (1974). A brief report on using a traditional social behavior scale with disturbed children. *Journal of Applied Behavior Analysis*, **7**, 345–348.

PART III

LEARNING DISABILITIES: CONCEPTS, COMORBIDITY AND HERITABILITY

Introduction

J.H. BEITCHMAN

The nature of dyslexia has long been the subject of controversy. In Chapter 10, Shaywitz and colleagues consider two prevailing views of dyslexia: dyslexia as a discrete categorical entity versus dyslexia as the exteme end of a normal continuum. Shaywitz and colleagues point out that these considerations can have profound implications especially if dimensionally distributed variables are treated as categorical then small shifts in scores can be interpreted as a qualitative change in status.

Using data from the Connecticut Longitudinal Study, Shaywitz and colleagues show that reading ability conforms to a normal distribution so there is a continuum of reading ability and reading disability. Children along this continuum differ by degree not by kind. Shaywitz argues that there is no "hump" in the distribution of reading ability. The trajectory shown by individual growth curve models of reading in two different groups of poor readers are qualitatively similar differing only in degree of severity. Shaywitz et al. conclude that poor readers whether they meet discrepancy criteria or not are united by a shared deficit in phonological processing. Over time, children who are at the lower end of the distribution, whether they meet discrepancy criteria or not, will continue to trail behind their nonreading disabled peers.

The thesis of a deficit in phonological processes as an underlying mechanism in developmental dyslexia (i.e., reading disability) is developed further in Chapter 11 by Vandervelden and Siegel. Phonological processes refer to a hierarchy of developing skills in making use of the systematic relationship between letters and phonemes (the smallest linguistic unit that signals a difference in word meaning) in learning to read and write an alphabetic script. The authors provide a developmental and integrated framework for understanding the role of phonological processing in the acquisition and use of reading and spelling. Vandervelden and Siegel propose that deficits in phonological analytical skill may be as much a consequence as the cause of reading and spelling problems. Also, they emphasize the need to use multiple measures that are developmentally appropriate in both basic research and the clinical/educational assessment of reading disabled children.

In Chapter 12, Faraone, Biederman, and Kiely explore the basis of the school failure and poor cognitive functioning common among ADHD children. Clinical heterogeneity complicates the comprehensive understanding of the cognitive deficits among ADHD children. Of particular interest to these investigators is the overlap between ADHD and learning disability (LD). The role of genetic factors in the emergence of LD among ADHD children is unknown. Faraone and colleagues examine cognitive impairment, school failure and LD among ADHD and normal control subjects and their relatives.

Using family-genetic data to clarify the relation between LD and ADHD by testing competing hypotheses of familial transmission, Faraone and colleagues concluded that these cognitive impairments were not due to co-morbidity. School failure and cognitive functioning among relatives was found to be higher than normal among the relatives of ADHD probands; the nonADHD relatives also showed an increased risk for school failure and cognitive dysfunction.

In examining the association between ADHD and LD, Faraone et al. conclude that these two conditions are etiologically independent but co-occur due to nonrandom mating. These authors believe that the ADHD − LD group show less evidence of school failure than the ADHD + LD group but significantly more school dysfunction than the normal comparison group. ADHD without LD has cognitive consequences that are exacerbated by the presence of LD.

Using data from the Colorado Reading Project, and employing a sophisticated multiple regression approach, DeFries and Light provide compelling evidence for a genetic etiology of reading disability. The heritability estimate suggests that about one-half of the reading performance deficits of probands is due to heritable influences. The authors define reading disabilities on the basis of a composite measure that includes reading recognition, reading comprehension, and spelling, and other diagnostic criteria including an IQ cut-off score of 90. The reading disabled twins studied had marked deficits on measures of phonological coding and segmenting skills. Given the known comorbidity between reading disabilities and ADHD, DeFries and Light also found that ADHD in their sample of reading disabled children was highly heritable. DeFries and Light cite studies showing a possible linkage of reading disability to markers on chromosome 6.

10 A conceptual model and definition of dyslexia: findings emerging from the Connecticut Longitudinal Study

SALLY E. SHAYWITZ, JACK M. FLETCHER, AND
BENNETT A. SHAYWITZ

Although not often discussed directly, the conceptual model describing a particular disorder will influence every aspect of how we think about that disorder and how we operationalize the care of affected individuals, including both how we first go about diagnosing the disorder and then how we go about treating the affected individuals (Shaywitz, Fletcher, & Shaywitz, 1994). What we eventually come to learn about dyslexia including its epidemiology and the characteristics of affected individuals, and how we then choose to address the critical issues of identification, treatment and prognosis will reflect the particular criteria used to define the disorder. How we define any disorder, including dyslexia, in turn reflects the conceptual framework used to think about the disorder. Thus the conceptual framework or model within which a disorder is considered will set the parameters for definition and will be inextricably linked both to the strategies chosen to investigate the disorder itself, and, ultimately, to the clinical care of affected individuals.

The purpose of this chapter is to provide a summary of some of the recent findings that relate to the development of a new conceptual model for reading disability (RD) that have emerged from an epidemiologic study of learning, the Connecticut Longitudinal Study (CLS). Beginning first with an overview of the models of reading disability that have been proposed, we describe how the availability of data from the CLS allowed us to consider each model and then to determine which model fits the data best. We review the various methodologies applied to the CLS data set including those based on general linear models (regression-based and multivariate analyses) and multilevel models of individual change. Reporting the results of each of the different analytic strategies individually, we then indicate how, together, these varied approaches provide convergent evidence that reading and reading disability are part of a continuum with no natural joints separating the two groups. Data from a complementary cross-sectional study of children specifically recruited because of a reading disability are reviewed to demonstrate how they reinforce the findings of the CLS, both in indicating the continuous nature of reading ability and reading disability and in providing insight into the basic underlying deficit responsible for the development of a reading disability. Based on a synthesis of these newer data, recommendations are provided for a definition of reading disability, with discussion of modifications relevant to specific subpopulations, that is bright young adults. Finally, to conclude our discussion of a conceptual framework for RD, we will review issues concerning the identification of reading disability in the context of recent data about the prevalence of reading disability in boys and girls and its relationship to school-identification procedures.

MODELS OF DYSLEXIA

Perhaps the most fundamental finding to emerge from the CLS concerns the basic conceptual model within which reading disability should be regarded. What we mean is whether reading disability represents the extreme of a normal distribution of reading ability so that there is an unbroken continuum from reading ability to reading disability, or, conversely, whether reading disability should be considered as an isolated entity qualitatively separate from normal reading ability. Embedded within this question is whether there are qualitative differences between poor readers who demonstrate a discrepancy between ability and achievement and those who are low achieving for age, but not for ability. The issue is an important one because, as we will discuss, for many years the belief that there were critical differences between these two groups of poor readers served as the rationale for making distinctions between groups of disabled readers, and then, based on these distinctions, for determining eligibility for special education services. Thus, the conceptual model of specific reading disability as a discrete categorical entity had important ramifications for the field, serving as the basis for scientific investigations into the biology of the disorder and also as the scientific rationale for common clinical practices relating to dyslexia including identification of, and provision of services to, children.

Traditional or categorical model

Traditionally, children who experience reading difficulties have been classified into two broad categories with the major interest centered on the group of affected children labeled as dyslexic. Within such a classification, dyslexia has been viewed as a specific categorical entity that affects a small circumscribed group of children, primarily male, who are often referred to as having specific reading retardation (SRR: Rutter, Tizard, & Whitmore, 1970). Thus the terms dyslexia, specific reading retardation and specific reading disability are often used interchangeably. Children with SRR are viewed as having characteristics that are qualitatively distinct from another group of poor readers, poor readers who are considered to have a more general cognitive impairment and thus are referred to as having general reading backwardness (GRB: Rutter et al., 1970), or as garden variety poor readers (Stanovich, 1988) or even more simply, as low achievers. Within such a view, discontinuities or distinct cut points or boundaries exist between the two groups of poor readers, SRR and GRB, so that there are qualitative differences in, for example, the underlying mechanisms and defining characteristics found in children with SRR compared to those with GRB.

The Isle of Wight series of surveys carried out in 1964 and 1965 and reported in the 1970s provided data that were interpreted at the time as providing a rationale as well as empirical support for the classification of SRR as a categorical entity (Rutter & Yule, 1975; Yule & Rutter, 1985). Within the population, these investigators used regression procedures to identify two groups of children with reading difficulty. One, a group of poor readers classified as SRR, manifest a severe discrepancy between observed reading and predicted reading based on age and short form WISC IQ; the other, a more diverse group of children experiencing reading problems, had reading scores below age expectations but not below ability. Since children with SRR read at a level below that predicted by their intelligence, they were referred to as having an unexpected failure to learn to read (Critchley, 1970). This notion of an unexpected failure to learn to read has served as the basis of the traditional definition of dyslexia, a definition often operationalized as a discrepancy between ability (IQ) and reading achievement. Within such a definition and view, other poor readers, that is children who do not manifest such a discrepancy between predicted and observed reading scores, are classified as having GRB and are often not eligible for special educational services.

When these two classifications of poor readers, SRR and GRB, were used to determine the prevalence of each type of reading impairment in the Isle of Wight sample, an overrepresentation (compared to the predicted prevalence rate) of observed children with SRR was reported and interpreted as providing support for the notion that "children with (specific reading retardation) form a 'hump' at the bottom of the normal curve" (Rutter & Yule, 1975, p. 447) (Figure 10.1). These findings then served as the basis for the argument that reading ability is bimodally distributed, with SRR representing the so-called lower hump in the distribution.

Dimensional models

The need to refer to disorders, even those that occur along a continuum, by a specific diagnostic label often obscures the fact that many, if not most disorders in nature, occur in gradations and thus conform to a dimensional rather than a categorical model. Occurring along a continuum, dimensional disorders blend into the normal distribution and require the imposition of, often arbitrary, cut-off points for identification (Figure 10.1). Hypertension and obesity represent two of the most common of the dimensional disorders. Blood pressure, like most physiological parameters (heart rate, temperature), occurs along a continuum; somewhere along the gradient of from low to

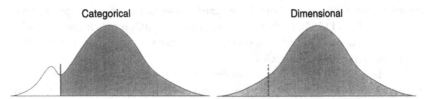

Figure 10.1. Classification models of dyslexia. The categorical models posits that there is a bimodal distribution with a sharply demarcated lower mode. Within the categorical model, this second, lower mode is considered to represent the cases of dyslexia. In contrast, within a dimensional model there is a unimodal distribution and no obvious cut-off point to separate one group of children from another. Within such a dimensional model, children with dyslexia are represented as the extreme lower tail of the distribution; there are no "natural joints" serving as cut-points. While cut-points may be imposed, these are arbitrary and do not necessarily represent a natural break in the distribution of readers. (From Shaywitz, Fletcher, & Shaywitz, 1994.)

high readings, a cut-point is arbitrarily imposed and individuals with values above that reading are considered to have hypertension. Such "hypertensive" individuals will differ in degree, but not necessarily in kind, from individuals on the other side of this cut-off point. Clearly, individuals just on the other side of the cut-point – although not labeled as hypertensive – will share many commonalities with those meeting clinical criteria for hypertension. Within such a dimensional model, there will be quantitative rather than qualitative differences in the characteristics of individuals who may or may not meet these arbitrary criteria. As a function of the normal distribution, there may also be variability in the diagnosis over time. Since individuals with the characteristic or quality in question are distributed along a continuum with no distinct or absolute boundary separating them, individuals may, from time to time, shift positions along the distribution and find themselves on one side or the other of an arbitrarily imposed boundary marker. If a dimensional disorder is clinically defined and treated as a categorical (all-or-none) entity, then small quantitative variations in scores may shift individuals to the other side of the cut-point which then may be misinterpreted as a qualitative change in status (Shaywitz, S.E., et al., 1992a). Such intraindividual variation has recently been described, not only for dyslexia, but also for blood cholesterol levels in children, leading to the conclusion that "the magnitude of within-person variability ... limits the ability to classify children into risk categories recommended by the National Cholesterol Education Program" (Gillman et al., 1992; p. 342). These findings emphasize the limitations of trying to use dimensionally distributed variables, whether they be blood lipids or reading achievement, to assign children to categorical groupings.

Thus, an alternative hypothesis to the categorical model considers dyslexia to represent the lower tail of a continuum of reading disability in which dyslexia blends imperceptibly with normal reading ability. As Blashfield (1984) has noted, such a notion is in contradistinction to the categorical view which rests on the concept of discontinuity. Kendell (1975), as quoted by Blashfield (1984), perhaps best captures the inherent discontinuity intended by the categorical classification model: "Classification is the art of carving nature at the joints, it should indeed imply that there is a joint there, that one is not sawing through bone" (p. 65). In contrast to the natural joint intended by the categorical classification model, the dimensional model of dyslexia posits that there is no natural break, no joint in nature separating dyslexics from children with GRB.

Implications

For many years dyslexia was conceptualized within such a categorical framework. As has been discussed in the above section of this chapter, such a conceptualization is dichotomous and does not encompass shades of gray. Children undergo clinical assessments and a determination is made that they are or are not dyslexic. Often, as we have indicated, based on such a categorical diagnosis, children will or will not receive special education services. Public policy for the provision of such services is formulated on an absolute basis supposed by the categorical model: a child either meets criteria for dyslexia or he or she does not. Like pregnancy, categorical conceptualizations of dyslexia do not have a provision for a touch of, or gradations of dyslexia. A major difficulty with this model occurs when investigators and clinicians attempt to apply this conceptualization to the actual care of children; very few children are either clearly dyslexic or nondyslexic but rather, not surprisingly, fit somewhere in between these two extreme categories. The categorical model does not recognize this group, and most importantly, makes no provisions for either their identification or their need to receive special attention for their reading difficulties. Within such a model, a child first has to fail and fall within the arbitrary cutpoint before becoming eligible for services. Children who fall within the arbitrary cutpoint receive services, those with similar characteristics who happen to fall just beyond the cutpoints, do not receive services. Since reading disability is viewed as a discrete separate entity apart from both other poor readers and normal readers, there is no perceived need for a continuum of services to reflect the continuum of the disability.

With concerns both about the basic theoretical foundation and the clinical infeasibility of the application of the categorical model serving as an impetus, we used the data from the CLS to test the hypothesis, that, rather than a categorical model, reading and reading disability are most appropriately considered within a dimensional framework. In the next sections of this chapter we consider the details of the CIS, and in particular, its design as an epidemiological study within a longitudinal framework, and then provide examples of how the data emerging from such an investigation can be applied to resolve basic questions relating to the conceptual model and definition for reading disability.

THE CONNECTICUT LONGITUDINAL STUDY

The Connecticut Longitudinal Study is an epidemiological study of learning carried out within a developmental framework. More specifically, the CLS is a longitudinal study of a probabilistic sample of Connecticut schoolchildren beginning at the time of kindergarten entry in 1983 and continuing on to the present (1994) time when the children are completing grade 10. These children have been studied annually within their school setting through direct individual assessment and by parent, teacher, and school reports.

The purpose of the CLS is to: (a) investigate the ontogeny of normal cognitive and behavioral development in a representative sample of school-children and (b) examine and gain an understanding of the various risk factors associated with the development of learning and attention problems in children. In particular, the aims of the study are to address questions related to conceptual models, definition, prevalence, demographic characteristics, and course over time of patterns of academic underachievement and attentional problems. Given the interest of our research group in the development of a broad classification system for this diverse group of disorders and our on-going studies of high-density disabled populations of children with learning and attention disorders, this sample is especially informative about the prevalence, stability, and representativeness of subtypes of reading and attention disorders in an epidemiological sample. While the high-density disabled populations of children serve as the basis for the development of a classification system (Morris & Fletcher, 1988; Fletcher, Morris, & Francis, 1992; Shaywitz, Shaywitz, & Fletcher, 1992c); the epidemiologic sample provides information on the generalizability or representativeness of any subtypes that may emerge from the studies of the referred samples.

PROCEDURES

Sample selection

The target population for the CLS was children attending Connecticut public kindergartens during the 1983–4 school year. The population was selected to represent the geographic and demographic diversity within the state. Children included in the study were selected by a two-stage probability sample. The process began with the stratification of the state into six regional areas reflecting educational administrative divisions that were already in place. Each of the 169 towns that exclusively as well as exhaustively partition the state falls within one and only one regional educational area. Twenty-three towns do not have their own school system, but have instead joined with a neighboring town or towns to form nine regional school districts at the elementary level. Therefore, there were 146 towns and nine regional districts, or 155 primary sampling units. Within each of the six regional areas, a systematic sample of a pair of towns (or town and district) was selected with probability proportional to size based on 1981 kindergarten enrollments. The second stage of sampling consisted of the selection of two kindergarten classes within each of the 12 selected communities, these classes were chosen by random numbers so that each class within a town had an equal probability of selection. All of the children in the 24 selected classes were invited to participate in the study. Exclusionary criteria were limited to English not being the primary language, significant sensory impairment and to serious psychiatric difficulty. Of the selected sample, 445 children representing 96.5% participated, including 235 girls (53%) and 210 boys (47%). The sample contained 375 Caucasian (84.3%), 50 African-American (11.2%), 4 Asian (0.9%), 9 Hispanic (2.0%), and 7 children whose race was unknown (1.6%). This racial distribution is comparable to the state of Connecticut for the 1980 census.

Measures

The children's ability and achievement were assessed individually; ability by the Wechsler Intelligence Scales for children (WISC-R) administered in alternate years beginning in grade 1 and achievement by the Reading and Math subtests of the Woodcock–Johnson Psycho-educational Battery (W–J) administered yearly. In the spring of the kindergarten year, a screening assessment was administered to each child using the Kindergarten Early Learning Profile (KELP). The KELP was developed after a review of the pertinent literature had indicated which measures both could be most reliably administered and offered some indication of predictive validity (Shaywitz, 1986). In addition, parents completed the Yale Children's Inventory (YCI: Shaywitz et al., 1986; Shaywitz et al., 1988; Shaywitz et al., 1992b) during the kindergarten year and an abridged form (containing a set of scales empirically derived from the full YCI) which was completed in grades 2 and 4. In the spring of each school year, teachers completed the Multigrade Inventory for Teachers (MIT: Agronin et al., 1992) which contains six empirically derived scales including Academic, Language, Dexterity, Attention, Activity and Behavior. In addition, teachers indicated the child's global classroom behavior, academic achievement and readiness to go on to the next grade and, more specifically, the child's performance relative to his or her peers in reading (decoding and comprehension), arithmetic (computation and problem solving), written expression and handwriting. Information was obtained directly from the school for each participant concerning whether the child has been identified as learning disabled, and, if so, what academic domain is involved (for example, reading or math), which specific educational services were provided and a tally of absences and tardiness.

Maintenance of the sample

The sample, the nature and range of the measures obtained and the longitudinal framework have made it possible to obtain data, unbiased through referral bias or other subject selection factors, concerning the epidemiology, definition, and course of reading disability. Contributing to the generalizability of the data has been the ability of the study to maintain its population relatively intact. In the 11 years since the inception of the study in 1983 the attrition rate has been minimal; currently, in 1994, 414 or 93% of the population are still participating. Thus, although the population has been peripatetic and now live, in addition to Connecticut, in 26 other states and in four foreign countries, the children and their families maintain their participation in the study. In this Chapter, the focus will be on children in the primary school years, from kindergarten to grade 5.

RESULTS

Normal distribution model

As discussed previously, at the time that the CLS population was recruited, the dominant thinking in the field conceptualized reading ability as occurring in a bimodal distribution with specific reading disability or dyslexia over-represented in the extreme lower tail. In contrast, we hypothesized that there was a continuum of reading and reading disability so that reading ability followed a normal distribution, with reading disability at the extreme lower tail of this continuum. Data provided by the CLS allowed a test of this hypothesis. Availability of an epidemiologic sample to whom a complete battery of ability and achievement measures had been administered over time allowed us to systematically and exhaustively test the assumptions underlying the normal model of reading ability and to confirm its validity. Results based on both empirical, graphic methods and more formal statistical tests indicated that a normal distribution model of dyslexia fit the data extremely well leading to the conclusion that "reading difficulties, including dyslexia, occur as part of a continuum that includes normal reading ability" (Shaywitz et al., 1992a, p. 145).

Differences between the Isle of Wight and the Connecticut studies

Several methodologic differences between the Isle of Wight and the Connecticut studies provide a possible explanation for the discrepant findings obtained by the two surveys (Table 10.1). Both the nature of the measures used and the testing procedures themselves offer some insight into the differences in results. Most saliently, the measure of reading used in the British study was selected to identify the poorest readers; several investigators have hypothesized that the reading test itself imposed a ceiling on reading ability and as a consequence skewed the reading scores to the left, causing the artifactual appearance of a hump or lower mode in the Isle of Wight data. Inspection of the distribution data from the Isle of Wight support the notion that rather than an overrepresentation of poor readers, there is an under-representation of good readers (van der Wissel & Zegers, 1985). In addition, although clearly of less importance, a shortened ability measure was used in the British study while the full WISC-R was given to all children in the Connecticut survey. Finally, the data from the Isle of Wight reflect group administered screening procedures while all the Connecticut data were obtained by individual administration of both the ability and the achievement measures. Rather than a two-stage procedure including preliminary screening of the population, in the Connecticut study all children in the selected classes were included and received invitations to participate. Thus, in the Isle of Wight surveys, 3468 children were screened and, of this group, 452 were examined individually; in the Connecticut survey, of the 461 children who were eligible and invited to participate, 445 children received individual assessments. The results of the CLS, based on an individually administered measure of reading which does not impose a ceiling on scores, are consistent with those obtained from other, more recent sample surveys, including those from New Zealand (Silva, McGee, & Williams 1985) and from Great Britain (Rodgers, 1983).

Ontogeny of reading ability

Multilevel models of individual change

Longitudinal data provide information not only on the distribution of reading ability, but also provide a measure of the actual developmental trajectory of reading over time. Such data can then be used as an additional powerful strategy to investigate both the nature of reading disability and the assumptions underlying different definitional models of reading and reading disability. In particular, the availability of a sample survey followed longitudinally allows the examination of the actual growth rates in reading manifest by different groups of readers within the population.

The idea of change, change in the rate of acquisition of a skill, is central to our conceptualization of both learning and learning disability so that failures of learning represent, at their most basic level, departures from the expected, ongoing process of change within the individual. If, indeed, what we are interested in is the learning that has taken, is taking, or will take place

Table 10.1. *Isle of Wight and Connecticut Surveys of Reading*

Isle of Wight	Connecticut Longitudinal Study
Group screening (n = 3468)	Each child individually tested
Examined individually (n = 452)	Examined individually (n = 445)
Reading test – ceiling imposed	Reading test – no ceiling imposed
Shortened ability measure	Full ability measure
Negatively skewed distribution	Normal distribution
Bimodal, artifactual appearance of "hump"	Normal distribution – unimodal

over time, measurement of change over time is the linchpin that holds together the twin concepts of learning and learning disability. What we mean here is not the usual outcome measure consisting of comparisons of discrete group age-standardized achievement scores at specified pre- and post-points in time, but rather the actual measurement of the rate of change as an on-going dynamic process over time (Francis et al., 1994; Shaywitz & Shaywitz, 1994). Such a measurement strategy based on the development of individual growth curves to chart the developmental trajectory of reading offers important advantages for the study and understanding of reading disability in children. The development of individual growth curves shifts the focus from change over time within a group to change over time within an individual and allows change to be viewed as an ongoing and continuous process rather than as an incremental process. Two fundamental assumptions underlie the development of such multilevel models of individual change: (a) that the rate of growth and development of reading varies across students and (b) that this variation will affect both the final level of reading performance, referred to as the *plateau*, and the *age* at which children reach this level of performance. Within such a conceptualization, the ontogeny of reading may differ according to: (a) the rate of change in reading skill (accelerations/decelerations); (b) the final level of reading performance achieved (plateau); and (c) the mathematical or developmental function that best fits the growth pattern, that is, whether it is linear or nonlinear and, if nonlinear, what specific model of growth (i.e., a quadratic growth curve to a plateau) best fits the data.

Discrepancy versus low achievement. The study design of the CLS: a large sample of children, each of whom received multiple assessments over time using the same measure, a measure (Woodcock–Johnson Psychoeducational Battery) providing interval scaling or *Rasch scoring*, met the requirements for the development of individual growth curve models. The availability of an epidemiological sample allowed us to identify different subpopulations, for example, groups meeting ability-achievement based and/or low achievement definitions of reading disability. The discrepancy based definition of reading disability conforms to the traditional categorical model of dyslexia or SRR, while the low achievement definition in which children's observed reading is below that predicted based on age, but not below that predicted based on ability, represents the group referred to as either GRB or garden variety poor readers.

Applying individual growth curve models to the CLS population data allows interindividual differences in intraindividual growth rates to be studied and compared. We can now consider the ontogeny of reading in different groups of poor readers, comparing one group of children classified on the basis of an ability-achievement discrepancy (dyslexic, SRR), to another group meeting criteria for low achievement in reading (GRB). For both groups, discrepant and low achieving, a model that incorporates a quadratic growth curve to a plateau fit the data extremely well. In fact, the shape of the growth curves describing the two reading-disabled groups were qualitatively similar, differing only in level of severity (Figure 10.2). These findings add further support to the notion that poor readers identified on the basis of criteria for SRR and GRB differ only in degree and not qualitatively, a view consistent with the hypothesis that reading ability/disability occurs along a continuum and that SRR represents the lower tail of this distribution (Shaywitz et al., 1992a).

Characteristics of discrepant compared to low achieving readers

Converging evidence from data using other methodological approaches brings further support for the notion that children with SRR and GRR differ in degree, but not in kind. For example, again using data from the survey sample but applying a different methodological strategy, Shaywitz et al. (B. Shaywitz, Fletcher, Holahan, & Shaywitz, 1992) demonstrated that there were more similarities than differences between two groups of poor readers, one meeting criteria for an ability-achievement discrepancy (n = 32), the other, conforming to a definition of reading disability based on low achievement (n = 38). In this series of analyses, the cognitive and behavioral characteristics of children meeting discrepancy based criteria were compared to those of children satisfying a low achievement definition of reading disability; with second grade as an anchor and using parent based, teacher based and child based measures, the groups were compared retrospectively in kindergarten and prospectively in fifth grade. Identification of children meeting criteria for each of the groups provided an indication of the relative degree of reading impairment of the discrepant compared to the low achievement group and quantification of the degree of overlap in prevalence between the two groups. As shown in Figure 10.3 where the standard score for reading and full scale IQ of each of the disabled groups and of a contrast group of nondisabled

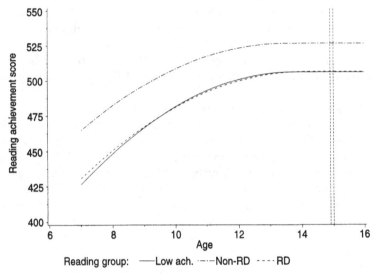

Figure 10.2. Mean achievement curves of three reading groups: children without reading disability ($\cdot\!-\!\cdot\!-$); those in the low achievement group (—); and those in the full scale IQ-achievement discrepant group (- - -). The figure demonstrates that the shape of the curve and the ultimate reading score (plateau) reached is very similar for both the low achievement group and the discrepant group. The nondisabled readers demonstrate a similar shape but reach a much higher level of reading achievement. (From Francis et al., 1994.)

children is plotted, 75% of the discrepant group have reading achievement scores below 90, and thus also meet the criterion for a definition of low reading achievement. Thus, three quarters of the group identified as discrepant would also meet criteria for low achievement in reading; in the remaining 25% of the discrepant group reading achievement scores are above 90 so that these children, while discrepant in reading are not also low achieving. These data, indicating that most children identified as meeting discrepancy criteria are also low achieving, are consistent with those obtained in the Isle of Wight survey where 76/86 (88%) of SRR children also met criteria for GRB (Rutter, Tizard, & Whitmore, 1970).

Comparisons of the performance of the two groups on the KELP, the kindergarten assessment survey, indicated no significant differences in any of five domains of function assessed, including motor and dexterity, language, finger agnosia, and laterality, visual perception, and sentence memory and coding. Parents' perceptions as reported on the Yale Children's Inventory (YCI) indicated that the two groups were also comparable in their histories of health problems, prior diagnoses, pre- and perinatal difficulties, and speech and language problems. The prevalence rate of attention deficit disorder

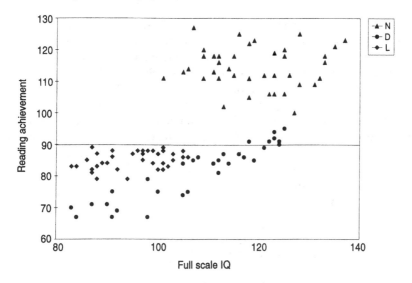

Figure 10.3. Full-Scale IQ and reading achievement in nondisabled children (N) and children with reading disability defined by either discrepancy (D) or low achievement (L) criteria. (From Shaywitz et al., 1992.)

defined by DSM-III (American Psychiatric Association, 1980) criteria using scales provided by the YCI was not significantly different when comparisons were made between the low achieving (56%) and the discrepant (46%) groups. For the most part, as reported on the MIT, teacher's perceptions of the children's in-class academic performance and behavior did not differ between the two groups. The only difference noted occurred in the fifth grade report where teachers viewed children identified as discrepant as having fewer problems with both math processes and math concepts when compared to their low achieving peers. Both in second grade and in fifth grade, there were no group differences in the frequency of identification by the school as requiring special education for reading.

However, while the two groups did not differ on most measures, there were some isolated differences observed; for example, mother's level of education of the low achieving group was significantly lower compared to the discrepancy group. Hypothesizing that the observed differences were a reflection of IQ (which defined the groups), a stepwise multiple regression was performed using group status as the dependent variable and the eight variables on which the groups differed as predictors. When these variables were placed into a discriminant analysis, IQ accounted for nearly all the variance between the two groups with the other variables not adding any significant variance to the discrimination. Thus the most salient differences between poor readers defined on the basis of an ability-achievement discrepancy or simply on the basis of low achievement in reading related to their intellectual ability, a characteristic inherent in the initial definitions of the groups. A number of investigations have now clearly demonstrated that children meeting discrepancy criteria have higher verbal, performance and full scale IQ scores compared to low achieving children (Rutter et al., 1970; Silva et al., 1985; Jorm et al., 1986); however, given how a discrepancy is determined, it is not surprising that children meeting such criteria should have higher IQ scores. In the CLS, the additional use of discriminant analysis demonstrated that other observed group differences were also explainable on the basis of IQ alone. These findings, together with those based on individual growth curve models, support what Stanovich (1991) termed "the correct null hypothesis that there are no qualitative differences between dyslexic and garden-variety poor readers" (p. 23).

CONVERGING EVIDENCE FROM OTHER LINES OF INVESTIGATION

Cognitive profiles of discrepant compared to low achieving readers

Differences in degree, but not in kind

The results of the Connecticut survey coincide with data derived from an investigation based on a different strategy, one in which the sample was specifically selected to address issues of definition and classification of reading disabilities. In this study, children meeting criteria for reading disability (n = 149) were further subdivided into groups meeting either discrepancy or low-achievement definitions (Fletcher et al., 1994). This large and diverse sample of reading disabled children allowed us to further examine the validity of differentiating poor readers on the basis of discrepancy versus low achievement definitions. Comprehensive test batteries using a range of linguistic and parallel non-linguistic measures were administered to each of the subjects. Detailed examination of the resulting cognitive profiles of these groups of disabled readers indicated that there were no qualitative differences between the two groups, the differences that were noted were either small or not significant.

Phonology represents the core deficit in discrepant and low achieving readers

Of particular significance was the finding that deficiencies in phonological processing represented the most severe and consistent deficit in children with reading disability, irrespective of how reading disability was defined. These data are consonant with those obtained by Stanovich & Siegel (1994) who report comparable performance of poor readers, with and without an ability-achievement discrepancy, on measures of phonological processing. Thus, not only are there no qualitative differences in the cognitive profiles of reading disabled children identified on the basis of a discrepancy or a low achievement definition, the two groups share in common what many have hypothesized to be the "core deficit" in reading disability: inadequately developed phonological processing (Liberman et al., 1974; Liberman, Shankweiler, & Liberman, 1989; Goswami & Bryant, 1990; Brady & Shankweiler, 1991; Perfetti, 1991; Vellutino, 1991; Gough, Ehri, & Treiman, 1992). Thus, overwhelming evidence indicates that poor readers have difficulty in appreciating that the orthography of print represents or maps onto the sound structure or phonological elements of spoken language. To read, the beginning reader must develop an awareness that the graphemes he or she sees on the printed page are related to the sounds he or she hears in spoken words. Gradually and over time, the novice reader becomes aware first, of the segmental nature of speech and then, of the internal phonological structure of words. A realization is made that the alphabetic transcription represents speech, and, indeed, has the same number of elements and the same sequence as speech. At last, the ready reader comes to the understanding that the structure of the printed word is related to the phonological structure of the spoken word it represents. Once the beginning reader has made this connection, he or she is said to have mastered the alphabetic principle. These findings that the correlates of reading achievement, linguistic and specifically, phonological processing skills, are similar at all levels of ability provide converging evidence that there are no clear boundaries separating nondisabled and disabled groups and no line of demarcation differentiating disabled readers identified on the basis of a discrepancy or a low achievement criterion. These results thus lend additional support to a dimensional model of reading where both reading ability and disability occur along the same continuum.

CONCLUSION

The nature and definition of reading disability

Deficits in phonological processing define reading disability

What then should be the definition of a reading disability? For too many years, the road to the identification of a reading disability has been littered with artificial barriers requiring children (and adults) to meet arbitrarily imposed criteria such as those requiring an ability-achievement discrepancy. Moreover, and of most concern, we now know that these definitions more often served administrative needs than reflected valid biological underpinnings. Before much was known of the nature of reading disability, there was little choice. Definitions reflected the state of the art, and were therefore distant from and unrelated to the fundamental processes responsible for creating the state of disability in reading. Now that there is an overwhelming consensus that reading disability is related to reading and further that reading reflects language, the opportunity exists for the development of a definition of reading disability that reflects the core deficit affecting disabled readers: phonological processing. As a result of this lower level deficit within the language system, affected individuals experience a predictable range of difficulties in both written and oral language. Thus the effects of the phonological deficit emanate up through the language system and may affect such diverse but phonologically based linguistic processes as decoding, spelling, writing, word naming and retrieval, verbal memory, speech perception, speech production, and listening. The approach of the astute diagnostician of today will very much reflect that first described by Critchley (Critchley, 1981) in searching for the signs of a language disorder in all of its forms. Such indications of a history of a language disorder, particularly one reflecting a deficiency in phonological processing, are much more informative than any statistical gyrations that must be invoked involving the child's scores on a reading and an intelligence test. A recent definition developed by a group of investigators, clinicians, representatives of advocacy groups and representatives from the National Institutes of Health avoids the inadequacies and arbitrary nature of the discrepancy based definition while incorporating newer knowledge about the basic or core deficit underlying reading disability.

Dyslexia is one of several distinct learning disabilities. It is a specific language based disorder of constitutional origin characterized by difficulties in single word decoding, usually reflecting insufficient phonological processing abilities. These difficulties in single word decoding are often unexpected in relation to age and other cognitive and academic abilities; they are not the result of generalized developmental delay or sensory impairment. Dyslexia is manifest by variable difficulty with different forms of language, often including, in addition to problems reading, a conspicuous problem with acquiring proficiency in writing and spelling (Operational definition of the Orton Dyslexia Society Research Committee, 18 April 1994).

The importance of the history in the diagnosis of reading disability

Although there is a tendency to focus on measures rather than the actuality of the life history; for reading disability, a developmental history of difficulties with language, particularly phonologically based components of language, often provides the clearest and most reliable indication of a reading disorder (Shaywitz & Shaywitz, 1994). Phonological processing has been conceptualized as encompassing at least three different components: phonological awareness; phonological recoding in lexical access; and phonetic recoding in working memory (for a comprehensive review, see Wagner & Torgesen, 1987) and the direct measurement of each of these components represents a rational goal of assessment for reading disability. However, while progress is being made, particularly for the assessment of specific phonological components in younger children (Torgesen et al., 1992), the availability of a standardized and reliable test of phonological processing, appropriate for older children and young adults and for very bright individuals, is still more of a goal than a reality. And it is particularly young adults, who are often bright and who have worked extremely hard to compensate for their phonological deficiencies, for whom standard testing and assessment procedures are inadequate. Such individuals will often compensate so that they are accurate in identifying words but will do so at a cost, their decoding skills lack automaticity and thus they decode and read very slowly (Lefly & Pennington, 1991). For these individuals especially, the history is paramount; thus a history of early and continuing difficulties in oral language, for example, in pronouncing words, in reading new or unfamiliar words, in spelling and in writing will represent the distinct diagnostic signature of a reading disability. Speech punctuated by hesitancies and dysfluencies, spelling difficulties, slow and laborious reading and writing represent rich historical data that together provide evidence of a core deficit in phonological processing resulting in the expression of a reading disability. The requirement of excessive amounts of time in relation to the relatively high level of competency achieved represents the hallmark of a reading disability in a compensated dyslexic.

Pending the development of appropriate and sensitive measures of phonological processing applicable to readers of all ages and all levels of intelligence, the history, for clinical purposes, represents the most sensitive and accurate indicator of a reading disability. In younger children, the finding of either a discrepancy and/or low achievement in reading supports the diagnosis of a reading disability. However, as children mature, the brighter ones will learn to compensate and simple reading tests will not be adequate to demonstrate the difficulties that such an individual has in decoding or the energy requirement accurate decoding demands. For these reasons, a history of phonologically based language difficulties, of laborious reading and writing, of poor spelling, of requiring additional time in reading and taking tests, provides indisputable evidence of a deficiency in phonological processing which, in turn, serves as the basis for, and signature of, a reading disability.

Further insights into the identification of disabled readers

Gender differences

Traditional notions of dyslexia not only envisioned a categorical model, but also considered the disorder to affect primarily boys. In fact, the perceived male prevalence in dyslexia was often invoked to support the biological basis for the disorder. While dyslexia is undoubtedly biologically based, it is neither necessary, nor correct to invoke either a categorical model or an excess of affected boys, to support this view. Data emerging from the CLS demonstrate that reading disability is as prevalent in young girls as in young boys (Shaywitz et al., 1990) and, at the same time, provide insights into factors contributing to the once widely held perception that dyslexia is primarily a disorder affecting males.

Reading disability represents a unique disorder. While biologically based, reading disability is most typically manifest and expressed within the context of the classroom. Consequently, the identification of children as reading disabled is often dependent on educational processes and procedures. Children identified as reading disabled through such school-identification processes are those who eventually go on to receive special education services, and are also those who represent the target population from which most research samples are constituted. Hypothesizing that results indicating a higher prevalence of dyslexia in boys compared to girls in school-identified samples of reading disabled children may reflect a bias in sample-selection, we investigated the prevalence of reading disability in two groups of boys and girls within the CLS population: one, research-identified on the basis of individual assessment of reading skills; the other, school-identified through the usual school-based identification procedures. Our findings indicated that, in the early primary grades (second and third grade), four times as many boys as girls are identified as reading disabled by their schools, a finding consonant with other reports in the literature which were also based on such school-identified populations (Finucci & Childs, 1981). However, data based on research-identification procedures, procedures in which all children in the CLS population were each individually assessed for a reading disability, indicated that there were no significant differences in the prevalence of reading disability in boys compared to girls (Shaywitz et al., 1990). Most recently, these results have been replicated in a study of 708 first and third grade students attending 26 midwestern schools (Flynn & Rahbar, 1994). Comparable to the Connecticut survey, these investigators report the absence of a gender effect on categories of reading disability in grades one and three with gender ratios falling between 1.1 to 1.4:1 for boys compared to girls meeting criteria for reading disability. In contrast, at both grades, teachers identified more than twice as many boys as girls as requiring remedial services in reading.

Our initial report on reading performance and behavioral ratings for boys and girls encompassed the very early primary grades, grades 1–3 (Shaywitz et al., 1990); in this section, we extend these findings up through the fifth grade. For these analyses, the CLS sample was again divided into two groups: a reading disabled group (RD) who met a Full Scale IQ (WISC-R) reading achievement (Woodcock-Johnson Psychoeducational Battery, reading cluster) regression-based discrepancy and a non-reading-disabled group (nonRD) who did not meet these criteria. We found no gender effects for reading, but a significant main effect for RD status. Thus reading scores of boys and girls were comparable in these grades, while the RD group performed significantly more poorly when compared to the nonRD group. Parents' and teachers' ratings of the subjects indicated that parents of sons, compared to parents of daughters, perceived their children as having more behavioral difficulties. Specifically, boys were rated as demonstrating more difficulties in the following scale domains of the YCI: Activity, Attention, Impulsivity, Aggression and Manageability. There were no significant gender effects apparent for ratings on scales that either reflected cognitive performance or internalizing behaviors: Academics, Language, Socialized Conduct Disorder and Negative Affect. There was consistency, in most areas, between parent and teacher ratings. Thus, on the MIT, teachers also rated boys compared to girls as showing higher activity levels, inattention and behavior problems, and as having poorer dexterity. When compared to nonRD subjects, RD subjects were rated as functioning more poorly in the areas of academics, attention, language and dexterity.

These data indicate that there are significant differences between the most visible and perhaps, most intrusive behaviors manifest by normal boys compared to normal girls. In general, boys compared to girls tend to exhibit higher levels of externalizing behaviors that are most likely to be disruptive in class and to attract their teacher's attention. There are no significant (RD) group differences in any of the highly externalizing behaviors; thus these behaviors should not be considered as characteristic of children with reading disability. Rather, school-identification procedures are often based on these behaviors so that as a result, populations of such school-identified disabled readers are reported as exhibiting more behavior problems. For example, in a previous report (Shaywitz et al., 1990), we noted that behavioral problems significantly differentiate reading-disabled children who are and are not identified by their schools. These data indicate that teachers' perceptions of what constitutes inappropriate behavior enter into the school-identification process for reading disability, and that, in particular, increased levels of activity and behavior problems are likely to be disruptive to a classroom and to influence decisions about such children.

A symptom complex for reading disability

These findings provide yet another level of information in directing approaches for the most appropriate and targeted identification of reading disabled individuals. Together with the results of the cognitive profiles of the large population of reading disabled children (Fletcher et al., 1994), we now know both where to look and where not to look for indications of a reading disability. Yes, there is a symptom complex characterizing reading disability; however, such symptoms emerge from the cognitive, and not, the behavioral domain. Reading disability is primarily a disorder of language, and thus the pathognomonic signs of a reading disorder will reflect phonological deficits, not only in reading, spelling and writing, but within a symptom complex of oral language and listening difficulties. Children who should be identified as at-risk for a reading disability are those who demonstrate evidence of an underlying phonological deficit having permeated the varied components of their language performance. Behavioral difficulties and increased activity levels should not be considered as part of a syndrome of reading disability, although these behavioral problems may, at times, co-occur with RD. We emphasize, the absence of behavioral difficulties should not be taken as an indication that a child does not harbor a reading disability. These findings are especially important for the identification of reading disability in girls. Data from several lines of investigation now clearly indicate that girls are no less at-risk for reading disability than are boys. Girls who demonstrate difficulties with phonologically based language skills should be referred for a possible reading disability; it is no longer acceptable to neglect and to under-identify girls who may be reading disabled, but quiet in class.

SUMMARY

These converging series of data now provide a much clearer conceptual model of the nature of reading disability, and further provide important information concerning approaches to the definition of reading disability. The belief that there were qualitative differences between poor readers who did and did not demonstrate a significant ability-achievement discrepancy was at the very heart of the most widely used definition of reading disability, and went even further in providing a scientific rationale for a public policy which provides special education for poor readers meeting discrepancy criteria, but not for other poor readers. Evidence now from several lines of investigation and using varied methodologies are all converging to indicate that the basic assumptions underlying the categorical model of reading disability are not receiving empirical support.

Reading ability conforms to a normal distribution model so that there is a continuum of reading ability and reading disability. Children along this continuum differ by degree but not in kind. Cut points may be instituted to segment this continuous distribution but these will be arbitrary and will not reflect any natural joints in nature; there is no second mode or "hump" in the distribution of reading ability. This continuity of reading ability and disability across the population is further demonstrated by the developmental trajectory shown by individual growth curve models of reading in two different groups of poor readers; the developmental functions fitting these trajectories are qualitatively similar, differing only in degree of severity. Similarly, the addition of a developmental perspective indicates that, over time, children who are at the lower end of the distribution – whether they meet discrepancy criteria or not – will continue to trail behind their non-reading disabled peers. Further, when the behavioral and cognitive characteristics of discrepant and low achieving poor readers are compared, the only meaningful differences are those that can be accounted for by the initial IQ disparity, a disparity which is inherent in the definitions of the two groups. These data obtained by complementary methodologies applied to a sample survey followed longitudinally are supported by data obtained from much more detailed assessments of samples explicitly recruited for meeting different definitional criteria for reading disability.

In addition to what they reveal about the basic nature of reading disability, these data are important, too, for what they tell us about where to look for a more fuller understanding of the mechanisms responsible for reading disability. The normal model of reading and reading disability indicates that reading disability is related to reading, that there is a seamless transition from one to the other. Awareness of this relationship is critical to our approach to understanding the basis of reading disability. Rather than reading disability representing a totally deviant and separate process apart from normal reading ability, we now appreciate that there is a continuum of reading skills which embraces both superior and average readers as well as poor readers, both discrepant and low achieving. This finding means that the large body of theoretical and practical knowledge that has been gained about reading can now be applied to the study of reading disability.

From a more clinical perspective, the notion of a continuum of reading and reading disability offers insight into the instructional needs of a range of readers. This view of reading brings a sense of unity and consistency to the approach to children who experience reading difficulty, for it indicates that struggling readers, no matter what side of an arbitrary cutpoint they may happen to find themselves, require help and require help for a quite similar pattern of deficiencies – those involving phonological processing. Thus interventions directed at the deficits in phonological processing would be beneficial to problem readers whether or not they meet discrepancy criteria. There is no scientific basis to deny a child who is experiencing difficulties reading either educational support or accommodations as reading disabled because that child does not meet discrepancy criteria for reading disability. It is also important to note that children who do meet discrepancy criteria but who are not low achieving, often children with higher IQs, also require assistance. Furthermore, there is now overwhelming evidence that phonological processing represents the basic core deficit in reading disability. Poor readers, whether they meet discrepancy criteria or not, are united by a shared deficit in phonological processing. This basic deficit in phonological processing drives the identification process, provides a template for understanding the associated symptomology of poor readers and indicates a direction for intervention for disabled readers along the continuum. Awareness of the phonological basis of reading and reading disability is particularly critical for the identification of older bright dyslexics, who may decode accurately but at a great cost in time. For these individuals, the signature of a reading disability will be found in the history, a history of phonologically based language difficulties involving both spoken and written language.

ACKNOWLEDGMENTS

This research was supported by grants from NICHD (POı HD21888 and P50 HD25802).

The authors wish to thank the parents, children and educators whose participation in the Connecticut Longitudinal Study has contributed so much to furthering our understanding of reading and reading disability. The contributions of Abigail Shneider, MA in coordinating the study and John Holahan, PhD in managing the data are also acknowledged.

REFERENCES

Agronin, M.E., Holahan, J.M., Shaywitz, B.A., & Shaywitz, S.E. (1992). The Multi-Grade Inventory for Teachers (MIT): Scale development, reliability, and validity of an instrument to assess children with attentional deficits and learning disabilities. In S.E. Shaywitz & B.S. Shaywitz (eds) *Attention Deficit Disorder Comes of Age: Toward the Twenty-first Century*. Austin, TX: Pro-Ed (pp. 89–116).

American Psychiatric Association (1980). *Diagnostic and Statistical Manual of Mental Disorders,* 3rd edn *(DSM III)*. Washington, DC: American Psychiatric Association.

Blashfield, R.K. (1984). *The Classification of Psychopathology: NeoKraepelinian and Quantitative Approaches*. New York: Plenum Press.

Brady, S.A. & Shankweiler, D.P. (eds) (1991). *Phonological Processes in Literacy: A Tribute to Isabelle Y. Liberman*. Hillsdale, NJ: Lawrence Erlbaum.

Critchley, M. (1970). *The Dyslexic Child*. Springfield, IL: Charles C. Thomas.

Critchley, M. (1981). Dyslexia: An overview. In G.T. Pavlidis & T.R. Miles (eds) *Dyslexia Research and its Applications to Education*. Chichester: John Wiley (pp. 1–11).

Finucci, J.M. & Childs, B. (1981). Are there really more dyslexic boys than girls? In A. Ansara, N. Geschwind, M. Albert, & N. Gartrell (eds) *Sex Differences in Dyslexia*. Towson, MD: Orton Dyslexia Society (pp. 1–9).

Fletcher, J.M., Morris, R.D., & Francis, D.J. (1992). Methodological issues in the classification of attention-related disorders. In S.E. Shaywitz & B.S. Shaywitz (eds) *Attention Deficit Disorder Comes of Age: Toward the Twenty-first Century*. Austin, Texas: Pro-Ed (pp. 13–28).

Fletcher, J.M., Shaywitz, S.E., Shankweiler, D.P., Katz, L., Liberman, I.Y., Stuebing, K.K., Francis, D.J., Fowler, A.E., & Shaywitz, B.A. (1994). Cognitive profiles of reading disability: comparisons of discrepancy and low achievement definitions. *Journal of Educational Psychology, 86*, 6–23.

Flynn, J.M. & Rahbar, M.H. (1994). Prevalence of reading failure in boys compared with girls. *Psychology in the Schools, 31*, 66–71.

Francis, D.J., Shaywitz, S.E., Stuebing, K.K., Shaywitz, B.A., & Fletcher, J.M. (1994). The measurement of change: assessing behavior over time and within a developmental context. In G. Reid Lyon (ed.) *Frames of Reference for the Assessment of Learning Disabilities: New Views on Measurement Issues*. Baltimore, MD: Paul H. Brookes (pp. 29–58).

Gillman, M.W., Cupples, L.A., Moore, L.L., & Ellison, R.C. (1992). Impact of within-person variability on identifying children with hypercholesterolemia: Framingham Children's Study. *Journal of Pediatrics*, **121**, 342–347.

Goswami, U. & Bryant, P. (1990). *Phonological Skills and Learning to Read*. Hillsdale, NJ: Lawrence Erlbaum.

Gough, P.B., Ehri, L.C., & Treiman, R. (eds) (1992). *Reading Acquisition*. Hillsdale, NJ: Lawrence Erlbaum.

Jorm, A.F., Share, D.L., Maclean, R., & Matthews, R. (1986). Cognitive factors at school entry predictive of specific reading retardation and general reading backwardness: a research note. *Journal of Child Psychology and Psychiatry*, **27**, 45–54.

Kendell, R.E. (1975). *The Role of Diagnosis in Psychiatry*. Oxford: Blackwell Scientific Publications.

Lefly, D.L. & Pennington, B.F. (1991). Spelling errors and reading fluency in compensated adult dyslexics. *Annals of Dyslexia*, **41**, 143.

Liberman, I.Y., Shankweiler, D., Fischer, F.W., & Charter, B. (1974). Explicit syllable and phoneme segmentation in the young child. *Experimental Child Psychology*, **18**, 201–212.

Liberman, I.Y., Shankweiler, D., & Liberman, A.M. (1989). The alphabetic principle and learning to read. In D. Shankweiler & I.Y. Liberman (eds) *International Academy for Research in Learning Disabilities Monograph Series: Number 6. Phonology and reading disability, Solving the reading puzzle*. Ann Arbor: University of Michigan Press (pp. 1–33).

Morris, R.D. & Fletcher, J.M. (1988). Classification in neuropsychology: a theoretical framework and research paradigm. *Journal of Clinical and Experimental Neuropsychology*, **10**, 640–658.

Perfetti, C.A. (1991). On the value of simple ideas in reading instruction. In S.A. Brady & D.P. Shankweiler (eds) *Phonological Processes in Literacy, A tribute to Isabelle Y. Liberman*. Hillsdale, NJ: Lawrence Erlbaum (pp. 211–218).

Rodgers, B. (1983). The identification and prevalence of specific reading retardation. *British Journal of Educational Psychology*, **53**, 369–373.

Rutter, M., Tizard, J., & Whitmore, K. (1970). *Education, Health, and Behavior*. London: Longman.

Rutter, M. & Yule, W. (1975). The concept of specific reading retardation. *Journal of Child Psychology and Psychiatry*, **16**, 181–197.

Shaywitz, B.A., Fletcher, J.M., Holahan, J.M., & Shaywitz, S.E. (1992). Discrepancy compared to low achievement definitions of reading disability: results from the Connecticut Longitudinal Study. *Journal of Learning Disabilities*, **25**, 639–648.

Shaywitz, B.A. & Shaywitz, S.E. (1994). Learning disabilities and attention disorders. In K.F. Swaiman (ed.) *Pediatric Neurology*, 2nd edn. St. Louis, MO: Mosby (pp. 1119–1151).

Shaywitz, B.A., Shaywitz, S.E., & Fletcher, J.M. (1992c). The Yale Center for the Study of Learning and Attention Disorders. *Learning Disabilities*, **3**, 1–12.

Shaywitz, S.E. (1986). Early Recognition of Educational Vulnerability-EREV. Technical report. Hartford, CT: Connecticut State Department of Education.

Shaywitz, S.E., Escobar, M.D., Shaywitz, B.A., Fletcher, J.M., & Makuch, R. (1992a). Evidence that dyslexia may represent the lower tail of a normal distribution of reading ability. *New England Journal of Medicine*, **326**, 145–150.

Shaywitz, S.E., Fletcher, J.M., & Shaywitz, B.A. (1994). A new conceptual model for dyslexia. In A.J. Capture, P.J. Accardo, & B.K. Shapiro (eds) *Learning Disabilities Spectrum: ADD, ADHD, and LD*. Timonium, MD: York Press (pp. 1–15).

Shaywitz, S.E., Holahan, J.M., Marchione, K.E., Sadler, A.E., and Shaywitz, B.A. (1992b). The Yale Children's Inventory: normative data and their implications for the diagnosis of attention deficit disorder in children. In S.E. Shaywitz & B.A. Shaywitz (eds) *Attention Deficit Disorder Comes of Age: Toward the Twenty-first Century*. Austin, TX: Pro-Ed (pp. 29–67).

Shaywitz, S.E., Schnell, C., Shaywitz, B.A., and Towle, V.R. (1986). Yale Children's Inventory (YCI): an instrument to assess children with attentional deficits and learning disabilities I. Scale development and psychometric properties. *Journal of Abnormal Child Psychology*, **14**, 347–364.

Shaywitz, S.E., Shaywitz, B.A., Fletcher, J.M., & Escobar, M.D. (1990). Prevalence of reading disability in boys and girls: results of the Connecticut longitudinal study. *Journal of the American Medical Association*, **264**, 998–1002.

Shaywitz, S.E., Shaywitz, B.A., Schnell, C., & Towle, V.R. (1988). Concurrent and predictive validity of the Yale Children's Inventory: an instrument to assess children with attentional deficits and learning disabilities. *Pediatrics*, **81**, 562–571.

Silva, P.A., McGee, R., & Williams, S. (1985). Some characteristics of 9-year-old boys with general reading backwardness or specific reading retardation. *Journal of Child Psychology and Psychiatry*, **26**, 407–421.

Stanovich, K.E. (1988). Explaining the differences between the dyslexic and the garden-variety poor reader: the phonological-core variable-difference model. *Journal of Learning Disabilities*, **21**, 590–604.

Stanovich, K.E. (1991). Discrepancy definitions of reading disability: has intelligence led us astray? *Reading Research Quarterly*, **26**, 7–29.

Stanovich, K.E. & Siegel, L.S. (1994). Phenotypic performance profile of children with reading disabilities: a regression-based test of the phonological-core variable-difference model. *Journal of Educational Psychology*, **86**, 24–53.

Torgesen, J.K., Wagner, R.K., Bryant, B.R., & Pearson, N. (1992). Toward development of a kindergarten group test for phonological awareness. *Journal of Research and Development in Education*, **25**, 113–120.

van der Wissel, A. & Zegers, F.E. (1985). Reading retardation revisited. *British Journal of Developmental Psychology*, **3**, 3–9.

Vellutino, F.R. (1991). Introduction to three studies on reading acquisition: convergent findings on theoretical foundations of code-oriented versus whole-language approaches to reading instruction. *Journal of Educational Psychology*, **83**, 437–443.

Wagner, R.K. & Torgesen, J.K. (1987). The nature of phonological processing and its causal role in the acquisition of reading skills. *Psychological Bulletin,* **101**, 192–212.

Wechsler, D. (1991). *Wechsler Intelligence Scale for Children,* 3rd edn. San Antonio, TX: Harcourt, Brace, Jovanovich.

Woodcock, R.W. & Johnson, M. B. (1989). *Woodcock-Johnson Psycho-educational Battery – Revised.* Allen, TX: Developmental Learning Materials.

Yule, W. & Rutter, M. (1985). Reading and other learning difficulties. In M. Rutter & L. Hersov (eds) *Child and Adolescent Psychiatry: Modern Approaches,* 2nd edn. Oxford: Blackwell Scientific (pp. 444–464).

11 Phonological recoding deficits and dyslexia: a developmental perspective

MARGARETHA C. VANDERVELDEN AND LINDA S. SIEGEL

Research indicates a persuasive role for phonological processing in the acquisition and use of written language. Phonological processing refers to "the use of phonological information (i.e., the sounds of one's language) in processing written and oral language" (Wagner & Torgesen, 1987, p. 197). It pertains to the articulatory/acoustic characteristics of language and the limited set of linguistic units, or phonemes, that are the basis for constructing the vocabulary of a language (e.g., Liberman & Shankweiler, 1985; Liberman et al., 1985). In this chapter we will discuss phonological processing in the acquisition of reading and focus on phonological processing deficits at the word level for several reasons. First, research consistently points to the word level to account for differences in reading skill, and fluency in word reading is fundamental to comprehension (e.g., Biemiller, 1977/1978; Gough & Tunmer, 1986; Lesgold & Curtis, 1981; Perfetti, 1985; Perfetti & Hogaboam, 1975; Rack, Snowling, & Olson, 1992; Stanovich, 1982, 1986a; Stanovich, Cunningham, & West, 1981). Biemiller (1970) found that differences in word level skill accounted for differences in comprehension as early as grade one. Secondly, research also indicates that differences in speed and accuracy in pseudoword reading most clearly differentiate skilled from less skilled readers (e.g., Perfetti & Hogaboam, 1975; Siegel, 1985, 1986, 1992; Siegel & Ryan, 1984, 1988, 1989; Stanovich, 1982, 1986b). Pseudowords are pronounceable combinations of letters, and speed and accuracy of pseudoword reading is an index of skill in using the systematic relationship between the letters in print and the phonemes underlying spoken language in reading unknown words. Such skill has variously been called "phonological recoding in lexical access" (Wagner & Torgesen, 1987), "pre-lexical phonological recoding" (e.g., Jorm & Share, 1983; McCusker, Hillinger, & Bias, 1981), and "cipher reading" (Gough & Hillinger, 1980). Ehri and Wilce (1987a) note that the still most prevalent term is "decoding," or "sounding out and blending." The present chapter will use "phonological recoding" as a superordinate term for a set of gradually developing skills in making use of the systematic relationship between letters and phonemes in learning to read and write an alphabetic script. If reading groups are defined in terms of word-reading skill, results of studies uniformly show that developmental dyslexia, or reading disability, is characterized by a deficit in phonological recoding and related phonological processing (see, e.g., Metsala & Siegel, 1992, for a review of issues in defining developmental dyslexia).

First, we will first address the role of phonological recoding in reading, discuss evidence for the relationship between phonological recoding deficits and reading disability, and present a developmental framework for viewing deficits in phonological recoding and their effects on the acquisition of a reading vocabulary. Next, we will address deficits in phonological recoding in terms of its component phonological processing skills: verbal coding and phoneme awareness. In this chapter, verbal coding refers to the use of known phonological information; that is, phonological information stored for letters, words, and syllables. For example, naming letters or pictures, or making judgments on rhyme between two or more visually presented stimuli, requires that a phonological (verbal) code for these stimuli is stored in memory that can be retrieved. Based on the definition proposed by Tunmer, Herriman, & Nesdale (1988), phoneme awareness is defined as recognition of the phoneme structure underlying spoken words and an ability to segment this structure. An example of an easy phoneme recognition task is: "Listen for /s/. /sick/. Does /sick/ have a /s/?" After presentation of a target phoneme and spoken word that may or may not contain the phoneme, the child responds "Yes" or "No" (Vandervelden & Siegel, 1995). An example of an easy segmentation task is asking children to articulate separately the initial consonant in spoken words: (e.g., "Say /sick/. What is the first sound in /sick/?") (see Lewkowicz, 1980, for a review of tasks). A common but more difficult segmentation task is deletion and segmentation: for example, "Say /sick/. Now say it again but instead of /s/ say /p/" (slashes will be used to indicate phonemes or spoken words and syllables and *italic* to indicate letters or spoken words and syllables).

PHONOLOGICAL RECODING

The strong relationship between pseudoword and word reading may seem to be in support of the theoretical position that words in reading are accessed in the internal lexicon (i.e., the hypothesized word store in memory) through a phonological pathway. However, there is evidence for the use of a direct visual or orthographic pathway also. For example, it is a well-documented finding that high-frequency words are read faster than low-frequency words with similar orthographic characteristics (e.g., *make*, a high-frequency word, would be read faster than *rake*, a low-frequency word) and that this difference in naming speed for printed words occurs relatively early in development (e.g., Barron & Baron, 1977; Bruck, 1988, 1990). Even so, skill in phonological recoding continues to develop throughout childhood (e.g., Backman et al., 1984). These two phenomena of normal development – that is, use of a visual pathway on the one hand, and, on the other hand, the importance of and continued development in phonological recoding – are captured in amalgamation theory (Ehri, 1978, 1980, 1984). In amalgamation theory, Ehri proposes that learning to read involves the acquisition of an orthographic form for words alongside already stored phonological and semantic/grammatical information. Once the orthographic form of a word has been acquired, direct visual access becomes possible. However, the orthographic form is acquired alongside the phonological form by making use of phonological recoding.

The important role of phonological recoding in the acquisition of a reading vocabulary is also indicated by differences in speed and accuracy in reading regular and exception words. Examples of regular words are *dog* and *take*, whose pronunciation is strongly predictable from the application of general letter (grapheme) to phoneme conversion (GPC) rules. General rule application has been suggested as one strategy for reading pseudowords or unknown words (Coltheart, 1978). In contrast to regular words, in exception words the application of GPC rules gives only some clues (e.g., *put, laugh, yacht*), minimal clues (e.g., *one*), or no clues (e.g., *eye*) to pronunciation. By definition, therefore, the reading of regular and exception words is differentially predicted by phonological recoding and this difference predicts that regular words are easier to learn than irregular words. Evidence for what is usually referred to as the regularity effect is particularly pronounced in the earlier grades and for low-frequency words (e.g., Siegel & Faux, 1989).

Deficits in phonological recoding and reading disability

The difference in naming speed between high- and low-frequency words that we noted earlier suggests that experience (i.e., the number of encounters with a printed word) also affects how words are processed. For that reason, deficits in phonological recoding in cases of reading disability are now usually investigated not only by comparing age-matched normal and disabled readers (who therefore differ in reading level), but also by comparing normal and disabled readers at the same reading achievement level, who therefore differ in age. These two kinds of comparisons between reader groups are referred to, respectively, as age-matched and reading level matched designs.

Rack et al. (1992) have presented an extensive review of studies which used a reading level match design in investigating the pseudoword reading deficit in reading-disabled children. The authors found that in the majority of the studies dyslexic readers performed more poorly in pseudoword reading than the reading level matched controls. Because these studies compared normal and disabled readers of equal reading skill, the results of these studies suggest that a comparatively large reading vocabulary may be acquired in spite of deficient phonological recoding skills. Bruck (1990) and Shafir & Siegel (1991) also report that although many adults with a reading problem may become reasonably accurate, they still continue to read words slowly and to have difficulties reading pseudowords. Bruck (1990) also observed that in spite of the continued deficit in pseudoword and word reading, dyslexics, in contrast to normal readers, continued to rely on phonological recoding, especially for multisyllable words. She explained the overreliance on phonological recoding on the one hand, and the continued deficit in word and pseudoword reading, on the other, by suggesting that dyslexic adults had failed to acquire accurate orthographic representations at the syllable level. It may be noted that syllable level orthographic representations (e.g., -*ake* or *bea* in *make* and *beak*, respectively) and their pronunciations are critical to an analogy strategy, which has been suggested as another way in which words (or pseudowords) can be read (e.g., Baron, 1977; Glusko, 1979; Kay & Marcel, 1981). Analogy may come to play a role in written word learning relatively early in normal development (e.g., Goswami, 1986, 1988, 1990; Goswami & Mead, 1992).

Evidence for a specific deficit in phonological recoding but not in specific word learning has also been found in studies which have used tasks other than pseudoword reading. For example, Olson et al. (1985) found that normal and reading-disabled children differed on a phonological but not on a lexical choice task (e.g., which of two identical-sounding letter strings *rain* and *rane* is the correct spelling for a word). Reading-disabled children also show a deficit in phonological recoding in spelling pseudowords (e.g., Siegel & Ryan, 1988; Waters, Bruck, & Seidenberg, 1985). They also have problems in matching a spoken pseudoword to its printed equivalent. For example, Siegel & Ryan (1984) used a subtest of the Gates–McKillop Test (Gates & McKillop, 1962) called recognizing the visual form of sounds. After hearing the pronunciation of the pseudoword, for example /whiskate/, subjects selected the correct version of the word from among four printed choices: *iskate, wiskay, whiskate,* and *whestit*. Although few of the 11–14-year-old normal readers made any errors on this task, most of the reading-disabled children made at least four errors and many made more. As Siegel and Ryan point out, since on this task children need only *recognize* the written form of a pseudoword they hear, the problem in phonological recoding is not limited to pseudoword reading, but includes recognition level recoding also.

Phonological recoding: developmental progression

One of the findings that emerges from the research is that phonological recoding is not an all-or-none phenomenon, but that it is a set of skills that develops over a time span which may include most of the elementary grades, even for normal readers (Siegel & Faux, 1989). If phonological recoding refers to a set of skills, research into reading disability must start to pay greater attention to developmental changes and what factors may determine development.

Developmental progression: orthographic complexity

Vellutino & Scanlon (1987) have suggested that poor readers are not sensitive to the structural regularities in complex representational systems such as English orthography. To investigate differences between normal and disabled readers in phonological recoding along a continuum of complexity for words and pseudowords, Siegel & Faux (1989) included simple consonant /vowel/ consonant (CVC) spellings, such as *dog*, or the pseudoword *mog*, as the easiest set. They also investigated accuracy in reading one-syllable words and pseudowords with blends, with spellings other than a single medial (short) vowel, and the reading of multisyllable words and pseudowords.

First, Siegel & Faux (1989) found that accuracy in reading the one-syllable words and pseudowords developed first. For the normal readers, this skill was at ceiling for the age group 9–10. However, the 11–14-year-old disabled readers attained the level of performance comparable to that of the normal 6–8-year-old. Although in word reading the 11–14-year-old disabled readers differed from normals by three years, in simple pseudoword reading the groups differed by as much as 5–6 years. Whereas accuracy in reading the one-syllable, one-vowel pseudowords with blends developed next in both groups, the reading-disabled group showed again a large developmental lag.

One consistent finding of the research is that inaccuracies in reading pseudowords in early normal development and in reading disability result from errors in vowel rather than consonant recoding (e.g., Fowler, Shankweiler, & Liberman, 1979; Vandervelden & Siegel, 1995; Weber, 1970). One explanation suggested for the greater difficulty of vowel recoding is that vowel phonemes are less clearly defined than consonant phonemes and are more subject to individual and dialect variations (Fowler, Liberman, & Shankweiler, 1977). However, the increased likelihood of vowel errors does not appear to be a result of inadequate perception of sounds or difficulties with speaking. When children were asked to repeat the words that they had been asked to read, Shankweiler & Liberman (1972) found that fewer errors occurred in vowels than consonants.

Another explanation for the relatively greater difficulty in vowel recoding is in terms of its complexity. First, each English vowel letter represents more than one phoneme, and accuracy in recoding the vowel letter in printed strings (words and pseudowords) depends on the orthographic context (i.e., the letters that follow the vowel). For example, the letter *a* in *cat* represents the same vowel phoneme in *cab* or *back*, but different phonemes in *bar* or *bake*. Thus, accuracy in reading even simply spelled consonant /vowel/ consonant (CVC) pseudowords involves complex rule application (i.e., short vowel sound, because the vowel letter is followed by one or more consonant letters and no other vowel). Alternatively, accuracy in pseudoword reading requires knowledge of syllable level orthographic representations, as suggested by

Bruck (1990) and applied in an analogy strategy (e.g., -*og* in *dog* to read *fog*). In a developmental study that investigated accuracy of vowel recoding on a pseudoword reading task with grade 2, 3, and 4 students, Fowler et al. (1979) found that most responses to vowels were not random but reflected the possible sounds for that vowel. Context-dependent responses (e.g., responses that reflected knowledge of orthographic patterns for short and long vowels) increased with age, but were evident in normal readers even after about one year of reading instruction.

Other studies confirm that reading-disabled children may have particular problems in the correct recoding of vowels in reading words and pseudo-words, but that the patterns of development are similar to those of normal readers. For example, Seidenberg et al. (1986) found that disabled readers made more vowel than consonant errors. Most of these errors involved incorrect lengthening or shortening of the vowel, indicating that the disabled readers made the same type of vowel errors reported for normal readers in the study by Fowler et al. (1979). However, the more severely disabled readers produced errors that involved substitutions of a totally different vowel (e.g., /lake/ for *like*). Also, whereas good readers tended to produce mispronuncia-tions of the target vowel on the exception words (e.g., *come*), and tended to regularize these (e.g., *come* pronounced to rhyme with /home/; or *says* with /days/), disabled readers were less likely to make such errors, indicating a difficulty with complex rule learning.

Furthermore, compared to consonants, orthographic representations of vowel phonemes more often than not involve considerable variability, including digraphs (i.e., two-letter spellings), and this may be another source of difficulty in vowel recoding. For example, Bryson & Werker (1989) have noted that disabled readers and younger normal readers, when attempting to read double vowels, sounded out the first letter and ignored the second. They also often assigned a vowel sound to the final -e (e.g., *sape* read as /sappy/).

Siegel & Faux (1989) also investigated orthographic complexity for vowels as a dimension in the development of accuracy in pseudoword and word reading and differences between normal and disabled readers. Their investiga-tion included, for example, final e (e.g., *take, hake*) and -r controlled vowels (e.g., *far, par*). These authors also investigated multiple-letter vowel forms with consistent (e.g., *coat, foat*) and inconsistent pronunciations (e.g., *down, pown; ow* in *pown* may be pronounced as in *down* or as in *own*). No major differences were found between reading level matched normal readers and disabled readers in the developmental patterns for accuracy in vowel recoding. Whereas normal 6–8-year-old readers attained an accuracy rate of 84% for reading one-vowel pseudowords, the percentage correct score for the pseudo-words with complex spellings for vowels ranged from 47 to 56%. For the reading-disabled 6–8-year-old group, percentage scores for reading the pseudowords with complex vowel spellings ranged only from 0 to 4%. Once again, the age-matched comparisons indicate a severe delay. It should be stressed that the difference in pseudoword reading skill between normal and disabled readers was never eliminated. The problems for learning arising from vowel complexity may further be seen from the finding that even at reading grade 6, scores on these sets of pseudoword reading tasks were well below ceiling and ranged for normals from 72 to 89% and for the reading-disabled group from 55 to 78%.

Siegel & Faux (1989) also identified number of syllables as another dimension in phonological recoding development. For example, even at reading grade level 6, only 67% of the two-syllable pseudowords and 50% of the three-syllable pseudowords were read correctly by the normal readers. However, only 33% of the three-syllable pseudowords were read correctly by the disabled group whose word-reading skill was at a reading grade 6 level.

To interpret differences in accuracy for word and pseudoword reading across a continuum from one- to three-syllable pseudowords, it may be noted, for example, that accuracy in reading multisyllable pseudowords or unknown multisyllable words almost always requires a shift from letter–phoneme relationships to relationships based also on semantic/grammatical, or morphemic, segments in words (e.g., Chomsky, 1971; Gillooly, 1972/1973; Henderson & Templeton, 1986; Liberman, 1983; Liberman, et al., 1980). For example, the reading (or spelling) of affixes, as in, for example, *nation* or *rotion*, is only marginally predictable from a relationship between single letters and phonemes. Instead, predictability derives from the stability between the written form *-ion* for /-tion/ as a suffix marker for nouns. Because English orthography is morphophonemic and the written form of affixes often only remotely reflects what words sound like, children must not only become aware of the semantic/grammatical constituents of words, but also develop memory for the syllabic units of written language that correspond to affixes (e.g., the sequence *-tion* or *-sion*).

In short, developmental patterns in word and pseudoword reading reflect the fact that English orthography is complex. Differences between normal and disabled readers suggest that abstracting the complex structure underlying the written form of words may be particularly problematic for reading-disabled children.

Developmental progression: phonetic cue reading

Accuracy in reading even simple pseudowords is not fully developed until well after children have acquired a first reading vocabulary (Siegel & Faux, 1989; Vandervelden & Siegel, 1995). For example, Siegel & Faux (1989) found that even at reading grade 2, the average and disabled group attained only a mean percentage correct score of 60% and 63%, respectively for reading the simple (CVC) pseudoword set.

Ehri & Wilce (1985) suggested that the finding that children may acquire a relatively large reading vocabulary even though they cannot read pseudowords has led to the hypothesis of a first stage in which word learning is not supported by making use of the systematic relationship between letters and phonemes (e.g., Gough & Hillinger, 1980; Mason, 1980). However, from their studies of early development in phonological recoding, Ehri & Wilce (1985, 1987a, and 1987b) concluded that the accurate use of sounding out and blending to retrieve the spoken form of unknown printed strings may be a separate and relatively advanced stage in the development of reading, which is preceded by a more rudimentary stage, phonetic cue reading. In phonetic cue reading, children use only some of the letters as cues to retrieve the spoken form. Ehri & Wilce (1985) found evidence that some form of phonetic cue reading is involved in the acquisition of a reading vocabulary from the outset.

The findings of Ehri & Wilce (1985) also suggest that phonetic cue reading refers to a complex of developing skill that may play a changing role in reading. For example, phonological recoding may start with partial *recognition* of the letter–phoneme match when children hear and see words simultaneously. A study by Ehri & Wilce (1987a) also confirmed the findings of earlier research (e.g., Chomsky, 1979) that children make use of phonological recoding in spelling unknown words before they are able to do so in reading. The authors also found evidence for a developmental link between early spelling and early word reading.

We (Vandervelden & Siegel, 1995) designed a study to investigate the role and development of phonological recoding in early reading prior to the ability to read accurately one-syllable, one-vowel pseudowords. Using a developmental approach, the measurement of phonological recoding was not confined to reading pseudowords, but also included a speech to print matching task to differentiate between *recognition* and *retrieval* in phonological recoding. On the speech to print matching task, the target word (e.g., /frog/) was pronounced before children selected its match in a set of three printed words (e.g., *sad, mitt, frog*). On this task, phonological recoding is therefore completely redundant for lexical retrieval, because the child need only *recognize* the match between a spoken and printed word. For purposes of investigating developmental progression in phonological recoding, redundancy was defined as the availability and ability to make use of information other than print to resolve problems of word reading. In contrast, in pseudoword reading, recoding of part (e.g., *sut* read as /sock/) or all of the letters in the printed string precedes pronunciation (i.e., *retrieval* of a spoken form, or verbal code), and phonological recoding is never completely redundant. In addition to speech to print matching and pseudoword reading, we also included a task that measured skill in using phonological recoding in spelling. As well, on each of these three tasks, recoding was measured from partial correctness, starting with correct first consonant recoding, to full correctness. That is, on the pseudoword reading and spelling task, it was also of interest how many letter–phoneme matches were correct and their position in substitutes. For example, reading /sock/ for *sut* or spelling /sut/ as *s* would indicate single letter–phoneme recoding of the initial consonant; reading /sit/ for *sut* or spelling /sut/ as *st* would indicate two letter–phoneme recoding for initial and last consonants. Thus, even though reading *sut* as /sock/ or spelling /sut/ as *s* is inaccurate, partial use of phonological recoding has contributed to these substitutions. On the speech to print matching task, it was of interest for what degree and position of overlap in letters in the printed word set, correct selection could be made. For example, correct selection of *sit* from the set *sit, milk, frog* or *sap, sink, sit* would indicate at least partial recoding skill, even though children may still be unable to select correctly from the set *sit, sat, sot*. We used the terms recognition, spelling, and retrieval to designate what we called the functions of phonological recoding operationalized in the speech to print matching, spelling, and pseudoword reading tasks, respectively.

First, like Ehri & Wilce (1985), we found evidence that phonetic cue reading underlies written word learning from the outset. For example, all children who did not show at least some skill on the speech to print matching task failed to attain criterion on a simple word-learning task. Children who read more than five beginning level words correctly on a word-reading task always showed skill in phonetic cue reading, including partial accuracy in pseudoword reading in most cases. Secondly, regular progression in phonetic cue reading was identified as follows. Use of phonological recoding (recognition) on the speech to print matching task developed before use of phonological recoding (retrieval) on the pseudoword reading task at each level of analysis; for example, the initial consonant was recoded first on the speech to print matching task before children showed evidence of initial consonant recoding skill on the pseudoword reading task (or in word reading). In most cases, a two-letter level of recoding (i.e., first and last) on the speech to print matching task coincided with initial consonant recoding on the pseudoword task. Some children, however, showed a two-consonant level of recoding on the speech to print matching task and still did not indicate any skill in initial consonant recoding in pseudoword or word reading. Comparisons between uses of phonological recoding on the speech to print matching and spelling tasks showed that recognition of the letter–phoneme match for the initial consonant and medial vowel developed before spelling of these phonemes in equivalent positions, but that last consonant recoding on these two tasks developed simultaneously. Comparisons between spelling and pseudoword reading showed that spelling of the initial and final consonant developed before correctly recoding these consonants in reading. On both these tasks, accuracy in recoding the vowel developed relatively late. Moreover, development from partial to full recoding was similar across the three tasks: initial consonant recoding developed first, followed by last consonant recoding, with medial vowel recoding developing last. Thirdly, although accuracy in reading simple pseudowords was found to be a relatively late-developing skill, skills assessed on the early measures of phonological recoding (i.e., speech to print matching and partial accuracy in spelling and pseudoword reading) were found to be strongly related to skill on a simple word-learning task and on the easier (high-frequency, one-syllable words) word-reading task. We concluded that the identification of a recognition level in phonological recoding that precedes even partial accuracy in pseudoword reading may explain how children start to notice the systematic relationship between spoken and printed words as they hear and see words simultaneously.

Summary and conclusion

In this section, we explained the role of phonological recoding in the acquisition of a reading vocabulary and reviewed differences between normal and reading-disabled groups in phonological recoding not only on pseudo-word reading, but also on lexical decision, spelling, and pseudoword recognition tasks. The word and pseudoword reading deficit which is characteristic of disabled readers was found to endure across development and into adulthood. Next, we reviewed evidence for developmental progression in phonological recoding. First, we discussed complexity in rule application as a factor affecting accuracy in vowel recoding and in reading multisyllable words and pseudowords. Furthermore, although disabled readers were found to show considerable delay, with some exceptions patterns in phonological recoding development were found to be similar to those of normal readers. Secondly, we discussed the developmental progression in phonetic cue reading; that is, the phase in phonological recoding development that precedes accuracy in reading simple pseudowords. We identified a regular developmental progression and found that the rudimentary skills of the phonetic cue reading stage related strongly to the acquisition of a first reading vocabulary.

In conclusion, findings of a developmental progression in phonological recoding indicate the need to measure phonological recoding along a developmental continuum. For example, pseudoword reading, as an index of skill in phonological recoding, may need to assess performance along a continuum of complexity with respect to vowel spellings and syllable structure. Furthermore, studies at reading grade 2 or below may need to include measures of the precursors of accuracy in pseudoword reading; that is, speech to print matching, and partial accuracy in spelling and pseudoword reading.

COMPONENT PHONOLOGICAL PROCESSES

Development, as well as deficits in phonological recoding in cases of reading disability, must be explained in terms of component phonological processing. For example, within the phonological domain, no or limited skill in phonological recoding may stem from sources as diverse as knowing and retrieving the phoneme associated with a particular letter (or letter digraph, e.g., *th*) to problems in relating a sequence of segmented phonemes to the phonological (verbal) code of syllables or words (e.g. /s/ /u/ /t/ to /sut/ or /s/ /i/ /t/ to /sit/). We referred to these phonological processing skills as verbal coding for letters, words, and syllables. On the other hand, no or limited skill in phonological recoding may also stem from limitations in phoneme recognition and/or segmentation skill, which we referred to as phoneme awareness.

Verbal coding

Verbal coding is an intrinsic aspect of all language function, including phonological recoding. For example, to name (e.g., /es/ for *s*) or sound a letter (e.g., /s/ for *s*) requires that the relevant code (i.e., name or sound) for that letter is stored in memory and that this information can be accessed and retrieved. Verbal coding is also required in the comprehension (i.e., recognition) of letters on selection tasks. For example, to select the letter *s* from a set of letters following the request "Which one is /s/?" requires knowing and recognizing *s* as /s/. However, in contrast to sounding, letter selection does not require retrieval of the target phoneme. With respect to the role of verbal coding for letters in learning to read, Ehri (1984) has suggested, for example, that letter names give children nameable referents with which to associate phonemes and knowledge of letter name codes may therefore be a first step in written word learning.

Verbal coding of words and syllables is also an intrinsic aspect of phonological recoding. For example, as we noted, in speech to print matching (recognition phonological recoding) retrieval of the spoken form of the word (i.e., the verbal code) precedes use of phonological recoding to make the correct speech to print match. Furthermore, the target word (or pseudoword) must be kept in memory until the print selection is completed. In pseudoword reading or in reading unknown words, the importance of verbal coding is based on the linguistic fact that letters map the phoneme structure underlying spoken words and syllables and not the surface form of speech directly. For example, all that can be recovered by recoding the letter sequence in *frog* is /f/ /r/ /o/ /g/ as isolated segments or, perhaps, /fr/ /og/ (the latter requires prior knowledge of the phoneme sequence associated with the initial consonant blend and of the pronunciation associated with the syllable *-og*). Even if segments larger than single phonemes and letter(s) are used, "sounding out" must be followed by making the connection with a known pronunciation (verbal code) of a word or syllable. The connection between the underlying phoneme sequence and the surface form of speech (e.g., /f/ /r/ /o/ /g/ and /frog/) will become transparent as a consequence of becoming literate (e.g., Liberman et al., 1985). Making the connection between the parts and the whole (e.g., between the separate phonemes /f/ /r/ /o/ /g/ and the word, /frog/) is called closure.

Evidence for the role of verbal coding for words and syllables in phonological recoding comes, for example, from training studies which have found a separate effect for "blending" as compared to "sounding out" on pseudoword or word reading (e.g., Fox & Routh, 1976, 1984; Lewkowicz, 1980). Chall, Rosswell, & Blumenthal (1963) define blending as accessing the sound form of a syllable or word from its segmented sequence. Lewkowicz describes instruction in blending as "helping children to supply the missing bonds between the sounds and how to induce that flash of recognition that blending requires" (1980, p. 696). Evidence for the role of verbal coding for words and syllables comes also from findings of a familiarity effect in phonological recoding or oral blending tasks. For example, substitutions in less skilled pseudoword reading are more often words than pseudowords; that is, children substitute the verbal codes of known words for the unknown verbal codes of pseudowords (Gough, Juel, & Roper/Schneider, 1983). Similarly, familiarity with the words or pseudowords used in blending training improved blending performance (Lewkowicz, 1980).

Further evidence for the role of verbal coding in early reading comes from findings of a relationship between performance on different naming tasks (accuracy and/or speed) and learning to read. For example, Scarborough (1990) found that children who later developed reading difficulties differed at age 2 years and 6 months in pronunciation accuracy of words produced in natural language production. At age 5, weaknesses in object naming remained one of their characteristics. Older reading-disabled children may also be less accurate than normal readers in naming pictures. For example, a picture of a volcano was labelled as /tornado/ in spite of knowing the meaning of these words (see e.g., Liberman & Shankweiler, 1995; Wagner & Torgesen, 1987; Wolf, 1991, for reviews). Although a deficit in naming accuracy is not found in all severe cases of reading disability, there is a considerable body of evidence that speed in naming letters, digits, colors, and pictures of common objects is strongly related to reading. For example, Blachman (1984) reports a strong relationship between letter-naming speed and word reading. Bowers, Steffy, & Swanson (1986) report a relationship between continuous naming speed and later performance in pseudoword reading. In contrast to measuring reaction time in one at a time (discrete) naming trials, continuous naming requires subjects to name repeatedly a limited set of stimuli and the score is the number of accurate responses within a given time. Following an extensive review of the literature, Wolf (1991) concluded that even though the evidence points to a changing relationship between naming and reading across development, the relationship endured "weaker but consistent across time" (p. 134).

Verbal coding may also play a role in pseudoword reading or in reading unknown words because the phoneme sequence must be kept "in mind" (short-term or working memory) until phonological recoding is completed (e.g., Wagner & Torgesen, 1987). There is considerable evidence that verbal coding is used to facilitate short-term memory (e.g., Baddeley, 1979 1982; Jorm, 1983) and that younger normal and older disabled readers show less efficiency in making use of verbal coding to facilitate short-term memory processing (e.g., Mann, Liberman, & Shankweiler, 1980; Shankweiler et al., 1979; Siegel & Linder, 1984).

Developmental progression

Vandervelden (1992) investigated developmental progression in letter naming, letter sounding, and in recognizing letter–phoneme correspondences. She reports that in kindergarten and grade 1, knowledge of consonant letter names exceeded knowledge of letter–phoneme correspondences (both recognition and sounding). Also, recognition (i.e., selection) following presentation of a phoneme developed before the ability to sound the ten consonant letters included in the testing. Moreover, in kindergarten, many children knew at least some letter names, but did not show necessarily concomitant development in letter–phoneme knowledge, even at a recognition (letter selection) level. A similar discrepancy between knowledge of letter name and letter–phonemes was found for a few children even in grade 1. Thus, some children may have problems in learning letter–phoneme correspondences as a second code (letter names being the first code), a problem somewhat similar to acquiring the multiple codes for vowels in later phonological recoding development.

It may be noted that phonemes, but not letter names, map onto the phonological structure underlying spoken words (e.g., /b/, but not /bee/, applies in recoding *bog* to /bog/). For that reason, although letters may provide nameable referents for learning letter–phoneme relationships, letter-naming skill is neither necessary nor necessarily facilitating in starting to use phonological recoding (e.g., Samuels, 1971; Vandervelden, 1992). For example, Vandervelden (1992) found that kindergarten children with letter name knowledge but no knowledge of letter–phoneme correspondences always failed the word-learning task and showed no skill in phonological recoding on any of the measures. Moreover, the relationship between letter naming and early reading was much weaker than that found for both letter–phoneme recognition and letter sounding.

Phoneme awareness

Phoneme awareness involves both phoneme categorization and abstracting the segmental nature of spoken language.

Phoneme categorization

Phoneme categorization within the context of reading and spelling refers to the ability to perceive phonemes as identical attributes of different words even though they may not be acoustically equivalent (e.g., Baron et al., 1980). For example, the spoken words /tuck/ and /truck/ start with the phoneme /t/ which is the reason why the first letter in both words is *t*. However, the articulatory and, hence, the acoustic features of the /t/ phoneme in /tuck/ differ from those in /truck/: /t/ followed by /r/ is affricated, whereas /t/ followed by a vowel is not. The /t/ in /tuck/ and the /t/ in /truck/ are said to be allophonic variations: that is, although both are instances of the phoneme /t/, they differ in their respective phonetic feature sets. These differences in the phonetic feature set for instances of the phoneme /t/ are determined by the articulatory context (i.e., whether an /r/ or a vowel follows the phoneme /t/). The term phoneme refers therefore to a category of sounds which signals a difference in meaning (e.g., /mad/ versus /sad/), whereas the term allophones (e.g., /t/ with or without affrication) refers to sounds that are functionally equivalent (e.g., Liberman, 1983; Liberman et al., 1985).

Phoneme categorization is one of the earliest developments in language acquisition, since without it comprehension and production of spoken language is not possible. However, immaturity in phoneme categorization may persist for some time as part of normal development. For example, children's early attempts at spelling based on how words sound may show sensitivity to the acoustic difference between /t/ with and without affrication, resulting in different spellings for the phoneme /t/. Research into children's early spellings shows, for example, a fairly frequent substitution of *ch* for /t/, as for example *chran* for *train* (e.g., Read, 1971, 1975; Treiman, 1985). Immaturity in phoneme categorization may thus affect what letters children choose to spell words.

Immaturity in phoneme categorization has also been found in cases of reading and/or spelling disability (e.g., Godfrey et al., 1981; Marcel, 1980).

Abstracting the segmental nature of spoken language

Phoneme awareness also includes the ability to analyze words and syllables in terms of their constituent phonemes. To cite an example from Liberman et al. (1985), although three phonemes underlie the spoken form of the word /big/, there is only one piece of sound. This is the case because the three phonological segments we write with the letters *b i g* are nearly simultaneously articulated (encoded) and for that reason are acoustically one sound segment. Encodedness within the speech stream may present a problem for the beginning reader. Although the written symbols map as a cipher onto the underlying phonological structure of words, speech does not map as a cipher onto the underlying phoneme structure. Inasmuch as the acoustic/articulatory unit of speech is approximately syllabic, syllables have, but phonemes do not have, a physical (acoustic/articulatory) reality as *separate* units within words.

In general, the research into phoneme awareness as a predictor of reading skill has focused on the analysis of words and syllables in terms of their constituent phonemes and it is this skill that is usually assessed in studies examining the relationship between phoneme awareness and early reading. This research has found a strong relationship between phoneme awareness and learning to read, and this relationship has been found for a wide variety of tasks and with subjects ranging from pre-kindergarten children to reading-disabled adults (e.g., Backman, 1983; Blachman, 1984; Bradley & Bryant, 1983, 1988; Calfee, Lindamood, & Lindamood, 1973; Fox & Routh, 1975, 1980, 1984; Juel, Griffith, & Gough, 1986; Liberman et al., 1974, 1977; Lie, 1991; Lundberg, Olofsson, & Wall, 1980; Share et al., 1984; Skelfjord, 1987; Stanovich, Cunningham, & Cramer, 1984; Torneus, 1984; Wagner & Torgesen, 1987; Yopp, 1988).

In spite of its strong relationship with reading and of findings that differences in phoneme awareness are found well before children receive formal instruction in reading, it is considerably more problematic how to interpret such findings. Whereas a causal relationship for phoneme awareness has often been assumed in the literature, there is evidence that phoneme awareness develops gradually and reciprocally with learning to read and spell. First, findings of research indicate that at least some levels of phoneme awareness do not develop independently from learning to read and write an alphabetic writing system. For example, in contrast to literate adults, illiterates were unable to learn a phoneme deletion task (Morais et al., 1979). Also, Japanese children in grades 1 to 6, whose literacy development initially focuses on a syllabic script, lagged behind US children and this difference was particularly noticeable in grade 1 (Mann, 1986). Moreover, Chinese adult readers, who knew only the logographic script, showed problems with phoneme awareness (Read et al., 1986). Secondly, spelling knowledge may play an important role in performing certain phoneme awareness tasks. For example, Ehri & Wilce (1980) found that in a study with fourth grade children, spelling knowledge affected judgments about the number of phonemes in spoken words and pseudowords (e.g., /rich/ and /pitch/ were judged as having respectively three and four phonemes even though they rhyme). Perin (1983) reports similar results in a study with adults.

Developmental progression and reciprocal development

To investigate developmental progression in phoneme awareness and its role in phonological recoding and in early literacy, we (Vandervelden & Siegel, 1995) used six tasks which measured skill from beginning to advanced levels.

First, children's performance across the six tasks indicated a regular developmental progression. For example, initial phoneme recognition and segmentation developed first (e.g., "Listen for /s/; /sock/. Does /sock/ have a /s/?") and before recognition and segmentation of the final consonant. The task children found most difficult included a series of phoneme deletion and substitution trials based on Rosner (1973, 1974); for example, "Say meat. Now say it again, but instead of /m/ say /f/."

Secondly, phoneme awareness increased concurrently, or reciprocally, with development in phonological recoding and in reading and spelling. For example, partial phoneme recognition and segmentation was most strongly related to, and increased commensurately with, early skill in phonological recoding (i.e., skill prior to accuracy in simple pseudoword reading) and reading (a word-learning and easy word-reading task). On the other hand, deletion and substitution were most strongly related to accuracy in pseudoword reading, to reading multisyllable and less common words, and to accuracy in spelling.

Summary and conclusion

In this section, we discussed the role of verbal coding and phoneme awareness in the development of phonological recoding in both normal and disabled readers. For example, we noted that letter naming is highly predictive of phonological recoding, but only if there is concurrent development in knowledge of letter–phoneme correspondences. With respect to the role of verbal coding for words and syllables, we noted, for example, the need for closure between a segmented phoneme sequence and the word or syllable represented by a letter string. Evidence in support of a relationship between verbal coding and reading was cited from training studies in blending, studies which have investigated the relationship between various naming and reading tasks, including pseudoword reading, and from studies which have investigated inefficient use of verbal coding in short-term memory in normal younger and in older reading-disabled children.

For phoneme awareness, we discussed two aspects: phoneme categorization, which pervades all language processing, and abstraction of the segmental nature of spoken language, which is specific to learning to read and write an alphabetic script. Although there is some evidence for immature phoneme categorization in cases of reading disability, by far the greatest research effort has been expanded on relationships between tasks that assess skills related to the segmental nature of language. Although the research indicates a strong relationship between phoneme awareness and progress in reading (and spelling), it also seems to be the case that phoneme awareness refers to a complex of developing skill that develops reciprocally with learning to read and spell. Consequently, it must be considered that deficits in phoneme awareness may be as much a consequence as a cause of reading and spelling problems.

In conclusion, findings of a gradual development in phoneme awareness and a strong but changing relationship with reading and with spelling along a developmental continuum emphasize the need for multiple tasks and appropriate task selection when investigating relationships with different levels of reading skill and with spelling.

CONCLUSION

Phonological recoding is a critical process in learning to read and write an alphabetic writing system and refers to a hierarchy of developing skills which seem to develop reciprocally with learning to read and write. Moreover, different levels of phonological recoding relate in specific ways to the component phonological processing skills of verbal coding and phoneme awareness. There is considerable evidence that phoneme awareness develops reciprocally with skill in phonological recoding and with learning to read and spell. These reciprocal relationships suggest that the severe developmental lag in phonological recoding found in cases of reading disability needs to be addressed early, particularly because, as Stanovich (1986b) emphasized, it results in large individual differences in essential reading practice that eventually affect all areas of learning.

Our purpose in this chapter has been to provide a developmental and integrated framework for understanding the deficits in phonological processing that characterize reading disability. In particular, our own research and that of others suggests the need for multiple measures and careful selection of tasks not only in basic research, but also in the clinical/educational assessment of reading-disabled children.

REFERENCES

Backman, J. (1983). The role of psycholinguistic skills in acquisition: a look at early readers. *Reading Research Quarterly*, **18**, 469–479.

Backman, J., Bruck, M., Hebert, M., & Seidenberg, M.S. (1984). Acquisition and use of spelling-sound correspondences in reading. *Journal of Experimental Child Psychology*, **38**, 114–133.

Baddeley, A.D. (1979). Working memory and reading. In P.A. Kolers, M.E. Wrolstad, & H. Bouma (eds) *Processing of Visible Language*, Vol. 1. New York: Plenum (pp. 355–370).

Baddeley, A.D. (1982). Reading and working memory. *Bulletin of the British Psychological Society*, **35**, 414–417.

Baron, J. (1977). Mechanisms for pronouncing pseudowords: use and acquisition. In D. Laberge & S.J. Samuels (eds) *Basic Processes in Reading: Perception and Comprehension*. Hillsdale, NJ: Erlbaum (pp. 175–216).

Baron, J., Treiman, R., Wilf, J.F., & Kellman, Ph. (1980). Spelling and reading by rules. In U. Frith (ed.) *Cognitive Processes in Spelling*. London: Academic Press (pp. 159–1893).

Barron, R. & Baron, J. (1977). How children get meaning from printed words. *Child Development*, **48**, 587–594.

Biemiller, A. (1970). The development of the use of graphic and contextual information as children learn to read. *Reading Research Quarterly*, **8**, 75–96.

Biemiller, A. (1977/1978). Relationships between oral reading, speed for letters, words, and simple text in the development of reading achievement. *Reading Research Quarterly*, **13**, 223–253.

Blachman, B. (1984). Language analysis skills and early reading acquisition. In G. Wallach & K. Butler (eds) *Language Learning Disabilities in School-Age Children*. Baltimore, MD: Williams & Wilkins (pp. 271–287).

Bowers, P.G., Steffy, R., & Swanson, L.B. (1986). Naming speed, memory, and visual processing in reading disability. *Canadian Journal of Behavioral Science*, **18**, 209–223.

Bradley, L. & Bryant, P.E. (1983). Categorizing sounds and learning to read: a causal connection. *Nature*, **30**, 419–421.

Bradley, L. & Bryant, P. (1988). *Rhyme and Reason in Reading and Spelling*. Ann Arbor: University of Michigan Press.

Bruck, M. (1988). The word recognition and spelling of dyslexic children. *Reading Research Quarterly*, **23**, 51–70.

Bruck, M. (1990). Word-recognition skills of adults with childhood diagnoses of dyslexia. *Developmental Psychology*, **26**, 439–454.

Bryson, J.F. & Werker, J.E. (1989). Toward understanding the problem in severely disabled children, Part I: Vowel errors. *Applied Psycholinguistics*, **10**, 1–12.

Calfee, R., Lindamood, P., & Lindamood, C. (1973). Acoustic-phonetic skill and reading-kindergarten through twelfth grade. *Journal of Educational Psychology*, **64**, 293–298.

Chall, J., Rosswell, F.G., & Blumenthal, S.H. (1963). Auditory blending ability: a factor in success in early reading. *Reading Teacher*, **17**, 113–118.

Chomsky, C. (1979). Approaching reading through invented spelling. In L.B. Resnick & Ph. A. Weaver (eds) *Theory and Practice of Early Reading*, Vol. 2. Hillsdale, NJ: Erlbaum (pp. 43–66).

Chomsky, N. (1971). Phonology and reading. In H. Levin & J. Williams (eds) *Basic Studies on Reading*. New York: Basic Books (pp. 3–18).

Coltheart, M. (1978). Lexical access in simple reading tasks. In G. Underwood (ed.) *Strategies of Information Processing*. London: Academic Press (pp. 151–216).

Ehri, L.C. (1978). Beginning reading from a psycholinguistic perspective: amalgamation of word identities. In F.B. Murray (ed.) *The Recognition of Words*. Newark, DE: International Reading Association.

Ehri, L.C. (1980). The development of orthographic images. In U. Frith (ed.) *Cognitive Processes in Spelling*. London: Academic Press (pp. 311–388).

Ehri, L.C. (1984). How orthography alters spoken language competencies in children learning to read and spell. In J. Downing & R. Valtin (eds) *Language Awareness and Learning to Read*. New York: Springer Verlag (pp. 119–147).

Ehri, L.C. & Wilce, L.S. (1980). The influence of orthography on readers' conceptualization of the phoneme structure of words. *Applied Psycholinguistics*, **1**, 371–385.

Ehri, L.C. & Wilce, L.S. (1985). Movement into reading: is the first stage of printed word learning visual or phonetic? *Reading Research Quarterly*, **20**, 163–179.

Ehri, L. & Wilce, L.S. (1987a). Cipher versus cue reading: an experiment in decoding acquisition. *Journal of Educational Psychology*, **79**, 3–13.

Ehri, L. & Wilce, L.S. (1987b). Does learning to spell help beginners to read words. *Reading Research Quarterly*, **21**, 41–65.

Fowler, C., Liberman, I.Y., & Shankweiler, D. (1977). On interpreting the error pattern in beginning reading. *Language and Speech*, **20**, 162–173.

Fowler, C., Shankweiler, D., & Liberman, I. (1979). Apprehending spelling patterns for vowels: a developmental study. *Language and Speech*, **22**, 243–251.

Fox, B. & Routh, D.K. (1975). Analyzing spoken language into words, syllables, and phonemes: a developmental study. *Journal of Psycholinguistic Research*, **4**, 331–341.

Fox, B. & Routh, D.K. (1976). Phonemic analysis and synthesis as word attack skills. *Journal of Educational Psychology*, **68**, 70–74.

Fox, B. & Routh, D.K. (1980). Phonemic analysis and severe reading disability in children. *Journal of Psycholinguistic Research*, **9**, 115–118.

Fox, B. & Routh, D.K. (1984). Phonemic analysis and synthesis as word-attack skills: revisited. *Journal of Educational Psychology*, **76**, 1059–1064.

Gates, A.I. & McKillop, A.S. (1962). *Gates–McKillop Reading Diagnostic Tests*. New York: Teachers College Press.

Gillooly, W.B. (1972/1973). The influence of writing system characteristics on learning to read. *Reading Research Quarterly*, **8**, 167–198.

Glusko, R. (1979). The organisation and activation of orthographic knowledge in reading aloud. *Journal of Experimental Psychology, Human Perception and Performance*, **5**, 674–691.

Godfrey, J.J., Syrdal-Laskey, A.K., Millay, K.K., & Knox, C.M. (1981). Performance of dyslexic children on speech perception tests. *Journal of Experimental Child Psychology*, **32**, 401–424.

Goswami, U. (1986). Children's use of analogy in learning to read: a developmental study. *Journal of Experimental Child Psychology*, **42**, 73–83.

Goswami, U. (1988). Orthographic analogies and reading development. *Quarterly Journal of Experimental Psychology*, **40A**, 239–268.

Goswami, U. (1990). A special link between rhyming skills and the use of orthographic analogies by beginning readers. *Journal of Child Psychology and Psychiatry*, **31**, 301–311.

Goswami, U. & Mead, F. (1992). Onset and rime awareness and analogies in reading. *Reading Research Quarterly*, **27**, 153–162.

Gough, P.B. & Hillinger, M.L. (1980). Learning to read: an unnatural act. *Bulletin of the Orton Society*, **30**, 179–205.

Gough, P.B. & Tunmer, W.E. (1986). Decoding, reading, and reading disability. *Remedial and Special Education*, **7**, 6–10.

Gough, P.B., Juel, C., & Roper/Schneider, D. (1983). Code and cipher: a two-stage conception of initial reading acquisition. In J.A. Niles and L.A. Harris (eds) *Searches for Meaning in Reading/Language Processing and Instruction: Thirty-second Yearbook of the National Reading Conference*. Rochester, NY: National Reading Conference (pp. 207–211).

Henderson, E.H. (1981). *Learning to Read and Spell: The Child's Knowledge of Words*. DeKalb, IL: Northern Illinois University Press.

Henderson, E.H. & Templeton, Sh. (1986). A developmental perspective of formal spelling instruction through alphabet, pattern, meaning. *Elementary School Journal*, **86**, 305–316.

Johnston, R. (1982). Phonological coding in dyslexic readers. *British Journal of Psychology*, **73**, 455–460.

Jorm, A.F. (1983). Specific reading retardation and working memory: a review. *British Journal of Psychology*, **74**, 311–342.

Jorm, A.F. & Share, D.L. (1983). Phonological recoding and reading acquisition. *Applied Psycholinguistics*, **4**, 103–147.

Juel, C., Griffith, P., & Gough, P.B. (1986). Acquisition of literacy: a longitudinal study of children in first and second grade. *Journal of Educational Psychology*, **78**, 243–255.

Kay, J. & Marcel, A. (1981). One process, not two, in reading aloud: lexical analogies do the work of non-lexical rules. *Quarterly Journal of Experimental Psychology*, **33**A, 397–413.

Lesgold, A.M. & Curtis, M.E. (1981). Learning to read words efficiently. In A. Lesgold & C. Perfetti (eds) *Interactive Processes in Reading*. Hillsdale, NJ: Erlbaum (pp. 329–360).

Lewkowicz, N. (1980). Phonemic awareness training: what to teach and how to teach it. *Journal of Educational Psychology*, **72**, 686–700.

Liberman, A.M. (1982). On finding that speech is special. *American Psychologist*, **37**, 148–167.

Liberman, A.M., Copper, F.S., Shankweiler, D., & Studdert-Kennedy, M. (1967). Perception of the speech code. *Psychological Review*, **74**, 431–461.

Liberman, I.Y. (1983). A language oriented view of reading and its disabilities. In H. Myklebust (ed.) *Progress in Learning Disabilities*, Vol. 5. New York: Grune & Stratton (pp. 81–102).

Liberman, I.Y. & Shankweiler, D. (1985). Phonology and the problems of learning to read and write. *Remedial and Special Education*, **6**, 8–17.

Liberman, I.Y., Liberman, A.M., Mattingly, I., & Shankweiler, D. (1980). Orthography and the beginning reader. In J.F. Kavanagh & R.L. Venezky (eds) *Orthography, Reading, and Dyslexia*. Baltimore: University Park Press (pp. 137–153).

Liberman, I.Y., Rubin, H., Duques, S., & Carlisle, J. (1985). Linguistic ability and spelling proficiency in kindergarteners and adult poor spellers. In D.B. Gray & J.F. Kavanagh (eds) *Biobehavioral Measures of Dyslexia*. Parkton, MD: York Press (pp. 163–176).

Liberman, I.Y., Shankweiler, D., Fisher, F.W., & Carter, B. (1974). Explicit syllable and phoneme segmentation in the young child. *Journal of Experimental Child Psychology*, **18**, 201–210.

Liberman, I.Y., Shankweiler, D., Liberman, A.M., Fowler, C., & Fisher, F.W. (1977). Phonetic segmentation and recoding in the beginning reader. In A.S. Reber & D.L. Scarborough (eds) *Toward a Psychology of Reading*. Hillsdale, NJ: Erlbaum (pp. 207–225).

Lie, A. (1991). Effects of a training program for stimulating skills in word analysis in first-grade children. *Reading Research Quarterly*, **26**, 234–250.

Lundberg, I., Olofsson, A., & Wall, S. (1980). Reading and spelling skill in the first school years predicted from phonemic awareness skills in kindergarten. *Scandinavian Journal of Psychology*, **21**, 159–173.

Mann, V.A. (1986). Phonological awareness: the role of reading experience. *Cognition*, **24**, 65–92.

Mann, V.A., Liberman, I., & Shankweiler, D. (1980). Children's memory for sentences and word strings in relation to reading ability. *Memory and Cognition*, **8**, 329–335.

Marcel, T. (1980). Phonological awareness and phonological representation: investigation of a specific spelling problem. In U. Frith (ed.) *Cognitive Processes in Spelling*. London: Academic Press (pp. 372–404).

Mason, J. (1980). When do children begin to read: an exploration of four-year-old children's letter and word reading competencies. *Reading Research Quarterly*, **15**, 203–227.

McCusker, L.X., Hillinger, M.L., & Bias, R.G. (1981). Phonological recoding and reading. *Psychological Bulletin*, **89**, 217–245.

Metsala, J. & Siegel, L.S. (1992). Patterns of atypical reading development attributes and underlying reading processes. In S. Segalowitz & I. Rapin (eds) *Handbook of Neuropsychology*, Vol. 7. Amsterdam: Elsevier (pp. 187–210).

Morais, J., Cary, L., Alegria, J., & Bertelson, P. (1979). Does awareness of speech as a sequence of phonemes arise spontaneously? *Cognition*, **7**, 323–331.

Olson, R.K., Kleigl, R., Davidson, B.J., & Foltz, G. (1985). Individual and developmental differences in reading disability. In G.E. MacKinnon & T.G. Waller (eds) *Reading Research: Advances in Theory and Practice*, Vol. 4. New York: Academic Press (pp. 1–64).

Perfetti, C.A. (1985). *Reading Ability*. New York: Oxford University Press.

Perfetti, C.A. & Hogaboam, T. (1975). The relationship between single word decoding and reading comprehension skill. *Journal of Educational Psychology*, **67**, 461–469.

Perin, D. (1983). Phonemic segmentation and spelling. *British Journal of Psychology*, **74**, 129–144.

Rack, J.P., Snowling, M.J., & Olson, R.K. (1992). The nonword reading deficit in developmental dyslexia: a review. *Reading Research Quarterly*, **27**, 28–53.

Read, Ch. (1971). Preschool children's knowledge of English phonology. *Harvard Educational Review*, **41**, 1–34.

Read, Ch. (1975). Children's categorization of speech sounds in English. *NCTE Research Report 17*, Educational Resources Information Center.

Read, Ch., Zhang, Y.F., Nie, H.Y., & Ding, B.Q. (1986). The ability to manipulate speech sounds depends on knowing alphabetic writing. *Cognition*, **24**, 31–44.

Rosner, J. (1973). *Perceptual Skills Curriculum: Auditory Motor Skills Training*. New York: Walker Book Corp.

Rosner, J. (1974). Auditory analysis training with prereaders. *Reading Teacher*, **27**, 379–381.

Samuels, S.J. (1971). Letter-name versus letter-sound knowledge in learning to read. *Reading Teacher*, **24**, 604–608.

Scarborough, H.S. (1990). Very early language deficits in dyslexic children. *Child Development*, **61**, 1726–1743.

Seidenberg, M.S., Bruck, M., Fornarolo, G., & Backman, J. (1986). Who is dyslexic? Reply to Wolf. *Applied Psycholinguistics*, **7**, 77–84.

Shafir, U. & Siegel, L.S. (1991). Cognitive processes of subtypes of adults with learning disabilities. Unpublished manuscript.

Shankweiler, D. & Liberman, I.Y. (1972). Misreading: a search for causes. In J. Kavanagh & I. Mattingly (eds) *Language by Ear and by Eye.* Cambridge, MA: MIT Press.

Shankweiler, D., Liberman, I.Y., Mark, L.S., Fowler, C.A., & Fisher, F.W. (1979). The speech code and learning to read. *Journal of Experimental Psychology: Human Learning and Memory,* 5, 531–545.

Share, D.J., Jorm, A.F., Maclean, R., & Mathews, R. (1984). Sources of individual differences in reading achievement. *Journal of Educational Psychology,* 76, 466–477.

Siegel, L.S. (1985). Psycholinguistic aspects of reading disabilities. In L.S. Siegel & F.J. Morrison (eds) *Cognitive Development in Atypical Children.* New York: Springer Verlag.

Siegel, L.S. (1986). Phonological deficits in children with a reading disability. *Canadian Journal of Special Education,* 2, 45–54.

Siegel, L.S. (1992). Phonological processing deficits as the basis of a reading disability. *Developmental Review,* 13, 246–257.

Siegel, L.S. & Faux, D. (1989). Acquisition of certain grapheme-phoneme correspondences in normally achieving and disabled readers. *Reading and Writing: An Interdisciplinary Journal,* 1, 37–52.

Siegel, L.S. & Linder, B. (1984). Short-term memory processes in children with reading and arithmetic disabilities. *Developmental Psychology,* 20, 200–207.

Siegel, L.S. & Ryan, E.B. (1984). Reading disability as a language disorder. *Remedial and Special Education,* 5, 28–33.

Siegel, L.S. & Ryan, E.B. (1988). Development of grammatical sensitivity, phonological and short-term memory skills in normally achieving and learning disabled children. *Developmental Psychology,* 24, 28–37.

Siegel, L.S. & Ryan, E.B. (1989). Subtypes of developmental dyslexia: the influence of definitial variables. *Reading and Writing: An Interdisciplinary Journal,* 1, 257–287.

Skelfjord, V.J. (1987). Phoneme segmentation: an important subskill in learning to read. I. *Scandinavian Journal of Educational Research,* 31, 41–57.

Stanovich, K.E. (1982). Individual differences in the cognitive processes of reading: 1. Word decoding. *Journal of Learning Disabilities,* 15, 485–493.

Stanovich, K.E. (1986a). Explaining the variance in reading ability in terms of psychological processes: what have we learned? *Annals of Dyslexia,* 15, 67–96.

Stanovich, K.E. (1986b). Matthew effects in reading: some consequences of individual differences in the acquisition of literacy. *Reading Research Quarterly,* 21, 360–407.

Stanovich, K.E., Cunningham, A.E., & Cramer, B.B. (1984). Assessing phonological awareness in kindergarten children: issues of task comparability. *Journal of Experimental Child Psychology,* 38, 175–190.

Stanovich, K.E., Cunningham, A., & West, R.F. (1981). A longitudinal study of the development of automatic recognition skills in first graders. *Journal of Reading Behavior,* 13, 57–74.

Torneus, M. (1984). Phonological awareness and reading: a chicken and egg problem? *Journal of Educational Psychology,* 76, 1346–1358.

Treiman, R. (1985). Onsets and rhymes as units of spoken syllables: evidence from children. *Journal of Experimental Child Psychology,* 39, 161–181.

Tunmer, W.E., Herriman, M.L., & Nesdale, A.R. (1988). Meta-linguistic abilities and beginning reading. *Reading Research Quarterly,* 23, 134–159.

Vandervelden, M.C. (1992). Phonological recoding and phonological analytical skill in early literacy: a developmental approach. Doctoral dissertation, The Ontario Institute for Studies in Education (University of Toronto), Toronto, Canada.

Vandervelden, M.C. & Siegel, L.S. (1995). Phonological recoding and phoneme awareness in early literacy: a developmental approach. *Reading Research Quarterly*, **30**, 854–875.

Vellutino, F.R. & Scanlon, D.M. (1987). Phonological coding, phonological awareness, and reading disability: evidence from a longitudinal and experimental study. *Merril Palmer Quarterly*, **33**, 321–363.

Wagner, R.K. & Torgesen, J.K. (1987). The nature of phonological processes and its causal role in the acquisition of reading skills. *Psychological Bulletin*, **101**, 192–212.

Waters, G., Bruck, M., & Seidenberg, M. (1985). Do children use similar processes to read and spell words? *Journal of Experimental Child Psychology*, **39**, 511–530.

Weber, R. (1970). A linguistic analysis of first-grade reading errors. *Reading Research Quarterly*, **5**, 427–451.

Wolf, M. (1991). Naming speed and reading: the contribution of the cognitive neurosciences. *Reading Research Quarterly*, **26**, 123–142.

Yopp, H.K. (1988). The validity and reliability of phonemic awareness tests. *Reading Research Quarterly*, **23**, 159–178.

12 Cognitive functioning, learning disability, and school failure in attention deficit hyperactivity disorder: a family study perspective

STEPHEN V. FARAONE, JOSEPH BIEDERMAN,
AND KATHLEEN KIELY

Children with attention deficit hyperactivity disorder (ADHD) are at high risk for poor cognitive functioning as measured by grade repetitions, academic underachievement, placement in special classes, need for tutoring, and impaired performance on neuropsychological measures (Weiss et al., 1979; Silver, 1981; Levine et al., 1982; Edelbrock et al., 1984; Lahey et al., 1984; Cantwell, 1985; Campbell & Werry, 1986; Barkley et al., 1990; Biederman et al., 1990; Faraone et al., 1993a; Faraone et al., 1993b). These problems continue through adolescence into adulthood and are associated with chronic underachievement and school failure (Hoy et al., 1978; Feldman et al., 1979; Amado & Lustman, 1982; Gittelman et al., 1985; Weiss et al., 1985; Wender et al., 1985; Hechtman & Weiss, 1986; Greenfield et al., 1988; Mannuzza et al., 1991; Biederman et al., 1993; Spencer et al., 1994).

The poor cognitive functioning and school failure of ADHD children have been well documented, yet comparatively little is known about the cause of these impairments. Are they direct manifestations of a compromised central nervous system? Or, are they epiphenomena resulting from a syndrome of inattentiveness, impulsivity, and hyperactivity that is often associated with social disadvantage, low self-esteem, and poor motivation (Campbell & Werry, 1986)? The answers to these questions are equally important to researchers seeking to discover the causes of ADHD and to clinicians facing frequent referrals of ADHD children with learning problems.

Clinical heterogeneity complicates any comprehensive understanding of cognitive deficits among ADHD children. ADHD children frequently have conduct, mood, and anxiety disorders (Biederman et al., 1991). Such findings have been reported in both epidemiological (Anderson et al., 1987; Bird et al., 1988) and clinical samples (Biederman et al., 1987a; Biederman et al., 1987b; Biederman et al., 1991a; Biederman et al., 1991b; Biederman et al., 1991). Although the causes of comorbidity are not well understood, its consequences are not benign. Many studies find that comorbid symptoms and disorders lead to high morbidity and disability (Loney et al., 1981; Stewart et al., 1981; August et al., 1983; Kovacs et al., 1984; Brent et al., 1988; Kovacs et al., 1988; Frost et al., 1989; Mannuzza et al., 1989). Indeed, the co-occurrence of ADHD with certain comorbid disorders suggests that there may be subtypes of ADHD children at higher risk for psychiatric morbidity, social disability, and cognitive dysfunction than ADHD children without comorbidity (Biederman et al., 1991).

The overlap between ADHD and learning disability (LD) also complicates studies of ADHD. The proportion of ADHD children with learning disabilities may be as low as 5% to 10% (Halperin et al., 1984; Holborow & Berry, 1986) or as high as 92% (Silver, 1981). This lack of agreement among studies reflects variable selection criteria, sampling, measurement instruments, and definitions of ADHD and LD (Semrud-Clikeman et al., 1992). Although the finding in some studies that LD is almost universally found among ADHD children (Silver, 1981) may suggest that ADHD and LD are indistinguishable (Prior & Sanson, 1986), important differences exist between these disorders.

ADHD is a behavioral syndrome with characteristic symptoms of inattentiveness, impulsivity, and hyperactivity. In constrast, LD refers to a group of cognitive disorders thought to reflect circumscribed perceptual handicaps in one or more basic cognitive processes that are manifested as disorders of language, reading, writing and spelling, or arithmetic. Since not all LD children have ADHD and many ADHD children achieve adequately, it may be that the two disorders are independent but can co-occur in some individuals (Interagency Committee on Learning Disabilities, 1987).

The work of August and Garfinkel (1989) suggested that ADHD can be divided into behavioral and cognitive subtypes; both types exhibit inattention, impulsivity, and hyperactivity, but differ concerning the degree of behavioral disruption and academic underachievement. Similarly, a factor analytic study was consistent with the presence of independent dimensions of hyperactivity and learning disabilities (Lahey et al., 1978).

The role that genetic factors play in the emergence of LD among ADHD children is unknown. Family-genetic studies consistently find relatives of ADHD probands to be at increased risk for ADHD (Cantwell, 1972; Biederman et al., 1986; Barkley et al., 1990; Biederman et al., 1992; Faraone et al., 1991a; Faraone et al., 1991b; Faraone & Biederman, 1994; Faraone, Biederman, & Milberger, 1994; Faraone et al., 1995) and there is strong evidence that some forms of LD have a genetic etiology (DeFries et al., 1987; Smith et al., 1990). Since the etiologies of ADHD and LD are both known to have familial and, possibly, genetic components, the examination of relatives of ADHD children may provide insights into the relationship between the two conditions.

For example, a recent twin study of ADHD and LD concluded that the two conditions are genetically independent (Gilger et al., 1992). In this chapter, we describe our work examining cognitive impairment, failure in school and learning disability among the ADHD and normal control subjects and their relatives (Faraone et al., 1993a; Faraone et al., 1993b). We sought to (1) describe the pattern of cognitive deficit and school failure among ADHD children; (2) demonstrate the effects of comorbid psychiatric disorders on the cognitive functioning of ADHD children; (3) determine if the non-ADHD relatives of ADHD subjects are at risk for school failure and impaired intellectual functioning; and (4) use family-genetic data to clarify the relationship between learning disabilities and ADHD by testing competing hypotheses based, in part on models of familial transmission proposed by Pauls et al. (Pauls et al., 1986a; Pauls et al., 1986b) and Reich et al. (Reich et al., 1972; Reich et al., 1979).

METHOD

Subjects

We studied two groups of index (proband) boys: 140 ADHD probands and 120 normal controls. These groups had 454 and 368 first degree biological relatives respectively. All probands were Caucasian, non-Hispanic males between the ages of 6 and 17. Potential probands were excluded if they had been adopted, or if their nuclear family was not available for study. We excluded probands if they had major sensorimotor handicaps (paralysis, deafness, blindness), psychosis, autism, or a Full Scale IQ less than 80. Subjects from the lowest socioeconomic class, SES VI (Hollingshead, 1975), were excluded to minimize the potential confounds of social adversity. All of the ADHD probands met diagnostic criteria for current ADHD at the time of the clinical referral; at the time of recruitment they all had active symptoms of the disorder for which they were receiving treatment.

Two independent sources provided the index children. We selected psychiatrically referred ADHD probands from consecutive referrals to the Pediatric Psychopharmacology Unit at the Massachusetts General Hospital (MGH). This service is not a tertiary care clinic since approximately 50% of new referrals have never been diagnosed or treated before. Parents, pediatricians, and schools had referred these children for psychiatric evaluations. The pediatrically referred ADHD probands consisted of pediatric patients from the Harvard Community Health Plan, a large Health Maintenance Organization (HMO). Within each setting, we selected normal controls from active outpatients at pediatric medical clinics.

A three-stage ascertainment procedure selected the probands. For ADHD probands, the first stage was the patient's referral to a psychiatric or pediatric clinic resulting in a clinical diagnosis of ADHD by a child psychiatrist (N = 154) or pediatrician (N = 238) as recorded in the clinic record. Since these diagnoses had been made by many different clinicians using different clinical standards of diagnosis, we included a second, systematic screening using DSM-III-R criteria. This second stage confirmed the diagnosis of ADHD by screening all children positive at the first stage using a telephone questionnaire with their mother. The questionnaire asked about the 14 DSM-III-R symptoms of ADHD and questions regarding race, ethnicity, age, sex and social class (study entry criteria). Of the referred pool of patients, 48% (N = 74) at MGH and 66% (N = 156) at the HMO were ineligible or unreachable. Of those remaining and meeting study entry criteria, 4% (N = 3) at MGH and 15% (N = 12) at the HMO refused participation. Eligible subjects meeting study entry criteria who consented to participate were recruited for the study and received a comprehensive assessment battery as described below. This assessment battery collected data for the final DSM-III-R diagnoses reported in this paper. Only patients who received a positive diagnosis at all three stages were included in the final analysis. Of the pool of patients who received this comprehensive assessment, 1% (N = 1) at MGH and 9% (N = 6) at the HMO did not receive a positive diagnosis of ADHD at this stage and were therefore not included in the final sample. The final ADHD sample consisted of 76 subjects at the MGH site and 64 at the HMO site.

We also screened potential normal controls in three stages. First, we ascertained them from referrals to medical clinics at the MGH (N = 282) and the HMO (N = 261) sites for routine physical examinations. Second, we administered the same DSM-III-R ADHD telephone questionnaire and the questions regarding race, ethnicity, age, sex and social class as those asked for the ADHD subjects to the mothers of referred controls. Of the referred pool of normal controls, 83% (N = 233) at MGH and 60% (N = 157) at the HMO were ineligible or unreachable. Of those remaining and meeting study criteria, 20% (N = 10) at MGH and 19% (N = 20) at the HMO refused participation. Eligible subjects who consented to participate were recruited for the study and received the same assessment battery as that used for the ADHD sample as described below. Control subjects were included only if they were not diagnosed with ADHD at any of the three stages and met sociodemographic study criteria. Of those who reached this stage, 3% (N = 1) at MGH and 2% (N = 2) at the HMO were diagnosed with ADHD and were therefore not included in the final sample. The final sample of normal controls consisted of 38 subjects at the MGH site and 82 at the HMO site.

Procedures

All diagnostic assessments were made using DSM-III-R-based structured interviews. Psychiatric assessments of probands and siblings were made with the Kiddie SADS-E, Epidemiologic Version (Orvaschel, 1985). Diagnoses were based on independent interviews with the mothers and direct interviews of probands and siblings, except for children younger than 12 years of age who were not directly interviewed. Diagnostic assessments of parents were based on direct interviews with each parent using the Structured Clinical Interview for DSM-III-R, SCID (Spitzer et al., 1990). To assess childhood diagnoses in the parents, we administered an addition to the SCID, consisting of unmodified modules from the Kiddie-SADS-E covering childhood DSM-III-R diagnoses.

All assessments were made by interviewers who were blind to proband diagnosis (ADHD or control) and ascertainment site (MGH or HMO). All efforts were made to sequence the mothers' interviews about their children after the direct interview with the mother about herself had been completed. Also, different interviewers were obtained to conduct the direct interviews of the siblings and the interviews with mothers about their children. Interview data were collected on all siblings in both the ADHD and control families. At MGH, 89% of the parents were directly interviewed and at the HMO, 93% were directly interviewed. Ninety-five percent of all uninterviewed cases were fathers. When a parent was not available for interviewing, information was obtained by administering the SCID about the absent spouse to the available spouse. Information from one HMO control father could not be obtained. The diagnostic data from absent spouses were used in the analyses reported in this paper. All parents signed a written consent form for participation in the study.

Interviews were conducted by five interviewers with undergraduate degrees in psychology who had been trained to high levels of interrater reliability. The training consisted of familiarization with psychiatric nosology (DSM-III-R) and the structured interviews. Interviewers in training first observed interviews carried out by experienced interviewers and clinicians. They subsequently conducted at least six practice (non-study) interviews and at least two study interviews while observed by senior interviewers before rating independently. Interviewers were supervised by the senior investigator (JB). Kappa coefficients of agreement were computed between raters and three experienced, board certified child and adult psychiatrists who listened to audiotaped interviews made by the raters. Based on 61 interviews, all kappas were higher than 0.82 with the exception of alcohol abuse which was 0.75. The mean Kappa was 0.90. Kappas of 1.0 were obtained for ADHD (95% confidence interval: 0.8–1.0), substance abuse (0.7–1.0), and substance dependence (0.7–1.0). Full information regarding kappa coefficients are available upon request.

Diagnoses were considered positive if, based on the interview results, DSM-III-R criteria were unequivocally met. All diagnostic uncertainties were resolved by a committee of four board-certified child and adult psychiatrists who were blind to the subject's ascertainment group, ascertainment site, all data collected from other family members, and all non-diagnostic data (e.g. cognitive functioning). Diagnoses were considered positive only if criteria were met to a degree that would be considered clinically meaningful. As suggested by others (Gershon et al., 1982; Weissman et al., 1984), the diagnosis of major depression was made only if the depressive episode was associated with marked impairment. Since the anxiety disorders comprise many syndromes with a wide range of severity, we also report results for two or more anxiety disorders to index the presence of a clinically meaningful anxiety syndrome (Biederman et al., 1990; Rosenbaum et al., 1991). For children older than 12, data from direct and indirect interviews were combined by considering a diagnostic criterion positive if it was endorsed in either interview. Since the structured interviews generate diagnostic information about both past and current disturbances, the rates of illness reported here are lifetime prevalence figures.

Our interviewers assessed academic achievement with the Arithmetic Subtest of the Wide Range Achievement Test and the Gilmore Oral Reading Test. For subjects younger than 17, they assessed cognitive functioning with the vocabulary, block design, arithmetic, digit span and coding subtests of the Wechsler Intelligence Scales for Children-Revised (WISC-R). For subjects 17-years-old and older, they assessed cognitive functioning with the vocabulary, block design, arithmetic, digit span, and digit symbol subtests of the Wechsler Adult Intelligence Scales-Revised (WAIS-R). Using the methods of Sattler (1988), we estimated Full Scale IQ from the vocabulary and block design subtests and computed the Freedom From Distractibility IQ from the other subtests. All of our analyses of the Wechsler subtests use age-corrected scaled scores. Our interviewers were trained to administer these tests by a child clinical psychologist with extensive experience with the psychological assessment of children. The psychologist supervised the interviewers throughout the study.

The definition of Learning Disabilities under Public Law 94–142 requires a significant discrepancy between a child's potential and achievement (Federal Register, 1977). These guidelines do not define the magnitude of discrepancy to be considered "significant." Reynolds (1984) provides a thorough review of measurement issues involved in the definition of learning disabilities. We used the procedure recommended by him and others (e.g., Frick et al., 1991) as follows. We first converted the estimated Full Scale IQ, and achievement scores to the Z-scores Z_{IQ} and Z_A. We then estimated the expected achievement scores Z_{EA}, by the regression equation

$$Z_{EA} = r_{IQA} \times Z_{IQ}$$

where r_{IQA} is the correlation between the IQ and achievement tests. Then, the discrepancy score is $Z_{EA} - Z_{IQ}$ and its standard deviation is $\sqrt{1 - r_{IQA}^2}$. Thus, we defined as learning disabled any subject who had a value greater than 1.65 on the standardized discrepancy score:

$$\frac{Z_{EA} - Z_{IQ}}{\sqrt{1 - r_{IQA}^2}}$$

We also used this procedure to define significant discrepancies in estimated verbal and performance IQ scores.

Table 12.1. *Percent of probands with school failure*

	ADHD N = 140	Control N = 120
Problem	%	%
Academic tutoring[2]	56	25
Repeated a grade[1]	30	13
Placed in special class[2]	35	2
Reading disability[2]	18	4
Arithmetic disability[1]	21	8

Note: [1] $p \leq 0.01$, [2] $p \leq 0.001$ by Fisher's Exact Test.
Source: This table was used with permission from the American Psychological Association for the article by Faraone et al., "Intellectual performance and school failure in children with attention deficit hyperactivity disorder and in their siblings," *Journal of Abnormal Psychology*, **102**(4), 616–623.

The ADHD families came from somewhat lower socioeconomic strata than the control families (Hollingshead, 1975): SES 1.8 ± 1.0 vs. 1.5 ± 0.7, $\chi^2 = 12.4$, $p = 0.002$. Thus, we present all statistical analyses with and without corrections for SES. For categorical variables, we used the Cochran–Mantel– Haenszel General Association statistic to control for SES. As suggested by a number of researchers (Chapman & Chapman, 1978, 1989; Saykin et al., 1991), we adjusted continuous variables for SES as follows. First, we used the control data to estimate the regression equation predicting the variable from SES. Then we used this equation to compute predicted scores for each variable. The difference between the predicted and observed scores (i.e., the residual) was used as the adjusted score in the analyses that corrected for SES.

RESULTS

School failure and cognitive functioning in probands

As indicated by Table 12.1, the ADHD probands exhibited significantly more school failure in all areas assessed. More than half had required tutoring and a third had been placed in special classes or had repeated a grade. The rates of learning disabilities were low among ADHD probands (18% for reading and 21% for arithmetic) but were significantly higher than the 4% and 8% rates observed among controls. Moreover, each of these findings remained significant after statistically controlling for socioeconomic status.

Table 12.2. *Percent of school failure among ADHD probands with comorbid psychiatric disorders*

	ADHD+CD N = 30	ADHD+MDD N = 40	ADHD+ANX N = 39	ADHD only N = 64
Academic tutoring	50	45	49	63[3]
Repeated a grade	20[1]	28[1]	26[1]	34[2]
Placed in special class	57	53	51	20[3]
Reading disability	25	14	21	17[2]
Arithmetic disability	21	24	21	20

Note: CD = conduct disorder; MDD = major depressive disorder; ANX = two or more anxiety disorders; [1] $p \leq 0.01$ for effects of comorbid disorders among ADHD probands; [2] $p \leq 0.01$; [3] $p \leq 0.001$ compared with normal controls in Table 12.1.
Source: This table was used with permission from the American Psychological Association for the article by Faraone et al., "Intellectual performance and school failure in children with attention deficit hyperactivity disorder and in their siblings," *Journal of Abnormal Psychology*, **102**(4), 616–623.

Table 12.2 presents the rates of failure in school among ADHD probands stratified by the presence of conduct disorder (CD), major depression (MDD), and two or more anxiety disorders (ANX).[1] We compared these comorbid subgroups with ADHD probands having none of these disorders (ADHD only). Forty-six percent of the ADHD probands are in this latter group; only 3.6% have all of these disorders. As Table 12.2 indicates, the three comorbidity groups do not differ among themselves. The only significant pairwise difference between each comorbidity group and the noncomorbid group is for placement in special classes. The rate of placement in special classes is two and half times higher among the comorbid groups compared to ADHD probands with no comorbidity. These differences remain significant after statistically controlling for SES.

Compared with controls, ADHD probands were significantly more impaired on the vocabulary, block design, arithmetic, digit span, and coding subtests of the Wechsler Intelligence Scale for Children – Revised (WISC-R; Table 12.3). They also had significantly lower estimated Full Scale and Freedom from Distractibility IQs (Table 12.3). To estimate the difference between verbal and performance IQs, we subtracted the block design scaled score from the vocabulary scaled score and adjusted this for the correlation between the variables. For ADHD probands, this difference was negative indicating higher scores on block design than vocabulary. In the controls, the difference was

---

[1] We have used two or more anxiety disorders in this and other publications to characterize a group of patients with substantial evidence of clinically relevant anxiety (Biederman et al., 1990, 1991a; Rosenbaum et al., 1990, 1991b).

Table 12.3. *WISC-R scores for ADHD and control probands*

	ADHD N = 140		CONTROL N = 120	
Test score (p ≤ 0.0001)	Mean	SD	Mean	SD
Vocabulary	11.1	3.2	13.0	2.7
Block design	13.1	3.8	15.2	3.3
Arithmetic	10.6	3.1	12.4	2.9
Digit span	8.9	2.8	10.8	2.8
Coding	9.9	3.5	11.8	2.6
FFDIQ	98.8	15.8	111.1	13.3
Estimated FSIQ	109.5	13.5	118.4	10.2

Note: WISC-R = Wechsler Intelligence Scale for Children-Revised; FFDIQ = Freedom From Distractability Intelligence Quotient; FSIQ = Full Scale Intelligence Quotient. *Source:* This table was used with permission from the American Psychological Association for the article by Faraone et al., "Intellectual performance and school failure in children with attention deficit hyperactivity disorder and in their siblings," *Journal of Abnormal Psychology*, **102**(4), 616–623.

positive, indicating higher scores on the vocabulary than block design; the difference between the two groups was significant. In a categorical analysis, the performance IQ was significantly greater than the verbal IQ for 6% of the ADHD probands and 3% of the control probands but the difference between groups was not significant (FET p = 0.23). The performance IQ was significantly lower than the verbal IQ for 4% of the ADHD probands and 6% of the control probands but the difference between groups was not significant (FET p = 0.58).

Each of the findings in Table 12.3 remains significant after statistically controlling for socioeconomic status. We note that the scores for control probands are all greater than their expected means (10 for scaled scores, 100 for IQ scores). This is consistent with our exclusion criteria, which excluded subjects with a Full Scale IQ lower than 80 and those from the lowest social class. Additionally, our method of ascertainment excluded potential controls who had a diagnosis of ADHD.

Table 12.4 presents cognitive test results after stratifying ADHD probands by psychiatric comorbidity. ADHD probands with conduct disorder (CD) performed significantly more poorly than other ADHD probands on the block design subtest of the WISC-R, even after correction for SES. They also had a lower estimated Full Scale IQ but did as well as other ADHD probands on other measures of cognitive functioning. Compared with ADHD probands without MDD, those with MDD tended to have *higher* test scores but the differences were not significant. ADHD probands with comorbid anxiety disorders (ANX) were more impaired on the coding subtest of the

Table 12.4. *WISC-R scores and comorbidity among ADHD probands*

Test score	ADHD + CD N = 30 Mean	SD	ADHD + MDD N = 40 Mean	SD	ADHD + ANX N = 39 Mean	SD	ADHD only N = 64 Mean	SD
Vocabulary	10.7	3.1	11.4	3.2	10.2	3.4	11.1[3]	3.0
Block design	11.5[1]	2.9	14.1[1]	3.8	12.1[1]	4.4	13.2[2]	3.7
Arithmetic	10.4	2.8	10.6	3.1	10.6	3.3	10.6[2]	3.4
Digit span	8.8	2.7	9.1	2.4	8.6	2.9	8.9[3]	2.9
Coding	9.1	3.8	9.6	3.1	8.8	3.3	10.3	3.7
FFDIQ	96.5	16.0	98.7	14.1	95.5	15.8	99.5[3]	16.9
Estimated FSIQ	103.8	13.0	112.3[1]	13.0	104.9[1]	15.8	109.4[3]	12.3

Note: CD = Conduct Disorder; MDD = Major Depressive Disorder; ANX = Two or more anxiety disorders; WISC-R = Wechsler Intelligence Scale for Children – Revised; FFDIQ = Freedom From Distractability Intelligence Quotient; FSIQ = Full Scale Intelligence Quotient; [1] p ≤ 0.01 for effects of comorbid disorders among ADHD probands; [2] p ≤ 0.01; [3] p ≤ 0.001 compared with normal controls in Table 12.3.

Source: This table was used with permission from the American Psychological Association for the article by Faraone et al., "Intellectual performance and school failure in children with attention deficit hyperactivity disorder and in their siblings," *Journal of Abnormal Psychology,* **102**(4), 616–623.

Table 12.5. *School failure among relatives of ADHD and control probands*

Problem	Adult relatives of ADHD probands N = 320		Adult relatives of control probands N = 273		Without ADHD relatives	
	N	%	N	%	FET	FET
Academic tutoring	83	26.5	35	13.0	0.000[3]	0.005[1]
Repeated a grade	63	19.9	34	12.5	0.019	0.023
Placed in special class	9	2.8	2	0.7	0.071	0.068
Reading disability	3	1.1	0	0.0	0.25	0.25
Arithmetic disability	4	1.4	2	0.8	0.69	1.0

Problem	Siblings of ADHD probands N = 134		Siblings of control probands N = 95		Without ADHD relatives	
	N	%	N	%	FET	FET
Academic tutoring	53	39.6	22	23.2	0.01[1]	0.024
Repeated a grade	26	19.4	5	5.3	0.002[2]	0.018[1]
Placed in special class	12	9.0	2	2.1	0.047	0.131
Reading disability	13	10.5	2	2.2	0.027[1]	0.107
Arithmetic disability	9	7.1	5	5.3	0.78	0.34

Note: FET = Fisher's Exact Test; [1] $0.01 < p \leq 0.05$, [2] $0.001 < p \leq 0.01$, [3] $p \leq 0.001$ after controlling for SES.

WISC-R, but the difference lost statistical significance after controlling for SES.

School failure and cognitive functioning in relatives

Table 12.5 compares the adult (age ≥ 17) and non-adult (age < 17) first degree relatives of ADHD and control probands. Age seventeen is a meaningful cut point because it separates subjects given the WISC-R from those given the WAIS-R. All of the nonadult relatives are siblings and most of the adult relatives are parents.

Compared with siblings of control probands, those of ADHD probands were significantly more likely to have repeated a grade, to have required academic tutoring, to have been placed in special classes, and to have a reading disability. Only the comparison for special classes lost significance after controlling for SES. The findings for adult relatives are similar (Table 12.5). However, the effects for placement in special classes and reading disabilities are not significant. Also, among the adult relatives without ADHD, only the effect for tutoring remained significant after correcting for SES.

Table 12.6. *Cognitive functioning among relatives of ADHD and control probands*

Test score	Adult relatives of ADHD probands N = 320		Adult relatives of control probands N = 273		Without ADHD relatives
	Mean	SD	Mean	SD	P-value	P-value
WAIS-R Vocabulary	11.9	2.7	13.0	2.6	0.0001*	0.0001*
WAIS-R Block design	11.6	2.8	12.3	2.7	0.0018	0.0029
WAIS-R Arithmetic	11.3	2.9	12.0	2.6	0.0029	0.0069
WAIS-R Digit span	10.6	2.6	11.3	2.7	0.0013*	0.0031*
WAIS-R Digit symbol	11.4	2.2	12.0	2.4	0.0046*	0.01
WAIS-R FFDIQ	104.3	12.8	108.5	12.7	0.0002*	0.0007*
WAIS-R estimated FSIQ	108.7	11.5	113.1	10.4	0.0001*	0.0001*
Vocabulary-Blocks	1.1	2.5	1.7	2.6	0.0043	0.0038

Test score	Siblings of ADHD probands N = 134		Siblings of control probands N = 95		Without ADHD relatives
	Mean	SD	Mean	SD	P-value	P-value
WISC-R Vocabulary	11.3	3.1	12.4	3.0	0.0087	0.02
WISC-R Block design	13.4	3.2	14.5	3.4	0.015	0.11
WISC-R Arithmetic	12.0	2.8	12.6	2.9	0.17	0.31
WISC-R Digit span	10.0	3.0	10.6	3.4	0.19	0.54
WISC-R Coding	11.3	2.9	12.3	2.9	0.01*	0.06
WISC-R FFDIQ	107.4	13.6	112.0	15.4	0.02	0.12
WISC-R estimated FSIQ	111.0	12.0	115.7	11.6	0.003	0.019
Vocabulary-Blocks	−0.3	2.9	0.3	2.8	0.13	0.09

Note: WISC-R = Wechsler Intelligence Scale for Children, Revised; WAIS-R = Wechsler Adult Intelligence Scale, Revised; FFDIQ = Freedom From Distractability Intelligence Quotient; FSIQ = Full Scale Intelligence Quotient; Vocabulary-Blocks: Vocabulary score minus block design score; *0.01 < p ≤ 0.05 after correcting for SES.

Since we have reported elsewhere that the relatives of ADHD probands have higher rates of ADHD than the relatives of control probands (Biederman et al., 1992), we repeated these analyses after excluding any relative with ADHD from the analysis. For these analyses (Table 12.5) the only significant differences are for requiring tutoring and repeating a grade and only the latter remains significant after controlling for SES.

The relatives of ADHD probands performed worse than relatives of controls on all of the administered subtests of the Wechsler Intelligence Scales: vocabulary, block design, arithmetic, digit span, and digit symbol/coding (Table 12.6). For the adult relatives, each of these differences was statistically significant and the effects for WAIS-R vocabulary, digit span, digit symbol, freedom from distractibility IQ, and estimated Full Scale IQ remained significant after controlling for SES. With the exception of the digit symbol subtest, each of these retained significance after we excluded all ADHD relatives and statistically controlled for SES.

For the child and adolescent relatives (Table 12.6), the only difference that remained significant after controlling for SES was WISC-R coding. There were statistically significant differences between the nonADHD siblings of ADHD probands and controls for WISC-R vocabulary and Full Scale IQ. However, these were not statistically significant after controlling for SES.

Association between ADHD and learning disability

We stratified the ADHD probands by the presence (ADHD + LD) or absence (ADHD − LD) of a Learning Disability (LD) in either reading or arithmetic. There were 40 ADHD + LD probands having 122 relatives; there were 93 ADHD − LD probands having 265 relatives. Compared with ADHD probands without LD (ADHD − LD), those with LD (ADHD + LD) were more likely to have repeated a grade (53% vs. 19%, Fisher's Exact Test [FET] p < 0.001), and been placed in special classes (50% vs. 28%, FET p = 0.02). They were not significantly more likely to have required academic tutoring (68% vs. 52%, FET p = 0.13). Both groups show more evidence of school failure than the normal comparisons. For the ADHD + LD probands, all contrasts with normal comparisons are significant (FET, all p's < 0.001). For the ADHD − LD probands, only the effects for tutoring and placement in special classes were significant (FET, both p's < 0.001).

We compared six competing hypotheses about the etiologic association between ADHD and LD (Reich et al., 1972; Reich et al., 1979; Pauls et al., 1986a; Pauls et al., 1986b).

Hypothesis 1: posits that ADHD and LD are etiologically independent and co-occur due to chance. If this is so, we should find equally high rates of ADHD in relatives of the ADHD − LD and ADHD + LD children but LD should be increased only among relatives of ADHD + LD children. Also, the two conditions should not cosegregate in families of ADHD + LD probands. In other words, the two disorders should be independently transmitted within these families such that the presence of ADHD in relatives does not increase their risk for LD.

Hypothesis 2: is that ADHD + LD is a distinct familial subtype. Thus, we should find high rates of ADHD in relatives of ADHD − LD and ADHD + LD children but LD should be increased only among relatives of ADHD + LD children. This is the same pattern as Hypothesis 1. However, we should also find strong evidence for cosegregation. Thus, among relatives of children with ADHD + LD, the presence of one disorder should predict the presence of the other; cases of ADHD without LD and LD without ADHD should be rare.

Hypothesis 3: posits that ADHD and LD are etiologically independent and that they co-occur due to nonrandom mating (i.e., the spouses of ADHD individuals have higher rates of LD than spouses of nonADHD individuals). This predicts the same pattern of familial transmission as Hypothesis 1, but we should also find evidence of nonrandom mating in the parents.

Hypothesis 4: states that ADHD + LD is a more severe familial form of ADHD − LD. Thus, we should find a higher risk for both ADHD and LD among relatives of ADHD + LD children compared to those of ADHD − LD children. Relatives of both types should have higher risks for each disorder compared with normal comparisons.

Hypothesis 5: states that ADHD children with and without LD share common familial etiologic factors but differ due to environmental effects. We should then find similar rates of ADHD and LD in the relatives of both subgroups.

Hypothesis 6: posits that the LD among ADHD children is secondary to the cognitive and social impairments associated with ADHD. It predicts no familial transmission of LD in the families of ADHD probands, although some increase in LD might be found among the ADHD relatives of ADHD probands.

In comparing these hypotheses, the most dramatic finding is that LD in the absence of ADHD is found more frequently among the relatives of ADHD + LD probands compared with relatives of ADHD − LD and normal comparison probands (Table 12.7). In contrast, ADHD is equally familial in ADHD + LD and ADHD − LD families. Clearly, hypotheses four, five and six are not tenable. To discriminate among hypotheses one, two, and three, we tested for cosegregation and nonrandom mating.

To test for cosegregation among the 122 relatives of ADHD + LD probands, we compared the 24 relatives with ADHD with the 98 without ADHD to determine if ADHD and LD were independently transmitted in these families. Those with ADHD had higher rates of learning disabilities but the difference was not significant (21% vs. 18%, p = 0.80). However, both of these rates were significantly greater than the 5% rate of LD among the normal comparison relatives (p's < 0.01). Overall, these findings do not suggest substantial cosegregation between ADHD and LD.

To test for nonrandom mating, we tested for associations between ADHD and LD in the parents of the ADHD probands. Among the 13 mothers with ADHD, 15% had husbands with a reading disability compared with 1% of the mothers with no history of ADHD (FET, p = 0.04). Among the 16 fathers with ADHD, 13% had wives with a reading disability compared with 0% for the non-ADHD fathers (FET, p = 0.02). There was no association between ADHD in the mother and arithmetic disability in the fathers or between ADHD in the father and arithmetic disability in the mother.

Table 12.7. *Familial distribution of ADHD and learning disabilities alone and combined in relatives of probands with (ADHD + LD) and without (ADHD − LD)*

	Proband diagnosis					
	ADHD + LD Proband N = 40 Adult relatives N = 79 Siblings N = 43		ADHD − LD Proband N = 93 Adult relatives N = 188 Siblings N = 77		Control Proband N = 120 Adult relatives N = 243 Siblings N = 93	
Relative's diagnosis	N	%	N	%	N	%
Adult relative's diagnosis (Parents and siblings ≥ 17 years)						
ADHD + LD	2	3	2	1	1	0.4
ADHD − LD	11	14†††	22	12†††	5	2
LD	9	12**†††	5	3	4	2
Sibling's diagnosis (Siblings < 17 years)						
ADHD + LD	3	7	5	6	2	2
ADHD − LD	8	19†	8	10	4	4
LD	9	21*	5	6	9	10

Note: For Adult table: $\chi^2(6) = 42.2$, $p < 0.0001$; for Sibling table: $\chi^2(6) = 18.0$, $p = 0.006$. $*$ p < 0.05; $**$ p < 0.01 by FET compared with ADHD − LD. † p < 0.05; †† p < 0.01; ††† p < 0.001 by FET compared with controls.

Source: This table is used with permission from the American Psychiatric Association for the article by Faraone et al., "Evidence for the independent familial transmission of attention deficit hyperactivity disorder and learning disabilities: Results from a family genetic study," *American Journal of Psychiatry,* **150,** 891–895.

Fifteen percent of the male relatives of ADHD probands had ADHD − LD; 3.8% had ADHD + LD and 9.2% had LD only. For females these rates were 10.8%, 2.5% and 5.4% respectively. Although the rates for each category are greater for males, the difference was not significant ($\chi^2(3) = 4.6$, p = 0.2). Among male relatives of normal comparisons, 3.9% had ADHD − LD, 1.9% had ADHD + LD and 3.2% had LD only. For females these rates were 1.6%, 0.0% and 4.4% respectively. The differences between males and females were not significant ($\chi^2(3) = 5.4$, p = 0.1). The percent of male relatives did not differ significantly between relatives of ADHD − LD (45%), ADHD + LD (53%) and normal comparison probands (46%; $\chi^2(2) = 2.5$, p = 0.3).

DISCUSSION

School failure and cognitive functioning in probands

We were not surprised to find more evidence of school failure and cognitive impairment among our ADHD probands compared with our normal control probands. Indeed, the presence of such problems is one of the most reproducible findings in studies of the ADHD syndrome (Semrud-Clikeman et al., 1992). In our sample, compared to normal controls, ADHD probands were more likely to have had histories of learning disabilities, repeated grades, placement in special classes and need for academic tutoring. They were also significantly more impaired on subtests of the Wechsler Intelligence Scale for Children-Revised (WISC-R). Of course, these significant differences should not obscure our finding that the mean levels of intellectual functioning on the WISC-R were well within the normal range. Although this is partly due to our selection criteria (i.e., Full Scale IQ greater than 80, not from the lowest social class), it also confirms the clinical observation that many ADHD children have average or above average WISC-R scores yet do poorly in school.

Our results are consistent with other published work in indicating the presence of two types of ADHD-related cognitive dysfunction that have clinical and educational implications. First, for many ADHD children, school achievement is significantly discrepant from estimates of ability derived from the WISC-R or other measures (Lambert & Sandoval, 1980; August & Holmes, 1984; Halperin et al., 1984; McGee et al., 1984; Barkley, 1990; Frick et al., 1991; Semrud-Clikeman et al., 1992). Second, ADHD children may have lower scores on standard measures of intelligence (e.g., Singer et al., 1981; Campbell & Werry, 1986; McGee et al., 1989; McGee et al., 1987; Werry et al., 1987; Schaughency et al., 1989). Thus, the absence of a discrepancy between estimates of achievement and ability may occur because *both* have been impaired by the disorder.

Our results indicate that the cognitive impairments of our ADHD sample are due to the ADHD syndrome itself; they do not appear to be accounted for by psychiatric comorbidity. Among ADHD probands, comorbid conduct, major depressive and anxiety disorders were associated with placement in special classes but not with tutoring, repeated grades or learning disabilities. Psychiatric comorbidity also had limited influence on WISC-R scores. Among ADHD probands, conduct disorder was significantly associated with poor block design scores and there was a trend for anxiety disorders to be associated with poor coding scores. Our results are similar to those of Frick et al. (1991) who examined academic underachievement in children with ADHD, conduct disorder and both disorders. They found that an apparent association between school failure and conduct disorder was due to the comorbidity of conduct disorder with ADHD. Frost et al. (1989) examined neuropsychological functioning in an unselected cohort of young adolescents. They found evidence of neuropsychological impairment among children with ADHD. However, in the absence of comorbid ADHD, children with conduct disorder or depression were similar to non-disordered controls. Children with multiple disorders were the most impaired.

Overall, these results suggest that psychiatric comorbidity affects school *placement* more than it affects school *failure* or WISC-R measures of ability. Similar results were reported by Sandoval and Lambert (1984–5). They found that hyperactivity and aggression were significant predictors of placement in special education classes. Also, Barkley et al. (1990) concluded that among ADHD children the presence of antisocial behaviors predicted placement in programs for behaviorally disturbed students rather than programs for learning disabled students. Although psychopathology should influence educational placements, it should do so in the context of a comprehensive assessment of psychiatric comorbidity and psychoeducational dysfunction.

Our comorbidity results also provide indirect evidence for the validity of the ADHD syndrome, *per se*. Although our noncomorbid ADHD subjects are not afflicted with the emotional and behavioral disruptions that accompany conduct, depressive, and anxiety disorders, 63% require tutoring, 34% had repeated a grade, 20% had been placed in special classes, 17% had a reading disability and 20% had an arithmetic disability. Thus, uncomplicated ADHD is associated with a serious risk for school failure; it may be less disruptive than its comorbid counterparts, but should not be ignored in educational settings.

As Shaywitz & Shaywitz (1989) note, these findings also have a methodological implication for research. Since comorbidity affects school placement, the selection of ADHD subjects from special education classes or other educationally specialized classes is likely to skew the psychiatric composition of a sample. Also, studies of children with conduct, anxiety and major depressive disorders have found some deficits in intellectual ability and achievement to be associated with these disorders (e.g., Cole, 1990; Hodges & Plow, 1990). However, results from such studies will be difficult to interpret if the comorbidity of these disorders with ADHD is not taken into account.

For example, others have shown that an observed association between conduct disorder and academic underachievement could be accounted for by the comorbidity of conduct disorder and ADHD (Frick et al., 1991).

School failure and cognitive functioning in relatives

Given that we and others have shown ADHD to be a familial disorder (Morrison & Stewart, 1971; Cantwell, 1972; Welner et al., 1977; Morrison, 1980; Stewart et al., 1980; Biederman et al., 1986; Barkley et al., 1990; Biederman et al., 1991), we were not surprised to find higher than normal rates of school failure and intellectual impairment among the biological relatives of our ADHD probands. Although these findings are mostly accounted for by the relatives having ADHD, some interesting patterns emerged when we limited the analyses to relatives without ADHD.

The nonADHD child and adolescent relatives of ADHD probands were more likely to have repeated a grade and required tutoring but, compared with controls they did not have higher rates of learning disabilities or placement in special classes. The findings for adult relatives without ADHD were similar. Thus, both classes of relatives show moderate signs of school dysfunction even though they do not have ADHD. We found a similar pattern for scores from the Wechsler Intelligence Scales. Compared with control relatives, the WAIS-R vocabulary and digit span scores were significantly lower among the nonADHD adult relatives of ADHD probands. All WISC-R subtest scores were lower among the nonADHD siblings of ADHD probands. However, none were significant after controlling for socioeconomic status.

The increased risk for school failure and cognitive dysfunction among the nonADHD relatives has implications for clinicians and educators. The presence of cognitive dysfunction and school failure among nonADHD relatives suggests that the siblings of ADHD children may be a high risk group deserving of special psychological or educational attention. Further work is needed to determine if this high risk status is predictive of subsequent problems. If so, it would be of interest to assess the utility of early intervention with these high risk children.

Association between ADHD and learning disability

We found that: (1) relatives of ADHD probands with and without LD had significantly higher risks for ADHD than did relatives of normal comparison probands; (2) the risk for LD was elevated only among relatives of ADHD + LD probands; (3) ADHD and LD did not cosegregate among the relatives of ADHD + LD probands and (4) there was nonrandom mating between ADHD and LD spouses. These findings suggest that the two conditions are etiologically independent (hypothesis 1) but co-occur due to nonrandom mating (hypothesis 3). Our results are not compatible with the idea that ADHD and LD are manifestations of a single disorder (hypotheses 4 and 5) or with the hypothesis that ADHD + LD patients are ADHD children who develop LD secondary to the symptomatology of ADHD (hypothesis 6). Our data are also not consistent with the hypothesis that ADHD + LD is etiologically distinct from ADHD − LD (hypothesis 2).

Our finding of independent transmission between ADHD and LD is consistent with a recent twin study of these conditions (Gilger et al., 1992). The cross concordances between ADHD and LD were 44% for monozygotic twins and 30% for dizygotic twins. The small difference between monozygotic and dizygotic twins led the authors to conclude that ADHD and LD were, primarily, genetically independent.

In concluding that ADHD and LD are independent conditions, we do not assert that ADHD − LD is without consequences for school functioning. Although ADHD + LD probands showed more evidence of school failure than the ADHD − LD probands, when contrasted with normal comparisons, the ADHD − LD probands show significantly more school dysfunction. Thus, their school and cognitive performance are intermediate between the ADHD + LD and normal comparison probands. This is consistent with the idea that ADHD without LD has cognitive consequences that are exacerbated by the presence of LD.

CONCLUSION

In conclusion, like others, we found ADHD to be associated with learning disabilities, repeated grades, placement in special classes and need for academic tutoring. In addition, compared with controls our ADHD probands did more poorly on subtests of the WISC-R. Among ADHD probands, comorbid conduct, major depressive and anxiety disorders were associated with placement in special classes but not with tutoring, repeated grades or learning disabilities. Psychiatric comorbidity also had limited influence on WISC-R scores. In the absence of psychiatric comorbidity, ADHD was associated with school failure and cognitive dysfunction. This provides indirect evidence for the validity of the ADHD syndrome, *per se*. We found higher than normal rates of school failure and intellectual impairment among the biological relatives of our ADHD probands, even when relatives with ADHD were excluded from the sample. The presence of cognitive dysfunction and school failure among nonADHD relatives suggests that these relatives may be a high risk group deserving of special psychological or educational attention.

Also, although ADHD itself is associated with cognitive impairment and school failure, it is likely to be etiologically independent from LD. One source of the comorbidity between ADHD and LD is nonrandom mating of parents with histories of ADHD. Researchers concerned with creating homogeneous samples should not consider using one of these conditions as an alternative manifestation of the other. Additionally the clinical approach to ADHD should attend to each disorder. It may be counterproductive to treat one with the hope that the other will remit as a consequence.

ACKNOWLEDGMENTS

This work was supported, in part, by grants from the Charlupski Foundation (JB), as well as USPHS (NIMH) grant R01 MH-41314-01A2 (JB). Requests for reprints should be sent to Joseph Biederman, Pediatric Psychopharmacology Unit (ACC 625), Massachusetts General Hospital, Fruit Street, Boston, MA 02114.
Material for this chapter was used with permission from the American Psychiatric Association for the article "Evidence for the independent familial transmission of attention deficit hyperactivity disorder and learning disabilities: Results from a family genetic study," published in the *American Journal of Psychiatry*, June 1993, pp. 891–895 and the American Psychological Association for the article "Intellectual performance and school failure in children with attention deficit hyperactivity disorder and in their siblings," published in the *Journal of Abnormal Psychology*, 1993, pp. 616–623.

REFERENCES

Amado, H. & Lustman, P.J. (1982). Attention deficit disorders persisting in adulthood: a review. *Comprehensive Psychiatry*, **23**(4), 300–314.

Anderson, J.C., Williams, S., et al. (1987). DSM-III disorders in preadolescent children: Prevalence in a large sample from the general population. *Archives of General Psychiatry*, **44**, 69–76.

August, G.J. & Garfinkel, B.D. (1989). Behavioral and cognitive subtypes of ADHD. *Journal of the American Academy of Child and Adolescent Psychiatry*, **28**(5), 739–748.

August, G.J. & Holmes, C.S. (1984). Behavior and academic achievement in hyperactive subgroups and learning-disabled boys. *American Journal of Diseases of Children*, **138**, 1025–1029.

August, G.J., Stewart, M.A., et al. (1983). A four-year follow-up of hyperactive boys with and without conduct disorder. *British Journal of Psychiatry*, **143**, 192–198.

Barkley, R.A. (1990). *Attention Deficit Hyperactivity Disorder: A Handbook for Diagnosis and Treatment*. New York: The Guilford Press.

Barkley, R.A., DuPaul, G.J., et al. (1990). Comprehensive evaluation of attention deficit disorder with and without hyperactivity as defined by research criteria. *Journal of Consulting and Clinical Psychology*, **58**(6), 775–798.

Biederman, J., Faraone, S.V., et al. (1992). Further evidence for family-genetic risk factors in attention deficit hyperactivity disorder (ADHD): patterns of comorbidity in probands and relatives in psychiatrically and pediatrically referred samples. *Archives of General Psychiatry*, **49**(9), 728–738.

Biederman, J., Faraone, S.V., et al. (1990). Family-genetic and psychosocial risk factors in DSM-III attention deficit disorder. *Journal of the American Academy of Child and Adolescent Psychiatry*, **29**(4), 526–533.

Biederman, J., Faraone, S.V., et al. (1991a). Familial association between attention deficit disorder (ADD) and anxiety disorder. *American Journal of Psychiatry*, **148**, 251–256.

Biederman, J., Faraone, S.V., et al. (1991b). Evidence of familial association between attention deficit disorder and major affective disorders. *Archives of General Psychiatry*, **48**, 633–642.

Biederman, J., Munir, K., et al. (1987a). Conduct and oppositional disorder in clinically referred children with attention deficit disorder: a controlled family study. *Journal of the American Academy of Child and Adolescent Psychiatry*, **26**(5), 724–727.

Biederman, J., Munir, K., et al. (1987b). High rate of affective disorders in probands with attention deficit disorder and in their relatives: a controlled family study. *American Journal of Psychiatry*, **144**(3), 330–333.

Biederman, J., Munir, K., et al. (1986). A family study of patients with attention deficit disorder and normal controls. *Journal of Psychiatric Research*, **20**(4), 263–274.

Biederman, J., Newcorn, J., et al. (1991). Comorbidity of attention deficit hyperactivity disorder with conduct, depressive, anxiety, and other disorders. *American Journal of Psychiatry*, **148**(5), 564–577.

Biederman, J., Rosenbaum, J.F., et al. (1990). Psychiatric correlates of behavioral inhibition in young children of parents with and without psychiatric disorders. *Archives of General Psychiatry*, **47**, 21–26.

Biederman, J., Faraone, S.V., et al. (1993). Patterns of psychiatric comorbidity, cognition and psychosocial functioning in adults with attention deficit hyperactivity disorder. *American Journal of Psychiatry*, **150**(12), 1792–1798.

Bird, H.R., Canino, G., et al. (1988). Estimates of the prevalence of childhood maladjustment in a community survey in Puerto Rico. *Archives of General Psychiatry*, **45**, 1120–1126.

Brent, D.A., Perper, J.A., et al. (1988). Risk factors for adolescent suicide: a comparison of adolescent suicide victims with suicidal inpatients. *Archives of General Psychiatry*, **45**(6), 581–588.

Campbell, S.B. & Werry, J.S. (1986). *Attention Deficit Disorder (Hyperactivity): Psychopathologic Disorders of Childhood*. New York: John Wiley.

Cantwell, D.P. (1972). Psychiatric illness in the families of hyperactive children. *Archives of General Psychiatry*, **27**, 414–417.

Cantwell, D.P. (1985). Hyperactive children have grown up. *Archives of General Psychiatry*, **42**, 1026–1028.

Chapman, L.J. & Chapman, J.P. (1978). The measurement of differential deficit. *Journal of Psychiatric Research*, **14**, 303–311.

Chapman, L.J. & Chapman, J.P. (1989). Strategies for resolving the heterogeneity of schizophrenics and their relatives using cognitive measures. *Journal of Abnormal Psychology*, **98**(4), 357–366.

Cole, D.A. (1990). Relation of social and academic competence to depressive symptoms in childhood. *Journal of Abnormal Psychology*, **99**(4), 422–429.

DeFries, J.C., Fulker, D.W., et al. (1987). Evidence for a genetic etiology in reading disability of twins. *Nature*, **329**, 537–539.

Edelbrock, C., Costello, A.J., et al. (1984). Empirical corroboration of attention deficit disorder. *Journal of the American Academy of Child and Adolescent Psychiatry*, **23**(3), 285–290.

Faraone, S., Biederman, J., et al. (1993a). Evidence for the independent familial transmission of attention deficit hyperactivity disorder and learning disabilities: results from a family genetic study. *American Journal of Psychiatry*, **150**(6), 891–895.

Faraone, S.V., Biederman, J., et al. (1993b). Intellectual performance and school failure in children with attention deficit hyperactivity disorder and in their siblings. *Journal of Abnormal Psychology*, **102**, 616–623.

Faraone, S. & Biederman, J. (1994). Genetics of attention-deficit hyperactivity disorder. *Child and Adolescent Psychiatric Clinics of North America*, **3**, 285–302.

Faraone, S., Biederman, J., & Milberger, S. (1994). An exploratory study of ADHD among second-degree relatives of ADHD children. *Society of Biological Psychiatry*, **35**, 398–402.

Faraone, S.V., Biederman, J., Chen, W.J., Milberger, S., Warburton, R.M., & Tsuang, M.T. (1995). Genetic heterogeneity in attention deficit hyperactivity disorder: Gender, psychiatric comorbidity and maternal ADHD. *Journal of Abnormal Psychology*, **104**, 334–345.

Faraone, S.V., Biederman, J., Keenan, K., & Tsuang, M.T. (1991a). A family-genetic study of girls with DSM-III attention deficit disorder. *American Journal of Psychiatry*, **148**, 112–117.

Faraone, S.V., Biederman, J., Keenan, K., & Tsuang, M.T. (1991b). Separation of DSM-III attention deficit disorder and conduct disorder: evidence from a family-genetic study of American child psychiatric patients. *Psychological Medicine*, **21**, 109–121.

Federal Register (1977). *Assistance to States for Education for Handicapped Children: Procedures for Evaluating Specific Learning Disabilities*. Bethesda, MD: US Department of Health, Education, and Welfare.

Feldman, S., Denhoff, E., et al. (1979). The attention disorders and related syndromes: outcome in adolescent and young adult life. *Minimal Brain Dysfunction: A Developmental Approach*. New York: Masson (pp. 133–148).

Frick, P.J., Lahey, B.B., et al. (1991). Academic underachievement and the disruptive behavior disorders. *Journal of Consulting and Clinical Psychology*, **59**(2), 289–294.

Frost, L.A., Moffitt, T.E., et al. (1989). Neuropsychological correlates of psychopathology in an unselected cohort of young adolescents. *Journal of Abnormal Psychology*, **98**(3), 307–313.

Gershon, E.S., Hamovit, J., et al. (1982). A family study of schizoaffective, bipolar I, bipolar II, unipolar and normal control probands. *Archives of General Psychiatry*, **39**, 1157–1167.

Gilger, J.W., Pennington, B.F., et al. (1992). A twin study of the etiology of comorbidity: attention deficit hyperactivity disorder and dyslexia. *Journal of the American Academy of Child and Adolescent Psychiatry*, **31**(2), 343–348.

Gittelman, R., Mannuzza, S., et al. (1985). Hyperactive boys almost grown up. *Archives of General Psychiatry*, **42**, 937–947.

Greenfield, B., Hechtman, L., et al. (1988). Two subgroups of hyperactives as adults: Correlations of outcome. *Canadian Journal of Psychiatry*, **33**(6), 505–508.

Halperin, J.M., Gittelman, R., et al. (1984). Reading-disabled hyperactive children: A distinct subgroup of attention deficit disorder with hyperactivity. *Journal of Abnormal Child Psychology*, **12**(1), 1–14.

Hechtman, L. & Weiss, G. (1986). Controlled prospective fifteen year follow-up of hyperactives as adults: non-medical drug and alcohol use and anti-social behaviour. *Canadian Journal of Psychiatry*, **31**, 557–567.

Hodges, K. & Plow, J. (1990). Intellectual ability and achievement in psychiatrically hospitalized children with conduct, anxiety, and affective disorders. *Journal of Consulting and Clinical Psychology*, **58**(5), 589–595.

Holborow, P.L. & Berry, P.S. (1986). Hyperactivity and learning difficulties. *Journal of Learning Disabilities*, **19**(7), 426–431.

Hollingshead, A.B. (1975). *Four Factor Index of Social Status*. New Haven: Yale University, Department of Sociology.

Hoy, E., Weiss, G., et al. (1978). The hyperactive child at adolescence: Cognitive, emotional and social functioning. *Journal of Abnormal Child Psychology*, **6**(3), 311–324.

Interagency Committee on Learning Disabilities (1987). Learning Disabilities: a Report to Congress.

Kovacs, M., Feinberg, T.L., et al. (1984). Depressive disorders in childhood: I. A longitudinal prospective study of characteristics and recovery. *Archives of General Psychiatry*, **41**(3), 229–237.

Kovacs, M., Paulauskas, S., et al. (1988). Depressive disorders in childhood: III. A longitudinal study of comorbidity with and risk for conduct disorders. *Journal of Affective Disorders*, **15**(3), 205–217.

Lahey, B.B., Schaughency, E.A., et al. (1984). Are attention deficit disorders with and without hyperactivity similar or dissimilar disorders? *Journal of the American Academy of Child and Adolescent Psychiatry*, **23**(3), 302–309.

Lahey, B.B., Stempniak, M., et al. (1978). Hyperactivity and learning disabilities as independent dimensions of child behavior problems. *Journal of Abnormal Psychology*, **87**(3), 333–340.

Lambert, N.M. & Sandoval, J. (1980). The prevalence of learning disabilities in a sample of children considered hyperactive. *Journal of Abnormal Child Psychology*, **8**(1), 33–50.

Levine, M.D., Bush, B., et al. (1982). The dimension of inattention among children with school problems. *Pediatrics*, **70**, 387–395.

Loney, J., Kramer, J., et al. (1981). The hyperactive child grows up: predictors of symptoms, delinquency and achievement at follow-up. *Psychosocial Aspects of Drug Treatment for Hyperactivity*. Boulder, CO, Westview Press (pp. 381–416).

Mannuzza, S., Gittelman-Klein, R., et al. (1991). Young adult mental status of hyperactive boys and their brothers: a prospective follow-up study. *Journal of the American Academy of Child and Adolescent Psychiatry*, **30**(5), 743–751.

Mannuzza, S., Gittelman-Klein, R., et al. (1989). Hyperactive boys almost grown up: IV. Criminality and its relationships to psychiatric status. *Archives of General Psychiatry*, **46**, 1073–1079.

McGee, R., Williams, S., et al. (1984). Behavioral and developmental characteristics of aggressive, hyperactive and aggressive-hyperactive boys. *Journal of the American Academy of Child Psychiatry*, **23**(3), 270–279.

McGee, R., Williams, S., et al. (1987). A comparison of girls and boys with teacher-identified problems of attention. *Journal of the American Academy of Child and Adolescent Psychiatry*, **26**(5), 711–717.

McGee, R., Williams, S., et al. (1989). A comparison of 13-year-old boys with attention deficit and/or reading disorder on neuropsychological measures. *Journal of Abnormal Child Psychology*, **17**, 37–53.

Morrison, J. (1980). Adult psychiatric disorders in parents of hyperactive children. *American Journal of Psychiatry*, **137**, 825–827.

Morrison, J.R. & Stewart, M.A. (1971). A family study of the hyperactive child syndrome. *Biological Psychiatry*, **3**, 189–195.

Orvaschel, H. (1985). Psychiatric interviews suitable for use in research with children and adolescents. *Psychopharmacology Bulletin*, **21**(4), 737–745.

Pauls, D.L., Hurst, C.R., et al. (1986a). Gilles de la Tourette's syndrome and attention deficit disorder with hyperactivity. Evidence against a genetic relationship. *Archives of General Psychiatry*, **43**, 1177–1179.

Pauls, D.L., Towbin, K.E., et al. (1986b). Gilles de la Tourette's syndrome and obsessive-compulsive disorder: evidence supporting a genetic relationship. *Archives of General Psychiatry*, **43**(12), 1180–1182.

Prior, M. & Sanson, A. (1986). Attention deficit disorder with hyperactivity: a critique. *Journal of Child Psychology and Psychiatry*, **27**, 307–319.

Reich, T., James, J., et al. (1972). The use of multiple thresholds in determining the mode of transmission of semi-continuous traits. *Annals of Human Genetics*, **36**, 163–183.

Reich, T., Rice, J., et al. (1979). The use of multiple thresholds and segregation analysis in analyzing the phenotypic heterogeneity of multifactorial traits. *Annals of Human Genetics*, **42**, 371–389.

Reynolds, C.R. (1984). Critical measurement issues in learning disabilities. *Journal of Special Education*, **18**, 451–476.

Rosenbaum, J.F., Biederman, J., et al. (1991). Further evidence of an association between behavioral inhibition and anxiety disorders: results from a family study of children from a non-clinical sample. *Journal of Psychiatric Research*, **25**(1/2), 49–65.

Sandoval, J. & Lambert, N.M. (1984–1985). Hyperactive and learning disabled children: who gets help. *Journal of Special Education*, **18**(4), 495–503.

Sattler, J.M. (1988). *Assessment of Children's Intelligence*. San Diego, CA: Jerome M. Sattler.

Saykin, A.J., Gur, R.C., et al. (1991). Neuropsychological function in schizophrenia: selective impairment in memory and learning. *Archives of General Psychiatry*, **48**(7), 618–624.

Schaughency, E.A., Lahey, B.B., et al. (1989). Neuropsychological test performance and the attention deficit disorders: clinical utility of the Luria-Nebraska neuropsychological battery-children's revision. *Journal of Consulting and Clinical Psychology*, **57**(1), 112–116.

Semrud-Clikeman, M.S., Biederman, J., et al. (1992). Comorbidity between ADHD and learning disability: A review and report in a clinically referred sample. *Journal of the American Academy of Child and Adolescent Psychiatry*, **31**, 439–448.

Shaywitz, S.E. & Shaywitz, B.A. (1989). Critical issues in attention deficit disorder. In *Attention Deficit Disorder Clinical and Basic Research*. Hillsdale, NJ: Lawrence Erlbaum (pp. 53–69).

Silver, L.B. (1981). The relationship between learning disabilities, hyperactivity, distractibility, and behavioral problems. *Journal of the American Academy of Child Psychiatry*, **20**, 385–397.

Singer, S.M., Stewart, M.A., et al. (1981). Minimal brain dysfunction: differences in cognitive organization in two groups of index cases and their relatives. *Journal of Learning Disorders*, **14**(8), 470–473.

Smith, S.D., Pennington, B.F., et al. (1990). Familial dyslexia: use of genetic linkage data to define subtypes. *Journal of the American Academy of Child and Adolescent Psychiatry*, **29**(2), 204–213.

Spencer, T., Biederman, J., et al. (1994). Is attention deficit hyperactivity disorder in adults a valid disorder? *Harvard Review of Psychiatry*, **1**(6), 326–335.

Spitzer, R.L., Williams, J.B., et al. (1990). *Structured Clinical Interview for DSM-III-R-Non-Patient Edition (SCID-NP, Version 1.0)*. Washington, DC, American Psychiatric Press.

Stewart, M.A., Cummings, C., et al. (1981). The overlap between hyperactive and unsocialized aggressive children. *Journal of Child Psychology and Psychiatry*, **22**, 25–45.

Stewart, M.A., deBlois, C.S., et al. (1980). Psychiatric disorder in the parents of hyperactive boys and those with conduct disorder. *Journal of Child Psychology and Psychiatry*, **21**(4), 283–292.

Weiss, G., Hechtman, L., et al. (1985). Psychiatric status of hyperactives as adults: a controlled prospective 15-year follow-up of 63 hyperactive children. *Journal of the American Academy of Child Psychiatry*, **24**, 211–220.

Weiss, G., Hechtman, L., et al. (1979). Hyperactives as young adults: a controlled prospective ten-year follow-up of 75 children. *Archives of General Psychiatry*, **36**, 675–681.

Weissman, M.M., Gershon, E.S., et al. (1984). Psychiatric disorders in the relatives of probands with affective disorders. *Archives of General Psychiatry*, **41**, 13–21.

Welner, Z., Welner, A., et al. (1977). A controlled study of siblings of hyperactive children. *Journal of Nervous and Mental Disorders*, **165**, 110–117.

Wender, P.H., Reimherr, F.W., et al. (1985). Stimulant therapy of "adult hyperactivity". *Archives of General Psychiatry,* **42**, 840.

Werry, J.S., Elkind, G.S., et al. (1987). Attention deficit, conduct, oppositional, and anxiety disorders in children: III. Laboratory differences. *Journal of the American Academy of Child and Adolescent Psychiatry*, **15**(3), 409–428.

13 Twin studies of reading disability

J.C. DeFRIES AND JACQUELYN GILLIS LIGHT

Previous twin studies of behavioral characters have been of two major types: (1) comparisons of identical (monozygotic, MZ) and fraternal (dizygotic, DZ) twin correlations to quantify the heritable nature of individual differences within the normal range of variation; and (2) comparisons of MZ and DZ twin concordance rates to assess the extent to which behavioral disorders are due at least in part to genetic influences. More recently, DeFries and Fulker (1985, 1988) have advocated a multiple regression analysis of data from selected twin pairs that facilitates an alternative test of the genetic etiology of deviant scores. This methodology may also be employed to assess the etiology of comorbid conditions (e.g., a learning disability and attention deficit hyperactivity disorder), and to test for differential etiology as a function of both continuous and dichotomous variables such as age and gender.

In the present chapter, previous twin studies of reading disability will be briefly reviewed. The multiple regression analysis of twin data will then be outlined and used to assess the etiology of reading performance deficits of children tested in our ongoing twin study of reading disability. This statistically powerful and highly flexible method will also be employed in this chapter to explore three current issues in the field of learning disabilities: the relevance of IQ to the definition of learning disabilities (Siegel, 1989); the etiology of covariation between measures of reading performance and phonological coding (Olson et al., 1989); and comorbidity between a learning diability and attention deficit hyperactivity disorder (Stevenson et al., 1993). Lastly, research on the chromosomal location of the individual genes that may cause reading disability will be reviewed, and results of these analyses will be compared to those obtained employing a recent adaptation of the multiple regression analysis of twin data.

CONCORDANCE RATES

Previous twin studies of reading disability used a comparison of MZ and DZ concordance rates as a test for genetic etiology (for a recent review, see DeFries and Gillis, 1991). A pair is concordant if both members of the pair are affected, but discordant if only one member expresses the condition.

Table 13.1. *Concordance or discordance of twin pairs*[a]

Number of pairs	Twin 1	Twin 2
C	+	+
D	+	−
D	−	+

[a] + or − indicates that a member of a twin pair is affected or not affected for a condition such as reading disability.

Because members of MZ twin pairs are genetically identical, whereas those of DZ pairs share only one-half of their segregating genes on average, MZ concordance should exceed DZ concordance if a condition is due at least in part to heritable influences.

Although the concept of twin concordance is deceptively very simple (the percentage of probands with affected cotwins), its estimation depends upon the manner in which the sample was ascertained. As shown in Table 13.1, both members of a twin pair may be affected (+ +), or only one may be affected (+ − or − +). If Twins 1 and 2 are arbitrarily specified (e.g., the members of the pair born first and second, respectively), there are two ways in which pairs may be discordant (+ − and − +) and we expect such pairs to be equally frequent in the population. When a sample of twins is selected in which at least one member of each pair is affected, two different types of ascertainment may be employed: (1) "single selection," in which only one member of a pair could be selected as a proband; and (2) "truncate selection," in which both members of a concordant pair could be ascertained as probands (Thompson & Thompson, 1986).

To illustrate the difference between single and truncate selection, assume that only first-born twins (Twin 1) are tested and that pairs are included in our sample if Twin 1 is affected. Thus, with such single selection, only twin pairs in the first two rows of Table 13.1 would be ascertained, resulting in a sample size of C + D. The "pairwise" concordance rate (DeFries & Gillis, 1991) estimated from this sample would be C/(C + D). However, if both members of each pair were tested, the third row in Table 13.1 would also be included in the sample. In order to correct for the greater number of discordant pairs in samples of twins ascertained using truncate selection (C + 2D), "probandwise" concordance should be computed where each concordant pair is counted twice, once when Twin 1 is the proband and once in which Twin 2 is the proband (DeFries & Gillis, 1991). This "double entry" of concordant pairs ascertained by truncate selection effectively increases the sample size to 2C + 2D, thereby resulting in a probandwise concordance rate

Table 13.2. *Probandwise concordance rates for reading disability*

Study	Number of pairs		Concordance (%)	
	Identical	Fraternal	Identical	Fraternal
Zerbin-Rüdin (1967)	17	34	100	52
Bakwin (1973)	31	31	91	45
Stevenson et al. (1987)	14–19	27–42	33–59	29–54

that is comparable to that of pairwise concordance with single selection, i.e., $2C/(2C + 2D) = C/(C + D)$. Because previous twin studies of reading disability ascertained samples using truncate selection, probandwise concordance rates will be reported in this review.

Probandwise concordance rates for each of the three previous twin studies of reading disability are presented in Table 13.2. The report by Zerbin-Rüdin (1967) was actually based upon a review of six case studies with "congenital word-blindness," a Danish twin study, and six pairs of twins included in Hallgren's (1950) classic family study. As shown in Table 13.2, the probandwise concordance rates for the 17 MZ and 34 DZ twin pairs included in this combined sample are 100% and 52%, respectively. Because case studies of concordant pairs are more likely to be reported than those of discordant pairs (Harris, 1986), the concordance rates estimated from the Zerbin-Rüdin (1967) review are probably inflated at least to some extent.

Bakwin (1973) ascertained a sample of 338 same-sex twin pairs through mother-of-twins clubs, and obtained reading history information via parental interviews, telephone calls and mail questionnaires. Defining reading disability "as a reading level below the expectation derived from the child's performance in other school subjects" (p. 184), Bakwin (1973) reported that the prevalence rates in the MZ and DZ twins were very similar, 14.0% and 14.9%, respectively. However, in the 31 pairs of MZ twins and 31 pairs of DZ twins in which at least one member of each pair was reading disabled, the probandwise concordance rates are quite different (91% and 45%, respectively). Thus, the results of Bakwin's (1973) twin study also suggest that reading disability may be highly heritable.

More recently, Stevenson et al. (1984; 1987) reported results from the first twin study of reading disability in which the subjects were administered standardized tests of intelligence, reading and spelling. The Schonell Graded Word Reading and Spelling Tests and the Neale Analysis of Reading Ability were used to diagnose reading or spelling "backwardness" or "retardation" in a sample of 285 pairs of 13-year-old twins living in London, England. Reading "backwardness" was defined as reading age 18 months below chronological age, whereas reading "retardation" was identified by marked underachievement relative to that predicted from IQ and chronological age. Using these different diagnoses, Stevenson et al. (1984) found that the prevalence of reading and spelling problems in DZ twins was unexpectedly higher than that in MZ twins (15.0% to 25.5% versus 8.9% to 14.2%). Nevertheless, as shown in Table 13.2, probandwise concordance rates employing these various criteria were somewhat higher for MZ twin pairs (33% to 59%) than for DZ twin pairs (29% to 54%). Thus, although concordance rates of MZ pairs exceed those of DZ pairs in each of the three previous twin studies of reading disability, substantial variation exists among the results of the individual studies.

THE PRESENT STUDY

Because of the paucity of previous twin studies of reading disability, a new twin study was initiated in 1982 as part of the on-going Colorado Reading Project (Decker and Vandenberg, 1985; DeFries, 1985). An extensive battery that includes the Wechsler Intelligence Scale for Children – Revised (WISC-R, Wechsler, 1974) or the Wechsler Adult Intelligence Scale – Revised (WAIS-R, Wechsler, 1981), the Peabody Individual Achievement Test (PIAT, Dunn and Markwardt, 1970), and several other psychometric tests, is being administered to MZ and DZ twin pairs in which at least one member of each pair manifested a school history of reading problems and to a comparison group of twins with a negative school history. In order to minimize the possibility of ascertainment bias, the sample is systematically obtained via cooperating school districts in Colorado. Without regard to reading status, all twin pairs in a school are identified by school administrators. Permission is then sought from parents to review the school records of each twin for evidence of reading problems (e.g., low reading achievement test scores, referral to a reading therapist because of poor reading performance). Twin pairs in which at least one member has a school history of reading problems are invited to complete a battery of psychometric tests in our laboratory at the University of Colorado. Data from the PIAT Reading Recognition, Reading Comprehension, and Spelling subtests are then used to compute a discriminant function score for each member of the pair. (Discriminant weights were estimated from an analysis of PIAT data from an independent sample of 140 reading-disabled and 140 control nontwin children ascertained by referral from local school districts and tested during an earlier phase of the project (DeFries, 1985).) Twin pairs are included in the proband sample if at least one member of the pair with a positive school history of reading problems is also classified as affected on the basis of his or her discriminant score, and has a Verbal or Performance IQ score of at least 90, is not diagnosed with neurological, emotional, or behavioral problems, and has no uncorrected visual or auditory acuity deficits. Control twins are matched to probands on the basis of age, gender, and school district, have a negative school history for reading problems, and are classified by the discriminant score as unaffected.

In order to diagnose zygosity of twin pairs, selected items from the Nichols & Bilbro (1966) Twin Zygosity questionnaire are administered. In doubtful cases, analyses of blood samples are employed to confirm zygosity. All twin pairs are reared in English-speaking middle-class homes, and range in age from 8 to 20 years at the time of testing.

As of 31 December 1992, a total of 149 pairs of MZ twins and 111 pairs of same-sex DZ twins met our criteria for inclusion in the proband sample. It is of interest to note that the numbers of male and female reading-disabled probands in the sample are 183 and 182, respectively. Because female MZ twin pairs are often overrepresented in twin studies (Lykken, Tellegen, & DeRubeis, 1978), this observed gender ratio of 1.01:1 may be due in part to a differential volunteer rate of male and female MZ twin pairs. In fact, the gender ratio in the sample of MZ probands (0.79:1) is lower than that for the same-sex DZ probands (1.48:1). However, both of these ratios are substantially lower than the ratio of three or four males to each female typically reported in referred and clinic samples. Shaywitz et al. (1990) also found a lower gender ratio in a research-identified sample of nontwin, reading-disabled children, than in a referred sample. Therefore, the preponderance of male subjects found in referred and clinic samples of reading-disabled children is almost certainly due, at least in part, to a referral bias (Finucci & Childs, 1981).

The number of affected twin pairs tested to date in the Colorado Reading Project exceeds the total number of reading-disabled twin pairs tested in the three previous studies. Thus, considerable confidence can be placed in the results of this single study. The probandwise concordance rates for MZ and DZ twin pairs tested in our study are 68% and 40%, respectively, thereby confirming the evidence obtained in previous twin studies that reading disability is due at least in part to heritable influences.

MULTIPLE REGRESSION ANALYSIS OF TWIN DATA

Although a comparison of concordance rates in MZ and DZ twin pairs provides a test of genetic etiology for dichotomous variables (e.g., presence or absence of a psychiatric illness), reading-disabled probands are ascertained because of deviant scores on continuous measures such as reading performance. In 1985, DeFries and Fulker noted that a comparison of the average scores of MZ and DZ cotwins facilitates an alternative test of genetic etiology.

When MZ and DZ probands have been ascertained because of deviant scores on a continuous measure, the scores of their cotwins are expected to regress toward the mean of the unselected population (μ). However, as shown in Figure 13.1, this regression towards the mean should differ for MZ

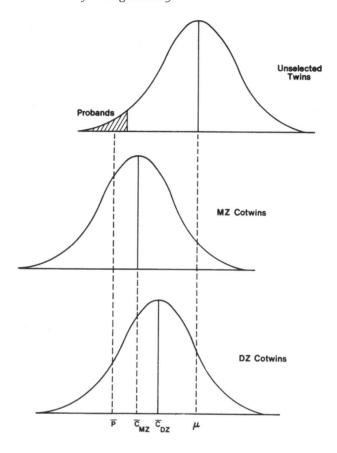

Figure 13.1. Hypothetical distributions for reading performance of an unselected sample of twins, and of the identical (MZ) and fraternal (DZ) cotwins of probands with a reading disability. The differential regression of the MZ and DZ cotwin means toward the mean of the unselected population (μ) provides a test of genetic etiology. (From: J.C. DeFries, D.W. Fulker, & M.C. LaBuda (1987). Evidence for a genetic aetiology in reading disability of twins. *Nature,* **329**, 537. Copyright © 1987 Macmillan Journals Ltd. Reprinted by permission.)

and DZ cotwins to the extent that the condition is due to heritable influences. Because members of MZ twin pairs are genetically identical, whereas members of DZ pairs share only about one-half of their segregating genes on average, scores of DZ cotwins should regress more toward the mean than those of MZ cotwins if reading disability is due at least in part to genetic factors. Therefore, if the MZ and DZ proband means ($\bar{P}$) are approximately equal, a simple t-test of the difference between the means of the MZ and DZ cotwins ($\bar{C}_{MZ}$ and $\bar{C}_{DZ}$) could be employed as a test of genetic etiology. However,

DeFries and Fulker (1985, 1988) have shown that fitting the following basic regression model to such data provides a more general, statistically powerful, and flexible test:

$$C = B_1 P + B_2 R + A \qquad (1)$$

where C is the cotwin's score, P is the proband's score, and R is the coefficient of relationship (R = 1.0 for MZ twin pairs and 0.5 for DZ pairs). B_1, the partial regression of cotwin's score on proband's score, is a measure of average MZ and DZ twin resemblance. Of greater interest for the purpose of this analysis, B_2 estimates twice the difference between the means of the MZ and DZ cotwins after covariance adjustments for any difference between the scores of the MZ and DZ probands. Thus, B_2 provides a direct and statistically powerful test for genetic etiology. Furthermore, when each score is expressed as a deviation from the mean of the unselected population and then divided by the difference between the proband and control means prior to regression analysis, B_2 directly estimates h_g^2, an index of the extent to which the deficit of probands is due to genetic factors.

To illustrate the multiple regression analysis of twin data, the basic model was fitted to discriminant function score data from the 260 pairs of probands and cotwins tested in the Colorado Reading Project. Because truncate selection was employed to ascertain this sample of affected twins, concordant pairs were double entered, in a manner analogous to that used for computation of the probandwise concordance rates. Standard error estimates and tests of significance provided by conventional computer regression programs have been adjusted accordingly.

The average discriminant scores of the 149 MZ and 111 DZ probands and their cotwins, expressed as standardized deviation units from the mean of 454 individuals included in the control sample, are presented in Table 13.3. From this table it may be seen that the means of the MZ and DZ probands are highly similar, over 2.5 standard deviations below the mean of the control twins. In addition, it may be seen that the MZ cotwins have regressed only 0.23 standard deviation units toward the control mean, whereas the DZ cotwins have regressed 0.90 standard deviations. Thus, when equation 1 was fitted to these data, $B_2 = -1.42 \pm 0.26$ ($p < 0.001$, one tailed). When the same model was fitted to transformed data, $B_2 = h_g^2 = 0.51 \pm 0.10$ ($p < 0.001$), suggesting that about one-half of the reading performance deficit of probands, on average, is due to heritable influences. One can also obtain an estimate of c_g^2, a measure of the extent to which the proband deficit in reading is due to environmental influences shared by members of twin pairs. From this data, $c_g^2 = 0.41 \pm 0.10$, suggesting that approximately 40 percent of the proband reading deficit can be attributed to shared environmental influences.

Table 13.3. *Mean discriminant scores of 149 pairs of identical twins and 111 pairs of same-sex fraternal twins in which at least one member of the pair is reading-disabled.[a]*

	Proband	Cotwin
Identical	-2.77 ± 0.83	-2.54 ± 1.07
Fraternal	-2.65 ± 0.82	-1.75 ± 1.33

[a] Expressed as standardized deviations from the mean of 454 controls.

RELEVANCE OF IQ

The multiple regression analysis of twin data may be used to test hypotheses that are relevant to a number of current issues in the field of learning disabilities. For example, reading-disabled children are assumed to have a cognitive deficit that is specific to the reading task, an assumption that Stanovich (1986) has referrred to as the "assumption of specificity." In contrast to children with a low IQ (the "garden-variety poor reader") whose reading deficits are presumed to be due to their impaired general cognitive ability, reading-disabled children with IQ scores within the normal range (the specifically reading disabled) are assumed to have some unique deficit that is independent of general cognitive ability (Olson et al., 1991b). Within the past several years, this specificity assumption has been seriously challenged (Stanovich, 1986; Fletcher et al., 1989; Siegel, 1989).

Although most currently accepted definitions of reading disability are based on a discrepancy with measured intelligence (Stanovich, 1989), Siegel (1989) has argued that IQ test scores should be irrelevant. She noted that learning-disabled children have deficits in various skills measured by IQ tests (e.g., expressive language abilities, short-term memory, speed of processing information, speed of responding, and knowledge of specific facts); consequently, reading problems may cause lower IQ scores. Moreover, Siegel (1989) presented evidence that the cognitive processes of reading disabled children (as measured by various reading, spelling, language, memory, and arithmetic tests) do not vary as a function of IQ, a result that is contrary to that predicted by the specificity assumption. Thus, the reading deficits of children with a low IQ may not differ fundamentally from those of children with an IQ score within the normal range. This lack of evidence for the assumption of specificity clearly raises a serious problem for the use of IQ-reading discrepancy definitions. However, Siegel (1989) acknowledges that the field is not yet ready to abandon the use of IQ tests and proposes that a cut-off IQ score of 80 be used instead.

We agree that reading problems may cause lower IQ scores and, therefore, do not routinely employ discrepancy scores (either difference scores or regression-deviation scores) in our genetic analyses. However, because reading disability has traditionally been defined by significant difficulty in reading that is not due to mental retardation (Kirk & Bateman, 1962; Interagency Committee on Learning Disabilities, 1987), we have used an IQ cut-off score of 90 to ensure that our probands have general mental ability within the normal range. Recently, however, we have begun to test subjects with lower IQ scores in order to assess the relevance issue (Olson et al., 1991b).

Our analysis sample includes only 28 pairs of twins (17 MZ and 11 DZ) in which at least one member of each pair is reading disabled using the discriminant function score criterion, and has an IQ score (either verbal or performance) of 80 or above, but less than 90. Thus, a multiple regression analysis of reading performance data from this sample is too small to yield reliable parameter estimates. Nevertheless, when such an analysis was undertaken, the resulting estimate of h_g^2 (0.29 $\pm$ 0.25) did not differ substantially from that obtained when data were analyzed from the much larger sample (260 twin pairs) in which a 90 IQ cut-off was imposed ($h_g^2 = 0.51 \pm 0.10$). As expected, when data from the two samples were combined, the estimate of h_g^2 did not change appreciably (0.50 $\pm$ 0.09).

As recently noted by Olson et al. (1991b), the multiple regression analysis of twin data facilitates an alternative test of the specificity hypothesis. If the cognitive processes of reading-disabled children with high IQ scores differ from those with low IQ scores, then the etiology of reading deficits should also vary as a function of IQ. This hypothesis may be tested by fitting the following hierarchical model to the reading performance data of twins in our expanded data set:

$$C = B_6P + B_7R + B_8I + B_9PI + B_{10}RI + A \qquad (2)$$

where I symbolizes the proband's Full Scale IQ. In hierarchical multiple regression models (Cohen & Cohen, 1975), interactions are represented by the products of independent variables. Thus, the coefficients of the PI and RI interaction terms in equation 2 test for differential twin resemblance (B_9) and differential $h_g^2(B_{10})$ as a function of IQ.

When equation 2 was fitted to the discriminant function score data for the sample of 288 twin pairs in which at least one member of each pair is reading disabled and has a verbal or performance IQ 80 or greater, $B_9 = -0.0005 \pm 0.007$ ($p = 0.94$) and $B_{10} = 0.007 \pm 0.009$ ($p = 0.48$), suggesting that neither twin resemblance nor the genetic etiology of reading deficits vary systematically as a function of IQ. Thus, results of this genetic analysis also fail to provide evidence for the assumption of specificity (Fletcher et al., 1989; Morrison & Siegel, 1991; Olson et al., 1991b; and Stanovich, 1986, 1989).

READING AND LANGUAGE PROCESSES

The multiple regression analysis of selected twin data is a highly flexible methodology. In addition to testing for differential genetic etiology as a function of various dichotomous and continuous covariates (e.g., gender and IQ), equation 1 may also be generalized to assess the etiology of bivariate relationships. If probands are selected for some variable X, they will also deviate from the population mean for character Y to the extent that X and Y are correlated. Therefore, the differential regression toward the mean of MZ and DZ cotwins for character Y can be used to partition the observed phenotypic correlation into components due to genetic and environmental influences. A bivariate form of equation 1 can be fitted to such data in which each cotwin's score of character Y is predicted from the proband's character X and the coefficient of relationship. The resulting estimate of "bivariate h_g^2" provides an index of the extent to which the proband's deficit in character Y is due to the same genetic influences that cause deviant scores in the selected variable X. Our colleague, Richard K. Olson, has employed this approach to assess the etiology of covariation between measures of word recognition and two major component processes, phonological and orthographic coding (Olson et al., 1989; Olson et al., 1991b).

In addition to the psychometric test battery, twin pairs in the Colorado Reading Project are also administered tests of various language processes in Olson's laboratory. For example, a phonological coding task requires subjects to read aloud 85 nonwords of varying difficulty (e.g., int, tegwop, calch) as quickly and accurately as possible. In contrast, an orthographic task requires subjects to designate a word in each of 80 word-pseudohomophone pairs (e.g., rain vs. rane; sammon vs. salmon) as quickly as possible. Because the two letter strings in each pair are phonologically identical, the subject must recognize the specific orthographic pattern of the target word to make a correct choice.

When Olson et al. (1989) compared test scores from older reading-disabled children with those from younger normal readers matched on PIAT Reading Recognition, a striking difference in the pattern of their average phonological and orthographic coding scores was observed. The average score of the older disabled readers on the phonological task was 0.8 of a standard deviation below the mean of the younger normal group, a highly significant ($p < 0.01$) difference. In contrast, the disabled group's performance on orthographic coding was about 0.3 of a standard deviation *above* that of the younger comparison group. These and other results reviewed by Olson et al. (1989) suggest that most reading-disabled children have a deficit in phonological coding and related segmental language skills.

Olson and his colleagues recently fit equation 1 to word recognition, phonological coding, and orthographic coding data from twins tested in the Colorado Reading Project (for a recent review, see DeFries et al. 1991).

Table 13.4. *Genetic correlations (above diagonal) and specific environmental correlations (below diagonal) among Word Recognition (REC), Phonological Coding (PHON), and Orthographic Coding (ORTH) measures*

	REC	PHON	ORTH
REC	–	0.75	0.42
PHON	0.42	–	0.56
ORTH	0.21	0.20	–

Resulting estimates of h_g^2 for word recognition (0.54 ± 0.08) and phonological coding (0.54 ± 0.10) were somewhat higher than that for orthographic coding (0.28 ± 0.11). A bivariate form of equation 1 was then used to predict cotwins' coding scores from proband's word recognition scores. Resulting estimates of bivariate h_g^2 were 0.81 ± 0.14 and 0.27 ± 0.18 for the phonological and orthographic coding tasks, respectively. These results suggest that the word recognition and phonological coding deficits of probands are largely due to the same heritable influences.

Olson et al. (1991a) recently employed confirmatory factor analysis of twin data to test this hypothesis. PIAT Reading Recognition (REC), phonological coding (PHON), and orthographic coding (ORTH) data from 86 pairs of MZ twins and 73 pairs of DZ twins in which at least one member of each pair is reading disabled, and from 92 pairs of MZ twins and 59 pairs of DZ twins from the control sample, were subjected to multivariate genetic analysis. Resulting estimates of h^2 (a measure of the extent to which individual differences *within* the group are due to heritable influences) for REC, PHON, and ORTH were 0.59, 0.41, and 0.05 in the reading-disabled sample, and 0.35, 0.52, and 0.20, in the control sample. After dropping the nonsignificant shared-environmental parameters from the model, estimates of the genetic correlation (an index of the extent to which individual differences in two different measures are due to the same genetic influences) between REC and PHON and between REC and ORTH were 0.81 and 0.45 in the reading-disabled sample and 0.68 and 0.45 in the control sample. The genetic correlation between REC and PHON was significantly larger than that between REC and ORTH in the disabled sample ($p < 0.005$), marginally significant in the control sample ($p < 0.10$), and highly significant in the combined sample ($p < 0.001$).

Results of the combined analysis are summarized in Table 13.4. It may be seen that the genetic correlation between REC and PHON in the combined sample is 0.75, whereas that between REC and ORTH is 0.42. In contrast, the correlation due to non-shared environmental influences between REC and

PHON is 0.42, compared to 0.21 between REC and ORTH. Thus, results of this analysis also suggest that individual differences in word recognition are largely due to heritable variation in phonological coding.

ATTENTION DEFICIT HYPERACTIVITY DISORDER

As discussed elsewhere in this volume, children with learning disabilities often manifest symptoms of attention deficit hyperactivity disorder (ADHD) (Shaywitz & Shaywitz, 1991). Results of recent twin studies suggest that ADHD is highly heritable (Stevenson, 1992; Gillis et al., 1992) and that its comorbidity with learning disabilities may be due substantially to common genetic influences (Stevenson et al., 1993).

In the London twin study (Stevenson et al., 1984, 1987), children were administered an extensive test battery that included a measure of sustained attention (checking a page of randomly listed letters for the occurrence of the letter "e"), as well as the WISC-R and various tests of reading and spelling. In addition, continuously distributed measures of activity level were obtained from ratings by mothers and teachers. In order to assess the genetic etiology of hyperactivity, Stevenson (1992) subjected attention and activity data from selected twin pairs (17–31 MZ and 25–47 DZ) to multiple regression analysis (equation 1). For both mother and teacher ratings of activity, as well as two measures of attention, scores of DZ cotwins regressed more toward the mean than did those of MZ cotwins. Moreover, this differential regression to the mean was highly significant for the maternal ratings of activity and "e" scan attentiveness, with corresponding h_g^2 estimates of 0.75 and 0.76, respectively. Thus, these results suggest that ADHD symptoms may be highly heritable.

Results obtained from analyses of data from twin pairs tested in the Colorado Reading Project (Gillis et al., 1992) were highly similar to those reported by Stevenson (1992). Twin pairs (37 MZ and 37 DZ) in which at least one member of the pair met the ADD criteria of the Diagnostic Interview for Children and Adolescents – Parent Interview (Herjanic, Campbell, & Reich, 1982) were selected from the reading-disabled sample. Whereas the mean DICA scores of MZ and DZ probands were highly similar (both about 2.2 standard deviations below the mean of the control group), those of the MZ and DZ cotwins differed substantially. MZ cotwins regressed only 0.27 standard deviation units on average toward the control mean, compared to 1.32 standard deviations for DZ cotwins. This differential regression of DICA scores for the MZ and DZ cotwins is highly significant ($p < 0.001$), and the corresponding h_g^2 estimate of 0.98 again suggests that ADHD symptoms are highly heritable.

Subsequently, Stevenson et al. (1993) subjected data from the London and Colorado twin studies to a "bivariate" regression analysis in order to assess the etiology of comorbidity between ADHD and spelling disability. Twin pairs in which at least one number of each pair obtained a spelling test score more than one standard deviation below the control mean were selected from both samples. A bivariate form of equation 1 was then used to predict ADHD symptoms in cotwins (maternal ratings of activity for the Londom sample; DICA scores for the Colorado sample) from the spelling scores of probands. Although the individual estimates of bivariate h_g^2 obtained from the two samples were nonsignificant (0.21 and 0.32, respectively), results of a combined analysis indicated that two independent estimates were significant ($p < 0.02$) when considered jointly. These estimates of bivariate h_g^2 were then divided by their respective covariances to assess the extent to which the observed correlation between ADHD symptoms and spelling is due to heritable influences. Resulting estimates obtained from the London and Colorado studies were again highly similar, 0.84 and 0.69, respectively. Thus, to the extent that ADHD symptoms and spelling deficits are syndromic, genetic influences may be substantially involved.

GENETIC LINKAGE ANALYSES

Finding evidence that reading disability is due at least in part to heritable influences is only the first step towards a comprehensive genetic analysis. If reading disability is caused by genes with major effects, it may be possible to determine their location on specific chromosomes. Researchers could then use molecular biological techniques to clone the genes, determine what proteins they produce, and thereby learn about the disorder's primary cause and development (Kidd, 1991).

Genes that are located near each other on the same chromosome tend to be inherited together when they are transmitted from parent to child. In contrast, those that are far apart on the same chromosome, or on entirely different chromosomes, are inherited independently. Therefore, a gene can be localized to a specific chromosomal region if its transmission pattern is compared to that of marker genes whose locations are already known. Observed co-transmission between a putative gene for a disorder and a marker gene provides evidence that the gene is located near the marker.

Evidence of linkage between a gene of interest and a marker may be quantified by computing a LOD score from pedigree data. LOD is an acronym for the logarithm to the base 10 of the odds, where the "odds" is the conditional probability of co-transmission between the character and a marker, given the linkage, divided by the probability of co-transmission given independent assortment. Thus, a LOD score of zero indicates that the two events are equally likely, that is, it provides no evidence for or against linkage. In contrast, a LOD score of three is obtained when the probability of co-transmission given linkage is one thousand times greater than the probability that it is due to independent inheritance. However, because the prior probability of linkage to a given chromosomal marker is very low, the true probability of linkage given a LOD score of three is much lower than 1000:1 (Risch, 1992). For example, the prior probability that two randomly selected genes are located within 30 map units of each other on the same chromosome is only about 0.02. Therefore, the true odds for linkage, given a LOD score of three, equals 0.02 times 1,000:1 (the nominal odds indicated by the data), that is, 20:1. Consequently, a LOD score of three has a true alpha level of about 0.05. A negative LOD score indicates that the probability of co-transmission due to linkage is less than that due to independent assortment and, thereby, provides evidence against linkage. LOD scores are computed from data for individual families, assuming various possible linkage relationships, and then summed across families.

The first evidence that a hypothesized gene that causes reading disability may be linked to a specific chromosome was reported by Smith et al. (1983). Data were obtained from 84 individuals who were members of nine extended families in which reading disability had apparently been transmitted in an autosomal dominant manner. A psychometric test battery was administered in order to diagnose reading problems and to ensure that the disability was specific to reading and spelling. Diagnostic criteria for reading disability in children included a reading level at least two years below expected grade level and a Full Scale IQ greater than 90. Self reports were used to diagnose adults if there was a discrepancy between test results and a history of reading problems. Observed co-transmission between reading disability and a marker on chromosome 15 in these nine families yielded a total LOD score of 3.2. However, about 70% of this total score was due to co-transmission in only one family, and data from one of the other families yielded a large negative score. Thus, results of this first genetic linkage analysis of reading disability suggested that the condition may be genetically heterogeneous.

Smith et al. (1990) subsequently augmented their sample to include a total of 250 individuals in 21 families. With the inclusion of these additional families, as well as additional chromosomal markers, the total LOD score for linkage to chromosome 15 was reduced to 1.33. However, LOD scores varied widely among families. As shown in Figure 13.2, one family had a LOD score of almost three, whereas others had scores less than minus two.

Results of these analyses suggest that only about 20% of the families of children with reading disability manifest apparent linkage to chromosome 15. Therefore, to the extent that reading disability is heritable, most cases must be caused by one or more genes at other chromosomal locations, or possibly by the combined effects of several genes. More recent studies by Smith and her colleagues (see DeFries et al. 1991, for a review) are using markers on chromosome 6 to search for other possible linkage relationships. As shown in Figure 13.2, results of preliminary analyses indicate that some families manifest apparent linkage to chromosome 6, but not 15. Because the markers for chromosome 6 are within the human leucocyte antigen (HLA) region, this very tentative evidence for linkage suggests a possible relationship between

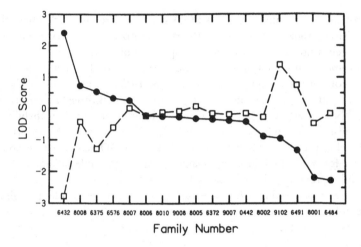

Figure 13.2. LOD scores for markers on chromosomes 15 (solid circles) and 6 (open squares) in families of children with reading disabilities. Families are listed in descending order of their LOD scores for chromosome 15. (After J.C. DeFries, R.K. Olson, B.F. Pennington, & S.D. Smith (1991). Colorado Reading Project: an update. In D. Duane & D.B. Gray (eds) *The Reading Brain: The Biological Basis of Dyslexia*. Parkton, MD: York Press. Copyright © 1991 York Press. Reprinted by permission.)

reading disability and genes that affect the immune system in a subgroup of reading-disabled children.

Evidence for the existence of yet another gene that may cause reading disability was recently reported by Rabin et al. (1993). Results of analyses of data from nine three-generation families provided suggestive evidence for linkage to markers on chromosome 1, but not to markers on chromosome 15. However, the maximum total LOD score for linkage to chromosome 1 in those families was only 2.33; thus, it is imperative that his tentative finding be confirmed in an independent study.

Linkage analyses of complex characters involving extended families have two serious limitations. First, it must be assumed that the condition is caused by a single gene that has a specific mode of inheritance (e.g., autosomal dominance). However, characters such as reading disability are likely to be influenced by genes at several chromosomal locations. Second, a diagnosis must be applied to each family member. Thus, accurate diagnosis is required across a wide age range, as well as across generations.

An alternative linkage analysis uses data only from sibling pairs (Haseman & Elston, 1972). This method does not assume a specific mode of inheritance, and only data from one generation are required. However, the sib-pair analysis is less powerful than the family study method;

thus, data may be required from more individuals to achieve statistical significance.

If a gene that causes reading disability is closely linked to a given chromosomal marker, then pairs of siblings that are concordant for reading disability will also tend to be concordant for the marker. In order to determine if a chromosomal marker carried by two siblings was inherited from the same parent, i.e., their markers are "identical by descent" (ibd), the parents of the siblings must also be genotyped. These data are then used to estimate the proportion (π) of the alleles two siblings share that are ibd at the marker locus. A pair of siblings can share either zero, one, or two alleles from their parents, with corresponding π values of 0, 0.5, and 1.0. The sib-pair linkage analysis of Haseman and Elson (1972) relates the square of the difference between the scores of siblings to their π value at each marker locus.

Smith, Kimberling, & Pennington (1991) first applied the sib-pair linkage method to reanalyze data from siblings included in their family study. Two different diagnostic criteria were used: (1) a qualitative diagnosis employed in their previous analyses; and (2) the continuous discriminant function score used in our study of reading disability. Although the two different diagnostic criteria yielded somewhat different results, the sib-pair analyses employing these criteria again detected possible linkages to markers on both chromosomes 6 and 15.

Fulker et al. (1991) employed an alternative analysis of sib-pair reading data to detect linkage of quantitative trait loci to chromosomal markers, a simple extension of the DeFries & Fulker (1985) multiple regression analysis of twin data. However, rather than using the coefficient of relationship (R) in equation 1, π is used to index ibd status at various marker loci. Fulker et al. (1991) suggest that this method has several advantages over the Haseman & Elston (1972) approach: (1) it is conceptually simple; (2) it can be applied using readily available computer programs; (3) it is applicable for the analysis of data from either selected or unselected samples; (4) it is very flexible, facilitating the analysis of interactions with variables such as age and gender; and (5) it is statistically powerful, especially when applied to data from selected samples (e.g., sibling pairs in which at least one member of each pair is reading disabled).

Fulker et al. (1991) used this multiple regression analyses to reanalyse discriminant function score data of siblings included in the Smith et al. (1991) family study. Several possible linkages to DNA markers on chromosome 15 were again detected, demonstrating the power of this method when applied to data from selected samples.

Because analyses of family data provided suggestive evidence for linkage to markers on chromosomes 6 and 15, a linkage analysis of data from fraternal twin pairs tested in the Colorado Reading Project was recently initiated. Analyses of data from this completely independent sample provide an important opportunity to confirm the previous evidence for linkage that was obtained in the family study. Results obtained from preliminary analyses of the twin data also suggest the possibility of linkage to markers on chromosome 6 (Cardon et al., 1994).

CONCLUSION

Results of twin studies reviewed in this chapter provide compelling evidence of a genetic etiology for reading disability. For example, in the Colorado twin study, data from 149 pairs of MZ twins and 111 pairs of DZ twins in which at least one member of each pair is reading disabled were subjected to multiple regression analysis. When a basic model that predicts the cotwin's score from the proband's score and the coefficient of relationship was fitted to these data, the resulting estimate of h_g^2 suggested that about one half of the reading performance deficit of probands, on average, is due to heritable influences. The results of this analysis also indicate that about 40% of the deficit is due to environmental influences that are shared by members of twin pairs, for example, prenatal factors, shared home and/or school experiences.

In accordance with Siegel's (1989) definition of learning disabilities, we do not routinely employ IQ discrepancy scores for diagnosing reading disability in our twin study. Instead, we employ a discriminant function score that provides a composite measure of three PIAT subtest scores: Reading Recognition, Reading Comprehension and Spelling. Other diagnostic criteria include a positive school history of reading problems, a Verbal or Performance IQ cut-off score of 90, and several exclusionary criteria including no diagnosed neurological, emotional or behavioral problems, and no uncorrected visual or auditory acuity deficits. As noted earlier in this chapter, Richard K. Olson has shown that the reading-disabled children in our twin sample also have marked deficits in measures of phonological coding and segmental language skills.

Pennington et al. (1992) recently compared groups of individuals in our twin study who were diagnosed for reading disability using either age- or IQ-discrepancy definitions. In brief, only very minimal differences were found with regard to etiology of deficit, gender ratio, clinical correlates, and neuropsychological profiles. Moreover, as described in the present chapter, results of an analysis of reading performance data from twins employing an IQ cut-off score of 80 provide little or no evidence for differential etiology as a function of IQ level.

The multiple regression analysis of twin data employed in the Colorado and London twin studies is a highly flexible methodology. In addition to providing a measure of the extent to which the deficit of probands is due to heritable influences, it can also be employed to test for differential etiology as a function of continuous covariates such as age (Wadsworth et al., 1989), or dichotomous variables such as gender (DeFries, Gillis, & Wadsworth, 1993). It can also be used to test the hypothesis that the etiology of deviant scores differs from that of individual differences within the normal range (DeFries & Gillis, 1991; Shaywitz et al., 1992), and bivariate applications may be employed to assesss the etiology of comorbidity for conditions such as learning disabilities and phonological coding deficits (DeFries et al., 1991) or ADHD symptoms (Stevenson et al., 1993). As also noted in this chapter, the method has even been adapted to determine the chromosomal location of the major genes or quantitative trait loci that cause reading disability (Fulker et al., 1991; Cardon et al., 1994). Thus, in addition to providing a statistically powerful test of genetic etiology, the multiple regression analysis of twin data may also be employed to test hypotheses that are relevant to a number of important current issues in the field of learning disabilities.

Finally, it should be noted that the Colorado Reading Project is the largest twin study of learning disabilities conducted to date. Although we recently initiated a small complementary twin study of mathematics disability, additional twin studies of learning disabilities and related language disorders are clearly warranted. Because of the apparent ascertainment biases inherent in both referred and clinic samples, twins with learning disabilities should be objectively and systematically ascertained for such studies using research criteria. About 1% of all births are twins, and their parents are usually very willing to participate in research because the children are obviously so special. Thus, twin studies are relatively easy to initiate, even by research groups with limited funding. Because of the statistical power provided by the multiple regression analysis of selected twin data, results of relatively small twin studies may be highly informative. Furthermore, collaborative analyses of combined data sets from two or more such twin studies could facilitate even more powerful tests of relevant hypotheses (e.g., DeFries et al., 1991). It is also the case that twin studies are fun – try one, and you may like it!

ACKNOWLEDGMENTS

This work was supported in part by program project and center grants from NICHD (HD-11681 and HD-27802) to J.C. DeFries. This report was prepared while J. Gillis Light was supported by NIMH training grant MH-16880. The invaluable contributions of staff members of the many Colorado school districts and of the families who participated in this study are gratefully acknowledged.

REFERENCES

Bakwin, H. (1973). Reading disability of twins. *Developmental Medicine and Child Neurology*, **15**, 184–187.

Cardon, L.R., Smith, S.D., Fulker, D.W., Kimberling, W.J., Pennington, B.F., & DeFries, J.C. (1994). Quantitative trait locus for reading disability on chromosome 6. *Science*, **266**, 276–279.

Cohen, J. & Cohen, P. (1975). *Applied Multiple Regression/Correlation Analysis for the Behavioral Sciences.* Hillsdale, NJ: Lawrence Erlbaum.

Decker, S.N. & Vandenberg, S.G. (1985). Colorado twin study of reading disability. In D.B. Gray & J.F. Kavanagh (eds) *Biobehavioral Measures of Dyslexia.* Parkton, MD: York Press (pp. 123–135).

DeFries, J.C. (1985). Colorado reading project. In D.B. Gray & J.F. Kavanagh (eds) *Biobehavioral Measures of Dyslexia.* Parkton, MD: York Press (pp. 107–122).

DeFries, J.C. & Fulker, D.W. (1985) Multiple regression analysis of twin data. *Behavior Genetics,* **15,** 467–473.

DeFries, J.C. & Fulker, D.W. (1988). Multiple regression analysis of twin data: etiology of deviant scores versus individual differences. *Acta Geneticae Medicae et Gemellogiae,* **37,** 205–216.

DeFries, J.C., Fulker, D.W., & LaBuda, M.C. (1987). Evidence for a genetic aetiology in reading disability of twins. *Nature,* **329,** 537–539.

DeFries, J.C. & Gillis, J.J. (1991). Etiology of reading deficits in learning disabilities: Quantitative genetic analysis. In J.E. Obrzut & G.W. Hynd (eds) *Neuropsychological Foundations of Learning Disabilities: A Handbook of Issues, Methods and Practice.* Orlando, FL: Academic Press (pp. 29–47).

DeFries, J.C., Gillis, J.J., & Wadsworth, S.J. (1993). Genes and Genders: a twin study of reading disability. In A.M. Galaburda (ed.) *Dyslexia and Development: Neurobiological Aspects of Extra-Ordinary Brains.* Cambridge, MA: Harvard University Press (pp. 187–204).

DeFries, J.C., Olson, R.K., Pennington, B.F., & Smith, S.D. (1991). Colorado Reading Project: an update. In D.D. Duane & D.B. Gray (eds) *The Reading Brain: The Biological Basis of Dyslexia.* Parkton, MD: York Press (pp. 53–87).

DeFries, J.C., Stevenson, J., Gillis, J.J., & Wadsworth, S.J. (1991). Genetic etiology of spelling deficits in the Colorado and London twin studies of reading disability. *Reading and Writing: An Interdisciplinary Journal,* **3,** 271–283.

Dunn, L.M. & Markwardt, F.C. (1970). *Examiner's Manual: Peabody Individual Achievement Test.* Circle Pines, MN: American Guidance Service.

Finucci, J.M. & Childs, B. (1981). Are there really more dyslexic boys than girls? In A. Ansara, N. Geschwind, A. Galaburda, M. Albert, & N. Gartell (eds) *Sex Differences in Dyslexia.* Towson, MD: Orton Dyslexia Society (pp. 11–19).

Fletcher, J.M., Espy, K.A., Francis, D.J., Davidson, K.C., Rourke, B.P., & Shaywitz, S. E. (1989). Comparisons of cutoff and regression-based definitions of reading disabilities. *Journal of Learning Disabilities,* **22,** 334–338.

Fulker, D.W., Cardon, L.R., DeFries, J.C., Kimberling, W.J., Pennington, B.F., & Smith, S.D. (1991). Multiple regression analysis of sib-pair data on reading to detect quantitative trait loci. *Reading and Writing: An Interdisciplinary Journal,* **3,** 299–313.

Gillis, J.J., Gilger, J.W., Pennington, B.F., & DeFries, J.C. (1992). Attention deficit disorder in reading-disabled twins: evidence for a genetic etiology. *Journal of Abnormal Child Psychology,* **20,** 303–315.

Hallgren, B. (1950). Specific dyslexia: a clinical and genetic study. *Acta Psychiatrica et Neurologica Scandinavia,* **65** (Suppl.), 1–287.

Harris, E.L. (1986). The contribution of twin research to the study of the etiology of reading disability. In S.D. Smith (ed.) *Genetics and Learning Disabilities.* San Diego, CA: College-Hill Press (pp. 3–19).

Haseman, J.K. & Elston, R.C. (1972). The investigation of linkage between a quantitative trait and a marker locus. *Behavior Genetics*, **2**, 3–19.

Herjanic, B., Campbell, J., & Reich, W. (1982). Development of a structured psychiatric interview for children: Agreement between child and parent on individual symptoms. *Journal of Abnormal Child Psychology*, **10**, 307–324.

Interagency Committee on Learning Disabilities (1987). *Learning Disabilities: A Report to the US Congress*. Washington, DC: US Government Printing Office.

Kidd, K.K. (1991). Trials and tribulations in the search for genes causing neuropsychiatric disorders. *Social Biology*, **38**, 163–178.

Kirk, S.A. & Bateman, B. (1962). Diagnosis and remediation of learning disabilities. *Exceptional Children*, **29**, 73.

Lykken, D.T., Tellegen, A., & DeRubeis, R. (1978). Volunteer bias in twin research: the rule of two-thirds. *Social Biology*, **25**, 1–9.

Morrison, S.R. & Siegel, L.S. (1991). Learning disabilities: A critical review of definitional and assessment issues. In J.E. Obrzut & G.W. Hynd (eds) *Neuropsychological Foundations of Learning Disabilities: A Handbook of Issues, Methods and Practice*. Orlando, FL: Academic Press (pp. 79–97).

Nichols, R.C. & Bilbro, W.C. (1966). The diagnosis of twin zygosity. *Acta Genetica et Statistica Medica*, **16**, 265–275.

Olson, R.K., Gillis, J.J., Rack, J.P., DeFries, J.C., & Fulker, D.W. (1991a). Conformatory factor analysis of word recognition and process measures in the Colorado Reading Project. *Reading and Writing: An Interdisciplinary Journal*, **3**, 235–248.

Olson, R.K., Rack, J.P., Conners, F.A., DeFries, J.C., & Fulker, D.W. (1991b). Genetic etiology of individual differences in reading disability. In L.V. Feagans, E.J. Short, & L.J. Meltzer (eds) *Subtypes of Learning Disability*. Hillsdale, NJ: Lawrence Erlbaum (pp. 113–135).

Olson, R.K., Wise, B., Conners, F.A., Rack, J.P., & Fulker, D.W. (1989). Specific deficits in component reading and language skills: genetic and environmental influences. *Journal of Learning Disabilities*, **22**, 339–348.

Pennington, B.F., Gilger, J.W., Olson, R.K., & DeFries, J.C. (1992). The external validity of age- versus IQ-discrepancy definitions of reading disability: lessons from a twin study. *Journal of Learning Disability*, **25**, 562–573.

Rabin, M., Wen, X.L., Hepburn, M., Lubs, H.A., Feldman, E., & Duara, R. (1993). Suggestive linkage of developmental dyslexia to chromosome 1p34–36. *Lancet*, **342**, 178.

Risch, N. (1992). Genetic linkage: interpreting lod scores. *Science*, **255**, 803–804.

Shaywitz, S.E., Escobar, M.D., Shaywitz, B.A., Fletcher, J.M., & Makuch, R. (1992). Evidence that dyslexia may represent the lower tail of a normal distribution of reading ability. *New England Journal of Medicine*, **326**, 145–150.

Shaywitz, S.E. & Shaywitz, B.A. (1991). Introduction to the special series on attention deficit disorder. *Journal of Learning Disabilities*, **24**, 68–71.

Shaywitz, S.E., Shaywitz, B.A., Fletcher, J.M., & Escobar, M.D. (1990). Prevalence of reading disability in boys and girls. *Journal of the American Medical Association*, **264**, 998–1002.

Siegel, L.S. (1989). IQ is irrelevant to the definition of learning disabilities. *Journal of Learning Disabilities*, **22**, 469–478.

Smith, S.D., Kimberling, W.J., & Pennington, B.F. (1991). Screening for multiple genes influencing dyslexia. *Reading and Writing: An Interdisciplinary Journal,* **3,** 285–298.

Smith, S.D., Kimberling, W.J., Pennington, B.F., & Lubs, H.A. (1983). Specific reading disability: Identification of an inherited form through linkage analysis. *Science,* **219,** 1345–1347.

Smith, S.D., Pennington, B.F., Kimberling, W.J., & Ing, P.S. (1990). Familial dyslexia: Use of genetic linkage data to define subtypes. *Journal of the American Academy of Child and Adolescent Psychiatry,* **29,** 204–213.

Stanovich, K.E. (1986). Cognitive processes and the reading problems of learning-disabled children: Evaluating the assumption of specificity. In J.K. Torgesen and B.Y.L. Wong (eds) *Psychological and Educational Perspectives on Learning Disabilities.* Orlando, FL: Academic Press (pp. 87–131).

Stanovich, K.E. (1989). Has the LD field lost its intelligence? *Journal of Learning Disabilities,* **22,** 487–492.

Stevenson, J. (1992). Evidence for genetic aetiology in hyperactivity in children. *Behavior Genetics,* **22,** 337–344.

Stevenson, J., Graham, P., Fredman, G., & McLoughlin, V. (1984). The genetics of reading disability. In C.J. Turner & H.B. Miles (eds) *The Biology of Human Intelligence.* Nafferton, Driffield, North Humberside: Nafferton Books Ltd. (pp. 85–97).

Stevenson, J., Graham, P., Fredman, G., & McLoughlin, V. (1987). A twin study of genetic influences on reading and spelling ability and disability. *Journal of Child Psychology and Psychiatry,* **28,** 229–247.

Stevenson, J., Pennington, B.F., Gilger, J.W., DeFries, J.C., & Gillis, J.J. (1993). Hyperactivity and spelling disability: testing for shared genetic aetiology. *Journal of Child Psychology and Psychiatry,* **34,** 1137–1152.

Thompson, J.S. & Thompson, M.W. (1986). *Genetics in Medicine.* Philadelphia, PA: Saunders.

Wadsworth, S.J., Gillis, J.J., DeFries, J.C., & Fulker, D.W. (1989). Differential genetic aetiology of reading disability as a function of age. *The Irish Journal of Psychology,* **10,** 509–520.

Wechsler, D. (1974). *Examiner's Manual: Wechsler Intelligence Scale for Children – Revised.* New York: The Psychological Corporation.

Wechsler, D. (1981). *Examiner's Manual: Wechsler Adult Intelligence Scale – Revised.* New York: The Psychological Corporation.

Zerbin-Rüdin, E. (1967). Kongenitale Wortblindheit oder spezifische dyslixic (congential word-blindness). *Bulletin of the Orton Society,* **17,** 47–56.

PART IV
BIOLOGICAL CONSIDERATIONS

Introduction

J. H. BEITCHMAN

With developments in neuroimaging technology the possibilities of anatomical and functional analyses of the brains of individuals with dyslexia and related conditions has never been greater. In Chapter 14, Logan reviews quantitative neuroimaging techniques and other newer approaches to the analysis of brain morphology and function. Although studies cited show evidence of anatomical differences between populations of language/learning disabled children and normals, Logan informs us that there are many examples in neurology in which structure and function are not always well correlated. Equally important, structural abnormality may not be localized, with many brain functions having a distributed or network representation in the brain instead. Interference, with any of the components of the network, Logan cogently argues, could disturb that cognitive capacity.

Selected findings from recent functional studies point to decreased frontal cortical activity in ADHD children and slower cognitive processing which was improved with stimulant medication. Studies of dyslexic children revealed that they required more time to process visual information for most tasks. Logan reminds us that ADHD and dyslexia are relatively subtle dysfunctions, compared to more severe developmental disorders such as cerebral palsy and mental retardation. Hence, more sensitive methods are required to demonstrate abnormal structure and or function in these conditions. Logan predicts that in the future techniques will become less invasive, less expensive and more accessible, and will lead to improved patient classification.

In Chapter 15, Halperin and colleagues examine the notion that comorbid aggressive behavior and or learning disabilities can be used to define meaningful subgroups of ADHD children with corresponding specific neurochemical correlates. Halperin and colleagues remind the reader that ADHD is not a unitary condition and questions on the neurochemical mechanisms associated with ADHD pathophysiology are best understood by examining distinct symptom dimensions in children with ADHD.

Halperin and colleagues examined ADHD children with and without reading disabilities and found them to differ on measures of noradrenaline (NA) function, whereas aggressive and non-aggressive ADHD children were found to differ on measure of 5-HT function (a serotonin metabolite). However because of the lack of normal controls, these authors are unable to say which groups show abnormal neurochemical responses. The authors conclude their chapter by raising questions on the specific neurochemical correlates of ADHD in children comorbid for aggressive behavior and or reading disabilities. Given the findings of Shaywitz et al. which suggested a dimensional view of reading disabilities, defining subgroups as categorical entities will need to be carefully examined.

Approaching issues of language from the point of view of memory, Krener provides a comprehensive and wide ranging overview of acquired disorders of memory in childhood in Chapter 16. Krener distinguishes between semantic (propositional) versus episodic (procedural) memory. Semantic memory is thought to be language based whereas the procedural is experiential and is difficult to describe in words. For example, riding a bicycle or typing, can be easily demonstrated motorically but is difficult to describe in words. Indeed, sometimes individuals are not entirely aware of their procedural memories.

Earliest memories are episodic consisting of the child's unique apprehension of personal perceptions and experiences. With the establishment of language, the child attains the capacity to convert events to narration which enables inner review of experiences, rehearsal and shared encoding of verbal representations. Around the age of 4 children exhibit autobiographical memory in describing their daily experiences. This is considered to be a form of episodic memory. Krener argues that the continuity between memories arising before language and those elaborated afterward is tenuous.

The author then proceeds to describe certain clinical syndromes of memory disorders in children, concurrently identifying the particular deficits in language and other cognitive processes. Krener concludes by noting that disorders of memory must be understood in the context of childhood development and developmental lines since the development of memory cannot be divorced from the development of language.

Studies of unusual clinical cases have had an honorable tradition in medicine because of their potential to reveal nature's secrets in ways not as apparent as for more common disorders. The studies of Williams syndrome patients described by Rossen and colleagues in Chapter 17 offers a look at an intriguing condition in which there is a juxtaposition of impaired and intact mental capacities, a factor accounting for researchers' fascination with them such as with autism. Core aspects of linguistic functioning are preserved while problem solving and visuospatial cognition are impaired. Areas of preservation exist in the visual-based domain, notably in face processing.

In free speech, Williams syndrome individual's use of language are characterized by the overproduction of unexpected or inappropriate words.

Interesting correlates of aberrant semantic processing in Williams syndrome are observable at the level of brain function since anomalous evoked potentials have been identified over the left temporal lobe in individuals with this syndrome. Rossen suggests that the language of Williams syndrome individuals may appear to be fluent but, because the cognitive competence that would support verbal fluency is missing, there is an unusual but superficially competent linguistic performance. Studies of unusual cases such as Williams syndrome patients are promising for the information they provide on brain mechanisms that underlie language and cognitive processes.

14 Neuroimaging and functional brain analysis

WILLIAM J. LOGAN

Most of our knowledge regarding localization of function in neurology and neuropsychology has derived from analysis of acquired brain lesions and the associated changes in cognitive function. Until the advent of neuroimaging techniques these correlations were made on postmortem material or at the time of brain surgery where the additional technique of electrical stimulation of the cortex provided further evidence of localization of function. Advances in neuroimaging, particularly with tomographic sectioning techniques, have permitted brain dissection in vivo concurrent with neurological and neuro-pyschological evaluation of these patients. This has confirmed much of what had been surmised from more traditional approaches but also has uncovered new structure/function relationships and has revised and/or extended previously held views in other areas. This review discusses quantitative neuro-imaging techniques and newer approaches to the analysis of brain function. There will be selected examples from the recent literature of the application of these techniques to the investigation of language, dyslexia and attention deficit hyperactivity disorder (ADHD).

QUANTITATIVE NEUROIMAGING

The developmental disorders of cognition and behavior have proven resistant to routine anatomical study since gross pathological abnormalities have not generally been found in these conditions or have been found inconsistently. One explanation for the lack of pathological correlation had been that the abnormality was in the organization of connections or, if on a structural basis, only on a submicroscopic level. Several years ago another view was proposed, promoting the concept that there were structural differences that could be measured using more precise neuroanatomical techniques (e.g. Hynd & Semrud-Clikeman, 1989). These changes for the most part were changes in size of volume or area that were demonstrable in postmortem material. Could they be detected in the living patient with new imaging techniques? The development of quantitative techniques has permitted an examination of this possibility. Computerized tomography (CT) of the head and more recently magnetic resonance imaging (MRI) of the brain are the techniques most frequently employed by investigators for this purpose.

The development of the CT permitted anatomical study of the living person. CT utilizes an X-ray beam and detector to construct an image of the brain. A CT scan can be obtained in a relatively short period and provides a fairly good representation of the anatomy of brain. Development of MRI has been a major advance in the study of brain structure. After exposure to a strong magnetic field and radio frequency excitation, tissue gives off a small but detectable signal which can be translated into an image of the brain. This image is superior to that of the CT scan for anatomical study. In addition there is no radioactivity exposure. Scanning time is generally longer than for CT and motion can produce a major artifact.

There has been considerable anatomical study, both postmortem and in vivo, of dyslexia, attention deficit disorder, autism, Rett syndrome, Tourette syndrome and other disorders of the developing nervous system (Hynd & Semrud-Clikeman, 1989; Filipek, Kennedy, & Caviness, 1992; Hynd et al., 1993; Kusch et al., 1993; Peterson et al., 1993; Reiss et al., 1993; Singer et al., 1993). For language in particular there have been consistent findings in postmortem brains of asymmetric development of language areas in normal subjects. These include a larger planum temporale (the posterior perisylvian area of the temporal lobe) on the left in most (65%) and on the right side in only a few (11%) cases. Other asymmetries have been reported including the anterior speech area (greater on the left) and others not clearly related to language (e.g. larger volume of right frontal cortex). There is some evidence that the asymmetries are not present or are reversed in some patients with dyslexia and microscopic abnormalities have been found in these language areas in other cases. Similar pathology has generally not been found in attention deficit disorder.

In order to document these abnormalities in vivo in patient groups, quantitative morphological studies have been performed using CT and MRI. The imaging techniques have evolved from one-dimensional evaluations of the length of a part of the brain to two-dimensional studies of areas of interest or identifiable structures in the brain. More recently three-dimensional volumetric analysis of brain structure using very sophisticated computerized techniques has been developed for identifying regions of interest and quantitating their volume (Damasio & Frank, 1992; Filipek et al., 1992; Jernigan et al., 1991). Many of these studies have demonstrated biological differences between groups of patients with specific abnormalities and controls. None are sufficiently discriminating for diagnosis in the individual patient.

SELECTED RECENT ANATOMICAL STUDIES IN ATTENTION DEFICIT AND DEVELOPMENTAL DYSLEXIA

Hynd and colleagues evaluated the MRI scans of 10 children with attention deficit disorder/hyperactivity (ADD/H), 10 with dyslexia and 10 normal controls. The dyslexic children all had a history of difficulty learning to read, a positive family history for learning problems and significant impairment of reading achievement on both word attack and passage comprehension on the Woodcock Reading Mastery Test – Revised. Their IQ (WISC-R) was normal and they had no behavioral symptoms of hyperactivity. The ADD/H children had behavior consistent with the DSM III definition of the disorder and had a history of a favorable response to stimulant medication. They had a normal IQ, no deficit in achievement and no family history of learning problems. Some subjects in both groups had codiagnoses such as anxiety, depression, and conduct disorder. The 10 normal children had no history of learning, behavioral, social, or emotional problems and had a normal IQ and school achievement. Thirty percent of dyslexics were judged to be left-handed, but all the ADD/H and control subjects were felt to be right-handed. The controls had a higher IQ than the other groups.

On a single axial section of the MRI, there was no difference in total brain area between the different groups. Both the dyslexic and ADD/H patients had smaller width of the right anterior region giving a loss of the normal R > L asymmetry seen in the control group (and previously reported by others). Dyslexics had significantly shorter insular regions bilaterally than controls. The results for the ADD/H patients fell somewhat between these groups and were not significantly different from either. Dyslexics had a shorter left planum temporale length. Seventy percent of both ADD/H and normal subjects had L > R planum temporale length asymmetry, but ninety percent of dyslexics had a reversal (i.e., R > L) of this.

These results are consistent with several other studies looking at asymmetrical brain development in patient populations. The finding of bilateral shortening of the insular region is new and unexplained. Although there has been a previously described, but little emphasized, association of left insular region with language, it is unclear why the authors picked this as a particular region of interest for this study. The presence of comorbidities and difference in handedness in the groups introduces important variables which need to be considered in explaining some of these results. When a single section of the brain is used it is difficult to always obtain the same slice position for comparable measurement. As the authors note, it was also not possible to obtain an area or volume of the planum temporale.

Using similar techniques, the same group has evaluated the corpus callosum and caudate in ADHD children. These patients also had recognized comorbidities. Hynd et al. (1991) reported smaller areas of the genu and splenium of the corpus callosum in ADHD patients. More recently Hynd et al. (1993) showed that normal children had an asymmetry of caudate area with the left side greater than the right in 72% of subjects. ADHD patients had a reversal of this asymmetry with the right side greater than the left in 64% of the patients. Thus this same group has shown that ADD/H patients have loss of the normal R > L asymmetry in the frontal region, and that ADHD patients have a smaller corpus callosum and a reversal of the normal L > R asymmetry of the caudate. Such results need to be replicated by other investigators using ADHD subjects without comorbidities and including volumetric measurements of the regions of interest.

MRI morphometry of language and learning impaired children (L/LI) was compared to that of control children by Jernigan et al. (1991). These were children who were identified as language impaired at age 4 years and followed longitudinally until age 8 or 9 years when the MRI study was done. Controls had slightly higher performance IQs and markedly higher language function but were otherwise matched for age, sex, handedness and socioeconomic status. The patients all had severe reading impairment but many had several other language and learning deficits and therefore would in several respects not be the same as patients in other studies of developmental dyslexia. Thus the authors refer to them as L/LI rather than dyslexic. Although the clinical MRIs did not show increased pathology in the patient group, because of these comorbid features (including IQ < 80 in three patients) the possibility of acquired brain damage in some of these patients must be considered.

Visual identification of the boundaries of various brain regions of interest is difficult and to a certain extent arbitrary. To obviate this problem and to ensure that the anatomical segmentation technique would be equally applicable to different subjects, the authors used a method which divided the brain into six well-defined volumes on each side. Control subjects had left/right asymmetries which confirmed previous reports and was consistent with hemispheric specialization. The inferior posterior volume, including the putative language areas, was greater on the left, whereas the superior volume was greater on the right. The L/LI children also had asymmetries but they were different. In the prefrontal zone, which was symmetrical in controls there was a right > left asymmetry in the L/LI subjects. For the superior posterior (parietal) area there was a reversal of the right > left asymmetry seen in controls. The inferior posterior volume which included the left posterior perisylvian region was reduced in the L/LI children compared to controls. This did not result, however, in a reversal of the left > right asymmetry seen in controls, presumably because there was a decrease (not statistically significant) in the right volume as well. The only other significant change in volume involved the right diencephalon which was reduced in the L/LI group.

The authors concluded that these results supported the concept of anomalous neuroanatomical development in the L/LI patients. They recognized that the subjects were not completely representative of a dyslexic population because of their comorbidities. Also, the subdivision of the brain was arbitrary and did not represent anatomically defined structures, but this approach did have the advantage of being consistent and reproducible and anatomical stuctures could be correlated with specific zones.

CRITIQUE OF ANATOMICAL STUDIES

There are several problems with these and other attempts to correlate structure with cognitive function. Perhaps the most important constraint and one which involves all studies of these patients is the heterogeneity of the diagnostic groupings. There is no gold standard for the diagnosis of most of these disorders. Even when the groups seem homogeneous from a neuropsychological perspective there are likely to be different causes for the same phenotype. In addition, it may be that investigators are looking for something that does not exist. There are many examples in neurology in which structure and function are not well correlated. Finally, the structural changes, if present, may not be obvious using current techniques and there are several possible explanations for this limitation.

It could be that the structural changes are sufficiently small that they do not exceed the wide range of variation seen in normal populations and may not be identifiable except when large numbers of subjects are examined or homogeneous groups are compared. It is possible that the structural abnormality may not be localized. It has been increasingly thought that many brain functions have a distributed or network representation in the brain rather than being highly localized. Thus while certain locations in the brain are recognized as essential for particular functions these areas may be part of a more widespread circuit interconnecting several other brain regions which are also essential for that cognitive function. Interference with any of the components could disturb that cognitive activity. In the visual system, for example, there are at least two different pathways, one for object recognition and another for spatial recognition; these are known as the "what" and "where" networks (Mishkin, Ungerleider, & Macko, 1983). The former involves a network with reciprocal connections from the occipital lobe through the temporal lobe to the frontal lobe. The latter involves the occipital, parietal, and frontal lobes in similar fashion. Selective disturbances in recognition can be produced by lesions in any of these different areas. Finally, the anatomical abnormality may be in the connecting pathways, the dendrites or the synaptic structures and not be detectable by current anatomical imaging techniques.

Table 14.1. *Functional brain analysis techniques*

ELECTROENCEPHALOGRAPHY (EEG)
Routine EEG, Computerized EEG
Sensory Evoked Potentials (EP)
Event Related Potentials (ERP)
MAGNETOENCEPHALOGRAPHY (MEG)
Computerized MEG
Sensory Evoked Potentials
Event Related Potentials
133 XENON REGIONAL CEREBRAL BLOOD FLOW (rCBF)
SINGLE PHOTON EMISSION COMPUTED TOMOGRAPHY (SPECT)
Blood Flow
POSITRON EMISSION TOMOGRAPHY (PET)
Glucose Metabolism, Oxygen Utilization
Blood Flow
Neurotransmitter Synthesis, Receptor Binding
MAGNETIC RESONANCE SPECTROSCOPY (MRS)
Metabolite Levels
FUNCTIONAL MAGNETIC RESONANCE IMAGING (fMRI)
Blood Flow

FUNCTIONAL BRAIN ANALYSIS

The possibility that the neurological substrate for developmental disorders of cognition and behavior may be physiologically based rather than structural has led investigators to seek methods of evaluating brain function in patients with these disorders. Early studies using electroencephalography (EEG) attempted to find EEG/cognitive correlations. While the routine EEG is sensitive to gross physiological (e.g. sleep) and pathological (e.g. encephalitis) changes in behavior, it has not been useful in more subtle changes as might be expected in the developmental disorders under consideration. More recently, however, there has been the rapid development of more sophisticated signal analysis of EEG as well as new methodologies for the study of other brain physiological functions (Table 14.1). These new capabilities for studying brain function open up new windows on the brain which hold great promise, but there are many assumptions, variables, and potential pitfalls in their application.

ELECTRO/MAGNETIC POTENTIALS

Electrical current and magnetic fields have a physical relationship in that they measure the same phenomenon. Of interest is the measurement of the very small electromagnetic currents produced by the brain and the identification of their electromagnetic fields. EEG, the simplest and oldest technique, has as its counterpart magnetoencephalography (MEG). The measured responses are waveforms which have different and varying frequencies (e.g. delta at 1–3 Hz, theta at 4–7 Hz, alpha at 8–12 Hz and beta at 13+ Hz) and amplitudes in microvolts. These electromagnetic potentials can be further processed and analyzed quantitatively and their distribution over the skull can be determined, producing a topographic map of brain electrical activity.

By summing the electrical (magnetic) responses to several identical stimuli, an evoked response to a primary sensory stimulus or an event related response to a more complex stimulus can be amplified sufficiently above background electrical activity to be identified as an evoked potential (EP) or an event related potential (ERP). This can be done using either EEG or MEG techniques. The EP and ERP responses have negative and positive waveform peaks which have been found to correlate with specific stages of neurological processing of sensory and cognitive activity. These peaks are labeled by their polarity (N-negative or P-positive) in the order in which they appear (e.g., N1, P1, N2, P2) after stimulation or by their usual latency of occurrence in milliseconds in adult normal subjects (e.g., P300, N400). Based on its appearance and variation with certain tasks, N2 has been considered to represent the cognitive processing related to the detection and discrimination of a stimulus. P3 represents information processing of the stimulus at a higher cognitive level and may have two recognizable components. P3a likely represents the response to any stimulus that is noticed whether attended to or not. P3b is produced by the appearance of a target stimulus that is anticipated (attended to) and may represent a confirmatory comparison with the memory of the stimulus.

The major assumption of all of these approaches when applied to cognitive studies is that the observed electro/magnetic activity has a recognizable relationship to the patient's brain function and behavior. In most cases this is assumed to be a fairly direct relationship. This assumption appears to be valid in cases of epileptic discharge where the electrophysiological and clinical correlation is high, but most brain function does not have such a dramatic spontaneous electrical correlate. EPs and ERPs, however, are responses which are directly related to a particular activity (the stimulus) and, if present, have a very high correlation with the brain processing of that activity. Electrical recording equipment is widely available and reasonable in cost. The routine EEG has not been very useful in cognitive and behavioral evaluation but there are many studies reporting the utility of more sophisticated computerized EEG techniques in the measurement of brain function (e.g. Galin et al., 1992). There are still many variables in technique, subject selection and paradigms used so it is not surprising that there are often differences in the results obtained. The value of electrophysiology in the detection of cognitive and behavioral disorders remains to be demonstrated.

MEG requires much more expensive equipment and specialized recording rooms because of the very low magnetic signal that is produced by the brain. It has an advantage over EEG because the signals are not as attenuated by the skull and scalp. Both techniques are non-invasive and they provide somewhat complementary information since they view the electromagnetic field from a different perspective. By use of computer modeling, the likely location of the neuronal activity producing an observed signal can be estimated. This provides some degree of anatomical localization which can be presented as a topographic map.

Evoked responses provide another dimension which investigators have found to be useful in dissecting brain function. These add the powerful aspect of determining brain processing time in milliseconds. To processing time or latency of the response can be added response intensity and its distribution over the brain surface which can be displayed using topographic mapping techniques. The evolution of the response temporally can be followed spatially over all brain regions. The anatomical resolution of electromagnetic signals is quite limited, however, due to the number of electrodes or probes routinely employed. Recently, investigators are using many more recording sites (128 +) to improve the anatomical resolution.

CEREBRAL BLOOD FLOW

Areas of increased electrical activity in the brain have increased metabolic activity as well as increased blood flow. The initial studies performed several years ago utilized similar principles to many of the techniques in use today. The subject's blood was labeled with a radioactive substance and entry into or exit from the brain could be evaluated by special detectors. The actual amount of blood flow could be determined based on several assumptions (models) and calculations. Because it could be measured at different sites over the skull surface, the distribution of the radioactivity could be determined. In early studies, the blood flow over the surface of the brain could be estimated using these techniques. An advance in methodology permitted tomographic sections or slices to be taken through the brain so that blood flow could be computed and visualized throughout the entire brain including subcortical regions. The specificity and accuracy of these localizations has been increased by having a larger number of detectors and by using different radioisotopes. If a sufficient number of tomographic sections are obtained they can be reassembled into a three-dimensional image of the brain.

The initial techniques for the study of blood flow used a limited number of detectors which could essentially only measure radioactivity in the directly underlying tissue. From these measurements the regional cerebral blood flow (rCBF) in the underlying cortex could be estimated. The radioactive substance (usually Xenon) is injected into the circulation or administered through inhalation. The more invasive injection into cerebral vessels provides for more selective intracranial perfusion and better cortical visualization. Blood samples are taken at intervals to determine the circulating radioactivity. The technique has been improved by obtaining three-dimensional computed tomographic measurements of the radioactivity thus allowing rCBF determination throughout a brain section (e.g., Lou et al., 1989). The single photon emission computed tomography (SPECT) scan uses a specific gamma emitting radiolabeled substance which passes from the blood into the brain in relation to the degree of blood flow. Since some of these substances remain in the brain parenchyma for a significant length of time, they can be given when detection of blood flow is of interest (e.g., during a cognitive task) and measured at some later time. This readily available technique presently has limited resolution and is not quantitative.

Positron emission tomography (PET) is an advance in technology which allows detection of specific radioactive elements which emit positrons. Since the frequently used elements have short radioactive half-lives, they must be generated by a cyclotron immediately before use. This requires the presence of a cyclotron on site or nearby. This technology provides improved anatomical resolution. For blood studies, 15 oxygen labeled water is most frequently used although there are other tracers available. Since 15 oxygen has a half-life of about 2 minutes, it has the added advantage that repeat studies can be performed in the same subject after several minutes. There is a limit to the number of repeat studies, however, because of the cumulative radioactive dosage. PET equipment, including a cyclotron, is expensive.

The most recent advance in detecting blood flow utilizes MRI. The obvious advantage to this technology is the lack of radiation exposure. Because the same study can be repeated in the same individual many times, there is improved resolution. Increased blood flow can apparently be detected without adding an exogenous agent because of a change in the paramagnetic properties of blood related to changes in oxygenation of hemoglobin. These changes occur during increased cerebral activity. This new technology is developing very rapidly and promises to provide a noninvasive method for determining changes in blood flow, presumably due to the increased neuronal activity associated with cognitive and behavioral function. There have not yet been reports on its use in children or in developmental disorders.

METABOLISM

With increased neuronal activity there is energy utilization and increased metabolism of the active tissue. Oxygen and glucose utilization and blood flow are increased. In addition to determining blood flow, PET techniques are available to measure both glucose and oxygen uptake. A glucose analogue, 2-deoxyglucose, which is taken up via a glucose transport mechanism is partially metabolized by phosphorylation and remains trapped in the cell unable to undergo further metabolism. This is fortuitous for the investigation of glucose metabolism for its accumulation reflects normal glucose uptake, and it can be determined when labeled with a positron emitting isotope such as 18F (fluoro-deoxyglucose). Because of the half-life of 18F and because of the persistence of deoxyglucose in the cell, it is generally only possible to determine glucose uptake a limited number of times. Usually, uptake is measured in a control and in an experimental state (e.g., during visual or other stimulation) separated by hours or days. Other repetitions are usually not possible during a single test period. An advantage of this technique for evaluation of brain function is that the cognitive or behavioral tasks can be performed in a more natural setting after injection of the deoxyglucose and the accumulation of glucose which occurs during the task can later be determined in the scanner.

OTHER FUNCTIONS

Any substance that can be labeled with a positron emitting element can theoretically be studied with PET (Roland, 1993). Other substances have been utilized in neurology such as L-dopa, the dopamine (DA) precursor, for evaluation of DA synthesis and other chemicals which bind to neurotransmitter (NT) receptors. DA synthesis in the caudate nucleus has been demonstrated using PET techniques. NT receptor agonists/antagonists can be labeled and their distribution and kinetic properties of receptor binding in brain regions can also be evaluated.

ACTIVATION STUDIES

While electromagnetic activity, blood flow and metabolism can be evaluated in subjects in the resting state this has not been informative in cognitive and behavioral studies. Of greater interest and utility is the investigation of these physiological parameters during activated brain function (Roland, 1993). Simple primary sensory stimulation (e.g., visual) has demonstrable effects on each of the parameters. The extension of these measurements to more complicated cognitive and behavioral tasks has been more difficult but also more rewarding. Even routine and apparently simple cognitive tasks utilize several different mechanisms and activate different neurological regions. Investigators have addressed this problem by simplifying the tasks and also by employing a subtraction technique to isolate the particular function they wish to study.

When a task involves several brain functions, by subtracting the initial processes from later processes, the latter can be evaluated. As an example, in a silent reading task, the response to viewing letters not in the form of words (visual perception) can be subtracted from the response to silent reading of words. This may determine what brain areas or processes are activated specifically by the act of reading. Other subtractions such as non-target response from target response in a visual recognition task may be used to dissect the various processes involved specifically in the recognition task. Subtraction works only when the same physiological measurements can be repeated for the two or more tasks in an otherwise identical setting.

CRITIQUE OF FUNCTIONAL STUDIES

There are several aspects to consider when evaluating functional analysis techniques and their application to cognition and behavior. These include patient (or subject), technical and experimental factors. More than with psychological testing, these techniques require subject cooperation, particularly when activation studies are being performed. Some of the techniques, such as blood flow studies, are quite confining. Certain patients may experience claustrophobia in the PET and MRI scanners. Unless the subject remains very still there is the likelihood of motion induced artifact; this is a major problem for the PET and MRI bloodflow techniques.

Technical issues including spatial and temporal resolution, invasiveness, cost, accessibility and ease of use are major considerations. Electromagnetic techniques provide better temporal resolution whereas blood flow and metabolic studies with PET and blood flow studies with MRI provide superior spatial resolution. EEG/MEG and MRI techniques are least invasive and there is no radiation. EEG (including EP) is least expensive and most accessible except for the more sophisticated and complicated computerized techniques. MRI will become more widely available but is still fairly costly. PET techniques are very expensive and of limited accessibility. SPECT scans are more widely available but somewhat limited technically at this time. With further development this technology is likely to provide the capability of measuring receptors, bloodflow and other functions with improved resolution. MEG techniques are found in only a few centers and are expensive to establish. MEG, PET and MRI require a team of experts from different disciplines (e.g., physics, engineering).

The major assumption underlying these investigations is that the particular physiological activity being measured actually represents the relevant cognitive and behavioral function one wishes to study. It is also often assumed that increased activity represents increased brain function and that these are directly proportional. Because of the many data points that are examined statistically for difference, there are likely to be several differences between experimental and control that occur just by chance. This can be minimized by statistical correction, by replication of the study or by examining a second cohort of subjects to determine which of the differences are consistent. Further, few reports contain information on the reproducibility and reliability of the results. Finally, since most studies require a subject to perform cognitive tasks, there should be some measure of how well and complete the task was performed, particularly if the task is silent or covert.

SELECTED RECENT FUNCTIONAL STUDIES IN ADHD

Quantitative EEG evaluation of children (aged 9 to 12) who had the clinical diagnosis of ADHD was reported by Mann et al. (1992). These were male patients who had no neurological impairment and who scored above 1.5 standard deviations on Connors parent and teacher rating scales. It appears that the authors studied a subpopulation of these patients who did not have the symptoms of hyperactivity, but it is not clear why this was done. Controls selected from the same school population were demographically matched. The patients, however, had significantly lower scores on reading, arithmetic and WISC-R verbal tests. The spectra of the amplitude of the power in the different EEG frequency bands (low delta, high delta, theta, alpha, low beta and high beta) was determined. The spectra were obtained during three conditions, namely baseline visual fixation, silent reading and drawing (subjects copied figures from the Bender–Gestalt visual motor test). These tasks are rather complex but that may be necessary for evaluation of ADHD.

The principal findings were an increase in theta power amplitude in frontal regions, especially on the right side and a decrease in beta amplitude in the temporal areas during the cognitive tasks and these changes were greater for the drawing than for the reading condition compared to baseline. Using these findings, the investigators were able to retrospectively predict the proper group membership (ADHD or control) for 80% of the patients and 74% of the controls. They concluded that this supported a biological basis for ADHD, possibly decreased cortical activity frontally. A virgin cohort was not used to test these findings, however.

Event related potentials (ERP) were evaluated in ADHD patients by Taylor et al. (1993). Patients who met DSM III-R criteria for ADHD and controls were divided into two age groups, 7 to 9.9 and 10 to 12.9 years. All patients were known responders to stimulant medication. They were evaluated under four conditions, namely baseline, placebo, low dose methylphenidate (5 to 10 mgm.) and higher dose methylphenidate (10 to 15 mgm.) Controls were assessed at baseline only. ERPs were obtained at multiple electrode sites following the presentation of visual stimuli. Subjects were required to discriminate target letters from nontarget letters. This task produced ERPs with identifiable N2, P3a and P3b peaks.

Younger children had longer latency responses than older children. P3a and P3b latencies were significantly longer in ADHD patients compared to controls. When given methylphenidate, the ERP latencies decreased to normal but the corresponding reaction times were not significantly changed. In other studies ADHD children have usually been found to have longer reaction times than controls and methylphenidate has normalized these. In this study the reaction times of the patients were similar to controls but as the authors note this could be due to practice effect for the patients were tested four times and the controls only once. There were no effects of the drug on topographic distribution of the ERP, but only 13 active electrodes were used. It was concluded that ADHD patients have slower cognitive processing and that this was improved with stimulant medication in patients who were previously considered to be positive responders to these drugs. Controls were not given medication so it is not certain if this improvement in ERP processing time is specific to ADHD.

Xenon 133 Cerebral Blood Flow (CBF) was evaluated in ADHD patients by Lou et al. (1989). A heterogeneous group of 19 patients with ADHD including 13 with other Central Nervous System (CNS) dysfunction such as language disorder were studied using siblings of patients as controls. Therefore this group of ADHD patients may not be strictly comparable to those of other studies. Xenon 133 was administered by inhalation and three-dimensional regional CBF (rCBF) was determined by emission computed tomography. Only the middle tomographic slice of three slices was used for this study because the other slices had too much extracranial tissue activity. This slice included the central part of prefrontal cortex, striatum, the perisylvian region and occipital cortex but excluded large regions of the frontal cortex. The studies were obtained at rest; no cognitive tasks were performed. Quantitative rCBF was determined for each region of interest. Four of the children were studied before and after methylphenidate was given.

In the ADHD group there was hypoperfusion in the striatal regions which was significant for right striatum. The left sensorimotor/primary auditory cortex (a combined region of interest in this study) and the occipital lobe were significantly hyperperfused compared to control. Somewhat similar findings were noted in the ADHD group with other CNS abnormality. Methylphenidate produced an apparent increase in flow in the striatal areas especially on the left side. It was not clear why the right striatum which had more prominent hypoperfusion did not demonstrate a greater response to the drug than the left striatum but this may relate to the small numbers studied. It was concluded that striatal hypoperfusion, possibly reflecting decreased neuronal activity, appeared to be a feature of ADHD. Since many of the patients in this study had other evidence of CNS dysfunction or insult, this may have reflected acquired injury to the striatum. It is unfortunate that large areas of the frontal lobes were not included in this study.

PET evaluation of brain glucose metabolism in adult parents of ADHD children who themselves had a history of hyperactivity in childhood has been reported by Zametkin et al. (1990). Adults without an ADHD history served as controls. The scans used 18-F fluorodeoxyglucose and were obtained during an auditory attention task, namely a continuous performance test in which subjects had to respond to a specific tone. The isotope was administered during the task and then later the subjects were scanned to determine glucose uptake. A decrease in glucose metabolism, especially in the left frontal area, was found in the subjects compared to controls.

A subsequent study (Zametkin et al., 1993) evaluated glucose metabolism in adolescents with ADHD using the same technique and protocol. Most of the control subjects were siblings of patients with ADHD and matching was not ideal. In this study, the results were less impressive than in the first study in adults. Overall glucose metabolism was not different in the patient and control groups, however two regions in the left frontal area and two regions in the right temporal area had decreased metabolism in the ADHD patients compared to controls. One posterior left frontal area had increased metabolism in ADHD adolescents unlike the adults. The changes in left anterior frontal area, however, were the same in both studies. One of the most important aspects of this study according to the investigators is that PET studies such as this can be performed in adolescents.

SELECTED RECENT FUNCTIONAL STUDIES IN DYSLEXIA

ERPs of dyslexic children with a primary deficit in visual processing and in the ability to encode and read words were compared to age matched controls with no reading impairment (Taylor & Keenan, 1990). Three age ranges were evaluated. The dyslexic children had normal intelligence but ranged from 1.3 to 2.5 years below average in reading ability. The specific criteria used to differentiate these patients from other dyslexics was not given. The ERPs were elicited using a paradigm in which subjects were asked to identify specific symbol, letter or word targets which were infrequently presented visually in a series of other similar but more frequently presented nontargets (e.g., nonword letter strings). The N2 and P3 peaks were identified and their latencies and amplitudes were compared between groups. ERP nontarget responses were subtracted from target responses to obtain the difference which was considered to be due to visual discrimination.

Both N2 and P3 peaks had shorter latency responses in older subjects and for the easier discrimination tasks. There were shorter latency responses over the left hemisphere for the alphabet and symbol but not the word recognition tasks. Dyslexic subjects had longer latency N2 and P3 and lower amplitude P3 centrally and posteriorly but not frontally compared to controls. Because each of the age groups had the same degree of abnormality (i.e. showed no improvement with age) the authors felt this was not consistent with a delayed maturation cause of the differences between the groups. The same patients were not followed and tested longitudinally to prove this. It was concluded that dyslexic children required more time to process visual information for most tasks and that this was evident at the early stages of processing (N2, 300 to 400 msec.).

PET evaluation of brain glucose metabolism in adult dyslexic subjects was studied by Hagman et al. (1992). The patients who had been identified as dyslexic from childhood were otherwise not subgrouped. Dyslexia was defined by scores on the Gray Oral Reading Test and the Wide Range Achievement

Test that were 1.5 years behind grade level when tested during childhood. The subjects also scored 2 SDs below the mean on the Finucci test for adult reading disability. They were compared to controls who were matched except for reading ability and verbal IQ. The subjects performed an auditory continuous performance test (CPT) of speech discrimination in which they were to respond to a target syllable. 18-F fluorodeoxyglucose was administered during the task and uptake was later measured in the scanner.

The dyslexic subjects did less well on CPT performance accuracy. There were no differences in brain metabolic rates between the controls and dyslexics on the lateral cortical surface, but dyslexics had significantly higher metabolism in a localized part of the medial temporal lobe bilaterally. These findings were not tested in an additional cohort of dyslexics to confirm the findings and studies were not done in children. It was concluded that these results were consistent with a processing abnormality of auditory stimuli in dyslexic subjects which was not lateralized.

PET evaluation of cerebral blood flow was performed in adult dyslexics using 15 oxygen labeled water by Rumsey et al. (1992). The patients had severe developmental dyslexia with decoding skill abnormality and poor word recognition. Controls were matched except for reading ability and verbal IQ. Repeat scans were performed during two psychological tasks and a resting baseline. In a rhyming task, pairs of 1–3 syllable words were presented aurally and the subjects were to respond if the words rhymed. In the continuous performance test (CPT) a series of tones of different intensities were presented with the target being the lowest volume tone. During a 4.5-minute scan several tomographic slices were obtained while one of the cognitive tasks (or the baseline) was performed.

The rhyme task increased blood flow (activated) in the left temporoparietal, middle temporal and posterior frontal regions as well as in two right temporoparietal regions in control subjects. In the dyslexic individuals, it did not activate these areas but instead activated left anterior temporal and right temporal regions as well as the left Rolandic area. On the rhyming task, the dyslexics' psychological performance was less accurate than the controls, reflecting the difficulty of the task. The CPT activated right temporoparietal regions in both control and dyslexic subjects but also activated the same left anterior temporal region in dyslexics that the rhyming task had. It was concluded that there were subtle differences between controls and adult dyslexics, especially a failure in the latter group to show activation of left temporoparietal cortex. This was task specific and seen only with a rhyming paradigm.

FUTURE DIRECTIONS

ADHD and dyslexia are relatively subtle dysfunctions compared to more severe developmental disorders (e.g., cerebral palsy, mental retardation) and many acquired brain disorders (e.g., trauma, stroke). It is not surprising that more sensitive methods have been required to demonstrate abnormal structure and/or function in these conditions. Various combinations of the newer technologies with psychological advances in the evaluation of cognition and behavior should permit the identification of specific subgroups of these disorders. In addition to providing insight into their pathogenesis, a major goal would be to use the new technologies for diagnosis of these disorders in an individual patient. The areas which are promising in this regard are both clinical and technical.

All structural and functional studies will benefit from more precise clinical and psychological characterization of the patient groups. There are, in functional analysis particularly, opportunities for development of new applications of psychology. Most of the recent work evaluating cerebral blood flow has investigated normal function (e.g. language, attention) and has used paradigms and cognitive tasks appropriate for the adult. These need to be revised and validated for children of different ages before studies can be extended to controls and patients in these groups. Approaches must also be developed to prepare children for the testing procedure. This will require instruction in task performance and training in how to behave (e.g. not move) during the test procedure. Finally, there is much challenge, but also opportunity, in the development of simpler and more targeted cognitive tasks that will activate specific brain functions and regions of interest using the new functional techniques.

Structural assessment of ADHD and dyslexia should become more quantitative using noninvasive MRI. The recently reported abnormalities in these conditions discussed above need to be confirmed and extended using volumetric evaluation of specific structures. New approaches are available which will permit segmentation of various regions and nuclei and parcellation of specific regions of the cortex.

Electro/magnetic analysis of brain function at a large number of recording sites and coregistration with MRI will produce highly localized maps of brain activity. Specific stimuli can be used to selectively activate particular brain areas. SPECT scanning will have improved resolution and increased application. For blood flow studies in children, functional MRI (fMRI) will likely replace PET, but neither will be able to provide information on processing speed as well as the electro/magnetic methods can. Advances in fMRI will be directed to decreasing the testing time and number of artifacts produced and to developing methods for assessing less cooperative children.

CONCLUSION

There is an increasing array of methods that may be used to evaluate brain structure and function. These have been utilized to investigate cognitive and behavioral disorders including ADHD and dyslexia. There are several new techniques for the analysis of different functions of the brain. Some of these are effective at temporal resolution of cognitive processes whereas others are more effective in spatial localization. Using cognitive activation tasks, group differences between patients with ADHD or dyslexia and controls have documented biological abnormalities in these conditions. Most reports have not been confirmed by additional studies, and some have only included adult patients. As yet none of the techniques or approaches has been shown to be diagnostic for the individual patient with ADHD or dyslexia.

Major advances are likely to occur in several areas in the near future. Techniques will become less invasive, less expensive and more accessible. There will be improved spatial and temporal resolution for all techniques. Combination of methods of functional analysis (e.g., EEG and PET) will provide complementary information not otherwise available with individual techniques. More specific and appropriate tasks will be developed to activate brain function during investigation. Finally, analysis of brain function will not only benefit from better patient selection and clinical subgrouping but will itself lead to improved patient classification.

REFERENCES

Damasio, H. & Frank, R. (1992). Three-dimensional in vivo mapping of brain lesions in humans. *Archives of Neurology, 49,* 137–143.

Filipek, P.A., Kennedy, D.N., & Caviness, Jr., V.S. (1992). Neuroimaging in child neuropsychology. In F. Boller & J. Grafman (series eds); I. Rapin & S. Segalowitz (vol. eds) *Handbook of Neuropsychology; Vol. 6, Child Neuropsychology.* Amsterdam: Elsevier (pp. 301–329).

Galin, D., Raz, J., Fein, G., Johnstone, J., Herron, J., & Yingling, C. (1992). EEG spectra in dyslexic and normal readers during oral and silent reading. *Electroencephalography and Clinical Neurophysiology, 82,* 87–101.

Hagman, J.O., Wood, F., Buchsbaum, M.S., Tallal, P., Flowers, L., & Katz, W. (1992). Cerebral brain metabolism in adult dyslexic subjects assessed with positron emission tomography during performance of an auditory task. *Archives of Neurology, 49,* 734–739.

Hynd, G.W. & Semrud-Clikeman, M. (1989). Dyslexia and brain morphology. *Psychological Bulletin, 106,* 447–482.

Hynd, G.W., Semrud-Clikeman, M., Lorys, A.R., Novey, E.S., & Elipulos, D. (1990). Brain morphology in developmental dyslexia and attention deficit disorder/hyperactivity. *Archives of Neurology, 47,* 919–926.

Hynd, G.W., Semrud-Clikeman, M., Lorys, A.R., Novey, E.S., Eliopulos, D., & Lyytinen, H. (1991). Corpus callosum morphology in attention deficit hyperactivity disorder (ADHD); morphometric analysis of MRI. *Journal of Learning Disabilities, 24,* 141–146.

Hynd, G.W., Hern, K.L., Novey, E.S., Eliopulos, D., Marshall, R., Gonzalez, J.J., & Voeller, K.K. (1993). Attention deficit-hyperactivity disorder and asymmetry of the caudate nucleus. *Journal of Child Neurology, 8,* 339–347.

Jernigan, T.L., Hesselink, J.R., Sowell, E., & Tallal, P.A. (1991). Cerebral structure on magnetic resonance imaging in language- and learning-impaired children. *Archives of Neurology*, **48**, 539–545.

Jernigan, T.L., Trauner, D.A., Hesselink, J.R. & Tallal, P.A. (1991). Maturation of human cerebrum observed in vivo during adolescence. *Brain*, **114**, 2037–2049.

Kusch, A., Gross-Glenn, K., Jallad, B., Lubs, H., Rabin, M., Feldman, E., & Durara, R. (1993). Temporal lobe surface area measurements on MRI in normal and dyslexic readers. *Neuropsychologia*, **31**, 811–821.

Lou, H.C., Henriksen, L., Bruhn, P., Borner, H., & Nielsen, J.B. (1989). Striatal dysfunction in attention deficit and hyperkinetic disorder. *Archives of Neurology*, **46**, 48–52.

Mann, C.A., Lubar, J.F., Zimmerman, A.W., Miller, C.A., & Muenchen, R.A. (1992). Quantitative analysis of EEG in boys with attention-deficit-hyperactivity disorder: controlled study with clinical implications. *Pediatric Neurology*, **8**, 30–36.

Mishkin, M., Ungerleider, L.G., & Macko, K.A. (1983). Object vision and spatial vision; Two cortical pathways. *Trends in Neuroscience*, **6**, 414–417.

Peterson, B., Riddle, M.A., Cohen, D.J., Katz, L.D., Smith, J.C., Hardin, M.T., & Leckman, J.F. (1993). Reduced basal ganglia volumes in Tourette's syndrome using three-dimensional reconstruction techniques from magnetic resonance images. *Neurology*, **43**, 941–949.

Reiss, A.L., Faruque, F., Naidu, S., Abrams, M., Beaty, T., Bryan, R.N., & Moser, H. (1993). Neuroanatomy of Rett syndrome: a volumetric imaging study. *Annals of Neurology*, **34**, 227–234.

Roland, P.E. (1993). *Brain Activation*. New York: Wiley-Liss.

Rumsey, J.M., Andreason, P., Zametkin, A.J., Aquino, T., King, C., Hamburger, S.D., Pikus, A., Rapoport, J.L., & Cohen, R.M. (1992). Failure to activate the left temporoparietal cortex in dyslexia: an oxygen 15 positron emission tomographic study. *Archives of Neurology*, **49**, 527–534.

Singer, H.S., Reiss, A.L., Brown, J.E., Aylward, E.H., Shih, B., Chee, E., Harris, E.L., Reader, M.J., Chase, G.A., Bryan, R.N., & Denkla, M.B. (1993). Volumetric MRI changes in basal ganglia of children with Tourette's syndrome. *Neurology*, **43**, 950–956.

Taylor, M.J. & Keenan, N.K. (1990). Event-related potentials to visual and language stimuli in normal and dyslexic children. *Psychophysiology*, **27**, 318–327.

Taylor, M.J., Voros, J.G., Logan, W.J., & Malone, M. (1993). Changes in event-related potentials with stimulant medication in children with attention deficit hyperactivity disorder. *Biological Psychology*, **36**, 139–156.

Zametkin, A.J., Nordahl, T.E., Gross, M., King, A.C., Semple, W.E., Rumsey, J., Hamburger, S., & Cohen, R.M. (1990). Cerebral glucose metabolism in adults with hyperactivity of childhood onset. *New England Journal of Medicine*, **323**, 1361–1366.

Zametkin, A.J., Liebenauer, L.L., Fitzgerald, G.A., King, A.C., Minkunas, D.V., Herscovitch, P., Yamada, E.M., & Cohen, R.M. (1993). Brain metabolism in teenagers with attention-deficit hyperactivity disorder. *Archives of General Psychiatry*, **50**, 333–340.

15 Neurochemical correlates of academic achievement deficits and aggressive behavior in children with ADHD

JEFFREY M. HALPERIN, JEFFREY H. NEWCORN, AND
VANSHDEEP SHARMA

Few investigators or clinicians would argue with the notion that the behavior and cognitive functioning of children with attention deficit hyperactivity disorder (ADHD) is highly influenced by a host of environmental factors. Yet, most believe that the etiology of the disorder has, at least in part, a neurochemical basis. Despite this belief, there has been little success in consistently distinguishing children with ADHD from normal children on any measure of neurotransmitter function (for review, see Zametkin & Rapoport, 1987; Rogeness, Javors, & Pliszka, 1992).

Similarly, neuropsychological studies have yielded conflicting results. Some neuropsychological test data suggest the presence of right hemisphere deficits in children with ADHD (Malone, Kershner, & Siegel, 1988; Heilman, Voeller, & Nadeau, 1991), some indicate the presence of frontal lobe deficits (Chelune et al., 1986; for review, see Barkley, Grodzinsky, & DuPaul, 1992) and still other data highlight the importance of left hemisphere dysfunction (Swanson et al., 1991). Finally, an emerging literature using neuroimaging techniques has provided data suggesting possible structural and/or metabolic differences in the striatum (Lou et al., 1989), caudate nuclei (Lou, Henrickson, & Bruhn, 1984; Castellanos et al., 1993; Hynd et al., 1993), corpus callosum (Hynd et al., 1991; Giedd et al., 1994) and frontal regions (Hynd et al., 1990; Zametkin et al., 1990) in children with ADHD, but thus far the precise location and direction of the findings have been somewhat variable. Overall, neurochemical, neuropsychological, and neuroimaging data have yielded few consistent findings. Consequently, the precise nature of the neural dysfunction in ADHD has remained elusive.

This lack of consistency in research findings is not entirely surprising. Although ADHD is defined by the "core" symptoms of inattention, impulsivity, and hyperactivity, children with ADHD comprise an extremely heterogeneous group who vary considerably in their clinical presentation and long-term outcome. The diagnostic criteria for ADHD have recently undergone substantial revision, and the new criteria in DSM-IV (APA, 1994) contain specific symptom lists that are likely to generate more homogeneous subtypes. However, the DSM-III-R (APA, 1987) definition of ADHD, which has been the basis of most recent biological research, did not require impairment in all three symptom domains and was therefore applied to children with variable patterns of symptom clusters (Newcorn et al., 1989). In addition, ADHD children frequently present with one or more comorbid conditions (for review, see Biederman, Newcorn, & Sprich, 1991), further contributing to their heterogeneity. Among ADHD children, as many as 30% to 50% are reported to have comorbid conduct or oppositional disorders, approximately 25% meet criteria for at least one anxiety disorder, and 15% to 25% meet full diagnostic criteria for an affective disorder. In addition, depending upon how it is defined, anywhere from 9% to 56% may meet criteria for a learning disability (LD), although recent research suggests that when conservative criteria for LD are used, the figure is approximately 20% (Hinshaw, 1992).

Children with ADHD also vary considerably in their development and long-term outcome. Whereas most ADHD symptoms tend to decline with age, a substantial proportion of patients continue to exhibit at least some of the core symptoms of inattention, impulsivity and overactivity well into adolescence and adulthood (Weiss et al., 1985; Klein & Mannuzza, 1991; Fischer et al., 1993). A subgroup of these individuals develop disorders characterized by criminality and/or substance abuse. Furthermore, cognitive problems tend to persist in those with childhood LD (Loney, Kramer, & Milich, 1981), although these may go unnoticed if the demand for cognitive skills is reduced in adulthood.

While each of the comorbid conditions in children with ADHD may affect clinical presentation, treatment response, course and outcome, the majority of studies have focused on the associated features of aggressive conduct problems and academic underachievement. These data indicate that comorbid aggressive behavior and/or academic underachievement (or LD) may have a consistent and predictable impact on the clinical presentation and long-term outcome of children with ADHD, raising the possibility that diagnostically and etiologically distinct subgroups of children with ADHD can be identified. This chapter will initially review the literature supporting the notion that comorbid aggressive behavior and/or LD can be used to define clinically meaningful subgroups of children with ADHD. Subsequently, we will propose neurochemical etiologies for these ADHD subgroups and provide preliminary data supporting these biological dissociations.

DISSOCIATION OF ADHD SUBTYPES

Factor analytic studies have provided convincing evidence that the symptom dimensions of inattention/hyperactivity and conduct problems/aggression are separable, even though measures of these behaviors are consistently found to be highly intercorrelated (for review, see Hinshaw, 1987). However, despite their overlap, these dimensions appear to have distinct etiologic and prognostic features. Childhood aggression has been related to low socioeconomic status and a variety of familial factors, whereas inattention/hyperactivity appears more associated with learning disorders and cognitive dysfunction (Biederman, Munir, & Knee, 1987; Hinshaw, 1987; Lahey et al., 1988; Szatmari, Boyle, & Offord, 1989; Schachar & Wachsmuth, 1990). Although the predictors of long-term outcome have not been fully clarified, data suggest that the presence of early aggression predicts antisocial behaviors in adulthood (Loney, Kramer, & Milich, 1981; Loeber et al., 1993), while learning and cognitive problems often persist into adolescence and early adulthood (Loney et al., 1981).

Yet, our ability to distinguish inattention/hyperactivity from conduct problems/aggression in individual children has been limited, making it difficult to identify homogeneous groups of children. This difficulty stems in part from the fact that children with disruptive behavior disorders frequently do not exhibit symptoms during one-to-one interactions in the clinician's office. As a result, rating scales are commonly used to systematically gather information from parents and teachers to assist in differential diagnoses. Although a higher degree of confidence is generally placed upon the teacher's input, studies (Schachar et al., 1986; Abikoff et al., 1993) have shown that teachers frequently rate disruptive/aggressive children as inattentive and hyperactive even if they do not present with difficulties in these latter domains. Thus, teacher ratings of inattention and hyperactivity in children who are not disruptive are likely to be valid, but similar ratings in disruptive/aggressive children are often erroneous. This suggests that most teacher rating scales select children with a wide range of behavior disorders, rather than more specific symptom profiles.

As a result, many studies that have attempted to identify subgroups of children with ADHD, primarily through the use of rating scales, have failed to find meaningful distinctions. For example, one early set of British studies used rating scales to divide clinic-referred (Sandberg, Rutter, & Taylor, 1978) and nonreferred school children (Sandberg, Wieselberg, & Shaffer, 1980) into ADHD, conduct disorder (CD) and comorbid ADHD + CD. They found no significant group differences on a host of cognitive, biological and psychosocial measures. Yet, they did find evidence for the existence of a distinct, small group of nonaggressive children, characterized by deficits in attention and cognitive functioning. Similarly, a five-year follow-up of the Isle of Wight study (Schachar, Rutter, & Smith, 1981) found that a small group of nonaggressive "pervasive hyperactive" children showed a persistent pattern of cognitive impairments. Thus, early studies using rating scales generated some support for the notion that a small group of primarily nonaggressive children with attentional and cognitive impairments may be separable from the larger group of children with disruptive behavior disorders.

A series of studies by Stewart and colleagues, which used structured diagnostic interviews, rather than rating scales, provided further evidence for the dissociation of ADHD subgroups based upon the presence or absence of aggressive behavior and/or learning problems. These investigators (August & Stewart, 1982) found that "pure" ADHD children had lower IQ scores and more problems in academic achievement than those with mixed ADHD/ CD, although these subgroups did not differ on a variety of prenatal, perinatal, developmental, or neurological measures. Furthermore, a four-year follow-up of this sample (August, Stewart, & Holmes, 1983) found that none of the pure ADHD children received a subsequent diagnosis of CD, whereas the ADHD/CD group continued to exhibit both aggressive and hyperactive disturbances. Thus, nonaggressive ADHD may be a stable phenomenon with a distinct prognosis from aggressive ADHD. Subsequently (August & Stewart, 1983), the sample was redivided based upon parent symptomatology. ADHD children who had at least one parent diagnosed as having a disorder in the "antisocial spectrum" were more likely to have conduct disturbance, to have siblings with CD, and to come from broken homes. Contrary to this, the ADHD children without a parental history of antisocial behavior had more learning and academic problems, and had siblings with attentional and learning problems, without conduct disturbances.

More recent data further support the dissociation of ADHD subgroups based upon the presence or absence of learning problems. August and Garfinkel (1989) found that ADHD children with reading disabilities (RD) were characterized primarily by inattention, as measured using a continuous performance test (CPT), and poor performance on measures of linguistic and mnestic abilities. In contrast, ADHD children without RD had fewer cognitive impairments, but had a substantially higher rate of comorbid conduct disorder and disruptive behavior. Based upon these data, a distinction between "cognitive" and "behavioral" subtypes of ADHD children was proposed. Consistent with this, using laboratory measures, Chee et al. (1989) found evidence for attentional and cognitive dysfunction among ADHD children without comorbid CD; those with comorbid ADHD + CD appeared similar to normals on their measures. Furthermore, investigations comparing ADHD children with and without comorbid RD have reported group differences on neuropsychological measures of visual-motor integration (August & Garfinkel, 1990; Robins, 1992), verbal fluency (Felton et al., 1987) and delayed recall of nonverbal material (McGee et al., 1989).

Data also indicate a higher incidence of substance abuse and criminality, as well as family chaos and instability, in relatives of ADHD children with comorbid CD as compared to those without comorbid CD (Biederman, Munir, & Knee, 1987; Lahey et al., 1988), raising the possibility of etiological distinctions between the subgroups. Furthermore, recent work of Loeber et al. (1993) strongly suggests that increased risk for a developmental course characterized by severe conduct disturbance is specifically associated with early childhood ADHD + aggression, whereas nonaggressive ADHD children (as well as aggressive nonADHD children) are less likely to develop serious conduct problems. In contrast, however, Klein and Mannuzza (1991) found that the presence of CD symptoms in the adolescent outcome of ADHD could not be accounted for entirely by an early history of aggressive behavior. In this latter sample, the most consistent predictor of CD symptoms on follow-up was the persistence of ADHD symptoms into adolescence.

Our research provides further evidence for the distinction between aggressive and nonaggressive subgroups of ADHD children, and partial support for the hypothesized dissociation of "cognitive" and "behavioral" subtypes. In one study, nonreferred children were divided into hyperactive, aggressive, hyperactive/aggressive and control groups using teacher ratings on the IOWA Conners (Loney & Milich, 1982). The hyperactive group was found to be most inattentive, whereas the hyperactive/aggressive group was most impulsive, as measured using a CPT. There were no significant group differences on measures of academic achievement, but the pure hyperactive group tended to have lower reading scores (Halperin et al., 1990b).

A subsequent study (Halperin et al., 1990a), in a new sample of nonreferred children, examined the relationship of objectively assessed attentional dysfunction to ADHD. Subjects were divided into ADHD and nonADHD groups based on teacher's ratings of DSM-III-R symptoms, and into objectively assessed inattentive and noninattentive groups based upon CPT performance. Significantly more ADHD children were objectively assessed as inattentive (47.4% vs. 13.6%), but about half of the ADHD children were not found to be inattentive. Two-way (ADHD × CPT-Inattention) analyses of variance yielded interactions such that noninattentive ADHD children were rated as most aggressive by teachers and as having the most conduct problems by parents, whereas inattentive ADHD children had the lowest IQ scores.

The data from these studies challenge the notion that ADHD children comprise a unitary group whose central deficit is inattention, and were interpreted as providing support for the existence of inattentive/cognitive impaired and impulsive/aggressive ADHD subgroups. However, the findings that ratings of inattention (or as having ADHD symptoms) in aggressive children were not confirmed by an objective CPT measure of attention could be due to halo effects. Teachers may have rated aggressive children as inattentive and hyperactive even when they were not. However, halo effects cannot account for the low IQ scores in the inattentive ADHD subgroup and the high impulsivity scores in the hyperactive aggressive group.

More recently (Halperin et al., 1995), CPT and solid-state actigraphs were used to assess attention, impulse control and activity level in a clinic-referred sample of child psychiatric outpatients who were diagnosed using a best-estimate method following a comprehensive clinical evaluation. ADHD children characterized by a persistent pattern of physical aggression were found to be highly impulsive, but not inattentive, as measured by the CPT. In contrast, activity level, as measured using solid state actigraphs, was associated with the presence of ADHD, but did not vary as a function of aggressive behavior. Notably, in this latter sample, this pattern of high impulsivity and low inattention was associated with the presence of physical aggression in children with ADHD, but not with the categorical diagnoses of ODD or CD.

Taken together, these findings indicate that the use of an undifferentiated diagnosis of ADHD is likely to obscure many important relationships that become apparent only when these children are more precisely subdivided. This difficulty may be partially rectified by the DSM-IV definition of ADHD, which more clearly delineates inattentive and hyperactive/impulsive symptoms, and establishes subtypes based on presenting symptomatology.

NEUROBIOLOGICAL MODEL OF ADHD SUBTYPES

The principal neurotransmitter systems implicated in the pathogenesis of ADHD are the noradrenergic (NA) and dopaminergic (DA) systems, and to a lesser extent, the serotonergic (5-HT) system. However, attempts to distinguish ADHD and normal children on measures of these neurotransmitters and/or their metabolites have failed to yield replicable differences. Yet, since ADHD is diagnosed in a heterogeneous group of children with diverse symptomatology, it possible that no single neurotransmitter deficiency characterizes all ADHD children. Instead, the relative function or balance of all three systems may reflect the variability of symptoms seen in children with ADHD. It is possible that one neurotransmitter system is primarily affected, and that the others are altered via communicating pathways. Alternatively, more than one system could be equally affected and depending on which ones, the clinical presentation may appear as one subtype of ADHD or another.

These possibilities suggest that children with ADHD may not have a unitary neural pathogenesis. Rather, several neurotransmitter systems are likely to be differentially affected, resulting in different patterns of symptomatology. The remainder of this chapter will focus primarily upon the NA and 5-HT systems in an attempt to provide evidence that differences in these neurotransmitter systems are closely associated with the clinical manifestations of learning problems and aggressive behavior in children with ADHD, respectively. Although DA is likely to be involved in the pathogenesis of ADHD and the regulation of motor activity, it will not be discussed in depth because it is less clear how DA may vary as a function of comorbidity or associated features in children with ADHD.

Noradrenergic mechanisms

Support for the NA hypothesis of ADHD is obtained from three lines of research; animal models of attention, which posit a central role for NA in mediating the neural response to external stimuli, pharmacological treatment data, and studies examining NA and its metabolites.

Animal models have primarily focused on the role of the locus coeruleus

(LC) in the regulation of arousal, the orienting response, and vigilance (Aston-Jones, 1985). The LC, which is located in the brainstem near the floor of the fourth ventricle, provides NA innervation throughout the brain and provides the sole NA innervation to the neocortex. Single-cell recording studies indicate that LC firing is highly associated with state of consciousness. LC firing is actively inhibited during rapid eye movement (REM) sleep, whereas these neurons fire slowly during slow wave sleep and more rapidly during waking. As such, the state-dependent rate of LC firing may be related to the subject's availability to environmental stimulation.

However, the firing rate of LC neurons is not only related to level of arousal. During waking, LC discharge appears to be related to the degree to which the animal is attending to its environment. When engaged in automatic, repetitive behaviors, such as grooming or feeding, the LC is relatively quiescent. Increased LC activity occurs when the animal orients in response to external stimuli and begins to scan its environment. The highest rates of firing occur in response to stimuli which have behavioral or affective significance to the animal. Thus, low vigilance states are accompanied by a low firing rate of LC neurons. However, when attention is shifted to the external environment there is marked increase in LC activity which is associated with a state of high vigilance.

One effect of LC firing is the post-synaptic release of NA in cortical sensory areas. In these brain regions, NA has been found to inhibit the spontaneous discharge of neurons, which causes neurons to respond preferentially to their most significant inputs (Aston-Jones, 1985; Foote & Morrison, 1987). For example, NA inhibits the spontaneous discharge of auditory cortex neurons more than the firing of neurons driven by specific auditory stimuli (Foote, Friedman, & Oliver, 1975). This essentially enhances the "signal-to-noise" ratio for target cells (for review, see Foote, Bloom, & Aston-Jones, 1983).

Rostral to the LC are three areas that are closely associated with enhanced neuronal activity when a subject attends to the location of a visually presented target stimulus. These areas, which receive dense innervation by NA neurons, are the posterior parietal lobe (Mountcastle, 1978; Wurtz et al., 1980), the pulvinar nucleus of the thalamus (Peterson, Robinson, & Morris, 1987), and the superior colliculus (Morrison & Foote, 1986; Posner & Peterson, 1990). Injury to any of these areas leads to a disruption in attentional function. Taken together, these data provide compelling evidence for a central role for NA in the regulation of attention and cognitive functioning, although not necessarily for the clinically defined syndrome of ADHD.

The strongest support for the NA hypothesis of ADHD comes from pharmacological treatment data, which indicate that virtually all medications that are efficacious in ADHD children affect NA transmission and metabolism (Zametkin & Rapoport, 1987). The most commonly used medications, methylphenidate (MPH), amphetamine, and pemoline, all have primary effects upon both NA and DA mechanisms. However, the more selective NA-mediated antidepressants, imipramine (Rapoport et al., 1974) and desipramine (Garfinkel et al., 1983; Donnelly et al., 1986), also result in substantial improvement in the behavior of ADHD children. As is the case with amphetamine, administration of desipramine leads to a significant decrease in the excretion of 3-methoxy-4-hydroxyphenylglycol (MHPG), a metabolite of NA (Donnelly et al., 1986).

When interpreting the pharmacological data, one must consider the fact that normal, as well as ADHD children have improved attention in response to stimulant medication (Rapoport et al., 1980). One possible explanation for this finding is that all children "benefit" from stimulants, but only those with deviant function have substantial clinical improvement because of ceiling effects. A large literature has consistently demonstrated that approximately 80% of ADHD children have a positive response to MPH. However, the magnitude of response is quite variable. In a sample of 38 ADHD children treated with MPH (Halperin et al., 1986), 78% showed significantly improved behavior ratings. However, only 53% improved to the point of no longer meeting diagnostic criteria for the study. Thus, a large proportion of ADHD children improve with stimulants, but only about half have a normalization of symptoms. A somewhat smaller proportion of ADHD children have a strong positive response to the more selective NA-mediated antidepressant medications.

Taken together, the pharmacologic treatment data suggest an important role for NA in the pathophysiology of ADHD. However, the fact that ADHD children vary considerably in responsivity to medication is not consistent with a unitary NA hypothesis. Consistent with findings from animal studies, which suggest that central NA may be closely related to attentional function, we hypothesize that only ADHD children with primary deficits in attention/cognitive functioning have significant NA pathophysiology.

NA metabolite data also support the existence of distinct ADHD subtypes. As reviewed by Zametkin and Rapoport (1987), studies comparing urinary MHPG in ADHD and normal children have yielded inconsistent results; some report decreased MHPG in ADHD children (Yu-cun & Yu-feng, 1984; Shekim et al., 1977; 1979; 1983; 1987), some report no difference (Rapoport et al., 1978; Wender et al., 1971), and one study found increased MHPG in ADHD children (Khan & Dekirmenjian, 1981). However, a consistent shortcoming in the methodology in these studies involves the use of a short washout period. Four weeks of stimulant treatment in ADHD children decreases urinary MHPG excretion for at least two weeks after medication is discontinued (Zametkin et al., 1985). Yet, in most of these studies, children received a standard washout period of two weeks or less. Therefore, reductions (or lack of a difference) in MHPG may have been due to prior drug use. It is notable that the only study (Khan & Dekirmenjian, 1981) to find increased MHPG in ADHD children used a longer, three-week washout period.

It is also possible that the lack of consistent differences is due to heterogeneity among samples of ADHD children. Interestingly, those studies that report individual MHPG data (Khan & Dekirmenjian, 1981; Shekim et al., 1979) indicate that about half of the ADHD children had MHPG levels substantially higher than controls, while half had substantially lower levels, suggesting the presence of two distinct ADHD subgroups with regard to NA function. Although behavioral/cognitive data distinguishing these MHPG-related subgroups of ADHD children were not presented, we have hypothesized (Halperin, Newcorn, & Sharma, 1991) that this difference in NA function would be related to differences in attentional and cognitive function.

Yet, the relationship between MHPG level and central NA function remains uncertain. Since NA, like other neurotransmitters, is metabolized by monoamine oxidase (MAO) primarily in the presynaptic terminal, most investigators interpret MHPG levels to reflect some aspect of presynaptic function. However, this cannot be readily translated into a definitive statement regarding the overall functioning of the neurotransmitter system. It is likely that there is a normal range from which deviation in either direction (i.e., high or low MHPG) would reflect some form of dysregulation and potential impairment. Therefore, assessment of MHPG level may be useful for determining that there is a difference between groups in NA function, but the precise nature or specific mechanism involved cannot be specified.

Serotonergic mechanisms

Despite the paucity of data demonstrating a link between 5-HT and ADHD, studies with animals, children, and adults have all demonstrated an association between impulsive aggressive behavior and central serotonergic (5-HT) function. In rats, lesions and pharmacological manipulations that result in diminished 5-HT activity have been consistently reported to induce an increase in aggressive behavior (for review, see Soubrie, 1986), and low levels of the 5-HT metabolite, 5-hydroxyindoleacetic acid (5-HIAA), have been found in the cerebrospinal fluid (CSF) of more aggressive and socially dominant monkeys relative to their peers (Higley et al., 1992). Similarly, negative correlations have been reported between CSF 5-HIAA and lifetime aggression in adult personality disordered patients (Brown et al., 1982), and impulsive violence in criminals (Linnoila et al., 1983). Finally, the prolactin (PRL) response to acute challenge with the 5-HT releaser/uptake inhibitor fenfluramine (FEN), which is considered to be an index of overall central 5-HT function, is inversely correlated with measures of aggression, motor impulsivity, assault and irritability in personality disordered adults (Coccaro et al., 1989), and has been found to distinguish between aggressive and non-aggressive adult polysubstance abusers (Fishbein, Lozovsky, & Jaffe, 1989).

Although two open clinical studies using the 5-HT reuptake inhibitor, fluoxetine, have reported a positive treatment response in ADHD children (Barrickman, Noyes, & Kuperman, 1991; Gammon & Brown, 1993), there are virtually no laboratory data to suggest an important role for central 5-HT mechanisms in ADHD. Decreased blood levels of 5-HT in ADHD children relative to normal controls have been reported by some investigators, but others have been unable to replicate these findings, and differences in urinary 5-HIAA have not been found (for review, see Zametkin & Rapoport, 1987).

However, in a diagnostically heterogeneous group of boys with disruptive disorders, approximately 2/3 of whom had ADHD, reduced CSF 5-HIAA was associated with high aggression ratings at the time of assessment (Kruesi et al., 1990), as well as more severe physically aggressive behavior at two-year follow-up (Kruesi et al., 1992). Furthermore, a reduced number of ^{3}H-imipramine binding sites, a putative index of presynaptic 5-HT activity, was reported in one study that compared children with comorbid CD + ADHD diagnoses to normal controls (Stoff et al., 1987), but not in a different study that used a sample of primarily non-aggressive ADHD children (Weizman et al., 1988). These data suggest reduced presynaptic 5-HT function in aggressive, but not non-aggressive, children with disruptive behavior disorders. In contrast to these rather consistent findings, a recent pilot study (Stoff et al., 1992) reported no significant relationship between the PRL response to FEN and ratings of aggression in a small heterogeneous sample of children with disruptive disorders. Yet, the limited sample size and the heterogeneity of the sample with regard to diagnosis make these latter findings difficult to interpret relative to ADHD.

Taken together, an emerging literature is consistent with the notion that aggressive behavior is associated with a neurochemical deficit involving central 5-HT mechanisms. Data suggesting a role for 5-HT mechanisms in the pathophysiology of the more globally defined ADHD syndrome are less compelling. Yet, in view of the fact that ADHD appears to be a risk factor for subsequent aggressive behavior (Loeber et al., 1993), it is possible that central 5-HT dysregulation is present in aggressive ADHD children.

NEUROBIOLOGICAL DISSOCIATION OF ADHD SUBTYPES

Pharmacological dissociation

In an initial test of these hypotheses (Matier et al., 1992), a sample of clinic-referred ADHD children were divided into aggressive and nonaggressive subgroups based upon the presence or absence of a persistent pattern of physically aggressive behavior. Both groups were evaluated, along with normal controls, using objective CPT measures of attention and impulsivity, as well as an actigraph measure of activity level, prior to and following a single low dose (5 mg) of MPH. Unlike amphetamines and higher doses of MPH, a low dose of MPH has minimal MAO inhibitory action (Szporny & Gorog, 1961) and thus almost exclusively affects NA and DA, but not 5-HT. Therefore, it was hypothesized that the medication would result in less symptom change in the aggressive group, whose symptoms were believed to be due at least in part to 5-HT dysfunction, as compared to the nonaggressive group.

We found that the aggressive and nonaggressive ADHD subgroups responded differentially to a low dose of MPH, as did the objective measures of inattention, impulsivity and hyperactivity. Both ADHD subgroups demonstrated reduced CPT-inattention following the medication. However, neither group demonstrated a significant change in CPT-impulsivity, which was only elevated in the aggressive ADHD subgroup relative to normals. Finally, the nonagressive ADHD subgroup had a significantly greater reduction in objectively assessed activity level than the aggressive ADHD children, despite the fact that both ADHD subgroups were equally overactive relative to controls prior to the medication.

These data are consistent with the notion that impulsivity and overactivity in aggressive ADHD children may be related in part to noncatecholamine (CA) neurotransmitter systems, whereas CA systems are primarily involved in the regulation of attention. Taken in the context of the previously discussed findings, as well as data indicating that lesions to the 5-HT-rich raphe nuclei in rats cause persistent overactivity (Jacobs, Wise, & Taylor, 1974), these data are consistent with the hypothesis that central 5-HT dysfunction is associated with aggressive behavior in ADHD children, perhaps via its role in the regulation of impulse control and activity level. This raises the possibility that the symptom of hyperactivity in aggressive and nonaggressive ADHD children is phenotypically similar, but neurobiologically distinct. Specifically, hyperactivity in nonaggressive ADHD children, which appears to parallel inattention, may be related to an underlying CA dysfunction, whereas hyperactivity in aggressive ADHD children is more closely associated with impulsivity and nonCA (presumably 5-HT) mechanisms.

Neurochemical dissociation

To more directly assess the neurochemical model of ADHD subtypes, we recruited a new sample of 7 to 11-year-old boys who met DSM-III-R criteria for ADHD. As described below, these boys were subsequently divided into subgroups based upon the presence/absence of reading disabilities (Halperin et al., 1993) and aggressive behavior (Halperin et al., 1994).

NA turnover was assessed through plasma assays of MHPG. Despite the fact that there is a barrier preventing CNS NA from entering the periphery, plasma MHPG is likely to provide a reasonably accurate reflection of CNS NA metabolism. Significant correlations between plasma MHPG and MHPG levels in both CSF and several brain regions have been reported in animals

(Elsworth, Redmond, & Roth, 1982; Jimmerson et al., 1981). In addition, plasma and CSF levels of NA have been found to be closely related in humans (Lake et al., 1981; Ziegler et al., 1980). As stated previously, assessment of MHPG levels can be used to determine that the groups differ with regard to some aspect of NA function, but cannot determine the precise nature of NA dysregulation.

Central 5-HT function was assessed via the PRL response to acute challenge with the 5-HT releaser/uptake inhibitor FEN (Quattrone, et al., 1978). FEN is a centrally acting pharmacological agent which releases stores of pre-synaptic 5-HT, blocks re-uptake of synaptic 5-HT, and stimulates, both directly and indirectly, post-synaptic 5-HT receptors (Rowland & Carlton, 1986). The enhancement of central 5-HT activity, following the administration of FEN, is reflected in a dose-related plasma PRL enhancement, which is blocked by 5-HT receptor antagonists. Since it is known that PRL release is regulated by neurons in the hypothalamic-pituitary axis, the PRL response to FEN challenge serves as a dynamic measure that reflects "net" central 5-HT function in that region of the brain (Coccaro et al., 1989). Furthermore, this procedure is far less invasive than other methods for assessing CNS 5-HT function, such as measurement of 5-HIAA in the CSF.

Reading disabled versus non-reading disabled ADHD boys

The ADHD boys were divided into those with and without RD, with the hypothesis that these groups would differ in plasma MHPG (Halperin et al., 1993). A wide array of criteria have been used to categorize RD and nonRD children, and to date, no consensus has been reached. We used criteria suggested by Morrison & Siegel (1991), which take into consideration the recently elucidated problems inherent in the use of discrepancy scores (Morrison & Siegel, 1991; Shaywitz et al., 1992). Only subjects with Full Scale IQ (FSIQ) scores of at least 80 were included. Those with either a reading or spelling standard score below 80, as measured by the Wide Range Achievement Test – Revised (WRAT-R; Jastak & Wilkinson, 1984), were placed in the RD group (N = 11). The nonRD group (N = 13) consisted of children who had a score of at least 85 on all three WRAT-R subtests (i.e., reading, spelling and arithmetic), thus allowing a clear separation between the two groups.

The RD and nonRD ADHD subgroups did not differ (p > 0.10) in age, or parent or teacher ratings of hyperactivity. However, similar to the findings of August & Garfinkel (1989), the non-RD group was rated by parents as significantly more aggressive than the RD group. The groups also differed (p < 0.05) in Verbal IQ, but not in Performance IQ or FSIQ; by definition, the groups differed significantly on all measures of academic achievement.

Neurochemically, the RD group was found to have a significantly higher level of plasma MHPG than the non-RD group, but the groups did not differ in their PRL response to FEN. Pearson product moment correlations were used to further assess the relationship of MHPG to the cognitive and behavioral measures. Plasma MHPG was negatively correlated with reading and spelling scores ($r = -0.51$ and -0.48, respectively), but not with IQ scores. MHPG level was unrelated to all parent and teacher ratings of behavior.

These results indicate a substantial relationship between NA function, as assessed through plasma MHPG, and academic achievement in ADHD children, that could not be accounted for by comorbid depression and/or anxiety disorders. Plasma MHPG not only distinguished between RD and nonRD ADHD subgroups, but it was dimensionally related to measures of reading and spelling. The specificity of the relationship of central NA function and academic achievement to ADHD children, as compared to those without ADHD, remains unknown. However, these findings appear to have held up in a new, independent sample of ADHD children (Pick et al., 1994).

Aggressive versus nonaggressive ADHD boys

The sample was also divided into aggressive and nonaggressive subgroups (Halperin et al., 1994), based upon the presence or absence of a persistent pattern of physically aggressive behavior, in the following manner. The clinical material (i.e., rating scale and interview data, as well as previous clinical and school reports when available) for each child was independently reviewed by three investigators who were blind to the biological data. The reviewers classified each child as either aggressive, nonaggressive or "equivocal." Inter-reviewer concordance was excellent with discrepancies occurring only where a child was rated as equivocal by one or two clinicians; no child was rated as aggressive by one reviewer and nonaggressive by another. In the few cases of discrepant ratings, the clinical material was discussed and consensus was reached. This "best-estimate" procedure was used instead of more traditional rating scale cut-offs because parent and teacher aggression scales tend to assess oppositional/defiant behavior rather than physical aggression, and because there is frequently disparity between parent and teacher reports. The aggressive and nonaggressive ADHD groups did not differ ($p > 0.10$) in age, FSIQ, academic achievement scores, or parent or teacher ratings of hyperactivity. However, as expected, they differed significantly ($p < 0.001$) in both parent and teacher ratings of aggressive behavior.

Aggressive and nonaggressive ADHD children did not differ in baseline plasma levels of PRL (5.65 vs. 7.09 ng/ml, respectively). However, the aggressive group had a significantly greater change in PRL level following the FEN challenge (18.43 vs. 10.46 ng/ml), suggesting group differences in central 5-HT function. This group difference could not be accounted for by differential absorption or metabolism of the FEN. The aggressive and nonaggressive ADHD subgroups did not differ in plasma MHPG.

The fact that ADHD children with and without aggressive behavior had a different PRL response to a challenge dose of FEN is consistent with the hypothesis that aggression in these children is mediated, at least in part, through central 5-HT mechanisms. In this study, aggressive ADHD children had a larger PRL response than nonaggressive children. However, since there was no normal control group, it is impossible to know with certainty which patient group had the deviant response. Since normal adults who have undergone this procedure had PRL responses similar to that of the nonaggressive children (Coccaro et al., 1989; McBride et al., 1989), we provisionally interpreted the data to indicate that the PRL response in our sample of aggressive ADHD children was enhanced. Yet, this presumption must be considered tentative until normative child data become available.

This finding is in a different direction than that of Coccaro et al. (1989), who found a blunted PRL response in aggressive personality disordered patients, but similar to that of Fishbein, Lozovsky, & Jaffe (1989), who reported an enhanced PRL response to FEN in aggressive polysubstance abusers. It is possible that the relationship between aggression and the PRL response to FEN varies as a function of diagnostic status and/ or age.

Another interesting possibility is that the relationship between aggression and central 5-HT systems is altered specifically in the context of ADHD symptomatology. ADHD, and particularly the symptom of hyperactivity, is believed to be related primarily to CA mechanisms and at least in part to dopaminergic (DA) dysregulation (Wender et al., 1971; Shaywitz, Yager, & Klopper, 1976). Animal studies indicate that neonatal DA-depleting lesions, which result in hyperactivity (Shaywitz, Yager, & Klopper, 1976), cause sprouting of 5-HT terminals (Stachowiak et al., 1984; Snyder, Zigmond, & Lund, 1986). While compensatory mechanisms may partially obscure the detection of a DA dysfunction by metabolite measures, such a dysfunction, if present in ADHD, could conceivably result in increased 5-HT innervation and enhanced response to 5-HT challenge in some children. Thus, it is possible that the interaction between these neurotransmitter systems is different in ADHD and nonADHD children.

Because the PRL response to the FEN challenge represents "net" 5-HT function in the hypothalamic-pituitary axis (Coccaro et al., 1989), the specific mechanism of this 5-HT dysregulation cannot be elucidated. One possibility is that the increased PRL response in the aggressive group represents a post-synaptic enhancement due to either receptor supersensitivity or greater receptor density. This enhanced post-synaptic responsivity could be compensatory for diminished 5-HT release and availability.

The notion that the enhanced PRL response to FEN in the aggressive group represents a post-synaptic phenomenon is supported by recent data indicating a strong positive correlation between the PRL response to FEN and the more specific post-synaptic 5-HT receptor stimulator, *m*-chlorophenylpiperazine (m-CPP) (Coccaro, personal communication). Furthermore, an enhanced PRL response to FEN following destruction of presynaptic 5-HT terminals has been reported in animals (Kuhn et al., 1981). Finally, autopsy data indicate a reduction in presynaptic 5-HT re-uptake sites (Stanley, Virgilio, & Gershon, 1982), accompanied by increased post-synaptic 5-HT$_2$ receptors (Stanley & Mann, 1983), in the frontal cortex of violent suicide victims. Taken together, these findings all point to an association between aggressive behavior and a reduction in presynaptic 5-HT mechanisms accompanied by enhanced post-synaptic responsivity. However, this hypothesis must remain tentative until further data are gathered.

In summary, neurobiological studies consistently report associations between aggressive behavior and central 5-HT mechanisms. However, the nature of the relationship has been somewhat inconsistent. This may be due to any of a number of subject-related variables such as diagnosis, age or duration of disorder. Furthermore, it remains unclear whether central 5-HT mechanisms are associated with all types of aggressive behavior, aggression associated primarily with symptoms of impulsivity and/or hyperactivity, or whether this varies as a function of patient diagnosis.

CONCLUSION

Our reading of the existing literature, as well as our own findings, are consistent with the notion that ADHD is not a unitary disorder and that a fruitful approach to unraveling the neural mechanisms associated with ADHD pathophysiology may be to dissociate subgroups based upon specific symptom dimensions or patterns of comorbidity. Another, related approach, could be to evaluate neurobiologic correlates of distinct symptom dimensions in children with ADHD.

Although data from several descriptive and psychometric studies suggest a dissociation between inattention/cognitive impairment and impulsive/aggression in ADHD children, our findings do not fully support a dichotomous relationship. Yet, our data do indicate that the associated symptoms of RD and aggression may be explained by different underlying neurochemical mechanisms in children with ADHD. RD and nonRD ADHD children were found to differ on a measure of NA function, whereas aggressive and nonaggressive ADHD children were found to differ on a measure of central 5-HT function.

These data cannot answer the question as to whether the heterogeneity seen among children with ADHD is due to the presence of multiple comorbid conditions (or associated features) on top of an otherwise unitary and valid diagnostic condition, or whether subtypes of ADHD, based upon patterns of comorbidity/associated features, should be seen as distinct diagnoses. The fact that nonoverlapping subgroups could not be formed by subdivision based upon the presence of *both* aggressive behavior and learning problems indicates that diagnostic groupings formed by these comorbid conditions do not lead to mutually exclusive diagnoses.

One possibility is that ADHD symptoms, which can probably be caused by a variety of genetic or early environmental (pre- or post-natal) factors (Sprich-Buckminster et al., 1993), represent markers of vulnerability in children who are highly susceptible to other conditions. Which, if any, comorbid condition emerges could be dependent upon a host of intrinsic as well as environmental factors. This hypothesis would suggest that early identification of these high risk children, coupled with intervention in the form of providing a more protective and growth-promoting environment, could prevent the onset of additional conditions which are often more debilitating than the ADHD itself.

The neurobiology of childhood psychiatric disorders is a field that is currently in its infancy. Not surprisingly, our data generate more questions than answers, particularly with regard to the neurochemical profile in normal children and the uniqueness of these findings to children with ADHD. In terms of the relationship of NA mechanisms to learning and cognitive problems, it remains to be determined whether (a) relative to normals, ADHD children with RD have elevated MHPG levels or ADHD children without RD have reduced plasma MHPG; (b) plasma MHPG is related to measures of academic achievement in children without ADHD; and (c) there are specific cognitive/neuropsychological factors that mediate the relationship between NA turnover and academic achievement.

Similarly, there are several unanswered questions related to 5-HT function and aggression. It is unknown (a) whether the differential PRL response to FEN between aggressive and nonaggressive ADHD children is due to an enhanced response in aggressive ADHD children, a diminished response in nonaggressive ADHD, or an abnormality in both groups compared to normals; (b) whether the enhanced PRL response to FEN challenge in aggressive, relative to nonaggressive, ADHD children is related to an interaction between ADHD and aggression or is characteristic of aggressive behavior in children irrespective of ADHD; and (c) what the impact of other factors such as age, other comorbid conditions (e.g., affective or anxiety disorders), family history, environmental stressors, and duration of disorder is on the nature of the relationship of central 5-HT function to aggression.

Determining the answers to these, as well as numerous other questions, is a challenge for the future. Hopefully, further elucidation of the neurobiological correlates of behavior and cognitive function in children with ADHD will enhance our ability to provide early protective interventions for this large group of high risk children.

REFERENCES

Abikoff, H., Courtney, M., Pelham, Jr., W.E., & Koplewicz, H.S. (1993). Teachers' ratings of disruptive behavior: influence of halo effects. *Journal of Abnormal Child Psychology*, **21**, 519–534.

American Psychiatric Association (APA) (1987). *Diagnostic and Statistical Manual of Mental Disorders*, 3rd edn. Washington, DC: APA.

American Psychiatric Association (APA) (1994). *Diagnostic and Statistical Manual of Mental Disorders*, 4th edn. Washington, DC: APA.

Aston-Jones, G. (1985). Behavioral functions of locus coeruleus derived from cellular attributes. *Physiological Psychology*, **13**, 118–126.

August, G.J. & Garfinkel, B.D. (1989). Behavioral and cognitive subtypes of ADHD. *Journal of the American Academy of Child and Adolescent Psychiatry*, **28**, 739–748.

August, G.J. & Garfinkel, B.D. (1990). Comorbidity of ADHD and reading disability among clinic-referred children. *Journal of Abnormal Child Psychology*, **18**, 29–46.

August, G.J. & Stewart, M.A. (1982). Is there a syndrome of pure hyperactivity? *British Journal of Psychiatry*, **140**, 305–311.

August, G.J. & Stewart, M.A. (1983). Familial subtypes of childhood hyperactivity. *Journal of Nervous and Mental Disease*, **171**, 363–368.

August, G.J., Stewart, M.A., & Holmes, C.S. (1983). A four-year follow-up of hyperactive boys with and without conduct disorder. *British Journal of Psychiatry*, **143**, 192–198.

Barkley, R.A., Grodzinsky, G., & DuPaul, G.J. (1992). Frontal lobe functions in attention deficit disorder with and without hyperactivity: a review and research report. *Journal of Abnormal Child Psychology*, **20**, 163–188.

Barrickman, L., Noyes, R., Kuperman, S. et al. (1991). Treatment of ADHD with fluoxetine: a preliminary trial. *Journal of the American Academy of Child and Adolescent Psychiatry*, **30**, 762–767.

Biederman, J., Munir, K., & Knee, D. (1987). Conduct and oppositional disorder in clinically referred children with attention deficit disorder: a controlled family study. *Journal of the American Academy of Child and Adolescent Psychiatry*, **26**, 724–727.

Biederman, J., Newcorn, J., & Sprich, S. (1991). Comorbidity of Attention Deficit Hyperactivity Disorder with conduct, depressive, anxiety and other disorders. *American Journal of Psychiatry*, **148**, 564–577.

Brown, G.L., Ebert, M.H., Goyer, P.F., Jimerson, D.C., Klein, W.J., Bunney, W.E., & Goodwin, F.K. (1982). Aggression, suicide, and serotonin: relationships to CSF amine metabolites. *American Journal of Psychiatry*, **139**, 741–746.

Castellanos, F.X., Giedd, J.N., Eckburg, P., Marsh, W.L., Vaituzis, A.C., Hamburger, S.D., & Rapoport, J.L. (1993). Quantitative morphology of the caudate nucleus in attention-deficit hyperactivity disorder. Presented at the 32nd Annual Meeting of the American College of Neuropsychopharmacology, December 12–17, 1993, Honolulu, Hawaii.

Chee, P., Logan, G., Schachar, R., Lindsay, P., & Wachsmuth, R. (1989). Effects of event rate and display time on sustained attention in hyperactive, normal and control children. *Journal of Abnormal Child Psychology*, **17**, 371–391.

Chelune, G.J., Ferguson, W., Koon, R., & Disckey, T.O. (1986). Frontal lobe disinhibition in attention-deficit disorder. *Child Psychiatry and Human Development*, **16**, 221–234.

Coccaro, E.F., Siever, L.J., Klar, H., et al. (1989). Serotonergic studies of personality disorder: Correlates with behavioral aggression and impulsivity. *Archives of General Psychiatry*, **46**, 587–599.

Donnelly, M., Rapoport, J.L., Zametkin, A.J., & Ismond, D. (1986). Treatment of childhood hyperactivity with desipramine: plasma drug concentration, cardiovascular function, plasma and urinary catecholamine levels, and clinical response. *Clinical Pharmacology and Therapeutics*, **39**, 72–81.

Elsworth, J.D., Redmond, D.E., Jr., & Roth, R.H. (1982). Plasma and cerebrospinal fluid 3-methoxy-4-hydroxyphenylglycol (MHPG) as indices of brain norepinephrine metabolism in primates. *Brain Research*, **235**, 115–124.

Felton, R.H., Wood, F.B., Brown, I.S., Campbell, S.K., & Harter, M.R. (1987). Separate verbal memory and naming deficits in attention deficit disorder and reading disability. *Brain and Language*, **31**, 171–184.

Fischer, M., Barkley, R.A., Fletcher, K.E., & Smallish, L. (1993). The adolescent outcome of hyperactive children: Predictors of psychiatric, academic, social, and emotional adjustment. *Journal of the American Academy of Child and Adolescent Psychiatry*, **32**, 324–332.

Fishbein, D.H., Lozovsky, D., & Jaffe, J.H. (1989). Impulsivity, aggression, and neuroendocrine responses to serotonergic stimulation in substance abusers. *Biological Psychiatry*, **25**, 1049–1066.

Foote, S.L., Bloom, F.E., & Aston-Jones, G. (1983). The nucleus locus coeruleus: new evidence of anatomical and physiological specificity. *Physiological Review*, **63**, 844–914.

Foote, S.L., Friedman, R., & Oliver, A.P. (1975). Effects of putative neurotransmitters on neuronal activity in monkey cerebral cortex. *Brain Research*, **86**, 229–242.

Foote, S.L. & Morrison, J.H. (1987). Extrathalamic modulation of cortical function. *Annual Review of Neuroscience*, **10**, 67–95.

Gammon, G.D. & Brown, T.E. (1993). Fluoxetine and methylphenidate in combination for treatment of attention deficit disorder and comorbid depressive disorder. *Journal of Child and Adolescent Psychopharmacology*, **3**, 1–10.

Garfinkel, B.D., Wender, P.H., Sloman, L., & O'Neil, I. (1983). Tricyclic antidepressant and methylphenidate treatment of attention deficit disorder in children. *Journal of the American Academy of Child Psychiatry*, **22**, 343–348.

Giedd, J.N., Castellanos, F.X., Casey, B.J., Kozuch, P., King, A.C., Hamburger, S.D., & Rapoport, J.L. (1994). Quantitative morphology of the corpus callosum in attention deficit hyperactivity disorder. *American Journal of Psychiatry*, **151**, 1791–1796.

Goyette, C.H., Conners, C.K., & Ulrich, R.F. (1978). Normative data on revised Conners parent and teacher rating scales. *Journal of Abnormal Child Psychology*, **6**, 221–236.

Halperin, J.M., Gittelman, R., Katz, S., & Struve, F.A. (1986). Relationship between stimulant effect, EEG and clinical neurological findings in hyperactive children. *Journal of the American Academy of Child Psychiatry*, **25**, 820–825.

Halperin, J.M., Newcorn, J.H., Matier, K., Bedi, G., Hall, S., & Sharma, V. (1995). Impulsivity and the initiation of fights in children with disruptive behavior disorders. *Journal of Child Psychology and Psychiatry*, **36**, 1199–1211.

Halperin, J.M., Newcorn, J.H., Schwartz, S.T., McKay, K.E., Bedi, G., & Sharma, V. (1993). Plasma catecholamine metabolite levels in ADHD boys with and without reading disabilities. *Journal of Clinical Child Psychology,* Special Issue on Neuro-psychology, **22**, 219–225.

Halperin, J.M., Newcorn, J.H., & Sharma, V. (1991). Methylphenidate, diagnostic co-morbidity and attentional measures. In B.P. Osman & L. Greenhill (eds) *Ritalin: Theory and Patient Management.* New York: Liebert (pp. 15–24).

Halperin, J.M., Newcorn, J.H., Sharma, V., Healey, J.M., Wolf, L.E., Pascualvaca, D.M., & Schwartz, S. (1990a). Inattentive and non-inattentive ADHD children: Do they constitute a unitary group? *Journal of Abnormal Child Psychology,* **18**, 437–449.

Halperin, J.M., O'Brien, J.D., Newcorn, J.H., Healey, J.M., Pascualvaca, D.M., Wolf, L.E., & Young, J.G. (1990b). Validation of hyperactive, aggressive, and mixed hyperactive/aggressive disorders in children: A research note. *Journal of Child Psychology and Psychiatry,* **31**, 455–459.

Halperin, J.M., Sharma, V., Siever, L.J., Schwartz, S.T., Maiter, K., Wornell, G., & Newcorn, J.H. (1994). Serotonergic function in aggressive and non-aggressive boys with attention-deficit hyperactivity disorder. *American Journal of Psychiatry,* **151**, 243–248.

Heilman, K.M., Voeller, K.K., & Nadeau, S.E. (1991). A possible pathophysiologic substrate of attention-deficit hyperactivity disorder. *Journal of Child Neurology,* **6**(suppl.), S76–S81.

Higley, J.D., Mehlman, P.T., Taub, D.M., Higley, S.B., Suomi, S.J., Linnoila, M., & Vickers, J.H. (1992). Cerebrospinal fluid monoamine and adrenal correlates of aggression in free-ranging rhesus monkeys. *Archives of General Psychiatry,* **49**, 436–441.

Hinshaw, S.P. (1987). On the distinction between attention deficits/hyperactivity and conduct problems/aggression in child psychopathology. *Psychological Bulletin,* **101**, 443–463.

Hinshaw, S.P. (1992). Externalizing behavior problems and academic underachieve-ment in childhood and adolescence: Causal relationships and underlying mechanisms. *Psychological Bulletin,* **111**, 127–155.

Hynd, G.W., Hern, K.L., Novey, E.S., Eliopulos, D., Marshall, R., Gonzalez, J.J., & Voeller, K.K. (1993). Attention deficit hyperactivity disorder (ADHD) and asymmetry of the caudate nucleus. *Journal of Child Neurology,* **8**, 339–347.

Hynd, G.W., Semrud-Clikeman, M., Lorys, A.R., Novey, E.S., & Eliopulos, D. (1990). Brain morphology in developmental dyslexia and attention deficit disorder/hyperactivity. *Archives of Neurology,* **47**, 919–926.

Hynd, G.W., Semrud-Clikeman, M., Lorys, A.R., Novey, E.S., Elipopulos, D., & Lyytinen, H. (1991). Corpus callosum morphology in attention-deficit hyperactivity disorder: morphometric analysis of MRI. *Journal of Learning Disabilities,* **24**, 141–146.

Jacobs, B.L., Wise, W.D., & Taylor, K.M. (1974). Differential behavioral and neurochemical effects following lesions of the dorsal or median raphe nuclei in rats. *Brain Research,* **79**, 353–361.

Jastak, S. & Wilkinson, G.S. (1984). *Wide Range Achievement Test–Revised.* Wilmington, DE: Jastak.

Jimmerson, J.D., Ballenger, J.C., Lake, C.R., Post, R.M., Goodwin, F.K., & Kopin, I.J. (1981). Plasma and CSF MHPG in normals. *Psychopharmacology Bulletin,* **17**, 86–87.

Khan, A.U. & Dekirmenjian, H. (1981). Urinary excretion of catecholamine metabolites in hyperkinetic child syndrome. *American Journal of Psychiatry*, **138**, 108–112.

Klein, R.G. & Mannuzza, S. (1991). Long-term outcome of hyperactive children. *Journal of the American Academy of Child and Adolescent Psychiatry*, **30**, 383–387.

Kruesi, M.J., Hibbs, E.D., Zahn, T.P., Keysor, C.S., Hamburger, S.D., Bartko, J.J., & Rapoport, J.L. (1992). A 2-year prospective follow-up study of children and adolescents with disruptive behavior disorders: prediction by cerebrospinal fluid 5-hydroxyindoleacetic acid, homovanillic acid and autonomic measures? *Archives of General Psychiatry*, **49**, 429–435.

Kruesi, M.J.P., Rapoport, J.L., Hamburger, S., Hibbs, E., Potter, W.Z., Lenane, M., & Brown, G.L. (1990). Cerebrospinal fluid monoamine metabolites, aggression, and impulsivity in disruptive behavior disorders of children and adolescents. *Archives of General Psychiatry*, **47**, 419–426.

Kuhn, C.M., Vogel, R.A., Mailman, R.B., Mueller, R.A., Schanberg, S.M., & Breese, G.R. (1981). Effect of 5,7-dihydroxytryptamine on serotonergic control of prolactin secretion and behavior in rats. *Psychopharmacology*, **73**, 188–193.

Lahey, B.B., Piacentini, J.C., McBurnett, K., Stone, P., Hartdagen, S., & Hynd, G. (1988). Psychopathology in the parents of children with conduct disorder and hyperactivity. *Journal of the American Academy of Child and Adolescent Psychiatry*, **27**, 163–170.

Lake, C.R., Gullner, H.G., Polinsky, R.J., Ebert, M.H., Ziegler, M.G., & Barterr, F.C. (1981). Essential hypertension: Central and peripheral norepinephrine. *Science*, **211**, 955–957.

Linnoila, M., Virkkunen, M., Scheinin, M., Nuutila, A., Rimon, R., & Goodwin, F.K. (1983). Low cerebrospinal fluid 5-hydroxyindoleacetic acid concentrations differentiates impulsive from nonimpulsive aggressive behavior. *Life Science*, **33**, 2609–2614.

Loeber, R., Wung, P., Keenan, K., Giroux, B., Stouthamer-Loeber, M., Van Kammen, W.B., & Maughan, B. (1993). Developmental pathways in disruptive child behavior. *Development and Psychopathology*, **5**, 103–113.

Loney, J., Kramer, J., & Milich, R. (1981). The hyperkinetic child grows up: Predictors of symptoms, delinquency and achievement at follow-up. In K.D. Gadow & J. Loney (eds) *Psychosocial Aspects of Drug Treatment for Hyperactivity*. Boulder, CO: Westview Press (pp. 381–416).

Loney, J. & Milich, R. (1982). Hyperactivity, inattention and aggression in clinical practice. *Advances in Developmental and Behavioral Pediatrics*, **3**, 113–147.

Lou, H.C., Henrickson, L., Bruhn, P., Borner, H., & Nielsen, B. (1989). Striatal dysfunction in attention deficit and hyperkinetic disorder. *Archives of Neurology*, **46**, 48–52.

Lou, H.C., Henrickson, L., & Bruhn, P. (1984). Focal cerebral hypoperfusion in children with dysphasia and/or attention deficit disorder. *Archives of Neurology*, **41**, 825–829.

Malone, M.A., Kershner, J.R., & Siegel, L. (1988). The effects of methylphenidate on levels of processing and laterality in children with attention deficit disorder. *Journal of Abnormal Child Psychology*, **16**, 379–395.

Matier, K., Halperin, J.M., Sharma, V., Newcorn, J.H., & Sathaye, N. (1992). Methylphenidate response in aggressive and non-aggressive ADHD children:

Distinctions on laboratory measures of symptoms. *Journal of the American Academy of Child and Adolescent Psychiatry,* **31,** 219–225.

McBride, P.A., Anderson, G.M., Hertzig, M.E., Sweeney, J.A., Kream, J., Cohen, D.J., & Mann, J.J. (1989). Serotonergic responsivity in male young adults with autistic disorder. *Archives of General Psychiatry,* **46,** 213–221.

McGee, R., Williams, S., Moffitt, T., & Anderson, J. (1989). A comparison of 13-year-old boys with attention deficit and/or reading disorder on neuropsychological measures. *Journal of Abnormal Child Psychology,* **17,** 37–53.

Morrison, J.H. & Foote, S.L. (1986). Noradrenergic and serotonergic innervation of cortical, thalamic, and tectal visual structures in old and new world monkeys. *Journal of Comparative Neurology,* **243,** 117–138.

Morrison, S.R. & Siegel, L.S. (1991). Learning disabilities: a critical review of definitional and assessment issues. In J.E. Obrzut & G.W. Hynd (eds) *Neuropsychological Foundations of Learning Disabilities: A Handbook of Issues, Methods, and Practice.* San Diego, CA: Academic Press (pp. 79–97).

Mountcastle, V.B. (1978). Brain mechanisms of directed attention. *Journal of Research in Social Medicine,* **71,** 14–27.

Newcorn, J.H., Halperin, J.M., Healey, J.M., O'Brien, J.D., Pascualvaca, D.M., Wolf, L.E., Morganstein, A., Sharma, V., & Young, J.G. (1989). Are ADDH and ADHD the same or different? *Journal of the American Academy of Child and Adolescent Psychiatry,* **28,** 734–738.

Peterson, S.E., Robinson, D.L., & Morris, J.D. (1987). Contributions of the pulvinar to visual spatial attention. *Neuropsychology,* **25,** 97–105.

Pick, L.H., Halperin, J.M., Newcorn, J.H., & Schwartz, S.T. (1994). Relationship of plasma MHPG to cognitive functioning in children with ADHD. Presented at the 24th Annual Meeting of the Society for Neuroscience, Miami Beach, Florida, 13–18, November 1994.

Posner, M.I. & Petersen, S.E. (1990). The attention system of the human brain. *Annual Review of Neuroscience,* **13,** 25–42.

Quattrone, A., DiRenzo, G., Schettini, G., & Tedeschi, G. (1978). Increased plasma prolactin levels induced by d-fenfluroamine: Relation to central serotonergic stimulation. *European Journal of Pharmacology,* **49,** 163–168.

Rapoport, J.L., Buchsbaum, M.S., Weingartner, H., Zahn, T.P., Ludlow, C., & Mikkelsen, E.J. (1980). Dextroamphetamine: cognitive and behavioral effects in normal and hyperactive boys and normal men. *Archives of General Psychiatry,* **37,** 933–943.

Rapoport, J.L., Mikkelsen, E.J., Ebert, M.H., Brown, G.L., Weise, V.L., & Kopin, I.J. (1978). Urinary catecholamine and amphetamine excretion in hyperactive and normal boys. *Journal of Nervous and Mental Disease,* **66,** 731–737.

Rapoport, J.L., Quinn, P.O., Scribanic, N., & Murphy, D.L. (1974). Platelet serotonin of hyperactive school-age boys. *British Journal of Psychiatry,* **125,** 138–140.

Robins, P.M. (1992). A comparison of behavioral and attentional functioning in children diagnosed as hyperactive or learning disabled. *Journal of Abnormal Child Psychology,* **20,** 65–82.

Rogeness, G.A., Javors, M.A., & Pliszka, S.R. (1992). Neurochemistry and child and adolescent psychiatry. *Journal of the American Academy of Child and Adolescent Psychiatry,* **31,** 765–781.

Rowland, N.E. & Carlton, J. (1986). Neurobiology of an anorectic drug: fenfluramine. *Progress in Neurobiology*, **27**, 13–62.

Sandberg, S.T., Rutter, M., & Taylor, E. (1978). Hyperkinetic disorder in psychiatric clinic attenders. *Developmental Medicine and Child Neurology*, **20**, 279–299.

Sandberg, S.T., Wieselberg, M., & Shaffer, D. (1980). Hyperkinetic and conduct problem children in a primary school population: some epidemiological considerations. *Journal of Child Psychology and Psychiatry*, **21**, 293–311.

Schachar, R., Rutter, M., & Smith, A. (1981). The characteristics of situationally and pervasively hyperactive children: implications for syndrome definition. *Journal of Child Psychology and Psychiatry*, **22**, 375–392.

Schachar, R., Sandberg, S., & Rutter, M. (1986). Agreement between teacher ratings and observations of hyperactivity, inattentiveness and defiance. *Journal of Abnormal Child Psychology*, **14**, 331–345.

Schachar, R. & Wachsmuth, R. (1990). Hyperactivity and parental psychopathology. *Journal of Child Psychology and Psychiatry*, **31**, 381–392.

Shaywitz, S.E., Escobar, M.D., Shaywitz, B.A., Fletcher, J.M., & MaKugh, R. (1992). Evidence that dyslexia may represent the lower tail of a normal distribution of reading ability. *New England Journal of Medicine*, **326**, 145–150.

Shaywitz, B.A., Yager, R.D., & Klopper, J.H. (1976). Selective brain dopamine depletion in developing rats: An experimental model of minimal brain dysfunction. *Science*, **191**, 305–308.

Shekim, W.O., Dekirmenjian, H., & Chapel, J.L. (1977). Urinary catecholamine metabolites in hyperactive boys treated with d-amphetamine. *American Journal of Psychiatry*, **134**, 1276–1279.

Shekim, W.O., Dekirmenjian, H., & Chapel, J.L. (1979). Urinary MHPG in minimal brain dysfunction and its modification by d-amphetamine. *American Journal of Psychiatry*, **136**, 667–671.

Shekim, W.O., Javaid, J., Dans, J.M., & Bylund, D.B.N. (1983). Urinary MHPG and HVA excretion in boys with attention deficit disorder and hyperactivity treated with d-amphetamine. *Biological Psychiatry*, **18**, 707–714.

Shekim, W.O., Sinclair, E., Glaser, R., Horwitz, E., Javaid, J., & Bylund, D.B. (1987). Norepinephrine and dopamine metabolites and educational variables in boys with attention deficit disorder and hyperactivity. *Journal of Child Neurology*, **2**, 50–56.

Snyder, A.M., Zigmond, M.J., & Lund, R.D. (1986). Sprouting of serotonergic afferents into striatum after dopamine depleting lesions in infant rats: a retrograde transport and immunocytochemical study. *Journal of Comparative Neurology*, **245**, 274–281.

Soubrie, P. (1986). Reconciling the role of central serotonin neurons in human and animal behavior. *Behavioral Brain Science*, **9**, 319–364.

Sprich-Buckminster, S., Biederman, J., Milberger, S., Faraone, S.V., & Lehman, B.K. (1993). Are perinatal complications relevant to the manifestation of ADD? Issues of comorbidity and familiarity. *Journal of the American Academy of Child and Adolescent Psychiatry*, **32**, 1032–1037.

Stachowiak, M.K., Bruno, J.P., Snyder, A.M., Stricker, E.M., & Zigmond, M.J. (1984). Apparent sprouting of striatal serotonergic terminals after dopamine depleting lesions in neonatal rats. *Brain Research*, **291**, 164–167.

Stanley, M. & Mann, J.J. (1983). Increased serotonin-2 binding sites in the frontal cortex of suicide victims. *Lancet*, **1**, 214–216.

Stanley, M., Virgilio, J., & Gershon, S. (1982). Tritiated imipramine binding sites are decreased in the frontal cortex of suicides. *Science,* **216,** 1337–1339.

Stoff, D.M., Pasatiempo, A.P., Yeung, J.H., Cooper, T.B., Bridger, W.H., & Rabinovich, H. (1992). Neuroendocrine responses to challenge with dl-fenfluramine and aggression in disruptive behavior disorders of children and adolescents. *Psychiatry Research,* **43,** 263–276.

Stoff, D.M., Pollack, L., Vitiello, B., Behar, D., & Bridger, W.H. (1987). Reduction of ³H-imipramine binding sites on platelets of conduct disordered children. *Neuropsychopharmacology,* **1,** 55–62.

Swanson, J.M., Posner, M., Potkin, S.G., Bonforte, S. et al. (1991). Activating tasks for the study of visual-spatial attention in ADHD children: A cognitive anatomic approach. *Journal of Child Neurology,* **6**(suppl.), S119–S127.

Szatmari, P., Boyle, M., & Offord, D.R. (1989). ADDH and conduct disorder: degree of diagnostic overlap and differences among correlates. *Journal of the American Academy of Child and Adolescent Psychiatry,* **28,** 865–872.

Szporny, L. & Gorog, P. (1961). Investigations into the correlations between monoamine oxidase inhibition and other effects due to methylphenidate and its stereoisomers. *Biochemical Pharmacology,* **8,** 263–268.

Weiss, G., Hechtman, L., Milroy, T., & Perlman, T. (1985). Psychiatric status of hyperactives as adults: A controlled prospective 15 year follow-up of 63 hyperactive children. *Journal of the American Academy of Child and Adolescent Psychiatry,* **24,** 211–220.

Weizman, A., Bernhout, E., Weitz, R., Tyano. S., & Rehavi, M. (1988). Imipramine binding to platelets of children with attention deficit disorder with hyperactivity. *Biological Psychiatry,* **23,** 491–496.

Wender, P., Epstein, R.S., Kopin, I., & Gordon, E.K. (1971). Urinary monoamine metabolites in children with minimal brain dysfunction. *American Journal of Psychiatry,* **127,** 1411–1415.

Wurtz, R.H., Goldberg, M.E., & Robinson, D.L. (1980). Behavioral modulation of visual responses in monkeys. *Progress in Psychobiology, Physiology and Psychology,* **9,** 42–83.

Yu-cun, A. & Yu-feng, W. (1984). Urinary 3-methoxy-4-hydroxyphenylglycol sulfate excretion in seventy-three school children with minimal brain dysfunction syndrome. *Biological Psychiatry,* **19,** 861–870.

Zametkin, A.J., Nordahl, T.E., Gross, M., Kings, A.C., Semple, W.E., Rumsey, J., Hamburger, S., & Cohen, R.M. (1990). Cerebral glucose metabolism in adults with hyperactivity of childhood onset. *New England Journal of Medicine,* **323,** 1361–1366.

Zametkin, I.A. & Rapoport, J.L. (1987). Neurobiology of attention deficit disorder with hyperactivity: where have we come in 50 years? *Journal of the American Academy of Child and Adolescent Psychiatry,* **26,** 676–686.

Zametkin, A.J., Rapoport, J.L., Murphy, D.L., Linnoila, M., Karoum, F., Potter, W.Z., & Ismond, D. (1985). Treatment of hyperactive children with monoamine oxidase inhibitors: II. Plasma and urinary monoamine findings after treatment. *Archives of General Psychiatry,* **42,** 969–973.

Ziegler, M., Lake, C., Wood, J., & Brooks, B. (1980). Relationship between cerebrospinal fluid norepinephrine and blood pressure in neurologic patients. *Clinical and Experimental Hypertension,* **2,** 995–1008.

16 Acquired disorders of memory in childhood

PENELOPE KRENER

INTRODUCTION

Before the turn of the century, William James observed that memories are formed within the brain in relation to the contextual events occurring at the time in the rememberer's experience. His description forecasted today's theories of distributed cognitive functions. Memory, he wrote, is found within a "cloud of associates" ". . . each [of which] becomes a hook to which it hangs, a means to fish it up by when sunk beneath the surface. Together they form a network of attachments by which it is woven into the entire tissue of our thought" (James, 1950).

Memory is still an elusive topic. Memory processes are inseparable from cognitive processes overall (Kail & Hagen, 1982), and thus memory research is part of research into understanding cognitive functioning. To understand acquired disorders of memory in children, we must address theories of memory and three general questions: How can human memory be studied? How does memory develop? What is the relationship of memory to learning disorders and other clinical syndromes?

A principal problem with the study of human memory is the fact that memory is a complex construct which does not easily lend itself to simple operationalization. Moreover, it is a construct which is used in clinical reports, as well as in the literature of developmental psychology, neuropsychology, and cognitive psychology. Neither the developmental psychology concepts nor the clinical literature share terminology or methodology with the neuropsychology literature or the cognitive psychology models of memory. However all four fields converge upon a range of cognitive processes which develop during childhood and which are vulnerable if that development is interfered with or if the brain is injured. Memory disorders in childhood may result from loss of previously acquired function, or from factors which impinge upon maturation of memory systems. Acquired disorders of memory with neurological bases will be discussed, as will disorders resulting from experience. A particular child with disordered memory may have more than one cause for it, and the disorder may be circumscribed or extended. To provide a framework for discussion of memory disorders in childhood, current work on cognitive and neuroanatomic bases for multiple memory systems in childhood will then be discussed, but it should be noted that memory norms for children are relative not only to the child's age but also to what he has learned from the persons and experiences in his life. This contributes cultural, subcultural and psychological specificity to the confounds of measurement of memory in childhood. Encoding constraints particular to childhood will be presented, and the role of language and narrative in organizing and demonstrating memory will be discussed.

Clinical manifestations of memory disorders in children will be reviewed, including disorders of learning ranging from cognitive style to developmental learning disorder. The relationship of personal experience to memory, will be explored, particularly the effect of trauma upon recall. Finally, guidelines for assessing a child's memory will be suggested, including strategies for optimizing assessment of the child's recall, and for being aware of three confounds to memory assessment: attention, state, and motivation.

COGNITIVE AND NEUROANATOMIC BASES FOR MULTIPLE MEMORY SYSTEMS

More-cognitive and less-cognitive memory system theories

The concept of memory refers to many subjective experiences, these include the experience of task familiarity, facility in recall for handling information, and the personal experience of the self through time. Memory is frequently conceptualized dichotomously, as long-term memory vs. short-term memory, or as cognitive vs. less cognitive memory. The more-cognitive and less-cognitive retention processes have been termed respectively: semantic (propositional) vs. episodic (procedural), (Tulving, 1972, 1984), explicit vs. implicit (Schacter, McAndrews, & Moscovitch, 1988), declarative vs. procedural (Cohen & Squire, 1980) or experience based and language based (Pillemer & White, 1989). For example, if a person is asked to directly recall something (such as a telephone number or historical date), the recalled statement is evidence of explicit memory; if the person's behavior reveals that he has previous training and experience (such as more rapidly solving a familiar puzzle), this is evidence of implicit memory. These conceptualizations, which do not precisely correspond to each other, derive from personal experience and also clinical observation. The reader is referred to an extensive discussion by Tulving with open peer commentary by 20 authors (Tulving, 1984) for detailed elaboration of these theories. Selective losses point to less-cognitive and more-cognitive memory functions which have been described and named as shown in Table 16.1.

The more cognitive memory system is conscious, is associated with language, and is that which is lost with destruction of the cortico-limbic

Table 16.1. *Retention processes*

More cognitive		Less cognitive	
semantic	vs.	episodic	(Tulving, 1972)
explicit	vs.	implicit	(Schacter et al., 1988)
declarative	vs.	procedural	(Cohen & Squire, 1980)
language-based	vs.	experience-based	(Pillemer & White, 1989)

system and hippocampus. The less cognitive memory system consists of expressed or demonstrated knowledge which persons are not phenomenalogically aware of having (Dudai, 1989); it is based in the context of the experience which gave rise to it, and it is verbalized with difficulty. Long-term memory has been also described by Tulving (1984) as *procedural* and *declarative*. Procedural memory is the repository of acquired patterns of behavior, eluding introspection, which may have been learned without the person being aware that they were learning them. Declarative memory may be divided into *episodic* memory, which Tulving (1972, 1984) considers to be the associations of information events in time and the temporal-spatial relationships between them, and *semantic* memory, which is the encoding of experience into categories which can be described and retrieved with language. Saffran (1990) has further developed views of short-term memory and its impairment which incorporates assumptions from the levels-of-processing approach. Focusing on a particular task the memory span, or immediate serial recall task, as an index of impaired short-term memory function, she notes that this requires linguistic processes and representations.

Clinical evidence for neuroanatomic siting of memory functions

The function of anatomic structures crucial for memory is inferred from their dysfunction, which may result either from injury to the brain or from experimental obliteration by lesion or pharmacological agent. Memory assessment has been developed in adults to evaluate neuropathology, and clinical tools for the measurement of memory have historically been lesion driven. Memory has been assumed to be something which has already developed and which is damaged or lost when there is a brain insult. Brain lesions and disorders result in loss of functions, including memory functions (Harrington et al., 1990; Schwartz et al., 1992). Two general kinds of memory are differentially affected by lesions and organic brain conditions (Dennis et al., 1991a, 1991b), and to some extent their different and specific anatomic distributions in the brain have been delineated. However, they cannot be specifically differentiated by particular memory tasks except in the most rudimentary way. Invasive monitoring or post-factum tissue analysis provide further clues (Dudai, 1989). Anatomic correlates of some aspects of memory function are recognized (Mishkin & Appenzeller, 1987). Lesions causing conjoint damage to amygdala and hippocampus result in severe amnesia with preserved ability to learn only some new skills. Correlations to injuries to the brain of the developing child may be possible if Positron Emission Tomography (PET) scan or MRI techniques can be carefully correlated with behavioral and cognitive syndromes.

Amnesia patients, in whom perceptual linguistic and intellectual skills may be preserved, but who have selective inability to learn certain new information or to remember recent experiences, exhibit partial memory loss. Long-term memory may be preserved, but the patient may be incapable of forming new short-term memories and converting them to long-term memories. Implicit or procedural memory for recent experiences may be preserved, while explicit or declarative memory is obliterated (Cohen & Squire, 1980; Squire & Cohen, 1984). For example, an amnesia patient may increase his skill at executing a complex task on successive sessions (procedural memory), yet state each time that he has never seen the task before (declarative memory). Other neuro-psychiatric syndromes may bring about dissociation between implicit and explicit knowledge as well (Schacter et al., 1988). Selective losses of long-term, of short-term and of explicit memory have been described (Kosslyn & Koenig, 1993: Markowitsch, 1994). Lesions within the left hemisphere result in impairment of certain linguistic functions, lesions to hippocampus and medial temporal regions produce severe amnesia for recent events with preserved performance on tests of intelligence, perception and language; lesions in the right hemisphere result in impairment of spatial tasks. Hence, there is evidence that intactness of all of these anatomic areas allows full engagement in learning and the functions measured as memory. The actual functioning of these areas in the intact brain, using PET, is beginning to be explored (Kapur et al., 1994; Mazziotta et al., 1982; Tulving et al., 1994).

The concept of distributed memory systems

Therefore there is more than one kind of memory "system" or retention process, and different processes are clinically dissociable. Hence "memory" is not singular and types of memory in any discussion of memory loss must be specified. Indeed this statement also oversimplifies the situation. Brain structures which subserve perception, homeostasis and their integrations, and which allow adaption by the organism, are distributed, not localized (Squire et al., 1993). "Memory" refers to integration of information from many such areas.

Shiffrin & Schneider (1977) distinguish between controlled and automatic processing of skills which may be either recalled implicitly or explicitly. Automatic processing is attention-independent, placing only limited demands on the information processing system, while controlled processing is capacity limited, and requires focus and effort. Both may be impaired in brain injured patients (Levin et al., 1988).

Several authors hypothesize that conscious experience of more cognitive memory results from the integration of input from several specific processes or modules which transmit or modulate information in the brain (e.g., Reason, 1984). Patients with anticipatory behavior deficits have difficulty in situations where current behavior should be regulated on the basis of expected future consequences. Cicerone, Lazar, & Shapiro (1983) have found that patients with frontal lobe lesions fail to systematically explore a hypothesis, which calls upon general concept formation, and do not discard inappropriate hypotheses. They suggest that this deficit may be the result of a disturbance in attentional control mechanisms which monitor environmental feedback in an ongoing fashion, and sift relevant from irrelevant sources of information. This integrative modality has been characterized as a conscious processing system (Posner, 1978), a commentary system (Weiskrantz, 1978, 1987), selector input (Shallice, 1972) or as the output of a left brain interpreter (Gazzaniga, 1985). Schacter, McAndrews, & Moscovitch (1988) hypothesize that clinical amnesia results from the functional failure of specific processors to gain access to this conscious module. According to their model, explicit (or declarative or semantic) function is the integrated and articulated product of several processes. These processes (implicit, procedural or episodic), termed slave systems, have dedicated capacities of their own and carry out their functions at a more automatic level. Without the organization of the higher processing system, they are depicted as a degraded or disconnected form of explicit function. This concept resembles Baddeley's model (1986) of the central executive in working memory, an attention controlling, limited capacity system which carries out the conscious direction of activities of so-called slave systems.

MEMORY DEVELOPMENT

Developmental course: from plasticity to specialization

There is proliferating neurobiological knowledge of how information, or synaptic input, is received by neurons, and in turn how that information may affect the behavior and even the fate of cells. Kandel et al. (1983) have shown in *Aplysia* that short-term learning modifies the network that subserves the animal's behavior. Genes are activated in memory consolidation; patterns found in protein synthesis inhibition at the time of training suggest that second-messenger system may regulate both post-translational modifications of proteins and gene expression. (Dudai, 1989; Lynch & Baudry, 1984; Edelman, 1984; Henderson, 1987).

Studies of the neurobiology of memory have shown that there is no single mechanism of information or memory acquisition or storage. Multiple cellular mechanisms operate concurrently and integratively; extracellular signals trigger event successions within the membrane, the cytoplasm and the nucleus of the cell, events which modify cellular properties. These events occur on a time scale of seconds to years. Hence the traditional classification of memory into only two discrete phases, short and long term, is naïve (Dudai, 1989), and represents a conceptual dichotomy which miscategorizes an organic process.

Studies of memory development: the importance of language

Despite the recent major gains in molecular analysis of neuronal memory, the clinical phenomenon of memory, its individuality and content, cannot be explained by delineating molecular cascades, but requires consideration of parallel systems of circuits at higher levels of neuronal organization. Clues to the process lie in observing the ontogeny of memory in the developing human brain. Learning and memory are linguistically distinct but functionally inseparable in the developing child.

Habituation implies memory, and newborn infants have been shown to habituate. Moreover infants habituate more rapidly as development progresses. This has been studied using event-related potentials (Nelson, 1994), demonstrating that three-month-old babies can differentiate between familiar and novel stimuli. Preschoolers have accurate recognition memory, but rarely use mnemonic strategies (Kail & Hagen, 1982) and occasionally use physical gestures, such as touching or pointing, to assist themselves in remembering (Paris & Lindauer, 1982). By middle childhood, children begin to rehearse items to be remembered, and show reorganization, elaboration and inference as strategies for recall (Paris & Lindauer, 1982). However, careful review of the literature on memory strategy development (Kail & Hagen, 1982) shows it to be fraught with methodological problems and does not present a clear relationship between conceptual development and memory performance. This is consistent with the notion that there is no unitary memory skill; instead measured memory capacity interacts with cognitive style, gender, and psychosocial factors.

Nelson (Nelson, 1986), studying event memory of young children, identifies four features: first, young children's memory is rarely deliberate; second, early childhood memories consist primarily of events that were directly experienced by the child; third, most of the content of the very young child's memory is inaccessible to retrieval later in life; and fourth, memory may be identified in a variety of intentional behaviors. Children can remember more than they can report, and remembering and reporting are not coterminous phenomena.

The perceived relevance of the memory task affects recall, which accounts for age differences and also cross-cultural differences in production of recall (Cole &

Scribner, 1977). The child's contexts of experience may affect both the memory itself and the reporting process (Neisser, 1988). This clinical observation of the importance of context is substantiated by experimental findings, as discussed below. Pillemer & White (1989) theorize that there is a dual memory system in the child. The first memory system encompasses the memories that are organized and evoked by an infant's experience of persons, location, and emotion, images and behaviors. These memories are stimulated by situational and affective cues but are not verbally mediated and not easily reported outside the original stimulus context. A second, language-connected system develops in later childhood. This allows memories to be accessed intentionally and in contexts different than that where the original learning happened. Events are represented or processed in verbal symbolizations, and encoded in narrative. These two systems function separately throughout the life span; Pillemer & White (1989) posit that even after the language-based memory system is established, certain powerful experiences may be stored in the first memory system and may not be retrieved by a simple verbal interview.

This raises questions about whether language development itself is the constraint upon memory development. Bjorklund & Bernholtz (1986) found that when reading disabled children were compared with normal children on list recall, they performed just as well, if the list of items to be recalled was personally familiar to the poor readers. This supports the thesis that children may spontaneously use deliberate organizational strategies only if they are able to activate relations among the to-be-remembered items without using so much of their capacity that there is not enough left over to develop a mnemonic strategy.

Earliest memories are episodic; consisting of the child's unique apprehension of personal perceptions and experiences, into which his consciousness of a consistent self through time is rooted. Certainly a crucial developmental epoch begins with the establishment of language, as the child then attains the capacity to convert events to narration, which enables inner review of experiences, rehearsal, and shared encoding of verbal representations. During this period hippocampal maturation is ongoing (Jacobs & Nadel, 1985). Around age 4 children exhibit autobiographical memory in describing their daily experiences and self-recollection.

Autobiographical memory is considered to be a form of episodic memory. However, the continuity between the memories arising before language and those elaborated afterward is tenuous. Failure of verbal (semantic) recall of earliest (episodic) childhood experiences has been termed infantile amnesia in psychoanalytic language and was theorized to result from repression, although it is clinically recognized that such experiences are not forgotten and may be communicated nonverbally through play (Terr, 1990) and in the later reconstruction of new relationships according to the pattern of early ones (Clyman, 1991). Clyman and his group have shown that procedural memory can be demonstrated in how preschool children, with immature capacities to express themselves in language, consistently carry out in play complex enactments of events which they have experienced. In play, the child reconstructs the context and thus recaptures the memory of events which he cannot verbalize about in response to questions. These events are laid down in procedural memory, and present a clear picture of the child's experience, which the child can only partly express in words, but which can be corroborated by observations in the original context, the home.

Encoding constraints

Memory is rooted in the experiences from which it was encoded, including motor experiences (Lesny et al., 1990), and is constrained by attention (Liason & Richman, 1987). In child developmental literature, the term general event representation (GER) describes the acquisition of factual events into memory. This early categorization allows subsequent routine events to be linked in general event representation rather than be treated as novel experiences each time. However, memory reconstruction from general event representation may be fuzzy or confused (Hudson, 1986), because specificity of the event is blurred as it is merged into a category. Recognition memory can be remarkably accurate even for preschoolers (Kail, 1989), but if free verbal recall is called for, age differences appear (Nurcombe, 1986). This experimental observation is consistent with the dependence upon context for memory retrieval, more pronounced in the younger child. Preschool children are found to be more suggestible than school aged children or adults in the vast majority of studies reviewed by Ceci & Bruck (1993). Preschoolers also encode experiences in a personally specific way, because they are not able to carry out simultaneous narrative reclassification of experiences, taking multiple points of view into account. Hence, context is more dominant. This could affect the child's "forgetting" of an unusual experience after being told by a molesting adult that they must not remember or disclose what has happened between them. It may also affect the way a "lost" memory resurfaces.

Cases of corroborated repressed memories have been reported, but reports may also be of intervening memory of discussion of the supposedly repressed event (Loftus, 1993), or be brought about by suggestion (Ofshe, 1992) sometimes from zealous therapists (Loftus, 1993). False memories have been documented, as well (Piaget, 1951). This will be discussed further in the section on trauma and recall below.

Fischer & Rose (1994), reviewing the development of coordination of components in brain and behavior, state that neural networks supporting control systems follow the principles of parallel, distributed, resonant processing, and are therefore both general and specific. Because these systems are general, networks have similar properties of information processing; for example, working memory components in different cortical networks operate similarly. In addition, a given section of neural tissue participates in many networks, and the child has the capacity to shift functions from one hemisphere to another if there is a neural insult. An insult to a developing brain, therefore, will change the trajectory of skill acquisition, and thus has a different effect than the same brain insult occurring in adulthood.

Children are less well able than adults to attend broadly to episodic event information, and where possible, to do context-interactive encoding. In context-independent situations, selective attention may facilitate memory but not in context-interactive situations (Ackerman, 1986). Since these systems are specific, each network may contain its own working memory, and context contributes directly to the system's generality and specificity. This explains the variation in developmental level which a child shows for the same skill across contexts and affective states. Language development facilitates encoding. If input matches top-down control signals, the child exhibits excellent understanding, for example of a story about a social situation. This is termed "priming." However, if there is no contextual priming, the same child shows a lower level of understanding. Therefore a single parallel, distributed, resonant network may produce different levels of functioning, depending on contextual input. This work provides a neuropsychological foundation for important clinical observations, for example that even very young children's recall performance can be improved by instructing them to use an instructional strategy (Sodian, Schneider, & Perlmutter, 1986).

The role of language and narrative

Unrehearsed personal memories may dissolve. Rehearsal, or retelling in personal narrative, reshapes the experience, always in the context of the person's past and current experience, in an ever-changing way. McCabe, Capron, & Peterson (1991) have shown that adolescents and adults do not remember early child experience in the terms that young children do; rather they select for recall the details which are consistent with their current framework. Routinized and stereotyped experiences may be recalled in more structured ways, whereas children's personal narratives about variable events are more differentiated and detailed (Gee, 1991).

Two experiments demonstrating this are offered as examples. Hicks (1991) compares the way in which children from two socioeconomic backgrounds retold the story of The Red Balloon movie in three genres: newscast, on-line narration from the film, and stories. Culturally mainstream (white middle-class) children interpreted both on-line and story-telling modes as tasks, and generated an unembellished, temporally connected account of events, whereas African American children of lower socioeconomic status interpreted narrative modes more freely, using both description and forecast, with evaluative commentary and expressive intonation as integral part of the narrative. Gee (1991), comparing the narratives of children from different social groups, demonstrated the range of possible encoding, which itself reshapes experience.

The same cross-cultural pattern was found: one child, an African American, created patterns of contrast, contact, stress, and refrain within the stanzas of her story, another, a white middle-class child, made rapid and linear progress to the point. Gee notes that mainstream practices have "effaced the spatial and poetic workings of narrative, at least on a superficial level."

What do such findings tell us about evaluating a child's memory? First, the age of the child and his or her language development must be taken into consideration. Schooling progressively augments and modifies children's capacities for verbal representation and moves them toward mainstream patterns of encoding private experience. Second, the context offered will limit the recall. Structured test settings may access a narrow channel, not allowing children to recruit other cues from their own larger narrative context, hence yielding a limited assessment of their capacity for memory reconstruction of their experience.

CLINICAL MANIFESTATIONS OF MEMORY DISORDERS IN CHILDREN

Amnesia syndromes in childhood

Characterization of memory disorders in childhood must be made in relation to existing models of memory systems, recognizing that these are hypothetical models rapidly evolving in response to new neuropsychological findings. Memory disorders in childhood may result from loss of previously acquired function, or from factors which impinge upon maturation of memory systems. Evaluation of impaired memory in clinical settings may shed light on memory development.

Memory disturbance occurs along with the loss of some or all other cognitive functions in children with progressive neurological disorders. This measured deterioration of function occurs independent of the cause of the progressive disease, and has been described with multiple etiologies. Etiologies may be infectious, metabolic-genetic, toxic or idiopathic.

Correlates of amnesia in childhood: clinical and research reports

Trauma, infarct, infection, neoplasm, metabolic, and epilepsy may injure the developing brain. Examining reports of these in turn, may cast light on different facets of memory functions in children.

Head trauma and post-traumatic amnesia (PTA)

Memory loss has been described as a result of blunt or closed head injury and may be persistent (Tate et al., 1991). It is termed post-traumatic amnesia

(PTA), and it typically includes memory loss for events preceding and surrounding the injury and memory loss for events occurring since the injury. Following resolution of PTA deficits may be present in a number of cognitive domains. Memory and attention/information processing speed and task efficiency are typically most severely affected (Capruso & Levin, 1992). Memory deficit persisted at least one year after severe closed head injury in 58 pediatric admissions in three age ranges (Levin et al., 1988). Impairment of visual recognition memory was directly related to severity of injury in all three age groups. Verbal memory skills were found to be more severely affected for adolescents, which the authors ascribed to the rapid verbal development in adolescents, as compared with verbal immaturity in the younger group.

Vascular insults

Infarcts may destroy specific anatomic structures necessary for memory function. Markowitsch et al. (1990) documented verbal memory deterioration after unilateral infarct of the internal capsule in a 15-year-old boy. Significant verbal long-term memory disturbances were present when the young person was tested 9 months after the infarct. He had impaired memory of personal events for the previous five years and poor performance on all verbal tasks that required remembering items for longer than one hour. His performance was indistinguishable from controls on short-term memory tests, nonverbal learning and recognition tests (Markowitsch, 1994). Painstaking testing of patients with quite specific lesions can give important information about what Markowitsch terms "bottleneck" areas where fibers from distributed memory systems converge.

Infections, including HIV

Infectious dementing disorders of the gray matter are exemplified by subacute sclerosing panencephalitis or progressive rubella encephalopathy, and of the white matter by Jacob-Creutzfeld disease. Viral infections of the brain may cause damage ranging from specific to protean. Herpes simplex viral encephalitis demonstrates a predilection for localization in the temporal and orbitofrontal regions of the brain. To the extent that the infection interferes with the patient's performance on memory tasks, it gives information about another domain of distribution of memory function (Quart, Buchtel, & Sarnaik, 1988; Greer et al., 1989).

AIDS encephalopathy may affect both gray and white matter and will produce developmental plateauing and decline or severe dementia, usually in latter stages of the disease. AIDS dementia complex is well-described in HIV positive adults as well as those meeting criteria for AIDS; it also exists in children. In a study of HIV-1 seropostive asymptomatic patients

(Tran-Dinh et al., 1990), quantitative tomographic studies, together with MRI, EEG, psychometric tests, and laboratory analyses found abnormal cerebral perfusion in 88%; most commonly in the frontal region. Fifty-five percent of patients had impaired performance on psychometric tests, mostly in cognitive functions and memorization. Because the AIDS retrovirus directly infects neural tissue, AIDS dementia complex reveals the normal function of the developing brain as that function is compromised by the evolving infection, or as the infection is reversed by AZT treatment, and function returns.

Neoplasms

Brain tumors, even if treated aggressively, may obliterate functional tissue and alter cognitive capacities. Dennis et al. (1991a, 1991b) studied memory functions and neuroanatomy of deficits in memory in children and adolescents with brain tumors. Performance on an intelligence and memory battery was analyzed in relation to age at onset of tumor symptoms, duration of tumor, pretumor developmental disturbances, pretumor closed head injury, post-tumor anticonvulsant treatment and post tumor epileptic seizures. Developmental effects were seen, and evidence for neuroanatomical separation of dissociable memory systems was found when computerized tomography scans of brain regions were coded for type of brain damage and localization of damage. Non-overlapping focal neuroanatomical substrates were found for two forms of memory: memory for serial order of pictures, corresponding to heard words, and memory for a succession of heard words. Memory for semantically based word-picture associations was unaffected by tumors in several subcortical brain regions (Dennis, 1991b). These results support a model which is both distributed over many brain regions, and specific to particular regions, and which changes with development.

A high incidence of memory deficits, visual-spatial skill impairment, learning problems, and attention deficit disorders has been described in long term survivors of brain tumors and acute lymphoblastic leukemia (ALL), and has been shown to be related to the disease and its treatment (Jannoun & Chessels, 1987; Mulhern et al., 1988; O'Hare, Aitken, & Eden, 1988; Gamis & Nesbit, 1991). These memory impairments, particularly those in short-term memory, may be attributable to an underlying attentional deficit affecting the encoding stage of memory (Brouwers & Poplack, 1990).

Disorders of metabolism

Metabolic insults may result in impaired attention, learning, memory and slowing of sensorimotor reaction times. This has been seen with high lead exposure (Stollery et al., 1989), and heavy marijuana use (Schwartz, 1991a, 1991b). Memory disorders have been described in children with multiple sclerosis (Septien et al., 1991), Lyme disease (Logiagian, Kaplan, & Steere,

1990), and metabolic-genetic disorders which may afflict gray matter generally, (e.g., Tay-Sachs), the basal ganglia specifically (e.g., Wilson's disease), or white matter (e.g., metachromatic leucodystrophy, adrenoleukodystrophy). Neurocutaneous degenerative disorders include tuberous sclerosis, neurofibromatosis, and Sturge–Weber syndromes. In some instances, acquired disorders of memory in childhood may occur without identifiable etiology (Wong et al., 1991).

Seizures

Children with recurrent seizures are known to be at risk for disorders of attention, learning and memory. However, an underlying diathesis may produce seizures as a symptom in association with other brain dysfunction. Still electroconvulsive events alone are recognized to produce memory deficit, as when ECT is given for therapeutic treatment of major depression (Calev et al., 1991). Close scrutiny, with a comprehensive memory battery pre- and post-treatment, shows that both anterograde and retrograde memory deficits results from bilateral dosage-titrated ECT. Testing of delayed recall reveals more rapid forgetting and more impaired immediate memory after ECT than in the depression pre-ECT state. The authors suggest this is explained by frontotemporal electrode placement which adversely affects both pure memory and memory dependent on associative (organizational) ability.

The clinical application of this to the child with a seizure disorder indicates the importance of localizing seizure areas electrographically and by history. Complex partial epilepsy may present as a memory disturbance (Gallassi et al., 1988). While it is hoped that if seizures are well-controlled, intellectual deterioration will be minimal, it has also been observed that recurrent convulsive seizures, depending on severity, type, age of onset and frequency of toxic levels of anti-epileptic drugs may be associated with interictal cognitive changes (Brown, 1991). Deficits in verbal language and memory have been observed, especially in patients with complex partial seizure foci in the left (dominant) hemisphere. The memory deficits appear to affect new learning and retention of material; verbal deficits are more subtle, affecting word-finding, verbal fluency, and comprehension abilities. Antiepileptic drugs may affect cognitive functioning; this has been described (in descending order) in treatment with Phenobarbital, Phenytoin, Valporic acid and Carbamazapine. However in a multisite study of children with epilepsy, significant improvement on withdrawal of antiepileptic medication was found in only one cognitive test: psychomotor speed (Aldenkampt et al., 1993), and group differences between the epilepsy and control children baseline persisted after drug withdrawal. Recent research on subclinical interictal spike-wave phenomena has illuminated the intermittent nature of attention deficits and slowing of cognitive processes in patients with frontal or generalized seizure patterns.

Seizure foci may afflict quite specific anatomic brain areas. Also a particular paroxysmal event may be more or less generalized and may occur with various intensity and frequency. If this is understood, for example through the use of EEG videotelemetry, the patient's function during, after, and between seizures may offer another possibility for elucidating the contributions of specific brain regions to memory function.

Disordered learning: from cognitive style to developmental learning disorder

If memory and experience shape each other in recursive ways, it follows that children whose experiences are constrained by learning handicaps, will remember these experiences in different ways. The clinical finding that learning disabled children exhibit dissociation in recall ability, depending upon how the recall is elicited, illustrates this. On a picture-naming and item recognition task designed to enable the manipulation of both presentation format (pictures of words) and retention interval (immediate or one-day), the performance of a group of learning-disabled and nondisabled children was dissociated on explicit and implicit tests of memory (Lorsbach, Sodoro, & Brown, 1992). This parallels the dissociation of functions seen in adults with specific lesions, and it is important, because in the learning disabled youngster, it may point to areas of brain which have failed to develop functions. Bishop (1992) reviews the question of whether double dissociation between tasks involving neighboring brain areas might explain clinical syndromes such as autism. Dissociations have been found in only one direction; in Asperger's syndrome children are not impaired on executive function tasks (problem solving) but are impaired on tasks drawing upon theory of mind (predicting another's point of view) (Ozonoff et al., 1991a, 1991b). Hence the pattern of perceptions and inferences which allows understanding another human's thought process may require the intactness and proper functioning of even more distributed anatomic areas.

Learning disorders are heterogeneous and often no anatomic site can be inferred to localize the observed dysfunction. Still, cognitive functions may be profiled, including memory performance. Some investigators have found that memory processes are separable from language and reading skills (Lindgren, Richman, & Liason, 1986). Others (Swanson, 1988; Wood & Richman, 1988) find learning disabled readers to be predominantly inferior in performance on a memory classification battery of semantic, elaborative, and effortful encoding tasks. This finding suggests that individual differences in recall are related to general cognitive features, namely whether the child possesses semantic structural resources. Such capability consists of a lexical knowledge base, demonstrable recall capacity under high-effort encoding conditions, and ability to monitor his attentional and semantic resources. This is supported by the finding of Raine et al. (1991) that for speech-disordered children, verbal short-term memory is limited by the speed of articulatory coding, which was not a function of general intellectual test scores or motor speed. This work is consistent with that of Bjorklund & Bernholtz (1986) showing that the effort of labeling the to be recalled items with words may preempt the child's capacity for developing a strategy to remember a word list.

There is evidence that, independent of genetically determined neuroanatomy and neuropsychological function, the child's pattern of experience may affect the ways in which his brain encodes information and retrieves it. Attention and memory functions are improved in some emotional states and interfered with if the child is excessively anxious, depressed or distressed. There is scant research on the biochemistry of the effect of distress upon the memory of children. Unpublished data (Carrey et al., 1992) have shown that sexually and physically abused children performed more poorly on a neuropsychological battery than did normals, and they did not show normal physiological responsiveness (e.g., cardiac deceleration with focus on novel task). Since they also did not show an orienting-type response to a nonsignal condition requiring only attention, this finding was not ascribable only to test anxiety. This indicates that performance on cognitive tasks, including memory and recall tasks, requires more than the processing of "cold" information; it may require that the child's emotional or affective state be at the right "temperature" to facilitate motivation and cognitive engagement. Two models of the relationship between physiological distress, arousal, and memory are found in clinical observations of child abuse and in observations of children under stress because of events and procedures in medical settings, both discussed below under Trauma and Recall.

TRAUMA AND RECALL: THE QUESTIONS OF REPRESSION, DISSOCIATION, REVISION AND MASTERY

Is failure to remember trauma a disorder of memory? Perceptual narrowing of memory has been shown to occur in situations perceived as dangerous, an effect which declines as the individual reduces anxiety and habituates to the danger (Broadbent, Reason, & Baddeley, 1991), but also, the individual's performance improves if the situation is structured to allow him to believe that his response to the task will affect the outcome (Baddeley, 1972). Single-blow traumatic or overwhelming experiences, depicted by Terr (1990) as "karate-chop" in character, are retained with "amazingly clear and detailed" memory. Terr (1991) labels these Type I trauma. Recurrent (and recurrently dreaded) traumatic experiences are remembered differently. Type II trauma memories "appear to be retained in spots rather than in clear, complete wholes." The child deals with the necessity of living with impending trauma by developing a number of defensive strategies which might interrupt the formation of specific memories, such as self-numbing, self-hypnosis, denial, dissociation, and rage, co-occurring with extreme passivity. Terr typifies the child who has had a Type I trauma as repetitively reviewing the traumatic experience, in an effort at *post-hoc* mastery. This conversion of memory to narration, and rehearsal in words, consistent with Baddeley's observation of improved performance with augmented personal role, has the effect of priming and sharpening the memory for Type I trauma events. By contrast, the avoidant cognitive strategies of the child who has suffered Type II trauma limit rehearsal and capacity for reconstructing specific memories of specific events. That, added to the fuzzy recall of more routine events predicted by GER (general event representation) theory (Hudson, 1986), explains vague recall, often mistaken for lack of credibility when the traumatized child comes into the forensic system.

In medical settings, children may also suffer fear, pain, helplessness and the dilemma of being urged to do so without complaint by a loving parent who has brought them to the frightening situation. Lehmann, Bendebba, & DeAngelis (1990) interviewed 91 children aged 3 to 8 years about painful events. Older children's reports showed more consistency than did those of younger ones, but the scaling procedure devised by the authors did not elicit consistent responses, illustrating that methodological problems may arise in assessing trauma without independent confirmation from parents, staff, or medical records. A more rigorous study was carried out by Steward et al. (1991) of young children's memory of the visit to a pediatric outpatient clinic where they experienced a wide range of touch, procedures and experiences. Visits were videotaped and both children and staff were interviewed. The accuracy of children's reports was evaluated, and those who had experienced distress were examined in detail. This distress group was divided into two subgroups, one which reported their distress, with accuracy comparable to the rest of the children, and one subgroup who denied not only the distress, but even denied having had their bodies touched during the examination. Half of these distress denying children actually appeared to have experienced no pain or distress when the videotapes were reviewed. The experience of the other half of the distress-denying subgroup of children was characterized in the words of one child as "He didn't touch me and it didn't hurt!" Closer scrutiny of this subgroup shows that they were disproportionately male, and that they did not fit the expectations of the memory deficit seen in the repeatedly traumatized group defined by Terr (1991). Their memories of the persons in, and details of, the examining room were accurate. The authors hypothesize that the parents' expectations that the child be "brave" and the child's conviction that he should not allow himself to lose control of his feelings or express distress resulted in the assignment of severe anxiety to this part of his experience. Therefore he constructed a "narrative of omission" where the part which he could not assimilate was left out; that part was where he felt hurt, could not ask for rescue, and broke down and cried. The denial of unmanageable and unacceptable distress by these children is consistent with the shaping of personal memory by intense cultural expectations (Baddeley, 1972; Gee, 1991; Hicks, 1991), including the microculture of an abusive family (Terr, 1994).

How can the inability to voluntarily retrieve memories of trauma be explained? Loftus (1993) and others argue against the possibility that repression of memories of catastrophic events occurs, stating that there is not sufficient clinical evidence for it. The inability of children and of adults to report their memories of events occurring before the age of 30 to 36 months has been documented, using cases where careful corroboration of the non-remembered events is possible (Terr, 1988). This can be explained in relation to the immaturity of left-brain development and verbal capacity at the time of the events. However, the same small children who are unable to verbalize are able to show gesturally and in play that they have incorporated preverbal epoch experiences and can accurately reenact them (Terr, 1990; Clyman, 1991) from procedural or extrinsic memory.

Dissociation, an involuntary adaptation to overwhelming trauma, is known to occur in childhood and to persist in severely traumatized adults (Putnam, 1985) who go on to develop multiple personality disorder with several "alter" personae. When dissociation has developed, retrieval of specific memories is rigidified into state dependence, with one alter able to reconstruct memories and the other unable to do so (Kluft, 1985). The revisions, integrations and inner narration of memories, which are a part of the dynamic adaptive processes of the developing brain, enable later reconstructions of details which were perceived but not understood at the time of the experience. The same process may make the rememberer vulnerable to reworking of recall by interpersonal and cultural pressures (Steward, 1993). Dissociation, in combination with emotional factors and cultural pressure, may bring about the construction of false, plausible, memories which not only cannot be corroborated, but which can be shown to result from suggestion (Ofshe, 1992).

ASSESSMENT

Clinical presentation: memory assessment in the office

Memory cannot be evaluated as a solitary function, as it is inextricably involved with attention, perception, cognitive capacities and previous experience. Evaluation of the child should include assessment of genetic and biological factors, developmental trajectory, environmental programming or input and life events. Indeed, as memory is a conceptual rubric for many cognitive processes such as encoding, retrieval, search clustering, rehearsal, elaboration and narrative schematization, evaluation should consist of several measures and observations. First, the child's developmental stage must be

Table 16.2. *Tests allowing assessment of learning and memory in children*

Intelligence tests, including memory component
   McCarthy Scales of Children's Abilities
   Wechsler Intelligence Scale for Children-R
   Bayley developmental test
   Kaufmann (K-ABC)

Tests of visual memory
   Benton Visual Retention test
   Rey Osterreith Complex Figure test

Tests of kinesthetic and auditory memory
   Tactual performance test
   Seashore Rhythm test

Tests of verbal memory
   California Verbal Learning Test for children (CALVT)

Tests of language development
   Detroit Test of Psycholinguistic Abilities
   Clinical Evaluation of Language Function (CELF)

Tests of verbal, visual and computational memory
   Wide Range Assessment of Memory and Learning

assessed. Second, the child's personal context of educational and cultural experience must be surveyed. Baseline and follow-up testing by a child psychologist or neuropsychologist should carefully delineate the child's level of function. Traditional tests of memory which might be used in such an evaluation are shown in Table 16.2.

The memory of very young children, children with autism or developmental disorders, and children with language handicaps, may be evaluated by performance on parts of the Bayley developmental test, or by their performance on a games requiring recall, as devised by Sodian & Frith (1992).

Language assessment is a crucial part of evaluating cognitive capacities, including memory function. Children with language processing problems and verbal short-term memory deficits may be evaluated (Shelton, Martin, & Yaffee, 1992), with phonological test manipulations (such as phonological similarity, word length, matching span), lexical semantic test manipulations (such as recognition probe, recall of words versus non words), sentence comprehension (of sentences with varying semantic load and simple syntax or complex syntactic structures), and sentence repetitions (of sentences with varying semantic load and simple syntax or complex syntactic structures such as adverbial phrases), complements and conjoined sentences.

Cognitive (clinical) psychology investigations of memory and learning in the laboratory or hospital

Recent advances in neuroimaging support both anatomic specificity and a distributed model. Structural imaging has implicated structures within the diencephalic midline, the mammillary bodies and the dorsomedial thalamic nucleus (in Korsakoff's amnesia), as well as the medial temporal area, including the hippocampus, known clinically to be critical (Scoville & Milner, 1957). Common to both kinds of amnesia patients is a limited and disrupted acquisition of new information, severe vulnerability to distraction, and impairment in long-term or secondary memory (Shimamura, 1986; Shimamura & Squire, 1984; Squire, Shimamura, & Graf, 1985; Warrington & Weiskrantz, 1974). Stimulation studies of neuroimaging and memory (Mazziotta et al., 1982) corroborate clinical observations, and show different activity on PET scan, depending on how tasks are presented, implicating language areas. Squire (1987) has argued that skills and priming are expressed through the operation of a memory system (or systems) that does not allow explicit access to the contents of the knowledge base. He hypothesizes a neural system, damaged in amnesia, which participates in memory storage without itself being the site of storage. When it is intact, normal memory function is possible. When it is damaged, the learning of declarative information (facts, lists, and day-to-day remembering) is impaired, but skill, or procedural learning, e.g. mirror-reading, pursuit rotor tasks, puzzle completion, and preservation of priming, that is facilitation of performance by prior exposure, is preserved.

Application of the reported findings to the clinical investigation of children with developmental disorders of learning and memory is a challenging area of child neuropsychology research. It will demand integration of a careful clinical history, the use of tasks which tap specific functions, and deployment of neuroimaging techniques.

Test conditions: optimizing prediction of the patient's capacities, and the question of ecological validity

As noted, test conditions, or environmental staging, affects the recruitment of processes resulting in production of memories (Mazziotta et al., 1982). Because location of lesions affects impairment of certain linguistic functions (Cohen & Squire, 1980), the most accurate diagnostic tasks are those devised to tap specific functions. In addition, the test conditions should allow the investigator to distinguish between "knowing how and knowing that" (Cohen & Squire, 1980), that is, to ascertain whether the patient can carry out the task under more than one test condition. Can the task distinguish whether the patient shows dissociation of function, when the task requires direct explicit use of a function or when it is presented in a way that taps the impaired function indirectly, in an implicit manner? (Graf, Squire, & Mandler, 1984). The use of such tasks also illuminates the role of language in cueing and recall. Hence evaluation of the patient's function must inventory the specific skills required to adapt in actual settings, must also consider how the person is able to put the skills together (Reason, 1984; Freedman, Bleiberg, & Freedland, 1987), and ideally, how he uses language to assist his performance.

Ecological validity is the term used to describe whether testing conditions make the same demands upon, and recruit the same capacities from, the patient as do the real-life conditions about which the predictions of his capacities are to be made. Special educational approaches for a child whose abnormal memory performance is associated with developmental learning disorder should be tailored to his cognitive needs. For example, if he has perceptual problems with auditory information, cross-modal presentation of academic material, using visual reinforcers, should be offered. By analogy, rehabilitation of patients after injury should be tailored to their deficiency (Giles, 1992). Approaches used for memory rehabilitation after brain injury include rote learning, elaborative encoding strategies, visual mnemonics, external memory aids, and the method of vanishing cues. Accurate diagnosis should underlie special education or rehabilitation strategies (Leng & Copello, 1990). For example, a battery is available to screen levels of cognitive function necessary for planned actions, namely manual, goal-directed, and exploratory actions. This allows defining the level of cognitive disability before rehabilitation, important both to evaluate progress, and to avoid embarking upon a treatment program which is beyond the patient's capability (Allen, 1992).

Confounds: measuring attention, state and motivation

Several authors propose that the sum of functions which are described within the concept of memory result from integration of extended and parallel processes (Squire, 1987; Dudai, 1989). Brainerd & Reyna (1989) note that the individual's capacity for such integration may be compromised if his cognitive energy is deflected. They state that data from dual tasks support the hypothesis that individuals' resources are limited. Memory processes tax a finite pool of cognitive energy, which has been termed "attentional, mental effort, and working-memory capacity." They further suggest that dual-task deficits are instances of output interference between otherwise independent systems. These integrative functions, which result in the successful production of memory, are likely executed in part within the frontal lobes. This is corroborated by the clinical observation that frontal electrode placement has a worse effect on post-ECT amnesia (Squire, Slater, & Miller, 1981). Integrative functions depend upon factors which have a general distribution as indicated by the observation that they are modified by affective states (Squire & Zouzounis, 1988). Hence factors such as emotions, state, attention or other frontal lobe functions, will affect memory and memory performance.

As noted above, language development underlies memory consolidation for long-term memory. A phonological basis for short-term memory has also been proposed (Allport, 1985; Saffran, 1990). Allport (1985) proposed that neuropsychological impairments such as the short-term memory deficit in short-term memory impaired patients, exhibit "graceful degradation" of performance, with particular linguistic functions diminished, slowed or hesitant but not lost altogether. This is best accounted for in terms of connectionist/parallel distributed processing models, which deserve further research pursuit. This approach has also been applied to speech perception in a fashion which makes no sharp distinction between perceptual and mnestic processes. Connectionist models allow explaining short-term retention in terms of interaction of several information sources which each furnish partial information. Implications of this work for assessing memory in children are that tasks must be within the child's cognitive energy limit, that the child's motivational and emotional state and his context must be considered, and that tasks must be designed so that his language skills are not a constraint.

CONCLUSION

Acquired disorders of memory in children must be understood in the contexts of childhood neurodevelopmental and developmental lines, and genetic, experimental and cultural factors which operate at the time earlier experiences are encoded into memory. Numerous descriptive and explanatory models of memory exist, complicating comparisons of studies. Theoretical models of memory describe a continuum between less-cognitive and more-cognitive kinds of memory, termed variously experience-based and language based (intrinsic versus extrinsic, procedural versus declarative, episodic versus semantic) memory types. Models also have been posited to describe the higher integration of inputs from specific neural processes. Translation of clinical data into theoretical models is difficult. Assessment of memory in children as well as in adults, faces many confounds such as attention, state, motivation and affect.

Development of memory cannot be studied without studying the development of language, and thus is of a piece with the child's personal experience and his own pattern of state regulation. Older children are more able to use language to achieve independence from context, but just as context limits recall for the young child, language may constrain the way memories are recalled for older children and adults. The child's semantic structural resources will determine how he encodes experience. Hence assessment of language is a crucial component of evaluating cognitive capacities, including memory.

Damage to the developing brain, resulting in impairment of a child's memory performance, has multiple etiologies. Recent clinical reports have been surveyed above. More theoretically driven investigations of memory in children with neurological impairment are needed. In such investigations, both developmental theory as well as cognitive theory should be considered, even though the focus of both is different. However, to assess memory function or dysfunction in the particular child, his developmental status must be described, the effect of confounding influences such as attention and affect must be estimated, and the cultural and educational modifiers of his memory process must be considered. Although specific anatomic localization of memory dysfunctions has eluded diagnostic effort for many categories of developmental memory dysfunction in childhood, newer imaging techniques, coupled with tasks which dissect out particular functions, may offer promise. In the absence of anatomic localization, however, cognitive and memory functions may still be profiled carefully, using neuropsychological and linguistic test instruments. This should enable tailoring special educational or rehabilitative programs for the child with a memory disorder.

REFERENCES

Ackerman, B.P. (1986). The relation between attention to the incidental context and memory for words in children and adults. *Journal of Experimental Child Psychology*, **41**, 149–183.

Aldenkampt, A.P., Sipherts, W.C., Blennow, G., Elmqvist, D., Heijbel, J., Nilsson, H.L., Snadstedt, P., Tonnby, B., Wahlander, L., & Wosse, E. (1993). Withdrawal of antiepileptic medication in children – effects on cognitive function: the Multicenter Holmfrid Study. *Neurology*, **43**(1), 41–50.

Allen, C.K. (1992). Cognitive disabilities. In N. Katz (ed.) *Cognitive Rehabilitation: Models for Intervention in Occupational Therapy*. Boston, MA: Andover Medical Publishers (pp. 1–21).

Allport, D.A. (1985). Distributed memory, modular subsystems and dysphasia. In S. Newman & R. Epstein (eds) *Current Perspectives in Dysphasia*. Edinburgh: Churchill Livingston (pp. 32–61).

Baddeley, A.D. (1972). Selective attention and performance in dangerous environments. *British Journal of Psychology*, **63**, 537–546.

Baddeley, A.D. (1986). *Working Memory*. Oxford: Clarendon.

Bishop, D.V.M. (1992). Annotation: autism, executive functions and theory of mind: a neuropsychological perspective. *Journal of Psychology and Psychiatry*, **34**(3), 279–293.

Bjorklund, D.F. & Bernholtz, J.E. (1986). The role of knowledge base in the memory performance of good and poor readers. *Journal of Experimental Child Psychology*, **41**, 367–393.

Blachstein, H., Vakil, E., & Hoofien, D. (1993). Impaired learning in patients with closed-head injuries: an analysis of components of the acquisition process. *Neuropsychology*, **7**(4), 530–535.

Brainerd, C.J. (1991). Fuzzy-trace theory and cognitive triage in memory development. *Development Psychology*, **27**(3), 351–369.

Brainerd, C.J. & Reyna, V.F. (1989). Output-interference theory of dual-task deficits in memory development. *Journal of Experimental Child Psychology*, **47**(1), 1–18.

Broadbent, D.E., Reason, J.T., & Baddeley, A. (eds) (1991). *Human Factors in Hazardous Situations*. New York: Oxford University Press.

Brouwers, P. & Poplack, D. (1990). Memory and learning sequelae in long-term survivors of acute lymphoblastic leukemia: association with attention deficits. *American Journal of Pediatric Hematology-Oncology*, **12**(2), 174–181.

Brown, E.R. (1991). Interictal cognitive changes in epilepsy. *Seminars in Neurology*, **11**(2), 167–174.

Calev, A., Nigal, D., Shapira, B., Tubi, N., Chasan, S., Ben-Yehuda, Y., Kugelmass, S., & Lehrer, B. (1991). Early and long-term effects of electroconvulsive therapy and depression on memory and other cognitive functions. *Journal of Nervous and Mental Disease*, **179**, 526–533.

Capruso, D.X. & Levin, H.S. (1992). Cognitive impairment following closed head injury. *Neurological Clinics*, **10**(4), 879–893.

Carrey, N., Butter, H., Charbonneau, P., & Bastien, C. (1992). Psychophysiology of Learning in Abused Children. Presented at the 39th annual meeting of the American Academy of Child and Adolescent Psychiatry, October 1993, Washington, DC.

Ceci, S.J. & Bruck, M. (1993). Suggestibility of the child witness: a historical review and synthesis. *Psychological Bulletin*, **113**(3), 403–439.

Cicerone, K.D., Lazar, R.M., & Shapiro, W.R. (1983). Effects of frontal lobe lesions on hypothesis sampling during concept formation. *Neuropsychologia*, **21**, 513–524.

Clyman, R.B. (1991). The procedural organization of emotions: a contribution from cognitive science to the psychoanalytic theory of therapeutic action. In T.E. Shapiro & R.N. Emde (eds) *Affect: Psychoanalytic Perspectives, Vol. 39*, Supplement. *Journal of the American Psychoanalytic Association*. Madison, CT: International Universities Press Inc.

Cohen, N.J. & Squire, L.R. (1980). Preserved learning and retention of pattern analyzing skill in amnesia: dissociation of knowing how and knowing that. *Science*, **210**, 207–209.

Cole, M. & Scribner, S. (1977). Cross-cultural studies of memory and cognition. In R.V. Kail & J.W. Kagen (eds) *Perspectives on the Development of Memory and Cognition*. Hillsdale NJ: Lawrence Erlbaum.

Dennis, M., Spiegler, B.J., Fitz, C.R., Hoffman, H.J., Hendrick, E.B. et al. (1991a). Brain tumors in children and adolescents I: Effects on working associative and serial-order memory of IQ, age at tumor onset, and age of tumor. *Neuropsychologica*, **29**(9), 813–827.

Dennis, M., Spiegler, B.J., Fitz, C.R., Hoffman, H.J. et al. (1991b). Brain tumors in children and adolescents II: the neuroanatomy of deficits in working, associative and serial-order memory. *Neuropsychologica*, **29**(9), 829–847.

Dudai, Y. (1989). *The Neurobiology of Memory*. Oxford: Oxford University Press.

Edelman, G.M. (1984). Expression of cell adhesion molecules during embryogenesis and regeneration. *Experimental Cell Research*, **161**, 1–16.

Fischer, K.W. & Rose, S.P. (1994). Dynamic development of coordination of components in brain and behavior: a framework for theory and research. In Dawson, G. & Fischer, K.W. (eds) *Human Behavior and the Developing Brain*. New York: Guilford Press (pp. 3–66).

Freedman, P.E., Bleiberg, J., & Freedland, K. (1987). Anticipatory behavior deficits in closed head injury. *Journal of Neurology, Neurosurgery and Psychiatry*, **50**, 398–401.

Gallassi, R., Morreale, A., Lorusso, S., Pazzaglia, P., & Luagresi, E. (1988). Epilepsy presenting as memory disturbances. *Epilepsia*, **29**(5), 524–529.

Gamis, A.S. & Nesbit, M.E. (1991). Neuropsychologic (cognitive) disabilities in long-term survivors of childhood cancer. *Pediatrician*, **18**(1), 11–19.

Gazzaniga, M.S. (1985). *The Social Brain*. New York: Basic Books.

Gee, J.P. (1991). Memory and myth: a perspective on narrative. In A. McCabe & C. Peterson (eds) *Developing Narrative Structure*. Hillsdale, NJ: Lawrence Erlbaum (pp. 1–26).

Giles, G.M. (1992). A neurofunctional approach to rehabilitation following severe brain injury. In N. Katz (ed.) *Cognitive Rehabilitation: Models for Intervention in Occupational Therapy*. Boston, MA: Andover Medical Publishers (pp. 195–218).

Goodman, G.S. & Haith, M.M. (1987). Memory development and neurophysiology: accomplishments and limitations. *Child Development*, **58**(3), 713–717.

Graf, P., Squire, L.R., & Mandler, G. (1984). The information that amnesic patients do not forget. *Journal of Experimental Psychology: Learning Memory and Cognition*, **10**, 164–178.

Greer, M.K., Lyons-Crews, M., Mauldin, L.B., & Brown, F.R. (1989). A case study of the cognitive and behavioral deficits of temporal lobe damage in herpes simplex encephalitis. *Journal of Autism and Developmental Disorders*, **19**(2), 317–326.

Harrington, D.L., Haaland, K.Y., Yeo, R.A., & Marder, E. (1990). Procedural memory in Parkinson's disease: impaired motor but not visuoperceptual learning. *Journal of Clinical and Experimental Neuropsychology*, **12**, 323–329.

Henderson, C.E. (1987). Activity and the regulation of neuronal growth factor metabolism. In J.-P. Changeuz & M. Konishi (eds) *The Neuronal and Molecular Bases of Learning*. New York: John Wiley (pp. 99–118).

Hicks, D. (1991). Kinds of narrative: genre skills among first graders from two communities. In A. McCabe & C. Peterson (eds) *Developing Narrative Structure*. Hillsdale, NJ: Lawrence Erlbaum (pp. 55–87).

Howard, L. & Polich, J. (1985). P300 Latency and Memory Span development. *Development Psychology*, **21**(2), 283–289.

Hudson, J.A. (1986). Memories are made of this: general event knowledge and the development of autobiographical memory. In K. Nelson (ed.) *Event Knowledge: Structure and Function in Development*. Hillsdale, NJ: Lawrence Erlbaum.

Jacobs, W.J. & Nadel, L. (1985). Stress-induced recovery of fears and phobias. *Psychological Review*, **92**, 512–531.

James, W.J. (1950). *The Principles of Psychology, Vol. 1*. New York: Dover.

Jannoun, L. & Chessels, J.M. (1987). Long-term psychological effects of childhood leukemia and its treatment. *Pediatric Hematology – Oncology*, **4**(4), 293–308.

Kail, R.V. (1989). *The Development of Memory in Children*, 2nd edn. New York: Freeman.

Kail, R. & Hagen, J.W. (1982). Memory in childhood. In B.B. Wolman, G. Stricker, S.J. Ellman, P. Kieth-Spiegel, & D.S. Palermo (eds) *Handbook of Developmental Psychology*. Englewood Cliffs, NJ: Prentice-Hall (pp. 350–366).

Kandel, E.R., Brunelli, M., Byrne, J., & Castellucci, V. (1983). A common presynaptic locus for the synaptic changes underlying short-term habituation and sensitization of the gill-withdrawn reflexes in Aplysia. *Cold Spring Harbor Symposium on Quantitative Biology*, **48**, 465–482.

Kapur, S., Craik, F.I.M., Tulving, E., Wilson, A.A., Houle, S. & Brown, G.M. (1994). Neuroanatomical correlates of encoding in episodic memory: levels of processing effect. *Proceedings of the National Academy of Science*, **91**, 2008–2011.

Kluft, R.P. (1985). Childhood multiple personality disorder: predictors, clinical findings, and treatment results. In R.P. Kluft (ed.) *Childhood Antecedents of Multiple Personality*. Washington, DC: American Psychiatric Press.

Kosslyn, S.M. & Koenig, O. (1993). *Wet Mind: The New Cognitive Neuroscience*. New York: Macmillan Free Press (pp. 341–400).

Lehmann, H.P., Bendebba, M., & DeAngelis, C. (1990). The consistency of young children's assessment of remembered painful events. *Development and Behavioral Pediatrics*, **11**, 128–134.

Leng, N.R. & Copello, A.G. (1990). Rehabilitation of memory after brain injury: is there an effective technique? *Clinical Rehabilitation*, **4**(1), 63–69.

Lesny, I., Nachtmann, M., Stehlick, A., Tomankova, A., & Zajidkova, J. (1990). Disorders of memory of motor sequences in cerebral palsied children. *Brain Development*, **12**(3), 339–341.

Levin, H.S., Goldstein, F.C., High, W.M., & Williams, D. (1988). Automatic and effortful processing after severe closed-head injury. *Brain and Cognition*, **7**, 283–297.

Levin, H.S., High, W.M. Jr., Weing-Cobbs, L., Fletcher, J.M., Eisenberg, H.M., Minere, M.E., & Goldstein, F.C. (1988). Memory functioning during the first year after closed head injury in children and adolescents. *Neurosurgery*, **6**(1), 1043–1052.

Liason, M.J. & Richman, L.C. (1987). The Continuous Performance Test in learning disabled and non disabled children. *Journal of Learning Disabilities*, **20**(10), 614–619.

Lindgren, S.D., Richman, L.C., & Liason, M.J. (1986). Memory processes in reading disability subtypes. *Developmental Neuropsychology*, **2**(3), 173–181.

Loftus, E.F. (1993). The reality of repressed memories. *American Psychologist*, **48**(5), 518–537.

Logiagian, E.L., Kaplan, R.F., & Steere, A.C. (1990). Chronic neurologic manifestations of Lyme disease. *New England Journal of Medicine*, **323**(21), 1438–1444.

Lorsbach, T.C., Sodoro, J.A., & Brown, J.S. (1992). The dissociation of repetition priming and recognition memory in language/learning disabled children. *Journal of Experimental Child Psychology*, **54**(2), 121–146.

Lynch, G. & Baudry, M. (1984). The biochemistry of memory: a new specific hypothesis. *Science*, **224**, 1057–1063.

Markowitsch, H.J., von Cramon, D.Y., Hofmann, E., Sick, D.C., & Kinzler, P. (1990). Verbal memory deterioration after unilateral infarct of the internal capsule in an adolescent. *Cortex*, **26**(4), 597–609.

Markowitsch, H.J. (1994). Anatomical basis of memory disorders. In M.S. Gazzaniga (ed.) *The Cognitive Neurosciences*. Cambridge, MA: MIT.

Mazziotta, J.C., Phelps, M.E., Carson, R.E., & Kuhl, D.E. (1982). Tomographic mapping of human cerebral metabolism: auditory stimulation. *Neurology*, **32**, 921–937.

McCabe, A., Capron, E., & Peterson, C. (1991). The voice of experience: the recall of early childhood and adolescent memories by young adults. In McCabe, A. & Peterson, C. (eds) *Developing Narrative Structure*. Hillsdale, NJ: Lawrence Erlbaum (pp. 137–173).

McKoon, G., Ratcliff, R., & Dell, G.S. (1986). A critical evaluation of the semantic-episodic distinction. *Journal of Experimental Psychology: Learning, Memory and Cognition*, **12**(3), 295–306.

Mishkin, M. & Appenzeller, T. (1987). The anatomy of memory. *Scientific American*, **256**, June, 62–71.

Mulhern, R.K., Wasserman, A.L., Fairclough, D., & Ochs, J. (1988). Memory function in disease-free survivors of childhood acute lymphocytic leukemia given CNS prophylaxis with or without 1,800 cGy cranial irradiation. *Journal of Clinical Oncology,* **6**(2), 315–320.

Neisser, U. (1988). New vistas in the study of memory. In U. Neisser & E. Winograd (eds) *Remembering Reconsidered: Ecological and Traditional Approaches to the Study of Memory.* New York: Cambridge University Press (pp. 1–10).

Nelson, C.A. (1994). Neural correlates of recognition memory in the first postnatal year. In Dawson, G. & Fischer, K.W. (eds) *Human Behavior and the Developing Brain.* New York: Guilford (pp. 269–313).

Nelson, K. (1986). Event knowledge and cognitive development. In K. Nelson, *Event Knowledge.* Hillsdale, NJ: Lawrence Erlbaum (pp. 231–248).

Nurcombe, B. (1986). The child as a witness: competency and credibility. *Journal of the American Academy of Child and Adolescent Psychiatry,* **27**, 473–480.

Ober, B.A., Reed, B.R., & Jagust, W.J. (1992). Neuroimaging and cognitive function. In D.I. Margolin (ed.) *Cognitive Neuropsychology in Clinical Practice.* New York: Oxford University Press (pp. 495–531).

Ofshe, R.J. (1992). Inadvertent hypnosis during interrogation: false confession due to dissociative state, misidentified multiple personality and the satanic cult hypothesis. *International Journal of Clinical and Experimental Hypnosis,* **40**, 125–156.

O'Hare, A.E., Aitken, K., & Eden, O.B. (1988). Computerized psychometry screening in long-term survivors of childhood acute lymphoblastic leukemia. *Pediatric Hematology – Oncology,* **5**(3), 197–208.

Ozonoff, S., Pennington, B.F., & Rogers, J.J. (1991a). Executive function deficits in high-functioning autistic children: relationship to theory of mind. *Journal of Child Psychology and Psychiatry,* **32**, 1081–1105.

Ozonoff, S., Rogers, J.J., & Pennington, B.F. (1991b). Asperger's syndrome: evidence of an empirical distinction from high-functioning autistic children. *Journal of Child Psychology and Psychiatry,* **32**, 1107–1122.

Paris, S.G. & Lindauer, B.K. (1982). The development of cognitive skills during childhood. In B.B. Wolman, G. Stricker, S.J. Ellman, P. Kieth-Spiegel, & D.S. Palermo (eds) *Handbook of Developmental Psychology.* Englewood Cliffs, NJ: Prentice-Hall (pp. 333–349).

Piaget, J. (1951). *Play, Dreams, and Imitation in Childhood.* New York: Norton.

Pillemer, D.B. & White, S.H. (1989). Childhood events recalled by children and adults. In H.W. Reese (ed.) *Advances in Child Development and Behavior.* New York: Academic Press (pp. 297–340).

Posner, M. (1978). *Chronometric Explorations of Mind.* Hillsdale, NJ: Lawrence Erlbaum.

Putnam, F.W. (1985). Dissociation as a response to extreme trauma. In R.P. Kluft (ed.) *Childhood Antecedents of Multiple Personality.* Washington, DC: American Psychiatric Press (pp. 65–98).

Quart, E.J., Buchtel, H.A., & Sarnaik, A.P. (1988). Long-lasting memory deficits in children recovered from Reye's syndrome. *Journal of Clinical Neuropsychology,* **10**(4), 409–420.

Raine, A., Hulme, C., Cadderton, H.J., & Baily, P. (1991). Verbal short-term memory span in speech-disordered children: implications for articulatory coding in short-term memory. *Child Development,* **62**(2), 415–423.

Reason, J. (1984). Absent-mindedness and cognitive control. In J.E. Harris & P.E. Morris (eds) *Everyday Memory Actions and Absent-mindedness*. London: Academic Press (pp. 113–132).

Saffran, E.M. (1990). Short-term memory impairment and language processing. In A. Caramazza (ed.) *Cognitive Neuropsychology and Neurolinguistics: Advances in Models of Cognitive Function and Impairment*. Hillsdale, NJ: Lawrence Erlbaum (pp. 137–168).

Schacter, D.L., McAndrews, M.P., & Moscovitch, M. (1988). Access to consciousness: dissociations between implicit and explicit knowledge in neuropsychological syndromes. In L. Weiskrantz (ed.) *Thought Without Language*. Oxford: Clarendon Press.

Schwartz, B.I., Rosse, R.B., & Deutsch, S.I. (1992). Toward a neuropsychology of memory in schizophrenia. *Psychopharmacology Bulletin*, **28**(4), 341–351.

Schwartz, R.H. (1991a). Heavy Marijuana use and recent memory impairment. *Psychiatric Annals*, **21**(2), 80–82.

Schwartz, R.H., Gruenewald, P.H., Klitzner, M., & Fedio, P. (1991b). Short-term memory impairment in cannabis-dependent adolescents. *American Journal of Diseases of Children*, **143**(10), 1214–1219.

Scoville, W.B. & Milner, B. (1957). Loss of recent memory after bilateral hippocampal lesions. *Journal of Neurology, Neurosurgery and Psychiatry*, **20**, 11–21.

Septien, L., Bourgeous, M., Altaba, A., Breno, M., Giroud, M., Dumas, R., & Nivelon, J.L. (1991). Multiple sclerosis in children: impact of memory disorders. *Archives Françaises de Pédiatrie*, **48**(4), 263–265.

Shaffer, D.R. (1993). Learning and information processing. In D.R. Schaffer (ed.) *Developmental Psychology*. Pacific Grove, CA: Brooks-Cole (pp. 301–310).

Shallice, T. (1972). Dual functions of consciousness. *Psychological Review*, **79**, 383–393.

Shelton, J.R., Martin, R.C., & Yaffee, L.S. (1992). Investigating a verbal short-term memory deficit and its consequences for language processing. In D.I. Margolin (ed.) *Cognitive Neuropsychology in Clinical Practice*. New York: Oxford University Press (pp. 131–167).

Sherry, D.F. & Schacter, D.L. (1987). The evolution of multiple memory systems. *Psychological Review*, **94**, 439–454.

Shiffrin, R.M. & Schneider, W. (1977). Controlled and automatic information processing: II Perceptual learning, automatic attending, and a general theory. *Psychological Review*, **84**, 127–190.

Shimamura, A.P. (1986). Priming effects in amnesia: evidence for a dissociable memory function. *Quarterly Journal of Experimental Psychology*, **38A**, 619–644.

Shimamura, A.P. & Squire, L.R. (1984). Paired-associate learning and priming effects in amnesia: a neuropsychological study. *Journal of Experimental Psychology: General*, **113**, 556–570.

Sodian, B. & Frith, U. (1992). Deception and sabotage in autistic, retarded and normal children. *Journal of Child Psychology and Psychiatry*, **33**, 591–605.

Sodian, B., Schneider, W., & Perlmutter, M. (1986). Recall, clustering and metamemory in young children. *Journal of Experimental and Child Psychology*, **41**, 395–410.

Squire, L.R. (1987). *Memory and the Brain*. New York: Oxford University Press.

Squire, L.R. & Cohen, N.J. (1984). Human memory and amnesia. In J. McGaugh, G. Lynch, & N. Weinberger (eds) *Proceedings of the Conference on the Neurobiology of Learning and Memory*. New York: Guilford Press (pp. 3–64).

Squire, L.R., Shimamura, A., & Graf, P. (1985). Independence of recognition memory and priming effects: a neuropsychological analysis. *Journal of Experimental Psychology: Learning Memory and Cognition*, **11**, 37–44.

Squire, L.R., Slater, P.C., & Miller, P.L. (1981). Retrograde amnesia and bilateral electroconvulsive therapy. *Archives of General Psychiatry*, **38**, 89–95.

Squire, L.R. & Zouzounis, J.A. (1988). Self-rating of memory dysfunction: different findings in depression and amnesia. *Journal of Clinical Experimental Neuropsychology*.

Squire, L.R., Knowlton, B., & Musen, G. (1993). The structure and organization of memory. *Annual Review of Psychology*, **44**, 453–495.

Steward, M.S. (1993). Understanding children's memories of medical procedures: "He didn't touch me and it didn't hurt!" In C.A. Nelson (ed.) *Memory and Affect in Development: The Minnesota Symposia on Child Psychology Vol. 26*. Hillsdale, NJ: Lawrence Erlbaum.

Steward, M.S., Steward. D.S., Joye, N., & Reinhart, M. (1991). Pain judgements by young children and medical staff. *Journal of Pain and Symptom Management*, **6**, 202.

Stollery, B.T., Banks, H.A., Broadbent, D.E., & Lee, W.R. (1989). Cognitive functioning in lead workers. *British Journal of Industrial Medicine*, **46**(10), 698–707.

Swanson, H.L. (1988). Memory subtypes in learning disabled readers. *Learning Disability Quarterly*, **11**(4), 342–357.

Tate, R.L., Fenelon, B., Manning, M.L., & Hunter, M. (1991). Patterns of neuro-psychological impairment after severe blunt head injury. *Journal of Nervous and Mental Disease*, **179**(3), 117–126.

Terr, L. (1988). What happens to early memories of trauma? A study of 20 children under age five at the time of documented traumatic events. *Journal of the American Academy of Child and Adolescent Psychiatry*, **27**, 96–104.

Terr, L. (1990). *Too Scared to Cry*. New York: Basic Books (pp. 168–188).

Terr, L. (1991). Childhood traumas: an outline and overview. *American Journal of Psychiatry*, **148**, 10–20.

Terr, L. (1994). *Unchained Memories: True Stories of Traumatic Memories, Lost and Found*. New York: Basic Books (pp. 1–30).

Tran-Dinh, Y.R., Mamo, H., Cervoni, J., & Saimot, A.C. (1990). Disturbances in the cerebral perfusion of human immune deficiency virus-1 seropositive asymptomatic subjects: a quantitative tomography study of 18 cases. *Journal of Nuclear Medicine*, **10**, 1601–1607.

Tulving, E. (1972). Episodic and semantic memory. In E. Tulving & W. Donaldson (eds) *Organization of Memory*. New York: Academic Press.

Tulving, E. (1984). Elements of episodic memory. *Behavioral and Brain Sciences*, **7**, 223–268.

Tulving, E. (1986). What kind of a hypothesis is the distinction between episodic and semantic memory? *Journal of Experimental Psychology: Learning, Memory and Cognition*, **12**(3), 307–311.

Tulving, E., Kapur, S., Markowitsch, H.J., Craik, F.I.M., Habib, R., & Houle, S. (1994). Neuroanatomical correlates of retrieval in episodic memory: auditory sentence recognition. In *Proceedings of the National Academy of Science*, **91**, 2012–2015.

Warrington, E.K. & Weiskrantz, L. (1974). The effect of prior learning on subsequent retention in amnesic patients. *Neuropsychologica*, **12**, 419–428.

Weiskrantz, L. (1978). A comparison of hippocampal pathology in man and other animals. In *Functions of the Septo-hippocampal System*. Ciba Foundation Symposium, **58**, 373–387.

Weiskrantz, L. (1987). Neuroanatomy of memory and amnesia: a case for multiple memory systems. *Human Neurobiology*, **6**, 93–105.

Wong, V.C., Wong, M.T., Ng, T.H., Chang, C.M., & Fung, C.F. (1991). Unusual case of Kluver Bucy syndrome in a Chinese boy. *Pediatric Neurology*, **7**(5), 385–388.

Wood, K.M. & Richman, L.C. (1988). Developmental trends within memory-deficit reading-disability subtypes. *Developmental Neuropsychology*, **4**(4), 261–274.

Wright, D.B. (1993). Misinformation and warnings in eyewitness testimony: a new testing procedure to differentiate explanations. *Memory*, **1**(2), 153–166.

17 Interaction between language and cognition: evidence from Williams syndrome

MICHAEL ROSSEN, EDWARD S. KLIMA, URSULA BELLUGI,
AMY BIHRLE, AND WENDY JONES

INTRODUCTION

In describing her future aspirations, Crystal, a 16-year-old adolescent, states: "You're looking at a professional book writer. My books will be filled with drama, action, and excitement. And everyone will want to read them. I'm going to write books, page after page, stack after stack . . . I'll start on Monday." Crystal describes a meal as "a scrumptious buffet," an older friend as "quite elegant," and her boyfriend as "my sweet petunia"; when asked if someone could borrow her watch, she replies "My watch is always available for service." Crystal can spontaneously create original stories – she weaves a tale of a chocolate princess who changes the sun color to save the chocolate world from melting; she recounts with detail a dream in which an alien from a different planet emerges from a television. Her creativity extends to music; she has composed the lyrics to a love song.

In view of her facility with language, proclivity for flowery, descriptive terms, and professed focus on drama and action, her aspiration may seem plausible; but in fact, Crystal has an IQ of 49, with an IQ equivalent age of 8 years. At the age of 16, she fails all Piagetian seriation and conservation tasks (milestones normally attained in the age range of 7 to 9 years); has reading, writing and math skills comparable to those of a first or second grader, demonstrates visuospatial abilities of a 5-year-old, and requires a babysitter for supervision.

Crystal has Williams syndrome (WMS), a rare (1 in 25,000) genetically based neurodevelopmental disorder involving a specific heart defect, characteristic facies and other dysmorphic traits, and a distinctive profile of dissociations of higher cortical functioning. Most prominently, a disparity between preserved linguistic abilities and gravely impoverished nonlinguistic cognitive functioning is *characteristic* of WMS, and forms the substrate for the studies discussed in this chapter. Our interest in WMS lies in the exploration of the boundaries between language and nonlinguistic cognition that are laid open for study by this dissociation.

Much of the data that we have gathered on WMS, from spontaneous and structured language samples as well as from more specifically targeted experimental measures, suggest that a characteristic anomaly exists in the lexical semantic system of WMS individuals. After reviewing the profile of WMS across cognitive domains, this paper presents results from a set of studies with adolescents with WMS on semantics-related tasks.

The relationship between language structure and other aspects of cognitive functions remains a strongly debated theoretical issue, as empirical evidence is hard to gather. In particular, study of the extent to which language ability is mediated by language-specific processes is hindered by the close coupling of language and cognition in the general population. WMS, in which linguistic functioning is largely spared despite unquestionable mental retardation, provides a rare and powerful opportunity to observe the workings of language disengaged to a remarkable extent from the workings of other aspects of cognition.

SUBJECTS

Through a coordinated program of studies of over 200 subjects with WMS, we have been able to develop a characterization of the phenotype of WMS across cognitive domains and at the levels of brain structure and brain function. Subjects are tested across an array of measures designed to probe aspects of higher cognitive functioning including problem solving skills, visuospatial abilities, memory, and linguistic abilities. In addition, subjects of sufficient developmental maturity participate in electrophysiological studies of language-related brain function and MRI studies of brain structure. The WMS profile on all of these measures is contrasted with normal control subjects and subjects of another developmental disorder, Down syndrome (DNS: trisomy 21), where matching is obtained in terms of chronological and mental age, IQ, and socioeconomic background.

WMS was identified following a clinical study by J.C.P. Williams and his colleagues, who described four patients with supravalvular aortic stenosis (SVAS: a narrowing of the aorta) in association with "mental retardation" and a peculiar facial appearance that is often referred to as "elfin-like" or "pixie-like" (Williams, Barratt-Boyes, & Lowe, 1961). Typical facial features include medial eyebrow flare, depressed nasal bridge with anteverted nares, thick lips with an open mouth posture, and a stellate pattern in the iris (for blue eyes) (Jones & Smith, 1975). Vascular disorders, including systemic hypertension, are also associated with WMS (Hallidie-Smith & Karas, 1988). Typical adolescents with WMS are shown in Figure 17.1.

Other clinical features frequently cited include sleeping and eating disturbances, hyperacusis, and social disinhibition (Arnold, Yule, & Martin, 1985; Meyerson & Frank, 1987; Udwin, Yule, & Martin, 1987; Klein et al., 1990; Reilly, Klima, & Bellugi, 1990; Harrison, Reilly, & Klima, 1994). Infantile Hypercalcemia was associated with WMS in 1963 (Black & Bonham Carter, 1963) and a recent study has demonstrated that WMS subjects have

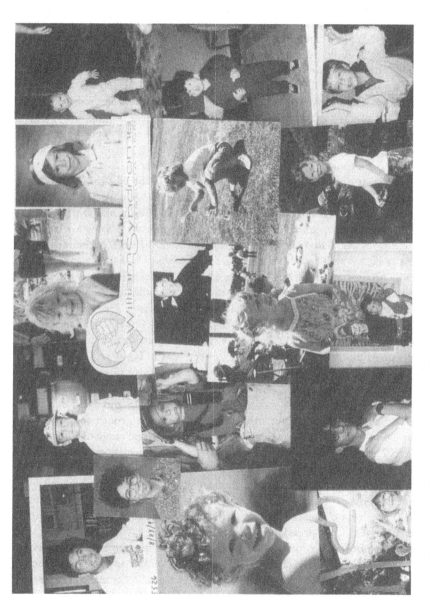

Figure 17.1. Pictures of subjects with WMS. Note that there are characteristic facial features for WMS.

abnormalities in both calcium and calcitonin metabolism (Culler, Jones, & Deftos, 1985). A pleasing gregarious friendlinesss typically marks the social behavior of WMS, although maladaptive social behavior can also result (Tomc, Williamson, & Pauli, 1990). In general Semel & Rosner (in press) is a good reference on the clinical and educational perspectives of WMS behavior.

Although WMS is predominantly sporadic in origin, a familial study in 1993 of three families, including one instance of father to son transmission, provided initial evidence of genetic etiology suggesting autosomal dominant transmission (Morris, Thomas, & Greenberg, 1993). More recently still, the application of fluorescent in situ hybridization techniques has revealed not only that WMS has a genetically based etiology, but that the preponderance of patients clinically diagnosed as having WMS possess a very specific genetic defect, a hemizygous microdeletion located on the long arm of chromosome 7 (7q11.23) that includes the gene for elastin (Ewart et al., 1993).

Our present discussion will focus on matched groups of WMS and DNS adolescents. All the subjects with WMS discussed in this article have been diagnosed by a medical geneticist as having WMS. Additionally, they have passed a minimum threshold for presentation of common medical and physical characteristics associated with WMS in medical studies (Jones & Smith, 1975; Morris et al., 1988). The DNS subjects are all diagnosed by karyotype analysis. We will discuss in detail results from six WMS adolescents and six DNS adolescents between the ages of 10 and 18 years. We will also discuss "within WMS" studies using larger groups of WMS adolescents. The "six and six" WMS and DNS groups are matched both in mean chronological age (CA) (WMS: 14.2 y; SD = 2.7; DNS: 13.7 y; SD = 2.9) and general intelligence as measured by WISC-R (Wechsler, 1974) (WMS: IQ = 50.8, SD = 5.8; equivalent test age (TA) = 7.1 y, SD = 0.7. DNS: IQ = 48.7, SD = 8.8, TA = 6.7 y, SD = 0.7).

Our subjects were chosen from a larger pool of WMS and DNS subjects that we have tested to obtain strict matching between groups (on age and IQ) and on the basis of their having participated in a broad range of laboratory studies. These have included the measures of lexical semantics that are the focus of this chapter, and also include measures of other language skills and measures of general intelligence, problem solving, and spatial cognition relevant to the overall WMS neurocognitive profile reviewed below and reported in detail elsewhere (Bellugi et al., 1992; Bellugi, Wang, & Jernigan, 1994; Wang et al., in press).

We have not found room to detail aspects of our three-dimensional in vivo MRI imaging studies which have suggested that WMS and DNS are each associated with a distinctive neuromorphologic profile. Whereas total cerebral volume is equally decreased in both syndromes, in WMS there is proportional preservation of neocerebellum, of temporal limbic areas, and perhaps also of anterior neocortex. In DNS, the volumes of the thalamus and of the lenticular nuclei are better preserved than in WMS. The distinct brain morphological stamp of WMS that is emerging may provide correlates for studies reported on in this chapter (Jernigan & Bellugi, 1990; Wang et al., 1992; Jernigan et al., 1993; Jernigan & Bellugi, 1994; Jones et al., 1995; Rossen et al., 1995).

General cognitive impairment

Because of the extent of language preservation typically found in adolescents with WMS, an observer of the casual conversation of a WMS adolescent could conceivably come to doubt that significant cognitive deficit – mental retardation – is a primary characteristic of WMS. For this reason alone one does well to re-emphasize the severity of impoverishment that we find in WMS throughout the subdomains of nonlinguistic cognition, including spatial cognition, analogical reasoning, problem-solving ability, and general cultural knowledge.

Full Scale IQ scores in WMS have been observed to fall predominantly within the mild to moderate mentally retarded range, from studies in our own laboratory and elsewhere (Bennett, LaVeck, & Sells, 1978; Arnold, Yule, & Martin, 1985). Even on the "verbal" section of the WISC-R, the performance of the WMS cohort attests to the cognitive limitations characteristic of WMS. For example, on the Similarities subtest of the WISC-R, when asked how beer and wine are alike, adolescent WMS subjects respond, "they both can fizz," "they both have screw tops," "they're both yellow," omitting that both are drinks. Similarly, when asked how a telephone and radio are alike, our subjects focus on similarities such as the fact that both devices have dials or speakers. The vocabulary subtest of the WISC-R highlights similar deficits in abilities of our WMS subjects. Although they produce significantly more relevant descriptions when presented with a target word than their DNS counterparts, WMS and DNS *scores* were not significantly different: WMS subjects do not seem to have the requisite cognitive (metalinguistic) ability to cast a description as a well-formed definition. In general on these two subtests, the WMS adolescents display considerable verbal facility, but typically focus on superficial likeness or scripts of personal experience, reflecting undeveloped conceptualization (Bellugi et al., 1988).

General problem solving impairment is severe in both the WMS and DNS populations (Bellugi et al., 1988). Both subject cohorts fail all Piagetian seriation and conservation tasks. Both cohorts also perform at the first grade level, on the average, on the WRAT-R sub-test for arithmetic. On the Reitan Indiana Category Test, a nonverbal test for analogical reasoning for 8 to 11-year-olds, both cohorts barely score in the normal range (i.e., not brain-damaged) according to norms for 8-year-olds, consistent with their WISC-R age equivalents.

Knowledge of general facts (as assessed by the Information subtest of the WISC-R) is also deficient in WMS and DNS. For example, five of the six subjects in the basic WMS cohort and all DNS subjects did not know common facts such as who discovered America and in what direction the sun sets, facts that an average 9 or 10-year-old would know.[1] None of the subjects could answer more difficult items (e.g., who invented the electric light bulb). Moreover, the WMS show an inability to appreciate social mores and exercise proper judgment. For example, when asked why we must put stamps on letters (Comprehension subtest of WISC-R), none of the adolescent WMS or DNS subjects gave a correct answer.

THE WMS PROFILE OF DISSOCIATIONS: AN OVERVIEW

Early reports on language functioning in WMS relied strongly on standardized measures, such as intelligence tests, which probe an amalgamation of diverse abilities (Kataria, Goldstein, & Kushnick, 1984; Udwin, Yule, & Martin, 1986; Meyerson & Frank, 1987; MacDonald & Roy, 1988). These studies produced inconsistent findings with respect to language.

Language itself is not a unitary phenomenon; rather, it is composed of distinct subcomponents whose separate workings can be seen most clearly with focused probes of specific linguistic processes. Our approach is to look beyond standard summary scores to critically assess performance on both standard tests and on finely-focused experimental probes to arrive at more precise characterizations of spared and impaired components of linguistic and nonlinguistic functioning.

Preserved grammar in Williams syndrome

The grammatical facility of WMS subjects, and their difference from matched DNS subjects, is apparent on formal tests of sentence comprehension and production (Bellugi et al., 1992). On a set of six such tasks developed to probe language development (Bellugi & Klima, 1966; Bellugi, 1971), adolescents with WMS are significantly better than their counterparts with DNS, and usually perform at or close to ceiling (Figure 17.2).[2] For example,

---

[1] Test item equivalent age assessed roughly from WISC-R equivalent test age table (Wechsler, 1974), assuming an ordering by increasing difficulty in test items.
[2] In the "Passives" test a subject must choose a picture to point to based on information within a passive construct in a sentence spoken by the experimenter. The "Negation" test requires the subject to transform a sentence spoken by the experimenter to an equivalent negative form. In the "Sentence Correction" test, each sentence spoken by the experimenter is grammatically incorrect in one of a variety of ways, and the subject must repeat the sentence with the grammatical violation corrected. For the sentence completion task, the subject must have competence in the same class of grammatical constructs to complete each partial sentence spoken by the experimenter. The "Conditionals: grammar" test follows a sentence completion format, but specifically probes the subjects ability to produce conditional forms. The "Conditionals: content" test probes a subject's ability to understand the meaning of sentences containing a conditional form. "Tag Questions" elicits the formation at the end of a sentence of common, but grammatically complex, "Tag" constructs such as "don't you?" or "is it?"

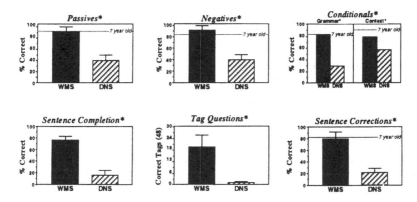

Figure 17.2. Spared linguistic processing in Williams syndrome vs. Down syndrome adolescents. WMS adolescents, unlike DNS adolescents, show preservation of production and comprehension of basic grammatical forms. *All tests significant, p < 0.01.

the WMS subjects, and not the DNS subjects, demonstrate an ability to comprehend and use full reversible passives appropriately. Some WMS subjects also can detect and correct anomalies in sentence syntax. This ability to reflect upon grammatical form suggests linguistic sophistication beyond the developmental level required for comprehension and production of basic grammatical constructions.

Linguistic affect and narrative in WMS

The grammar competence, rich vocabulary, relevant (if not exaggerated) affect, and coherent, fluent flow of conversation typical of WMS adolescents are observable on an experimental task we use where the subject is asked to tell a story from a picture book without words (Bamberg, 1987; Reilly et al., 1990). The picture book depicts a plot about a boy (with a dog) losing, looking for, and finding a runaway pet frog (Mayer, 1969). Figure 17.3 provides excerpts (from the end of transcript) from WMS subjects and matched DNS subjects. Among the complex grammatical constructions to be found in WMS narratives, but not DNS narratives, are subordinate clauses and appropriate use of conditional tense. In contrast, DNS narratives contain many grammatical errors and involve mostly simple grammatical constructions.

Exuberant and abundant use of linguistically encoded affect also seems to be a distinctive trait of WMS adolescents. WMS narratives include frequent comments on the affective state of characters ("And ah! he was amazed"), as well as the use of dramatic devices such as *sound effects* ("And BOOM, millions of bees came out"), *character speech*, and *audience hookers* ("Guess what happened next?" and "Suddenly"), as well as *embellishments* ("Lo and behold, they found him with a lady"). Both affective prosody and linguistically

Examples from Williams Syndrome	Examples from Down Syndrome
Age 13: And he was looking for the frog. What do you know? The frog family! Two lovers. And they were looking. And then he was happy 'cause they had a big family. And said "good bye" and so did the frogs. "Ribbit."	**Age 13:** There you are. Little frog. There another little frog. They in that . . . water thing. That's it. Frog right there. In a hand [cups right hand].
Age 17: They looked over the dog and him looked over. Suddenly when they found the frogs . . . there were two frogs, one female and one male frog. There was a whole family of frogs. Little ones . . . there was a mother and a father. And, ah, he was amazed. Then he, then he takes one of the little frogs home. So when the frog grows up . . . it will be his frog. The frog went back home with them. And the boy said "good bye, Mrs. Frog . . . good bye, Mr. Frog . . . good bye, many frogs. I might see you again if I come around again. Thank you Mr. Frog and Mrs. Frog, for letting me have one of you baby frogs to remember him." The end of the story.	**Age 18:** They're hiding; see the frogs . . . the baby frogs. Uh, the boy, and, and the dog saw the frogs. The frog's got babies. The boy saw the . . . no, the boy say good bye.

Figure 17.3. Excerpts from Frog story narratives by WMS and DNS adolescents.

encoded affective devices are used by these WMS subjects to a degree that is not only significantly greater than DNS subjects, but is also significantly more than comparable normal control subjects matched for mental age. We also found that some of these WMS subjects use the same level of expressivity regardless of how many times or to whom they told the story.

Further clues to the special social "personality" that may be characteristic of WMS come from several sources. One quantifiable feature is the ease and rapidity with which subjects initiate linguistic interactions. WMS subjects that come into our lab are often immediately friendly, running up to the examiner or to strangers, requiring little no "warm up" period. This behavior is unlike the matched DNS subjects. It is also unlike normal children in the same situation (Kagan, 1989). In addition, during biographical interviews, some WMS subjects manifest linguistic sociability by turning the tables and asking the experimenter questions, shifting the focus from the subject's life and experiences to those of the interviewer (Harrison et al., 1994; Reilly, Harrison, & Klima, 1994). In these respects, the sociability and extreme expressivity shown by WMS subjects may turn out to be a characteristic of the syndrome.

Equivalent global language delay in WMS and DNS toddlers

In contrast with the marked differences in language ability between WMS and DNS in studies with adolescents, evidence is accumulating that WMS and DNS arise from equivalent, global developmental delay. When CA-matched WMS and DNS toddlers (mean CA = 33 months) are compared using a parental questionnaire study of language development (Fenson et al., 1993), no difference in word production levels is found (Singer, Goodman, & Bellugi, 1992; Singer et al., in press). Only with older children do differences between WMS and DNS counterparts become apparent in this study. At a mean CA of 47 months, word production levels in WMS exceed those in CA-matched DNS children; moreover, when a match is made based on word production level, the WMS children show significant advantages in developmental measures of grammatical development including "mean length of utterance," number of auxiliary verb types produced, and sentence complexity.

Well-focused studies may in the future differentiate the two groups at increasingly early ages. Language differences between WMS and DNS at ages as early as 20 to 40 months have been observed through separate analyses of the language-related and nonlanguage-related portions of the standardized Mental Scales of Bayley (Bayley, 1969; Mervis & Bertrand, 1992; Mervis & Bertrand, 1994). When matched WMS and DNS toddlers are considered, the WMS toddlers perform better on the language-related items and the DNS toddlers on the nonlanguage-related items. Nevertheless, evidence remains that language is delayed in both populations, and it is only when language begins to develop that differences between the mental profiles of the two populations becomes apparent (Jones, Rossen, & Bellugi, 1994).

Visual based processing: a characteristic mode of failure

In contrast to their remarkable linguistic ability, unquestionable deficit is evident in individuals with WMS in the domain of visuospatial cognition. A WMS adolescent is characteristically unable to perceive gross distinctions in orientation or to draw or copy simple stick figures. For example, on a test of visuo-motor integration (Beery, 1982), WMS subjects score worse than their matched DNS counterparts and significantly below their WISC-R mental age level.

Furthermore, the characteristic WMS visuospatial deficit appears to be a highly specific one in which there is selective attention to details of a configuration at the expense of the whole. Moreover, DNS results in the opposite profile. The Block Design subtest of the WISC-R provides a

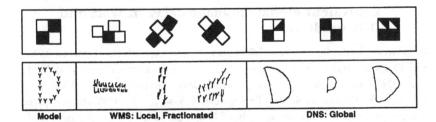

Figure 17.4. Hierarchical processing: distinct modes of failure. In block design (above)
and hierarchical drawing (below), WMS subjects show fractionated, local
processing, while DNS subjects show more global processing.

good example. The groups score equally poorly but fail in different ways.
DNS subjects are typically able to construct the overall configuration of
blocks (a simple 2 × 2 grid of blocks forming a square or diamond
shape), although they frequently make errors on internal design. In contrast,
not only do WMS subjects fail to reproduce internal details of a design,
they often cannot even construct the correct global organization. Blocks
are instead placed at odd angles to each other in a disjointed array
(Figure 17.4).

Further data characterizing the distinct modes of visuospatial deficit of
WMS and DNS comes from our experimental examination of processing of
hierarchical stimuli: stimuli in which local features are nested within a single
global feature (e.g., a large "D" made of small "L"s). In the copying
condition shown in Figure 17.4, the drawings of the DNS adolescents show
only the global level. The drawings of the WMS adolescents show precisely
the opposite failing: the local features are identifiable but their arrangement
on the page in no way resembles the global model.

Face processing: remarkable sparing in WMS

While the preponderance of WMS subjects show a severe spatial cognitive
deficit, most of these same individuals exhibit a remarkable ability in processing, discriminating, and remembering faces (Bellugi et al., 1988; Rossen
et al., 1994, 1995). This stands in intriguing contrast to their profound
impairment in other visually based cognitive tasks. This nested dissociation
may be observed in our results using two contrasting experimental probes of
visual based discrimination, one involving discrimination of faces (Benton
et al., 1978) and the other involving discrimination of oriented lines (Benton
et al., 1983). On the line orientation task, all subjects are in the range
considered "severely deficient" for adults; most WMS and DNS could not
even pass the pre-test. However, WMS (but not DNS) demonstrated a
dramatic ability to discriminate unfamiliar faces in pictures under different
angles and lighting conditions. On this task, WMS subjects performed

significantly better than DNS matches, and were as good as chronological-age matched normals; some WMS children as young as six years of age performed at the mean level for normal *adult* controls (Jones et al., 1993).

Unusually good WMS performance in face processing extends to other test paradigms. On a recognition memory test for faces (Warrington, 1984), WMS subjects performed significantly better than their DNS counterparts. Although norms are not available for adolescent ages, the performance of WMS adolescents approached the level for normal adult performance. This face memory ability in WMS has also been documented in other laboratories (Udwin & Yule, 1991). Yet another face processing paradigm in which a WMS advantage relative to DNS is apparent is The Mooney Face Classification test (Mooney, 1957). This task requires strong skills in contour closure and foreground/background segregation, skills in which WMS subjects show marked deficiencies. Nevertheless, WMS subjects score better on the Mooney Faces task than their DNS counterparts, despite the difficulties imparted by the visual closure processing demands (Bellugi et al., 1994). These findings together suggest that preservation of face processing in WMS is a general phenomenon observable across a varied array of paradigms probing multiple modes of processing.

Lexical semantics in WMS: a subdomain of preservation and anomaly

Lexical semantics in WMS presents a fascinating spectrum of results, indicating, at first glance, remarkable integrity of function, but under closer scrutiny, undeniable evidence of anomalous function. The anomalous lexical semantics profile of WMS is characteristically manifested by production of words that strike the listener as subtly "unusual" – although not always wrong in an obvious way – in the context of the conversation. Inappropriate lexical substitutions in frozen phrases, such as "He cried his eyeballs out," although lexically reasonable, hint at this type of dysfunction. Before addressing evidence on anomalous processing, however, we first discuss the evidence for the more salient characteristic of the WMS profile in lexical semantics: a remarkable wealth of word knowledge.

Word knowledge in WMS

WMS adolescents, unlike matched DNS adolescents, provide evidence of word knowledge at an age-equivalent level distinctly above the level that would be predicted by mental age. Examples can be startling: WMS individuals typically fail conservation tasks and cannot add two columns of numbers but yet can correctly pick out from an array the correct pictures relating to words denoting abstract concepts such as "abrasive" or "solemn." Quantitative data on the superior word knowledge of WMS adolescents,

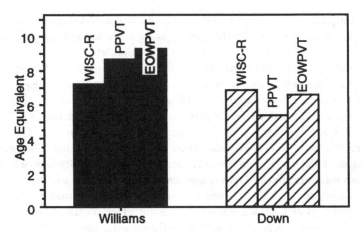

Figure 17.5. Relative preservation of word knowledge in Williams syndrome. WMS mental age on tests of word knowledge is higher than overall (WISC-R) mental age.

relative to DNS adolescents, come from tests of pure comprehension of meanings of words. We mention results from two such tests: (1) the Peabody Picture Vocabulary Test (PPVT-R) [48], a test of *receptive* word knowledge involving picture pointing; and (2) the Gardner Expressive One Word Vocabulary Test (EOWPVT) [55], a test of *experience* word knowledge involving naming of pictures (Figure 17.5). DNS adolescents that we have tested obtain word knowledge scores that trend below their WISC-R mental age, with the PPVT-R to WISC-R difference being significant at the (p = 0.05) level.

WMS adolescents, on the other hand, score significantly higher on word knowledge measures than on WISC-R (p < 0.05) and dramatically better than their DNS counterparts. Not only are PPVT-R scores of WMS adolescents significantly higher than their WISC-R scores; in addition, the correlation of PPVT-R to WISC-R in WMS is negligible: (r = 0.07) in contrast to our DNS subjects (r = 0.42) and in contrast to studies from the literature of normals and individuals with non-specific mental retardation (Altepeter & Handal, 1986; Mangiaracina & Simon, 1986; Altepeter & Johnson, 1989).

The relative preservation of word knowledge in WMS shown on these measures does, however, seem subject to delay. The results in Figure 17.5 involve subjects between the ages of 11 years and 19 years. Results from other laboratories suggest that differences between PPVT-R and WISC-R do not exist in pre-adolescent Italian WMS children (Volterra et al., 1994). In a cross-sectional study of a large population of individuals with WMS and DNS, we found that performance difference on PPVT-R between WMS and DNS subjects only begins to emerge in early adolescence (Jones et al., 1993).

The absence of evidence of "word finding difficulty" in either population is notable, such as would be evidenced by a depression of expressive word knowledge (EOWPVT) relative to receptive word knowledge (PPVT-R). In fact, the data show both WMS and DNS subjects trending higher on expressive word knowledge tests. One explanation is that PPVT-R, because it involves distractors pictures, probes the limits of the *specificity* with which a word is understood more explicitly than do expressive tests where no distractor stimuli are involved.

In this context, we may speculate that the above data on WMS suggests that words are learned readily by WMS individuals, but with a subtle *lack of specificity*. If true, this lack of specificity could conceivably be connected with several other characteristics of WMS: (1) production of "unexpected" (but in-category) words in fluency tests and in conversation; (2) unusual processing of the alternate meanings of homonyms; and (3) evidence of anomalous processing in electrophysiological (ERP) data from WMS subjects that are listening to sentences with "unexpected" words. These intriguing possibilities are pursued further below.

Preserved production within elementary categories

Typical WMS adolescents display a rich vocabulary and a fluent flow of speech in free conservation. These characteristics provide perhaps the most salient initial evidence of the unexpected preservations in WMS of semantic knowledge and of the ability to access semantic knowledge. Category production paradigms provide good initial experimental tools for revealing levels of fluency and command of semantic categories. The particular task we discuss requires a subject to generate verbally as many exemplars as possible in 60 seconds in each of two particular semantic categories (animals and food). Norms for this task are available (Semel & Wiig, 1986).

The WMS cohort produces significantly more in-category items (excluding repetitions) than the DNS cohort for each of these measures, with results significant at the (p < 0.01) level (Figure 17.6a). Additionally, while the DNS results are comparable to scores of *mental* age-matched normals, the WMS results are indistinguishable from standardized norms for their *chronological* age. This is relevant evidence against a hypothesis of general word finding difficulty being characteristic of the lexical semantic profile in the WMS population.

There is evidence for an age effect in WMS on this fluency task, as there is for the word knowledge measures discussed above. Recently, a study of category production using the "animals" category was conducted with younger groups of WMS and DNS subjects than we have been discussing. The study, which compared 10 WMS subjects 9 to 11 years in age, with CA- and MA-Matched DNS subjects (Scott et al., 1994), found no significant differences between WMS and DNS on the number of correct exemplars

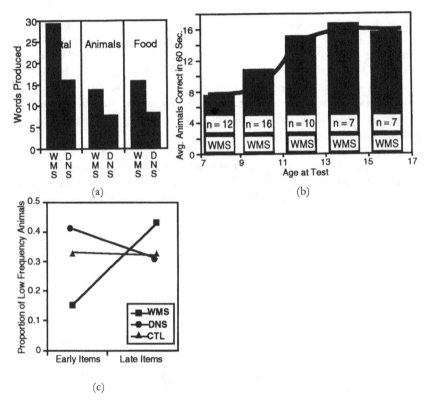

(a)

(b)

(c)

Figure 17.6. Category production in Williams syndrome and Down syndrome. (a) WMS subjects name many more category exemplars than subjects with DNS. (b) Fluency on this task increases dramatically in WMS around early adolescence. (c) WMS subjects also produce more low frequency exemplars late in the trial, relative to DNS or normal controls.

produced. It should be noted that the Scott et al. experiment did not employ a time limit, and so did not test fluency in the same way as ours does, which had a 60-second time limit. Nevertheless, it provides important evidence of an apparent lack of difference in category production between WMS and DNS at early ages. Figure 17.6b shows our own results from a study of 52 WMS subjects over a range of ages on our 60-second category production task with "animals" as the category. A sharp rise in production levels is apparent at 11 years of age. These results are consistent with the Scott et al. study; together the studies complement and extend our findings – that WMS language ability becomes evident after initial delay – to multiple paradigms probing different aspects of lexical semantics.

The atypicality of many of the responses by the WMS group is perhaps more remarkable than the quantity of responses. Example animal category responses include "unicorn," "pteranodon," "brontosaurus," "yak," "ibex," "water buffalo," "sea lion," "saber-tooth tiger," and "vulture." Unusual food exemplars from WMS subjects included "teriyaki," "pumpkin pie," and "chop suey." In pilot results with "birds" as the category, they included such responses as "shriek," "golden eagle," "blue heron," "spear hawk," "kite," "vulture," and "cockatoo." The unusualness lies at least partly in the high specificity of the exemplar in addition to its lack of typicality. This is taken up again below in the context of WMS language production in spontaneous speech.

As an initial measure of unusualness of the WMS productions, we have used a standardized empirical estimate of word frequency per million tokens in grade school text books (Carroll, Davies, & Richman, 1971). A cutoff value of 10 occurrences per million tokens was arbitrarily chosen to divide the responses within the "animal category" condition into high frequency words and low frequency words.[3] Nine 10 to 11-year-old normal subjects were also tested for this portion of the study. No significant differences were found among WMS, DNS, and normals on total production of low frequency exemplars.[4] However, significant (p < 0.014) differences were found *late in the trial* when a median split is performed allowing separate examination of the proportion of low-frequency items early (first seven exemplars) and late (after first seven exemplars) in a trial.[5] This interaction effect, as shown in Figure 17.6c, seems to reflect a tendency of WMS subjects to produce more low-frequency exemplars late in the trial, relative to DNS subjects and normals.

Why might this effect show up preferentially late in a trial? One speculative explanation is that the additional processing load late in the trial may be sufficient to uncover a subtle imbalance in interaction among excitatory and inhibitory effects in lexical semantic processing necessary to produce appropriate words and avoid repetitions and out-of-category responses. Being subtle, the imbalance results in production of unusual, rather than wrong, exemplars. Consistent with this line of reasoning is our observation that some WMS adolescents tend to produce exemplars in high speed bursts, in one case with 14 (correct) exemplars produced at four words per second. This trait was not at all apparent in the DNS subjects, and our informal observation suggests that even normal subjects do not tend to have such high frequency,

---

[3] By our definition (> 10 occurrences per one million words in corpus), high frequency words correspond, roughly, to the 5100 most frequent words in the total corpus of 86,741 words. Of the animal word types catalogued during scoring of all cohorts, 84 out of 142 were low frequency.
[4] Overall differences were significant in an earlier study, with WMS having more low frequency exemplars than DNS. Subjects were slightly older and 10 WMS and 10 DNS subjects were studied (Bellugi et al., 1994).
[5] This is roughly half the mean production for both WMS and the nine 10 to 11-year-old normal subjects who we tested for this portion of the study. Note that use of proportional production is especially important, since the DNS cohort produce many fewer late trial exemplars than do the WMS cohort or the CTL cohort. Only data from subjects producing more than seven words in the animal category were considered in this part of the analysis. WMS and DNS subjects were re-tested in the animal category, and the data from the session with highest production were used in the analysis.

prolonged bursts of responses. If we assume that response rate is normally controlled by a balance of excitatory and inhibitory activation, then these word bursts suggest some combination of increased excitation and/or anomalously low inhibition within the lexicon.

Homonyms and lexical ambiguity

Further data suggesting anomalous lexical semantics comes from our preliminary results in studies involving homonyms. Our homonyms battery examines relative salience of primary (high frequency) and secondary (low frequency) meanings of homonyms (Bihrle, Rossen, & Bellugi, 1992). We constructed a list of 22 homonyms, word forms with the same pronunciation but two distinct meanings. Each homonym was chosen so that one meaning (the primary meaning) was more prevalent than the other meaning (the secondary meaning), according to comprehensive norms for homonym word association by college students (Perfetti, Lindsey, & Garson, 1971).[6] A *word triad* was then constructed for each homonym, consisting of the homonym itself, a word related to the primary meaning and a word related to the secondary meaning. The word associated with the primary meaning was required to be a higher frequency associate of the homonym than the word associated with the secondary meaning, again according to the existing norms. An example triad is: "FALL – DOWN – AUTUMN." "Fall," the homonym, has a primary meaning relating to descent, for which "down" is an associate. The secondary meaning relates to seasons, and "autumn" is one of its associates. Words related to "descent" are associated with "fall" 1.7 more frequently than are words related to "seasons." "Down" is specifically associated with "fall" 1.2 more frequently than "autumn" is associated with "fall."

Three separate subtasks are used to assess how subjects understood the homonyms: free association, similarity judgment, and definitions. In the free association task, the homonyms are read to the subject in a prerandomized order, and the subject is asked for the first word that comes to mind after hearing each stimulus word. This task condition is similar to the task used to construct the homonym association norms. In the similarity judgment subtask, each word triad is read to the subject. The subject is asked to repeat the three words and "pick which 2 go best together." Both item order and triad word order within item were pre-randomized. As an example, the subject hears: "BANK – RIVER – MONEY." After repeating the three words, the subject might say: "RIVER – BANK," indicating the two words the subject thinks go together best. The homonym definition subtask elicits references

---

[6] Many homonyms have more than two senses. The stimuli for the present experiment were chosen so that the first two meanings dominated subjects' associations in the norming trials in Perfetti et al. (1971).

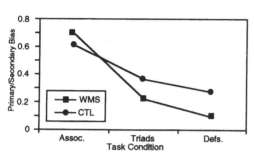

Meanings of homonyms

E: What does "nuts" mean?
DNS: "We crack nuts." (Probe)
"We eat nuts."
WMS: "There are two kinds of nuts, a peanut, and nuts and bolts."

E: What does "club" mean?
DNS: "Go to a club." (Probe)
"I'm in the key club."
WMS: "A secret kind of club, and a club with spurs – those pointy things for killing animals."

Figure 17.7. Anomalous semantic organization in Williams syndrome. On the homonyms battery, WMS subjects are no different from normals in free association, but are increasingly more secondary on the triads and definitions subtasks.

to alternate homonym senses with the cue: "tell me everything you know about what 'X' (homonym probe) means." If references to both meanings are not spontaneously produced, a second meaning is probed for: "Can you tell me anything else that 'X' means?" The definitions subtask allows observation of the relative ease of access of alternate homonym senses in an expressive task (unlike the triads condition) and when the subject is allowed a more or less exhaustive response (unlike the associations condition). Consequently, scoring is based on whether the response indicates access of each of the homonym's senses, regardless of "definitional quality."

Anomalies are apparent in WMS in the data from both the triads subtask and the definitions subtask (Figure 17.7). On the triads task, WMS subjects display a weaker primary bias[7] than do normal fourth grade controls (p < 0.06). A tendency for a weakened primary bias on the triads subtask is also seen for the small subset of our DNS subjects who we could test on this measure; however, the majority of our DNS subjects were not able to complete this task. On the homonym definitions subtask, the WMS subjects performed differently from both normal controls and DNS subjects. In particular, WMS subjects are just as likely to access primary senses as controls, but are in addition significantly more likely than normal controls (p < 0.02) or DNS subjects (p < 0.01) to access secondary meanings of a homonym. The WMS/normals contrast on this subtask is even stronger than with the triads task. Interesting in this context is that WMS subjects show a normal

---

[7] Primary bias is, percent primary responses – percent secondary responses, divided by total (correct) responses. This provides a consistent measure across subtasks.

bias for the primary homonym meaning on the free association subtask, with no differences from either DNS or normals.

An intriguing interpretation of these results can be obtained from a view of the relative task demands. The associations subtask, which is the least taxing, provides no population differences. The triads task is more taxing, requiring explicit comparisons, while the definitions task also has an additional task load: it uses open-ended free recall rather than explicit comparison to measure relative salience of alternate homonym senses. It is telling that this last task most definitively highlights WMS differences from both normal controls and DNS. Perhaps the unusual aspects in WMS lexical semantics are most evident in spontaneous, nonconstrained contexts that nevertheless require the subject to focus on specific topic categories.

Word usage in spontaneous speech of WMS

Unusual or anomalous word choice. Most WMS adolescents whom we have studied so far often use English words that are hardly commonplace, and use them appropriately, like "commentator," "sauté," "mince," "alleviate." Not infrequently, however, uncommon words are used incorrectly, for example, saying "evacuate the glass" for emptying a glass of water. The word includes the notion of emptying, but in ordinary usage the word implies the complete removal of all inhabitants or troops from a threatened structure or area. The word also has specialized meanings in medical and in chemical parlance, meanings which are also inappropriate in this context. The error would be an improper troponymic substitution in the terminology of Miller et al. (1990). Another error is the use of the word "concierge" to refer to an usher. The erroneously used words are typically in the right semantic ballpark, but they have semantic nuances not appropriate for the context, or imply specific features that the object or event does not manifest. For example, the use of "toucan" to refer to an ordinary parrot, shown in a photo, without the huge bill that distinguishes a toucan. Similarly, one WMS adolescent said "Two of them pigs TRAMPLED over me." The pigs were in fact merely stepping over the person; there was no indication of harshness, or of the person being injured or crushed. The following is another example of the incorrect use of a word with relatively restricted meaning where a semantically related word with a more general meaning would be appropriate: "I'll put the earrings in and you can BUCKLE them." Here the verb "fasten" would be more appropriate. The verb "buckle" does indeed involve the notion of fastening, but implies that a buckle or clasp is involved.

Idioms. In some instances, arbitrary constraints on words in an idiom or fixed expression are violated, as in "He cried his eyeballs out" (for "He cried his eyes out"); "When the clock HANDS strike midnight" (for "When the clock strikes midnight"); "You have to take the way she acts IN a grain of SAND" (for ". . . with a grain of salt"). With respect to the last error, it is revealing that at the end of the utterance, the subject, later in the conversation, produced the correct form: "So you have to take what she says with a grain of salt." *Overgeneralization.* There are cases where a perfectly reasonable and interpretable nonce form results from an overgeneralization of a morphological pattern, as in the following: "My dad doesn't want any BOTHERANCE." In English there does exist a derivational suffix "-ance" that derives nouns from certain verbs. In this way, "disturbance" is related to "disturb." But this morphological process is restricted to particular verbs and does not extend to the verb "bother," for which the verb root itself, without any suffix, serves also as the noun counterpart.

At this point we are still unable to determine to what extent the lexical anomalies are performance errors or knowledge errors. Performance-type anomalies might be related to a temporary "glitch" in lexical retrieval, due, perhaps, to an imbalance in excitation and inhibition in underlying processing. The "IN a grain of SAND" example above might represent a performance error of this type. Alternatively, anomalies might reflect incorrect or incomplete knowledge *of the world*. Another possibility is that they represent incomplete or incorrect knowledge of the *meaning of the word* in normal usage. The substitution of "TOUCAN" for "parrot," discussed above, is a likely candidate. Finally, some of the errors could also represent the internalization of an incorrect form. An example, observed in young normals, is internalizing and consistently using "taking for GRANITE" in place of "taking for granted."

WMS semantics and measures of brain function

In light of our behavioral evidence for anomalous lexical semantic processing in WMS, it is pertinent that data on brain function exist that bear strongly on this issue. These data come from our collaboration with the laboratory of Helen Neville, where measurements are made of event related potentials (ERP) from WMS subjects performing tasks involving sound stimuli and auditory word stimuli (Neville, Mills, & Bellugi, 1994).

The auditory investigation of perceptual functioning was motivated in part by evidence that WMS individuals have an unusual sensitivity to certain sounds, a condition sometimes called hyperacusis (e.g., Klein et al., 1990). While brain stem auditory evoked potentials showed no abnormality, anomalous signal morphology was evident at the cortical level in data from an auditory recovery paradigm (Bellugi et al., 1992; Neville, Holcomb, & Mills, 1989). In this experiment, subjects listen to 1500 Hz tones at fast (200 ms) or slow (1000 ms) repetition rates. Normal subjects show reduced N100-P200 signal amplitudes[8] at faster repetition rates. This reduction is

---

[8] N100 refers to the negative valued voltage measurement at approximately 100 ms after stimulus onset characteristically found, mostly prominently over the temporal lobe, in response to an auditory stimulus. P200 refers to a subsequent positive-going signal at 200 ms.

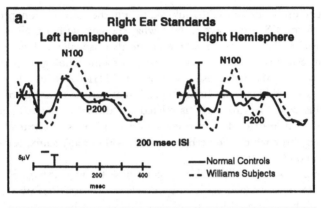

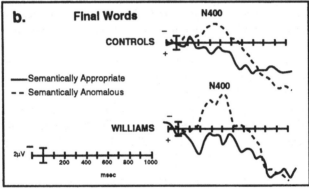

Figure 17.8. Neurophysiological (ERP) indices show anomalous auditory and language processing in WMS. (a) Auditory refractions period; (b) auditory sentences.

thought to be indicative of the operation of neurally based refractory processes in normal populations. WMS subjects, in contrast, do not show this reduced signal strength. Instead, their data show abnormality high amplitude N100 and P200 responses at fast repetition rates, unlike normal populations of any age (Figure 17.8). This result was found primarily over temporal cortex and only in the auditory modality. No amomalies were found for the DNS population in either the auditory or the visual modality. These data suggest that WMS individuals have brain activation responses to auditory stimuli that are less refractory and/or more excitable than those found in normals or in the DNS population.

Auditory word processing also gives rise to abnormal ERP signal morphology in WMS (Bellugi et al., 1992; Neville et al., 1994). When normals process auditory sentences, presented through headphones at one word per second, they show both a characteristic N100-P200 signal morphology and a characteristic N400 morphology, most prominently over temporal lobes. WMS adolescents, on the other hand, show signal *positivities* at both 100 ms and 200 ms (i.e., a P100 and a P200), diverging markedly from the N100-P200 signal seen in age-matched normals; moreover, this characteristic WMS waveform is unlike the 100 ms to 200 ms ERP waveform seen for normal subjects at any age.

Processing of *unexpected* words presented auditorially yields yet another ERP anomaly in the WMS population. When a sentence stimulus has an inappropriate final word, as in: "The sun was shining and the birds were CAMPING" (semantically *inappropriate*), normal subjects show a left temporal negativity at 400 msec (N400) that is particularly large relative to appropriate sentence-final words. WMS subjects' waveforms share this feature. However, preliminary results indicate that the WMS N400 for inappropriate or unexpected auditory words is even larger than in normal populations (Figure 17.8) (Neville et al., 1986; Neville et al., 1994).

This neurophysiological evidence suggests an anomalous mechanism associated with processing auditorially presented words, and unexpected words in particular. The coincidence in time course of the signal anomalies from the auditory recovery paradigm and the sentence processing paradigm may indicate the existence of a common basis for the WMS anomalies seen with these paradigms. Most important, however, is that these results represent emerging evidence of links across levels, providing insight on the connections of abnormal cognitive process in WMS lexical semantics to the underlying brain mechanism.

GENERAL DISCUSSION

Our multilevel investigations of the WMS profile strongly suggest that certain core aspects of language form an independent domain of cognition that can develop and function amidst grave deficits in nonlinguistic cognitive functioning. Language itself is not a unitary phenomenon, however, and in WMS there are, within the domain of language, patterns of spared and impaired abilities. In particular, within the subdomain of lexical semantics, fluency is excellent and word knowledge is distinctly above mental age levels, but anomalies are in evidence.

In the lexical semantic studies described above, anomalous WMS performance involved words that for the sake of generality may be called "unexpected" (low frequency in category production; secondary senses for homonyms; unusual or anomalous in spontaneous speech; semantically inappropriate in the ERP experiment). We presented evidence as to why word finding difficulty may not be at the root of this problem. Instead, our results suggest that anomalies characteristic of WMS semantics involve a subtle problem in specificity, or malspecificity, in lexical processing. We discussed the possibility that anomalous lexical processing was involved, perhaps a combination of reduced inhibitory activity and increased excitatory activity in response to the activation of a word or associated concept. ERP results underscored the likelihood that a processing anomaly is involved.

Further delineation of the nature of the hypothesized lexical processing anomaly may eventually be addressed by lexical priming studies that investigate the characteristics of distinct mechanisms of attention and lexical access underlying semantic processing (Brownell, 1988; Chiarello, 1988; Swinney & Prather, 1989). Studies of WMS using these paradigms are underway which, along with ERP studies and studies of neuropharmacological anomaly in WMS (Culler et al., 1985; August & Realmuto, 1989; Galaburda et al., 1994a; Galaburda et al., 1994b), may help to clarify the bases of the anomalous characteristics we have observed in the lexical semantics of the WMS population. While we are still far from a specific brain structure/brain function model of the WMS neuropsychological profile, the highly specific brain abnormalities in function and structure already found to underlie the distinctive behavioral profile of WMS provide strong motivation and direction for future research.

ACKNOWLEDGMENTS

We thank Dr Paul Wang for his helpful and comprehensive comments on this manuscript. This work was supported in part by National Institutes of Health grants R01 HD26022, P50 NS22343, and P01 DC01289; by a grant from the Oak Tree Philanthropic Foundation; and a grant from the March of Dimes Foundation to The Salk Institute for Biological Studies. The photographs of Williams Syndrome children are provided courtesy of the Williams Syndrome Association. We thank the National Williams Syndrome Association, several Regional Associations, the Canadian Association for Williams Syndrome, and the Parents of Down Syndrome Association. We are particularly grateful to subjects and their families for their participation in these studies. Illustrations copyright Ursula Bellugi, The Salk Institute for Biological Studies, La Jolla, California.

REFERENCES

Altepeter, T. & Handal, P.J. (1986). Use of the PPVT–R for intellectual screening with school-aged children: a caution. *Journal of Psychoeducational Assessment*, **4**(2), 145–154.
Altepeter, T.S. & Johnson, K.A. (1989). Use of the PPVT–R for intellectual screening with adults: a caution. *Journal of Psychoeducational Assessment*, **7**(1), 39–45.
Arnold, R., Yule, W., & Martin, N. (1985). The psychological characteristics of infantile hypercalcemia: a preliminary investigation. *Developmental Medicine and Child Neurology*, **27**, 49–59.
August, G.J. & Realmuto, G.M. (1989). Williams syndrome: serotonin's association with developmental disabilities. *Journal of Autism and Developmental Disorders*, **19**(1), 137–141.

Bamberg, M.G.W. (1987). *The Acquisition of Narratives: Learning to Use Language.* Berlin, Germany: Mouton de Gruyter.

Bayley, N. (1969). *Manual for the Bayley Scales of Infant Development.* San Antonio, TX: The Psychological Corporation.

Beery, K.E. (1982). *Revised Administration, Scoring, and Teaching Manual for the Development Test of Visual-Motor Integration.* Cleveland, OH: Modern Curriculum Press.

Bellugi, U. (1971). Some language comprehension tests. In C. Lavatelli (ed.) *Language Training in Early Childhood.* Urbana, IL: University of Illinois Press (pp. 157–169).

Bellugi, U., Bihrle, A., Neville, H., Jernigan, T., & Doherty, S. (1992). Language, cognition, and brain organization in a neurodevelopmental disorder. In M.R. Gunnar & C.A. Nelson (eds) *Developmental Behavioral Neuroscience.* Hillsdale, NJ: Lawrence Erlbaum (pp. 201–232).

Bellugi, U. & Klima, E.S. (1966). Syntactic regularities in children's speech. In J. Lyons & R. Wales (eds) *Psycholinguistic Papers.* Edinburgh, Scotland: Edinburgh University Press (pp. 183–208).

Bellugi, U., Marks, S., Bihrle, A., & Sabo, H. (1988). Dissociation between language and cognitive functions in Williams syndrome. In D. Bishop & K. Mogford (eds) *Language Development in Exceptional Circumstances.* London: Churchill Livingstone (pp. 177–189).

Bellugi, U., Wang, P., & Jernigan, T.L. (1994). Williams syndrome: an unusual neuropsychological profile. In S. Broman & J. Grafman (eds) *Atypical Cognitive Deficits in Developmental Disorders: Implications for Brain Function.* Hillsdale, NJ: Lawrence Erlbaum (pp. 23–56).

Bennett, F., LaVeck, B., & Sells, C. (1978). The Williams elfin facies syndrome: the psychological profile as an aid in syndrome identification. *Pediatrics,* **61**, 303–306.

Benton, A.L., Hamsher, K., Varney, N.R., & Spreen, O. (1983). *Judgement of Line Orientation.* New York: Oxford University Press.

Benton, A.L., Van Allen, M.W., Hamsher, K.D.S., & Levin, H.S. (1978). *Test of Facial Recognition, Form SL: Manual.* Department of Neurology, University of Iowa.

Bihrle, A., Rossen, M., & Bellugi, U. (1992). *Salk Homonyms Test.* La Jolla, CA: Laboratory for Cognitive Neuroscience, The Salk Institute for Biological Studies.

Black, J.A. & Bonham Carter, R.E. (1963). Association between aortic stenosis and facies of severe infantile hypercalcaemia. *Lancet,* **2**, 745–749.

Brownell, H.H. (1988). Appreciation of metaphoric and connotative word meaning by brain-damaged patients. In C. Chiarello (ed.) *Right Hemisphere Contributions to Lexical Semantics.* Heidelberg: Springer-Verlag (pp. 19–31).

Carroll, J.B., Davies, P., & Richman, B. (1971). *The American Heritage Word Frequency Book.* New York: American Heritage.

Chiarello, C. (1988). Semantic priming in the intact brain: separate roles for the right and left hemispheres? In C. Chiarello (ed.) *Right Hemisphere Contributions to Lexical Semantics.* Heidelberg: Springer-Verlag (pp. 59–67).

Culler, F., Jones, K., & Deftos, L. (1985). Impaired calcitonin secretion in patients with Williams syndrome. *Journal of Pediatrics,* **107**, 720–723.

Ewart, A.K., Morris, C.A., Atkinson, D., Jin, W., Sternes, K., Spallone, P., Stock, A.D., Leppert, M., & Keating, M.T. (1993). Hemizygosity at the elastin locus in a developmental disorder, Williams syndrome. *Nature Genetics,* **5**, 11–16.

Fenson, L., Dale, P.S., Reznick, J.S., Thal, D., Bates, E., Hartung, J.P., Pethick, S., & Reilly, J.S. (1993). *MacArthur Communicative Development Inventories: User's Guide and Technical Manual*. San Diego, CA: Singular Publishing Group.

Galaburda, A., Wang, P.P., Bellugi, U., & Rossen, M. (1994a). Cytoarchitectonic anomalies in a genetically based disorder: Williams syndrome. *Neuroreport*, 5, 753–757.

Galaburda, A., Wang, P.P., Rossen, M.L., & Bellugi, U. (1994b). Cytoarchitectonic and immunohistochemical findings in Williams syndrome. Presentation, Sixth National/International Conference of the Williams Syndrome Association, San Diego, CA.

Hallidie-Smith, K.A. & Karas, S. (1988). Cardiac anomalies in Williams-Beuren syndrome. *Archives of Disease in Childhood*, 63, 809–813.

Harrison, D., Reilly, J., & Klima, E.S. (1994). Unusual social behavior in Williams syndrome: evidence from biographical interviews. Presentation, Sixth National/International Conference of the Williams Syndrome Association, San Diego, CA.

Jernigan, T.L. & Bellugi, U. (1990). Anomalous brain morphology on magnetic resonance images in Williams syndrome and Down syndrome. *Archives of Neurology*, 47, 529–533.

Jernigan, T.L. & Bellugi, U. (1994). Neuroanatomical distinctions between Williams and Down Syndromes. In S. Broman & J. Grafman (eds) *Atypical Cognitive Deficits in Developmental Disorders: Implications for Brain Function*. Hillsdale, NJ: Lawrence Erlbaum (pp. 57–66).

Jernigan, T.L., Bellugi, U., Sowell, E., Doherty, S., & Hesselink, J.R. (1993). Cerebral morphological distinctions between Williams and Down syndromes. *Archives of Neurology*, 50, 186–191.

Jones, K.L. & Smith, D.W. (1975). The Williams elfin facies syndrome: a new perspective. *Journal of Pediatrics*, 86, 718–723.

Jones, W., Rossen, M.L., & Bellugi, U. (1994). Distinct developmental trajectories of cognition in Williams syndrome. Presentation, Sixth National/International Conference of the Williams Syndrome Association, San Diego, CA.

Jones, W., Rossen, M.L., Hickok, G., Jernigan, T., & Bellugi, U. (1995). Links between behavior and brain: brain morphological correlates of language, face and auditory processing in Williams syndrome. *Society for Neuroscience Abstracts*, 21(3), 1926.

Jones, W., Singer, N., Rossen, M., & Bellugi, U. (1993). Fractionations of higher cognitive functions in Williams syndrome: developmental trajectories. Presentation, ASHA National Convention, Anaheim, CA.

Kagan, J. (1989). *Unstable Ideas: Temperament, Cognition, and Self*. Cambridge, MA: Harvard University Press.

Kataria, S., Goldstein, D.J., & Kushnick, T. (1984). Developmental delays in Williams ("elfin facies") syndrome. *Applied Research in Mental Retardation*, 5, 419–423.

Klein, A.J., Armstrong, B.L., Greer, M.K., & Brown, F.R. (1990). Hyperacusis and otitis media in individuals with Williams syndrome. *Journal of Speech and Hearing Disorders*, 55, 339–344.

MacDonald, G. & Roy, D. (1988). Williams syndrome: a neuropsychological profile. *Journal of Clinical Experimental Neuropsychology*, 10, 125–131.

Mangiaracina, J. & Simon, M.J. (1986). Comparison of the PPVT-R and WAIS-R in state hospital psychiatric patients. *Journal of Clinical Psychology*, 42(5), 817–820.

Mayer, M. (1969). *Frog, Where Are You?* New York, NY: Dial Books for Young Readers.

Mervis, C. & Bertrand, J. (1992). Early cognitive and language development: toddlers with Williams syndrome. In *Williams Syndrome Association Professional Conference*, Chicago.

Mervis, C. & Bertrand, J. (1994). Early lexical development of children with Williams syndrome. Presentation, Sixth National/International Conference of the Williams Syndrome Association, San Diego, CA.

Meyerson, M. & Frank, R. (1987). Language, speech and hearing in Williams syndrome: intervention approaches and research needs. *Developmental Medicine and Child Neurology*, **29**, 258–262.

Miller, G.A., Beckwith, R., Feldbaum, C., Gross, D., & Miller, K. (1990). *Five papers on WordNet* (No. CSL Report 43). Cognitive Science Laboratory, Princeton University.

Mooney, C.M. (1957). Age in the development of closure ability in children. *Canadian Journal of Psychology*, **11**, 219–226.

Morris, C.A., Dilts, C., Demsey, S.A., Leonard, C., & Blackburn, B. (1988). The natural history of Williams syndrome: physical characteristics. *Journal of Pediatrics*, **113**, 318–326.

Morris, C.A., Thomas, I.T., & Greenberg, F. (1993). Williams syndrome: autosomal dominant inheritance. *American Journal of Medical Genetics*, **47**, 478–481.

Neville, H.J., Holcomb, P.J., & Mills, D.M. (1989). Auditory, sensory and language processing in Williams syndrome: an ERP study. In Symposium: neural correlates underlying dissociations of higher cortical functioning. *Journal of Clinical and Experimental Neuropsychology*, **11**(1), 52.

Neville, H.J., Kutas, M., Chesney, G., & Schmidt, A.L. (1986). Event-related potentials during initial encoding and recognition memory of congruous and incongruous words. *Journal of Memory and Language*, **25**, 75–92.

Neville, H.J., Mills, D.L., & Bellugi, U. (1994). Effects of altered auditory sensitivity and age of language acquisition on the development of language-relevant neural systems: preliminary studies of Williams syndrome. In S. Broman & J. Grafman (eds) *Atypical Cognitive Deficits in Developmental Disorders: Implications for Brain Function*. Hillsdale, NJ: Lawrence Erlbaum (pp. 67–83).

Perfetti, C.A., Lindsey, R., & Garson, B. (1971). *Association and Uncertainty: Norms of Association to Ambiguous Words* (No. 1971/17). University of Pittsburgh, Learning R&D Center.

Reilly, J., Harrison, D., & Klima, E.S. (1994). Emotional talk and talk about emotions. Presentation, Sixth National/International Conference of the Williams Syndrome Association, San Diego, CA.

Reilly, J.S., Klima, E.S., & Bellugi, U. (1990). Once more with feeling: affect and language in atypical populations. *Development and Psychopathology*, **2**(4), 367–391.

Rossen, M.L., Jones, W., Wang, P., & Klima, E.S. (1994). Face processing: remarkable sparing in Williams syndrome. Presentation, Sixth National/International Conference of the Williams Syndrome Association, San Diego, CA.

Rossen, M.L., Smith, D., Jones, W., Bellugi, U., & Korenberg, J. (1995). Spared face processing in Williams syndrome: new perspectives on brain-behavior links in a genetically based syndrome. *Society for Neuroscience Abstracts*, **21**(3), 1926.

Scott, P., Mervis, C.B., Bertrand, J., Klein, B.P., Armstrong, S.C., & Ford, A.L. (1994). Semantic organization and word fluency in older children with Williams syndrome. Presentation, Sixth National/International Conference of the Williams Syndrome Association, San Diego, CA.

Semel, E. & Rosner, S.R. (in press). *Williams Syndrome: Behavior Patterns and Interventions.* Oxford: Blackwell.

Semel, E.M. & Wiig, E.H. (1986). *Clinical Evaluation of Language Functions – Revised.* Columbus, OH: Charles E. Merrell.

Singer, N., Goodman, J., & Bellugi, U. (1992). Differentiating characteristics of early language and cognition. Presentation, 1992 Convention of the American Psychological Society, San Diego, CA: APS Monitor.

Singer, N.G., Jones, W., Rossen, M., Bellugi, U. (in press). Emerging language in two genetically based neurodevelopmental disorders.

Swinney, D. & Prather, P. (1989). On the comprehension of lexical ambiguity by young children: investigations into the development of mental modularity. In D. Gorfein (ed.) *Resolving Semantic Ambiguity.* New York: Springer-Verlag (pp. 4–5).

Tomc, S.A., Williamson, N.K., & Pauli, R.M. (1990). Temperament in Williams syndrome. *American Journal of Medical Genetics,* **36**(3), 345–352.

Udwin, O. & Yule, W. (1991). A cognitive and behavioral phenotype in Williams syndrome. *Journal of Clinical and Experimental Neuropsychology,* **13**(2), 232–242.

Udwin, O., Yule, W., & Martin, N. (1987). Cognitive abilities and behavioural characteristics of children with idiopathic infantile hypercalcaemia. *Journal of Child Psychology and Psychiatry,* **28**, 297–309.

Udwin, O., Yule, W., & Martin, N.D.T. (1986). Age at Diagnosis and Abilities in Idiopathic Hypercalcaemia. *Archives of Disease in Childhood,* **61**, 1164–1167.

Volterra, V., Sabbadini, L., Capirc, O., Pexxini, G., & Ossella, T. (1994). Language development in Italian children with Williams syndrome. Presentation, Sixth National/International Conference of the Williams Syndrome Association, San Diego, CA.

Wang, P.P., Doherty, S., Hesselink, J.R., & Bellugi, U. (1992). Callosal morphology concurs with neurobehavioral and neuropathological findings in two neuro-developmental disorders. *Archives of Neurology,* **49**, 407–411.

Wang, P.P., Doherty, S., Rourke, S.B., & Bellugi, U. (in press). Unique profile of visuo-perceptual skills in a genetic syndrome. *Brain and Cognition.*

Warrington, E.K. (1984). *Recognition Memory Test.* Windsor, England: NFER-Nelson.

Wechsler, D. (1974). *Wechsler Intelligence Scale for Children – Revised.* San Antonio, TX: The Psychological Corporation.

Williams, J.C.P., Barratt-Boyes, B.G., & Lowe, J.B. (1961). Supravalvular aortic stenosis. *Circulation,* **24**, 1311–1318.

PART V
INTERVENTION

Introduction

M. MARY KONSTANTAREAS

The four chapters of this section are addressing issues on treatment. As in the previous readings, they too take cognizance of such concepts as the notion of comorbidity, the need for a broader and multifaceted conceptualization of language and communication and how this translates into remediation and the importance of sound methodology.

Chapter 18 by Hechtman, Kouri, and Respitz addresses intervention with ADHD children comorbid for learning disabilities. The authors make the point that despite a normal intelligence, most ADHD children present with concomitant learning disabilities, and many may be destined for school failure. The children's less than optimal cognitive and information processing styles and inadequate or inappropriate social skills are partly responsible for these adaptational difficulties. After reviewing evidence on the advantages and limitations of pharmacotherapy, cognitive behavior therapy, social skills training, cognitive therapy, parent counseling, and individual psychotherapy, the authors conclude that any single one of these promising approaches is by itself inadequate to address the many and diverse needs of the ADHD child. They then offer the particulars of a multimodal intervention strategy currently in effect at the Montreal Children's Hospital. In this approach not only are the children's pharmacological and intrapersonal needs addressed, but their interpersonal and academic skills are also remediated. Parental counseling in understanding the disorder and in dealing with the child's needs as well as family therapy are included in the treatment configuration. Although still in the process, the study appears quite promising.

In Chapter 19, Gallagher provides a well-reasoned review of the currently popular social-interactional approaches to language intervention, a development that has capitalized on research in developmental pragmatics, peer acceptance and social effectiveness through communication. She outlines communication goals and procedures within this approach, linking them to literature and research on child discourse in the peer context and on social skill interventions. She then describes teaching communicative alternatives to socially penalizing behaviors, the use of "scripts," and the reasoned use of antecedents and consequences. To illustrate, she highlights a 10-week intervention strategy with a small group of Specifically Language Impaired preschoolers incorporating these elements. Gallagher concludes by reviewing the literature on the role of peers as models or as confederates in communication intervention and the use of a cooperative group context, capitalizing on these principles to promote positive peer interaction.

Hayden and Pukonen's contribution, Chapter 20, expands on Gallagher's chapter by addressing in some detail the intervention strategy they employ with the subgroup of language impaired children who present with pragmatic and social deficits. Their approach is predicated on the assumption that intervention is optimal when it addresses the deficits of homogeneous subgroups within this relatively large grouping. The underlying philosophy of the program and its main components are then presented, along with a description of an assessment battery used for arriving at subgrouping. One of the strong points of this chapter, much as of the one by Hechtman and coworkers (Chapter 18), is that the assessment battery, the goals of intervention, the procedures employed, and the materials used are presented in sufficient detail to allow replication. The authors provide a case presentation to highlight the program's goals and effectiveness, and inform us that group data will also be provided in due course.

Chapter 21 by Konstantareas addresses intervention with a more pervasively disturbed population, namely children with autistic disorder, whose diagnosis hinges critically on their inability to use speech and language in the typical fashion. She divides the material along two main theoretical positions, behavioral and cognitive. She then critically reviews the relative advantages and limitations of the work of Lovaas and his students that spans a 30-year period and the work of the cognitive functionalists whose interventions are more closely linked to the main stream of developmental psycholinguistics research. In view of the well-documented fact that as many as 50% of autistic individuals never develop useful spoken language, she also addresses the issue of modality of training, presenting evidence from her team's work and the work of others on the use of the main alternative to speech for the mute children, namely simultaneous communication training. She alerts us to the fact that, although the latter has been adopted extensively by front line workers, regrettably little conceptual and empirical work has been carried out to further elucidate its relevance and applicability. She concludes by offering an appraisal of recent trends in this area, including what some see as a recent rapprochement between the behavioral and cognitive positions.

18 Multimodal treatment of the hyperactive child with and without learning disabilities

LILY HECHTMAN, JOAN KOURI, AND CHAVA RESPITZ

This chapter addresses the comorbidity between attention deficit hyperactive disorder (ADHD) and learning disabilities (LD) and the effectiveness of a multimodal treatment approach for the learning disabled ADHD child. A description of remedial intervention as part of a multimodal approach to treatment is also provided. This is followed by recommendations for future intervention strategies.

LITERATURE REVIEW

Attention deficit hyperactive disorder (ADHD) is a condition which is characterized by symptoms of inattention, hyperactivity, and impulsivity. A child is said to have learning disabilities when there is a discrepancy of at least one standard deviation between the child or adolescent's potential intellectual (IQ) ability and his or her academic performance (Silver, 1989). The learning disabilities may take a number of forms such as auditory and visual processing (memory, discrimination, sequencing), figure ground relationships, encoding, comprehension of content, and contextual clues. Both conditions are thought to reflect some nervous system dysfunction. An overlap between attention deficit hyperactivity disorder and learning disabilities has been consistently reported in the literature. This overlap ranges from as low as 10% (August & Holmes, 1984) to as high as 92% (Silver, 1981). The usual co-morbid figure quoted tends to be 20–25% (Biederman, Faraone, & Lapey, 1992).

There is some evidence that this variability is most likely due to differences in selection criteria, sampling and modes of test presentation (i.e. timed versus untimed items). As well, there are numerous inconsistencies in the criteria used to define both ADHD and learning disabilities. However, regardless of the variability, it is clear that children with ADHD are being seen in significant numbers in classrooms for students with emotional, behavioral and learning disorders. The findings in some studies that learning disabilities are almost universally found among children with ADHD (Silver, 1981) has resulted in some authors suggesting that ADHD and learning disabilities may be indistinguishable (Prior & Sanson, 1986).

Hyperactivity is often considered a characteristic of learning disabilities (Anderson & Halcomb, 1976) and learning disabilities are often given symptoms of hyperactivity (O'Mally & Eisenberg, 1973). However, important differences exist in the defining characteristics of both disorders. Children with ADHD have difficulty with the processing of symbols because of attentional interference. Children with LD have difficulty in one or more of the basic psychological processes involved in understanding or in using language, spoken or written, which may manifest itself in an imperfect ability to listen, think, speak, read, write, spell, or do mathematical calculations. Not all children with learning disabilities have ADHD although some disabilities have been found to coexist with ADHD in about 20% to 25% of ADHD children (Biederman et al., 1992).

What is still unclear is whether difficulties in learning and/or school failure in ADHD children are related to inattention, hyperactivity and impulsivity; to cognitive deficits; to a combination of both sets of factors or to such factors as social disadvantage and consequent decline in motivation (Campbell & Werry, 1986). Children with ADHD are known to experience poor academic achievement, more tutoring, more grade repetitions and more frequent placement in special education classes (Edelbrock, Costello, & Kesler, 1984; Lahey et al., 1984; Silver, 1981; Weiss et al., 1979).

Follow up studies of children with hyperactivity generally substantiate that these children are destined for school failure and learning difficulties. For example, in a study by Hussey & Cohen (1976) half of the sample had experienced school failure by the time they had reached grade nine (Lambert & Sandaval, 1980). In another follow up study, Charles & Schain (1981) reported that the majority of pre-schoolers with hyperactivity when they entered school, tended to function below grade level in reading and mathematics.

More recently, Anderson et al. (1987) reported that 80% of 11-year-olds with ADHD were at least two years behind in reading, spelling, mathematics or written language. Thus, although there still appears to be uncertainty regarding the association of LD and ADHD, most studies support the hypothesis that academic difficulties and school failure are likely to be found in children with ADHD.

Several studies have also demonstrated that individuals with ADHD tend to have less efficient cognitive styles (Douglas, 1972, 1976; August & Garfinkel, 1990). The work of Douglas suggests that different types of cognitive disabilities may underlie the two disorders (ADHD and LD). Douglas suggests that children with ADHD have specific difficulties with the strategic problem solving skills that are necessary for learning (i.e., memory strategies). In contrast, learning disabled children measure normally on all perceptual and motor skills singly but have difficulty integrating them.

August & Garfinkel (1990) hypothesize that a subgroup of ADHD students with concurrent reading difficulty would show a more pervasive profile of cognitive impairment, including deficits in the encoding and retrieval of linguistic information as measured by tests of verbal intelligence and memory, rapid naming and word decoding. As hypothesized, the cognitively impaired ADHD group did perform worse than all other groups on such measures as rapid word naming.

Despite normal intelligence, ADHD children often underachieve in school. Their inappropriate activity, poor sustained attention, distractibility, impulsive cognitive style, low frustration tolerance and poor organization all contribute to academic difficulties. Furthermore, the disruptive activity, poor attention, impulsivity and low frustration tolerance result in significant interpersonal problems with family, peers and teachers. All the above difficulties, not surprisingly, give rise to poor self-esteem.

It is clear that attention deficit hyperactive disordered children often have multiple deficits which require multiple intervention. However, both in clinical practice and early studies, most of the children have received only stimulants. In short-term controlled studies, stimulants have been shown to decrease activity level and inattention (see review by Gittelman et al., 1980). They also positively affect rote learning, short-term memory (Stephens, Pelham, & Skinner, 1984) and classroom behavior (Rapport et al., 1985; Pelham et al., 1985).

All these positive short-term effects do not appear to result in significant gains in academic skill acquisition (Gadow & Swanson, 1985). Furthermore, follow-up studies of children treated with stimulants indicate that almost all continue to have significant academic, social and emotional problems in childhood (Riddle & Rapoport, 1976), adolescence (Weiss et al., 1975; Charles and Schain, 1981; Satterfield et al., 1982) and many in young adulthood (Hechtman, Weiss, & Perlman, 1984; Gittelman et al., 1985).

The first study of hyperactive children that provided multimodal treatment was done by Satterfield, Satterfield, & Cantwell in 1981. This study examined behavior, psychosocial adjustments, antisocial behavior, psychiatric evaluations of child and family, neurological evaluation, and intellectual functioning. Treatment included stimulant medication, behavior therapy, cognitive behavior therapy, social skills training, cognitive therapy in interpersonal problem solving skills, parent counseling and training, remedial tutoring, and individual psychotherapy. Results of the study suggested that a multimodality treatment plan to meet the needs of the child was partly responsible for the positive outcomes (Satterfield et al., 1981).

Stimulant medication is the most common intervention for ADHD children. However, stimulant medication cannot remediate specific learning disabilities. Therefore a multimodal treatment plan for ADHD learning disabled children was undertaken in this study.

TREATMENT MODALITIES

This section describes studies which have included such interventions as behavior therapy, cognitive training and cognitive behavior therapy, social skills training, cognitive therapy in interpersonal problem solving skills, parent training and counseling, remedial education and tutoring, and individual psychotherapy. Generally, the efficacy of these treatments is compared to that of medication alone and/or the combination of the intervention with medication. The review is presented to provide the rationale for which interventions were included in our multimodal treatment program.

Review of studies of treatment modalities other than medication

Behavior therapy

The results from controlled studies comparing medication, behavior therapy and their combination (reviewed by Pelham & Murphy, 1986; Rapport, 1983) have dampened the initial enthusiasm for behavior therapy based on operant principles used singly, as it was shown to be less potent than stimulants, and to have limited generalizability. Although most reports indicate that the combination produces the best results, its overall clinical utility is limited because of the absence of maintenance effects following treatment termination and the failure to enhance the development of self-regulatory skills. Cognitive training was designed to address these therapeutic deficits.

Cognitive training/cognitive behavior therapy (CBT)

There have been several reviews of CBT in ADHD children (see Abikoff, 1987; 1991; Gresham, 1985; Hinshaw & Erhardt, 1991). Overall, empirical support for the efficacy of CBT with these children is extremely limited. Moreover, the addition of CBT to medication has not produced incremental improvements in cognitive or academic performance, or in behavior. The possible short-term ceiling effects of stimulants, the narrowness of training, the failure to train for generalization, and questions regarding the theoretical underpinnings of self-instructional training for ADHD children have been suggested as explanations for the absence of positive results.

Social skills training

The social interactions of ADHD children are characterized frequently by intrusiveness, bossiness, aggressiveness, uncooperativeness, and noncompliance (see Whalen & Henker, 1985). Although their nature changes and they diminish somewhat over time (Cunningham & Siegel, 1987), follow-up studies attest to continuing social difficulties. The efficacy of clinical interventions on social difficulties has not been established and such studies are few in number. Stimulant medication has been associated with changes in social behavior (Whalen & Henker, 1991), but the magnitude of the effect has been limited.

Cognitive therapy in interpersonal problem-solving skills (ICPS)

ICPS has been largely unsuccessful in facilitating social competence, either in medicated or unmedicated children. Training in ICPS attempts to effect change by modifying maladaptive covert cognitions believed to mediate problematic social behavior. Despite early favorable reports (e.g., Spivak & Shure, 1974), subsequent studies have not documented gains in social behavior with ICPS (Abikoff & Gittelman, 1985; Gresham, 1985; Abikoff, 1987), and there is little indication that the skills are generalized so as to alter social behavior.

The deficient behavioral repertoires characteristic of at least some ADHD young people has prompted a call for treatment programs that focus on direct training in social skills (Guevremont, 1990; Hinshaw & Erhardt, 1991). However, such training alone is unlikely to counteract the social impairment of ADHD young people, and it has been argued that the best hope lies in combining training and pharmacotherapy (Pelham & Bender, 1982; Pelham & Milich, 1984).

Parent training and counseling

Mothers of ADHD children have been found to be more controlling, negative, and disapproving than mothers of normal control children (see Barkley et al., 1990). Mother–child interactions become more positive when the child is on a stimulant (Humphreys et al., 1978; Barkley & Cunningham, 1980), but the need to foster effective parenting remains. Few studies have addressed this issue. Firestone, Kelly, & Davey (1981) found no significant benefit from the addition of parent training to the administration of medication. However, training was limited (9 sessions) and no clear program was set up. Barkley (1981, 1987) describes a very detailed parent training program that has shown some success with a few (N = 3) school age ADHD children (Pollard, Ward, & Barkley, 1983). A controlled study with ADHD preschoolers (N = 48) (Pisterman, 1989), reported significant improvement in child compliance and parent/child interactions that were maintained at three months follow-up. However, there was no evidence of generalization to nontargeted child behaviors.

Remedial education and tutoring

The academic problems of ADHD children are well documented (Barkley & Cunningham, 1978; Cantwell & Satterfield, 1978). Stimulant medication alone improves academic productivity (Rapport et al., 1985; Douglas, Barr, O'Neill, & Britton, 1988), but does not eliminate academic handicaps, as suggested by a lack of improvement in long-term academic achievement (Gadow & Swanson, 1985; Pelham, 1986). A placebo controlled study compared the effects of tutoring and amphetamine in various combinations (Conrad et al., 1971), but medication compliance was very poor, rendering the results uninterpretable. The usefulness of remedial tutoring has been documented in reading disabled nonADHD children (Gittelman, Klein, & Feingold, 1983). Stimulants added little to reading performance, but arithmetic improved significantly. A multi-push program for ADHD children used by Satterfield, Satterfield, & Cantwell (1981) (described below), included "educational therapy," and resulted in greater than expected gains in achievement. Overall, these findings suggest that ADHD youngsters, who are often far behind academically, could benefit from remedial tutoring.

Individual psychotherapy

There are no controlled studies of the efficacy of individual psychotherapy for children with ADHD. However, in the long-term follow-up of hyperactive children into adulthood (Hechtman, Weiss, & Perlman, 1984), the adult hyperactives often reported that an important relationship with a therapist or adult who had faith in them had a significant long-term positive impact on their view of themselves and their optimism about their future, which positively affected their outcome.

Multimodal intervention

Clinical reports by Satterfield and colleagues document that multiple interventions may have far reaching short and long-term effects (Satterfield et al., 1981). In their multimodal treatment study all the hyperactive children received stimulant treatment; in addition, 41% received individual psychotherapy, 30% group therapy and 41% received education therapy. Of parents, 57% received individual counseling, 30% group counseling, and 48% family therapy. Children and families received any combination and any number of these interventions. When compared to other studies, the investigators showed that the outcome of this comprehensively treated group was unusually good. The multmodal treated children who had treatment for three years were functioning better academically and socially than those hyperactive children without such long-term treatment. This view was further supported in Satterfield's et al. (Satterfield, Satterfield, & Schell, 1987) study which compared the felony arrests and institutionalization records of hyper-actives who received drug treatment only and those who received multimodal treatment.

The drug-only group had significantly more arrests and institutionalization than the multimodal treatment group. These results do not come from systematic studies (i.e., treatment was not random, or controlled) but are suggestive of the superiority of multimodal treatment.

Summary and conclusions of pertinent literature findings

(1) Children with ADHD have multiple social, emotional, and academic problems.

(2) No single treatment has a satisfactorily broad therapeutic impact.

(3) Combined treatment strategies have been limited in scope and have invariably included two approaches only; typically stimulants and some form of psychosocial intervention. Here too, treatment efficacy has been limited and very disheartening.

(4) No controlled studies have used concurrent treatments for an extended time; treatment duration has ranged from two or three sessions to four months. "Booster" sessions to enhance maintenance effects have been rare.

(5) There is a need for well-controlled long-term studies to assess multimodal treatment which, at this time, is only promising. Others have increasingly noted this need, and have called for such clinical trials (Hinshaw & Erhardt, 1991; Horn et al., 1991; Whalen & Henker, 1991).

DESCRIPTION OF THE PRESENT STUDY

Based on the documented deficits of ADHD children and the clinical reports of Satterfield, we have included the following interventions in the multimodal treatment described below: medication, social skills training, academic skills training, remedial tutoring, parent training and counseling, and individual psychotherapy.

This is the first controlled study to investigate the efficacy of a multifaceted treatment program for ADHD children that is substantially broader in scope and time than treatment regimens used in previous studies. Our intent is to ascertain whether a comprehensive, integrated treatment approach will benefit ADHD children across multiple domains of functioning, and whether any gains are maintained during the year after intensive treatment termination.

The study involves 102 children, their mean age being 8.5 years old: 93% are boys and 7% are girls. Specifically, our goal is to compare the outcome in these 7 to 9-year-old ADHD children receiving methylphenidate and intensive (weekly) comprehensive interventions for one year, and monthly boosters in each of these interventions for a second year, to two control treatments. The first consists of methylphenidate and paraprofessional attention equal in time and type to the multimodal treatment (MMT) but not in the specific content. The second is the typical prevailing clinical treatment of ADHD consisting of stimulus medication, nonspecific clinical management and crisis intervention. The sample consisted of 102 children who were randomly assigned to these three treatment groups.

We hypothesize that, compared to controls, multimodal treatment will lead to:

(1) significantly better (a) social, (b) academic, and (c) overall functioning;
(2) a long-term post-treatment effect, beyond the period of intensive intervention;
(3) a significantly greater percentage of ADHD children who will be able to be maintained off medication after the first year of intensive treatment.

MULTIMODAL TREATMENTS OF STUDY

Setting

This multimodal treatment takes place in the context of an afterschool program, two afternoons per week, from 4pm to 6pm.

Medication

Generally stimulant medication (methylphenidate) is the drug of choice for ADHD children. As much as possible, titration is geared to optimize behavioral and cognitive functioning.

Cognitive titration

There are no established standards for the clinical utility of specific cognitive tests in titration procedures. There has been a movement away from laboratory measures of cognitive performance and an emphasis instead on academic performance in dose response studies. However, there is no consensus as to which academic skill(s) to titrate against (e.g., arithmetic, reading comprehension, decoding, oral reading, spelling) nor are there decision rules to follow if different doses maximize different academic skills. There is evidence, however, that arithmetic performance (productivity, accuracy) improves with stimulant medication (Douglas et al. 1986; Pelham, 1986). These arithmetic effects are incorporated into our titration procedures.

Children's arithmetic performance is evaluated during the titration phase, using Douglas et al.'s (1986) arithmetic task. Testing occurs weekly, corresponding to weekly increments in dose. Testing is carried out two hours after ingestion of the child's morning dose of methylphenidate.

Behavioral titration

This follows standard clinical practice. Children are seen weekly at the clinic during a four-week period, and dosages are increased gradually to a maximum of 50 mgs/day, based on parents' reports and teachers' impressions obtained via weekly phone contacts. Dosages are increased until the teacher reports no improvement, compared to the child's functioning during the previous week. At this point, the child is returned to the previous week's dosage. (Teacher or parent reports of an adverse response or side effects do, of course, also result in a return to a lower dose.)

Social skills training

Social skills training sessions are given with a view to establishing better interpersonal relationships as well as more appropriate behavior in daily experiences.

There is an extensive children's social training literature (see reviews by Hops et al., 1985; Ladd, 1984; Michelson et al., 1983) which includes several detailed training programs. Our review of the literature led us to choose two programs which have been tested empirically and have shown promise in improving children's social competency. Further, these programs also focus on social skills excesses and deficits that are especially relevant to ADHD children. Our intention is to utilize components of these established training programs, modifying them when necessary so as to increase the relevance to hyperactive children, as well as adding training features meant to enhance the generalizability of training effects.

The specific programs that are used in the study are the training manuals developed by Michelson et al. (1983), also described by Walker et al. (1983) and the Walker Social Skills Curriculum: The ACCEPTS Program. Both of these programs consist of a variety of techniques to alter social behavior and develop particular skills, via: direct instruction, modeling, behavioral rehearsal, feedback, reactions of others, and social reinforcement.

The sessions continue weekly for one year and then there are boosters once a month for a second year. They are conducted by a psychologist with social skills training experience. The weekly sessions for a year are needed to provide enough time for defining deficits, acquiring social skills, and generalizing these skills to naturally occurring settings. The booster sessions are required since many studies have shown that training gains are lost with time once training stops.

Parent training and counseling

Parents meet once weekly in a small group for approximately 12 weeks. They receive a parent effectiveness training program detailed by Barkley (1981). This program provides principles and strategies of behavioral management, reviews the particular problems hyperactive children have and which approaches would be best suited for them. Parents are assigned homework, keep behavioral and reinforcement charts and report on their efforts and experiences. Following the Parent Training program, parents meet three times a month with the therapist. The purpose of these individual family meetings is to help generalize the skills acquired in the Parent Training program. In the parent group, the technique focuses on the strategies of effective and more enjoyable parenting of the hyperactive child in his/her family. Once a month, the whole family is seen. The family meeting gives information to the therapist as to sibling relationships and how the family functions as a system. During these monthly family meetings, not only does the therapist acquire new information as to the individual family system, but he uses this information to point out and help the family change maladaptive interactions. For this, both a systems theory as well as behavior management approach are utilized. In the second year, there are monthly meetings with parents to reinforce gains made in the first year. Training programs are headed by a psychologist experienced in conducting parent effectiveness training groups.

Play or individual therapy of the child

Therapy is provided by a trained child psychiatrist with a background in psychodynamic understanding of a child's psychosocial development and experience in conducting child psychotherapy. Initially, the therapist establishes a positive therapeutic alliance with the child. Throughout the treatment, this alliance is the background against which problem solving is achieved by the child. Once this relationship is achieved, the therapy focuses on the following specific goals which relate to the known psychosocial difficulties of children with ADHD.

Self-esteem

In the context of the therapeutic alliance, all positive responses, whether verbal or in play, are commented upon and thus reinforced by the therapist. The respect and hope held for the child by the therapist becomes known to the child by verbal and nonverbal affective interchanges intended to enhance self-esteem. Negative statements about the self, or play symbolizing the above, are pointed out to the child as unrealistic and not helpful.

Promoting better understanding of the disorder

Hyperactive children, in our experience, vary from complete denial that anything is wrong with them (blaming others for the trouble they are in), to feeling that they are "bad," or "dumb." When the latter is observed, the children generally feel the problem is unchangeable. The therapist helps the child to delineate the difficulty he has realistically, counteracts that the problem is global and unchangeable, and helps create in the presence of the therapeutic alliance a climate for problem solving.

Changing the child's perception of his experienced rejection

Almost all hyperactive children have experienced rejection from parents, teachers, sibling, and peers. Therapy focuses on the chance that the rejection, while being real, is the direct result of certain behaviors which elicit a negative response in significant others. These negative responses are devastating to the child. For example, ADHD children at school are frequently nicknamed "contaminated," "dumb," etc., to the point that the child will only expose the hurt in a trusting relationship. Again, the emotional problem created will be changed to a problem solving one by directly linking certain behavior to rejection by others.

Enhancing self-effectiveness

Most hyperactive children feel that their difficulties are insoluble. At times, giving them medication can enhance this feeling by showing them that medication is required to change something about themselves. It is explained to each child that the medication is given to help the child effect changes in himself, but only he can really do this job. The child is taught by the therapist that his feelings of hopelessness about changing anything do not reflect reality and that he can indeed have control of his behaviors, particularly with the initial help of medication. The success thus experienced by the child also helps his self-esteem.

In addition to the above specific goals, it has been found clinically that each individual hyperactive child has unique psychological problem areas or conflicts. These will come out during the course of therapy and will be addressed appropriately.

What we will be describing next is the academic skills training and remedial intervention of the multimodal treatment. It is important to remember that the syndromes of hyperactivity and learning disabilities are different. A child may have one or the other disorder and at times both.

(1) The child may suffer only from perceptual deficits, cognitive impairments, and sensory motor integration difficulties. This is the primary LD child.

(2) The hyperactive child may be hyperactive, inattentive and impulsive. This may interfere with learning. This is the child whose learning problem is secondary to the hyperactivity. Such children can learn if their attention improved (Douglas, 1976).

(3) The hyperactive child may be hyperactive and may suffer from a perceptual, cognitive or integrative deficit. This child's learning disability implies both primary and secondary components, and treatment will need to recognize both of these.

DESCRIPTION OF ACADEMIC INTERVENTIONS

The first 16 weeks of the study focuses on the development of academic skills training and/or organizational strategies. This is followed by 29 weekly remedial sessions for which an individualized education plan (IEP) for each child is created in consultation with the respective teacher(s). Once the weekly academic skills training and the remedial sessions are complete, monthly booster sessions are held.

RATIONALE FOR ACADEMIC SKILLS TRAINING

Appropriate strategies for meeting the educational needs of a child with ADHD will differ from child to child. Forness & Walker (1991) have pointed out that the problems of any child with this diagnosis may vary considerably depending on age, presence or absence of associated problems, (i.e., Specific Learning Disabilities) and level of academic functioning. However, certain instructional strategies and classroom modifications have been found to be useful in the education of children with ADHD.

In terms of the educational impact, the ADHD may "adversely affect educational performance, to the extent that a significant discrepancy exists between a child's intellectual ability and that child's educational productivity with respect to listening, following directions, planning, organizing or completing academic tasks that require reading, writing, spelling or mathematical calculations" (PGARD: Professional Group for Attention Deficit Disorder and Related Disorders, 1991, p. 2).

Because ADHD children have difficulty in sustained attention, they may have secondary problems in processing visual and auditory stimuli. They also have difficulties in sequencing and classifying, in daily responsibilities requiring an awareness of time, and so on, all of which impede organizational strategies imperative to successful academic achievement.

Almost all children with ADHD suffer from difficulties with learning that are secondary to their limited attention span. These include impulsivity, poor handwriting, and poor fine motor skills. Because of poor organizational strategies, homework often becomes a battlefield. Moreover, the interpersonal difficulties that derive from an inability to behave appropriately in school

Table 18.1. *The remedial program*

Difficulty	Intervention
Age and grade differences	(a) The group is divided as equally as possible, either by age or grade, with one teacher per group (e.g., 1 teacher for 3 students; 1 teacher for 2 students). (b) In order that the students experience different teaching styles, the two teachers alternate in leading their groups after approximately 15 sessions.
Language instruction	In order to accommodate those children who are in a unilingual French or French immersion program, much of the remedial intervention is formulated in collaboration with the classroom teacher who provides class worksheets and/or textbooks. This is complemented by the project teacher providing individual instruction in reading, and written expression in French.
Differences in academic ability	As previously mentioned, individual educational plans, according to individual needs, are developed after consulting with the students' teacher(s).
Monthly boosters	Because it is considered unlikely to expect remedial gains based on monthly remedial sessions, the monthly booster sessions include discussions on various themes which lead to the completion of written projects.
Generalization of skills taught	In order to reinforce and supervise both organization and remedial skills in settings outside of the classroom, the students are taken to a local library. There, such skills as using the resources of a library, selecting books and writing book reports are reinforced. The children also participate in activities organized by the librarian. This allows the project teachers to observe their students in social interactions with children whom they did not know and in activities not exclusive to the project.
Crisis intervention as a result of uncontrolled behavior	In order to be prepared for possible behavior outbursts on the part of any student, there are always two teachers present during the part of the program dealing with academic skills training.

usually leads to an emotionally charged classroom milieu. This in turn leads to impaired learning (Weiss, 1992). Because of the diverse individual difficulties and because each of the students in the remedial program presents unique challenges, the remedial program, as outlined in Table 18.1 above, was adopted with a view to addressing these differences.

Table 18.2. *Academic skills training program*

Subskills	Target behaviors
Awareness of time	1. Punctuality 2. Completing tasks in the allotted time 3. Pre-planning and scheduling
Organization of written work	1. Spacing and utilization of the page 2. Legibility 3. Preparing text books, etc.
Attention	1. Blocking out external stimuli 2. Following instructions 3. Focusing and refocusing
Study skills	1. Reviewing directions 2. Finding key words 3. Note taking (for the older children) 4. Identifying relevant facts 5. Preparing for tests, i.e. where to study, time, scheduling
Self-evaluation	1. Monitoring one's own progress 2. Rating scales 3. Ability to identify own needs (teacher allowed students to select an area in which they chose to practice and to improve)

Description of academic skills training program

The target behaviors include organizational skills, identification and comprehension of task instructions, and checking work for accuracy and completeness (see Table 18.2). To increase the relevance of training to the children's daily experiences, training materials include the children's own classwork and homework. Notebook organization, note taking, recording and monitoring of homework assignments, clarity of work, studying for tests, and so on, are some of the subskills covered. A variety of training procedures are used, including modeling, direct instruction, self-monitoring and self-evaluation, and response cost for inaccurate self-evaluations.

Enhancers and their goals

The following enhancers complement the more specific subskill objectives:
1. *Relaxation.* To increase the ability to establish a state of mental and physical calm, necessary prerequisites to successful academic functioning.
2. *Free play.* To be used as a reward for fulfilling the goals set out. This also allows therapists an opportunity for observation in a less structured setting.

3. *Organization of time and materials.* To introduce "school survival skills" (i.e., coming to class prepared with necessary material, writing down homework assignments in an assignment calendar, turning in completed homework).

4. *Anticipating consequences.* To organize thinking in order to equip the child with multiple alternatives of behaviors and to consider the impact of his/her actions on himself/herself (i.e., not doing homework, calling out and not completing assignments).

5. *Inhibition and response delay.* To ensure inhibition and response delay skills as a basic part of a child's behavioral repertoire, with a view to enhancing long-term prospects for success in the classroom.

RATIONALE AND DESCRIPTION OF INDIVIDUAL EDUCATION PLAN (IEP)

One of the major components of the academic intervention of the study is the individualized education plan (IEP) which takes place following the 16-week organization study skills program.

The IEP is intended to be a tool for ensuring that the students' special learning needs are addressed. As a result of consultation between the teachers in the study and the students' classroom teachers, a program is set up which provides special teaching that the student requires. Because the students in the study do not have a repertoire of learning strategies, emphasis is placed on how the student learns as well as what the student learns. As pointed out by Lerner (1993), "Learning is strategic. Learning is more than simply remembering. People need strategies to learn."

Following the 16-week group study skills program, the children are seen individually for seven months of weekly remediation. These sessions, conducted by special education teachers, are individualized according to the academic needs of each student. All students, however, continue to receive training in organizational and study skills strategies. The emphasis in these sessions is on the student's current academic program, although supplementary training materials and tasks for specific subskills are available as needed.

Remedial tutoring is provided for students with specific academic skills deficits. Diagnostic assessments in reading, mathematics, language, and spelling is done for each student, and a prescriptive tutorial program is developed and implemented for each child. Some students are at grade level and do not require remediation. Training with these students continues to emphasize the organizational and study skills described previously. To address the needs of each student and to remediate specific academic difficulties, that is reading, reading for understanding, mathematics, spelling, written expression, handwriting, and so on, the following skills are reinforced.

Visual and auditory memory

To improve ability to remember and organize visual and auditory material and to reconstruct presented material through oral or written expression, the teacher requests of each student to:

(1) introduce a picture
(2) discuss the picture
(3) list everything he/she remembers about the picture
(4) write a story about the picture
(5) share the story with the group.

Figure ground auditory and visual processing

This strategy is meant to improve the ability to distinguish discreet parts of a stimulus arrangement from the remaining parts, to separate the stimulus that has relevance and to be able to ignore extraneous stimuli. Examples:

(1) Where's Waldo? (Finding a hidden picture.)
(2) Auditory Figure Ground Tapes and Worksheets.

Focusing and concentration

To improve ability to focus attention on a specific task, increase attention span, and concentrate on task directed activities, the teacher is expected:

(1) to present task in short work packages
(2) to time the activity
(3) at the end of the first work package to monitor and/or correct students' work
(4) to recognize so that the student achieves mastery before continuing with next work package.

Sequencing and ordering

(A) To improve ability to place things and events into time and space relationships, the teacher:
  (1) gives exercises related to seasons, holidays and personal experiences
  (2) have students prepare calendars with emphasis on sequential order of months, dates, and personal experiences.
(B) To increase the student's ability to accurately arrange and/or reproduce a sequence of auditory and/or visual stimuli, the teacher:
  (1) employs *Memory Games,* i.e., "I went on a trip and in my suitcase I packed..." (each item repeated by each group member in sequence).
  (2) asks students to read and follow recipes. Students are expected to create own recipes.

As a result of the above described remedial interventions, each of the students appeared to find the interventions beneficial. The teaching interventions were developed to address the specific cognitive function described. Such functions are often problematic for children with ADHD and learning disabilities. The following case study illustrates the above.

Case presentation

Douglas, who is of above average intelligence, was referred to the program by his classroom teacher. At the time of referral, Douglas, whose first language is English, was in Grade III in a unilingual French school. Major concerns were his restricted verbal and written expression in both English and French and his limited academic progress. As well, his progress in the development of reading skills, decoding and comprehension, was below expected for age and grade level. Douglas' teachers also reported that Douglas lacked friends and did not relate well to peers. Generally, his behavior was described as immature and forgetful.

During the first 16 weeks of the program, although the weaknesses in verbal and written expression were addressed, the emphasis was on helping Douglas to learn to relax, to preplan, to sustain attention to the task and to develop organizational strategies. As a result of relaxation exercises, Douglas' level of anxiety regarding academic tasks appeared to diminish. This was evidenced when Douglas himself reported that, when he used these exercises in class, he was less anxious and better able to perform.

During the second year of the program, the Individual Educational Plan devised for Douglas concentrated on improving communication skills, both expressive and written. For example, rather than first being expected to transcribe his thoughts on paper, Douglas dictated his ideas to the teacher; he then copied his output into his journal, following which he taped his composition. Douglas then listened to the tape in order to make personal comments which helped with verbal expression. As this drill continued, his speed and accuracy to detail as well as verbal and written expression improved. It is important to note that Douglas became responsible for monitoring his speed and accuracy on the above tasks.

As the sessions progressed, Douglas became more verbal, more confident and he developed better interpersonal skills. Toward the end of the second year of the program, Douglas succeeded in independently finding a "job" in a pet store. As well, his teacher's reports were much more positive than when he was first referred.

MONTHLY BOOSTER SESSIONS

During the second year of the project, the students return once a month for academic follow-up. Specific areas including historical reviews, biographies, ecology, current events are discussed with the students as possible themes for monthly projects. Following this, the students view a film related to the theme chosen by them, do introductory vocabulary exercises, discuss the content and then move towards projects relevant to the theme.

The monthly booster sessions are designed to reinforce and maintain academic and organizational skills developed in the first year of the academic intervention.

INDICATIONS FOR FUTURE INTERVENTION STRATEGIES

As a result of experimentation of the multifaceted approach to the ADHD learning disabled child, there are clear indications for future intervention strategies:

(1) more in-service training in schools regarding the ADHD syndrome
(2) more parent involvement in the academic aspect of the program and sensitization of the family (i.e., siblings) regarding the learning disabled – ADHD syndrome is strongly recommended
(3) more frequent consultation with all teachers involved.

CONCLUSION

Since the study is ongoing, specific statistical data are not available. However, we have the clinical impression that significant academic gains were made during the time that the children were in the program and that the multiple concurrent interventions were essential to this growth. It is important that the academic input was just one intervention in the multimodal treatment approach which also included stimulant medication, parent training, social skills training, and individual psychotherapy. The multimodal treatment group was compared to a group receiving stimulant medication and equal paraprofessional attention in the form of a parent support group, a peer activity group, help with homework group and individual time with an adult. Finally, the last comparison group was a conventionally treated group. These children received monthly stimulant medication visits and a total of eight crisis intervention sessions to deal with any family or school problems which might arise. Judging from the clinical indications to date, the results seem promising.

It is our hope that this multifaceted approach will meet the needs of the ADHD learning disabled child and will result in positive changes in his/her academic performance. Longer term prospective studies appear to be necessary in order to determine the most effective interventions or combinations of interventions for addressing the needs of the ADHD learning disabled child.

REFERENCES

Abikoff, H. (1987). An evaluation of cognitive behavior therapy for hyperactive children: a critical review. *Clinical Psychology Review*, **5**, 479–512.

Abikoff, H. (1991). Cognitive training in ADHD children; less to it than meets the eye. *Journal of Learning Disabilities*, **24**, 205–209.

Abikoff, H. & Gittelman, R. (1985). Hyperactive children maintained on stimulants: is cognitive training a useful adjunct? *Archives of General Psychiatry*, **42**, 952–961.

Ackerman, P., Dykman, R., & Peters, J. (1977). Teenage status of hyperactive and non-hyperactive learning disabled boys. *American Journal of Orthopsychiatry*, **47**, 577–596.

Anderson, J.C., Williams, S., McGeer, R., & Silva, P.A. (1987). DSM III disorders in pre-adolescent children. *Archives of General Psychiatry*, **44**, 69–76.

Anderson, R.P. & Halcomb, C.G. (1976). *Learning Disability/Minimal Brain Dysfunction Syndrome: Research Perspectives and Applications*. Springfield Publishers.

August, G.S. & Garfinkel, B.D. (1990). Comorbidity of ADHD and reading disability among clinic-referred children. *Journal of Abnormal Child Psychology*, **18**(1), 29–45.

August, G.S. & Holmes, C.S. (1984). Behavior and academic achievement in hyperactive subgroups and learning disabled boys. *American Journal of Diseases of Children*, **138**, 1025–1029.

Barkley, R.A. (1981). Training parents to cope with hyperactive children. In *Hyperactive Children: A Handbook for Diagnosis and Treatment*. New York: Guilford Press (pp. 271–365).

Barkley, R.A. (1987). *Defiant Children: A Clinician's Guide to Parent Training*. New York: Guilford Press.

Barkley, R.A., et al. (1990). Comprehensive evaluation of attention deficit disorder with or without hyperactivity defined by research criteria. *Journal of Consulting and Clinical Psychology*, **58**(6), 775–789.

Barkley, R.A. & Cunningham, C.E. (1978). Do stimulant drugs improve the academic performance of hyperkinetic children? A review of outcome research. *Clinical Pediatrics*, **17**, 85–92.

Barkley, R.A. & Cunningham, C.E. (1980). The parent-child interactions of hyperactive children and their modifications by stimulant drugs. In R. Knights & D. Bakker (eds) *Treatment of Hyperactive and Learning Disabled Children*. Baltimore: University Park Press.

Biederman, J., Faraone, S.V., & Lapey, K. (1992). Comorbidity of Diagnosis in attention deficit hyperactive disorder, attention deficit disorder. *Child and Adolescent Psychiatry Clinics of North America*, **2**, 335–361.

Biederman, J., Newcorn, J., & Sprich, S. (1991). Comorbidity of attention deficit disorder with conduct, depressive anxiety and other disorders. *American Journal of Psychiatry*, **148**(5), 564–577.

Campbell, S.B. & Werry, J.S. (1986). Attention deficit disorder (hyperactivity). In H.C. Quay & J.S. Werry (eds) *Psychopathologic Disorders of Childhood*. New York: John Wiley (pp. 1–35).

Cantwell, D.P. & Satterfield, J.H. (1978). The prevalence of academic underachievement in hyperactive children. *Journal of Pediatric Psychology*, **3**, 168–171.

Charles, L. & Schain, R. (1981). A four year follow up study of the effects of methylphenidate on behavior and academic achievement of hyperactive children. *Journal of Abnormal Child Psychology*, **9**, 495–505.

Conrad, W.G., Dworken, E.S., Shai, A., & Tobisen, J.E. (1971). Effects of amphetamine therapy and prescriptive tutoring on the behavior achievement of lower class hyperactive children. *Journal of Learning Disabilities*, **5**, 509–517.

Cunningham, C.E. & Siegel, L.S. (1987). Peer interaction of normal and attention deficit disabled boys during free play, cooperative tasks, and simulated classroom situations. *Journal of Abnormal Child Psychology*, **15**(2), 247–268.

Douglas, V.I. (1972). Stop, look and listen: the problem of sustained attention and impulse control in hyperactive and normal children. *Canadian Journal of Behavioral Science*, **4**, 259–282.

Douglas, V.I. (1976). Research on hyperactivity: stage two. *Journal of Abnormal Child Psychology*, **4**, 307–308.

Douglas, V.I., Barr, R.G., O'Neill, M.E., & Britton, B.G. (1986). Short-term effects of methylphenidate on the cognitive, learning and academic performance of children with attention deficit disorder in the laboratory and classroom. *Journal of Child Psychology and Psychiatry*, **27**, 191–211.

Douglas, V.I., Barr, R.G., O'Neill, M.E., & Britton, B.G. (1988). Dosage effects and individual responsivity to methylphenidate in attention deficit disorder. *Journal of Child Psychology and Psychiatry*, **29**, 453–475.

Doyle, R.B., Anderson, R.P., & Halcomb, C.G. (1976). Attention deficit and the effects of visual distraction. *Journal of Learning Disabilities*, **9**, 48–54.

Edelbrock, C., Costello, A.J., & Kesler, M.D. (1984). Empirical corroboration of attention deficit disorder. *Journal of the Academy of Child and Adolescent Psychiatry*, **23**, 285–290.

Firestone, P., Kelly, M.J., & Davey, J. (1981). Differential effects of parent training and stimulant medication with hyperactives. *Journal of the American Academy of Child Psychiatry*, **20**, 135–147.

Forness, S. & Walker, H.M. (1991). Classroom system. Strategies for attention deficit disorders (Part 1). *Challenge*, **5**(c), 1–4.

Gadow, K.D. & Swanson, H.E. (1985). Assessing drug effects on academic performance. *Psychopharmacological Bulletin*, **21**, 877–886.

Gittelman, R., Klein, D., & Feingold, I. (1983). Children with reading disorders: Effects of methylphenidate in combination with reading remediation. *Journal of Child Psychology and Psychiatry*, **24**, 193–212.

Gittelman-Klein, R., Abikoff, H., Pollack, E., et al. (1980). A controlled trial of behavior modification and methylphenidate in hyperactive children. In C. Whalen & B. Henker (eds) *Hyperactive Children: The Social Ecology Identification and Treatment*. New York: Academic Press (pp. 259–295).

Gittelman, R., Mannuzza, S., Shenkar, R., & Bonagura, N. (1985). Hyperactive boys almost grown up I: psychiatric status. *Archives of General Psychiatry*, **42**, 937–947.

Gresham, F.M. (1985). Utility of cognitive-behavioral procedures for social skills training with children. A critical review. *Journal of Abnormal Child Psychology*, **13**, 411–423.

Guevremont, D. (1990). Social skills peer relationship training. In R.D. Barkley (ed.) *Attention Deficit Hyperactivity Disorder: A Handbook for Diagnosis and Treatment*. New York: Guilford Press (pp. 540–572).

Hechtman, L., Weiss, G., & Perlman, T. (1984). Young adult outcome of hyperactive children who received long-term stimulant treatment. *Journal of American Academy of Child Psychiatry,* **23,** 261–269.

Hinshaw, S.P. & Erhardt, D. (1991). Attention deficit hyperactivity disorder. In P.C. Kendal (ed.) *Child and Adolescent Therapy: Cognitive-Behavioral Procedures.* New York: Guilford Press (pp. 98–130).

Hops, M., Finch, M., & McConnell, S. (1985). Social skills deficits. In P.H. Bornstein & A.E. Razdiw (eds) *Handbook of Clinical Behavior Therapy with Children.* Homewood, IL: Dorsey Press.

Horn, W.F., Islong, N.S., Pascoe, J.M., et al. (1991). Additive effects and self control therapy with ADHD children. *Journal of American Academy of Child and Adolescent Psychiatry,* **30,** 233–240.

Humphreys, T., Kinsbourne, M., & Swanson, S. (1978). Stimulant effects on cooperation and social interaction between hyperactive children and their mothers. *Journal of Child Psychology,* **19,** 13–22.

Hussey, H.R. & Cohen, A.H. (1976). Hyperactive behavior and learning disabilities followed over seven years. *Pediatrics,* **57,** 4–10.

Ladd, G.W. (1984). Social skill training with children: issues in research and practice. *Clinical Psychological Review,* **4,** 317–337.

Lahey, B., Shaughnessey, E.A., Strauss, C.C., & Fame, C.L. (1984). Are attention deficit disorders with and without hyperactivity similar or dissimilar disorders? *Journal of American Academy of Child Psychiatry,* **23,** 302–309.

Lambert, N.M. & Sandaval, J. (1980). The prevalence of learning disabilities in a sample of children considered hyperactive. *Journal of Abnormal Child Psychology,* **8,** 33–50.

Lerner, J.W. (1993). Learning disabilities. *Child and Adolescent Psychiatric Clinics of North America,* 309–321.

Michelson, L., Susgai, D.P., Wood, R.P., & Kazdin, A.E. (1983). *Social Skill Assessment and Training with Children.* New York: Plenum Press.

O'Mally & Eisenberg, L. (1973). *The Hyperkinetic Syndrome.* New York: Grame & Shatton.

Pelham, W.E. (1986). The effects of psychostimulant drugs on learning and academic achievement in children with attention-deficit disorders and learning disabilities. In J.K. Torgensen & B.Y.L. Wong (eds) *Psychological and Educational Perspectives in Learning Disabilities.* New York: Academic Press (pp. 220–295).

Pelham, W.E. & Bender, M.E. (1982). Peer relationships in hyperactive children: description and treatment. In K.D. Gadow & I. Bialer (eds) *Advances in Learning and Behavioral Disabilities,* Vol. 1. Greenwich, CT: JAI Press (p. 365).

Pelham, W.E., Bender, M.E., Caddell, J. et al. (1985). Methylphenidate and children with attention deficit disorder: Dose effects on classroom, academic and social behavior. *Archives of General Psychiatry,* **42,** 948–952.

Pelham, W.E. & Murphy, H.A. (1986). Behavioral and pharmacological treatment of attention deficit and conduct disorders. In M. Hersen & D.E. Bruening (eds) *Pharmacological and Behavioral Treatment: An Integrative Approach.* New York: John Wiley (pp. 108–148).

Pelham, W.E. & Milich, R. (1984). Peer relations in children with hyperactivity attention deficit disorder. *Journal of Learning Disabilities,* **17,** 560–567.

PGARD (Professional Group for ADD and Related Disorders) (1991). *Department of Education's Notice of Inquiry.*

Pisterman, S. (1989). Outcome of parent-mediated treatment of pre-schoolers with attention deficit disorder. *Journal of Consulting and Clinical Psychology*, **57**, 628–635.

Pollard, S., Ward, E.M., & Barkley, R.A. (1983). The effects of parent training and Ritalin on the parent–child interactions of hyperactive boys. *Child and Family Therapy*, **5**, 51–69.

Prior, M. & Sanson, A. (1986). Attention deficit disorder with hyperactivity: a critique. *Journal of Child Psychology and Psychiatry*, **27**, 307–319.

Rapport, M.D. (1983). Attention deficit disorder with hyperactivity: critical treatment parameters and their application in applied outcome research. In M. Hersen, R. Eisler, & P. Miller (eds) *Progress in Behavior Modification, Vol. 3*. New York: Academic Press (pp. 220–291).

Rapport, M.D., Stonar, G., DuPaul, G. et al. (1985). Methylphenidate in hyperactive children: Differential effects of dose in academic learning and social behavior. *Journal of Abnormal Child Psychology*, **13**, 227–244.

Riddle, D. & Rapoport, J. (1976). A 2-year follow up of 72 hyperactive boys. *Journal of Nervous and Mental Diseases*, **162**, 126–234.

Satterfield, J.H., Satterfield, B.T., & Schell, A.E. (1987). Therapeutic intervention to prevent delinquency in hyperactive boys. *Journal of American Academy of Child and Adolescent Psychiatry*, **26**, 56–64.

Satterfield, J.H., Satterfield, B.T., & Cantwell, D.P. (1981). Three-year multimodality treatment study of 100 hyperactive boys. *Journal of Pediatrics*, **98**, 650–655.

Satterfield, J.H., Cantwell, D.P., & Satterfield, B. (1979). *Archives of General Psychiatry*, **36**, 965–974.

Satterfield, J.H., Hoppe, C., & Schell, A.E. (1982). Prospective study of delinquency in 110 adolescent boys with attention deficit disorder and 88 normal adolescent boys. *American Journal of Psychiatry*, **139**, 795–798.

Silver, L.B. (1981). The relationship between learning disabilities, hyperactivity, distractibility and behavioral problems. *Journal of American Academy of Child and Adolescent Psychiatry*, **20**, 385–397.

Silver, L.B. (1989). Psychological and family problems associated with learning disabilities, assessments and interventions. *Journal of the American Academy of Child and Adolescent Psychiatry*, **28**, 314–325.

Spivak, G. & Shure, M.B. (1974). *Social Adjustment of Young Children: A Cognitive Approach to Solving Real-life Problems*. San Francisco, CA: Jossey-Bass.

Stephens, R.S., Pelham, W.E., & Skinner, R. (1984). State-dependent and main effects of methylphenidate and pemoline on paired-associate learning and spelling in hyperactive children. *Journal of Consulting Clinical Psychology*, **52**(1), 104–113.

Walker, H.M., McConnell, S., Holmes, D., Todis, B., et al. (1983). *The Walker Social Skills Curriculum: The Accepts Program*. Austin, TX.

Weiss, G., Kruger, E., Danielson, U., & Elman, M. (1975). Effect of long-term treatment of hyperactive children with methylphenidate. *Canadian Medical Association Journal*, **112**, 159–165.

Weiss, G., Hechtman, L., Perlman, T., Hopkins, J., & Werner, A. (1979). Hyperactives as young adults: A controlled prospective ten-year follow-up of 75 children. *Archives of General Psychiatry*, **36**, 675–681.

Weiss, G., Hechtman, L., Perlman, T., & Milroy, T. (1985). Psychiatric status of hyperactives as adults: A controlled prospective 15-year follow-up of 63 hyperactive children. *Journal of American Academy of Child and Adolescent Psychiatry*, **24**, 211–220.

Weiss, M. (1992). Psycho-educational intervention with children with ADHD. *Child and Adolescent Clinics in North America*, 467–479.

Whalen, C.K. & Henker, S.P. (1985). Cognitive-behavioral therapies for hyperactive children: Premises, problems and prospects. *Journal of Abnormal Child Psychology*, **13**, 391–403.

Whalen, C.K. & Henker, B. (1991). Therapies for hyperactive children: comparison combinations and compromises. *Journal of Consulting Clinical Psychology*, **59**, 126.

19 Social-interactional approaches to child language intervention

TANYA M. GALLAGHER

INTRODUCTION

Over the last decade, the most dramatic changes in speech-language pathology service delivery to children with language disorders have involved the development of social-interactional approaches to language intervention. This focus on intervention procedures is a sharp contrast to the language content focus that dominated the clinical intervention literature previously when major changes in the specification of semantic, syntactic, and phonological language intervention goals reflected the influence of generative linguistic theory. Since the 1960s, generative linguistic theory has provided the basis for major improvements in language assessment and intervention goal setting. Generative theories, however, provided little insight into the actual conduct of language therapy, that is, little insight into how best to achieve those goals (see Craig, 1983, for review). Recent additions to the literature, therefore, are to a large extent complementary to those that appeared earlier and address questions such as who should be involved in language intervention, what should be the focus of intervention and what techniques should be used.

The development of new approaches to the conduct of language intervention reflects the influence of pragmatic language theories (Searle, 1969; Bates, 1976). Pragmatic theories have increased speech-language pathologists' awareness of the social role of language by highlighting the interpersonal nature of communication. Language use is viewed as an inherently social phenomenon with interpersonal consequences.

Additional impetus for the development of new approaches has come from a growing literature indicating that there is a relationship between children's language skills and their social acceptability among peers. Skills such as the ability to adjust messages to the listener's needs, to initiate conversation successfully, to ask appropriate questions, to contribute substantively to ongoing conversation, to communicate intentions clearly, to address all participants when joining a group, and to present comments positively more often than negatively have been found to correlate with measures of peer acceptance and sociometric status (see Gallagher, 1993, for review). Even at the preschool level, children's preferred play partners were found to talk significantly more, share information more successfully, produce more related utterance sequences, produce more relevant responses, and use language more successfully in support of their interactions (Parker & Gottman, 1989; Hazen & Black, 1989).

Research on populations receiving speech and language intervention also has suggested a relationship between child language disorder and social interaction skills (Aram, Ekelman, & Nation, 1984; Schery, 1985; Silva, Williams, & McGee, 1987; Tallal, 1988; Tallal et al., 1991). These studies have reported significantly higher than expected frequencies of social interactional problems among language disordered children. Conversely, a higher than expected prevalence of language problems has been reported among psychiatric populations (Baker & Cantwell, 1982, 1987; Gualtieri et al., 1983; Beitchman et al., 1986; Beitchman, Hood, & Inglis, 1990) and behaviorally disordered populations (Camarata, Hughes, & Ruhl, 1988; Mack & Warr-Leeper, 1992).

Studies of the conversational features of language disordered children's peer interactions suggest why this may be the case. It is just those language skills that have been noted frequently to correlate positively with children's peer status and peer acceptability that have been found to be problematic in the conversations of language disordered children. These data have indicated that language disordered children are responsive but are more likely to be inappropriate or unrelated (Brinton & Fujiki, 1982); responsive but only with greater discourse support than required by age-matched peers (Craig & Gallagher, 1986); responsive but with greater difficulty framing responses specific to the conversational demands (Gallagher & Darton, 1978; Brinton et al., 1986); verbally interactive but more likely to use routines developed early in life even though they are no longer appropriate or effective (Gallagher & Craig, 1984; Loucks & Gallagher, 1988); other-directed in their speech less frequently than peers (Craig & Evans, 1989) and ignored by peers and responded to less frequently by peers (Craig & Gallagher, 1986; Hadley & Rice, 1991).

Fujiki & Brinton (1991) described the conversational interactions of a language impaired child with a number of partners including younger language-matched and age-matched peers. They observed that as the interactions progressed, normal language partners became more unresponsive to the language impaired child. This was true even when the partner was an adult. Since each of these partners behaved differently with the language impaired child than they did with other partners, Fujiki & Brinton concluded that it was the language impaired child's conversational style, which they described as intrusive, that had resulted in the lower frequencies of related partner responses.

Analyses of language disordered children's social interactions indicate an overall reduction in the quantity and quality of their relationships with peers. Craig & Washington (1993), for example, found that children with specific language impairments, language impairments without cognitive, neurological, emotional, or sensory etiologies, had greater difficulty entering peers' ongoing play than did age-matched peers and also greater difficulty than language-matched children who were younger in age but developing language normally. Hadley & Rice (1991) studied classroom interactions among children with and without language impairments and noted that even children at the preschool level "behave as if they know who talks well and who doesn't and they prefer to interact with those who do" (p. 1315). In a study of disputes among preschool specifically language impaired (SLI) children and children with normal language development, Loucks & Gallagher (1988) reported that the language impaired children's nonverbal behaviors led to disputes more often than those of their normal language peers, and that the language impaired children did not seem to be able to recognize or monitor the potentially negative social consequences of their interactional behaviors.

Given the important roles peers play in the development of language skills by providing linguistic and conversational role models, opportunities for practising language skills and opportunities for receiving naturally consequent communication feedback, as well as the roles they play in the development of cognitive and social-cognitive skills in general (Hartup, 1983), language structural goals are being increasingly integrated into more comprehensive communication intervention plans. These plans include conversational goals as well as social-interactional approaches to the development of language structural skills.

COMMUNICATION INTERVENTION PLANS

Communication intervention plans have been influenced by two major literatures, the child discourse literature, and the child social skill intervention literature. Specifications of communication goals have tended to reflect the former and intervention procedures have reflected the latter. Both goals and procedures have been expanded as a consequence.

Communication goals

Intervention goals have been expanded to include the development of discourse management skills such as topic initiation, topic maintenance, turn-taking, requesting, commenting, referencing presuppositions, narratives, and responding (see Gallagher, 1991; Craig, 1991, for reviews). Identification criteria have been expanded to include this new range of skills and assessment procedures modified to meet a broader mandate.

Spontaneous language sampling procedures were modified in several ways. As more was learned about the interactions among communication contexts and language structural features, it became clear that it was futile to attempt to control for context effects across all children. Previous attempts to define a "standardized" language sampling context that could be used across all children were replaced with procedures to accommodate inevitable language use variability. Pre-assessment, a procedure by which information is obtained about the child prior to language sampling to permit individualized contextual configurations to elicit optimal language structural performance (Gallagher, 1983; Lund & Duchan, 1988), was included as a component of the assessment protocol. Another modification was sampling in more than one context.

Language analysis procedures were expanded to include nonverbal as well as verbal behaviors, and some behaviors were analyzed from multiple perspectives. Gaze and pauses are examples of communicatively relevant nonverbal behaviors that are now being assessed. Assessing questions within the broader framework of requesting, which can include other sentence types also serving that communicative function, as well as in terms of the formal syntactic features of question formation, is an example of analyses from multiple perspectives.

Pragmatic profiles also have been introduced (Prutting & Kirchner, 1983, 1987; Roth & Spekman, 1984; Penn, 1988). These solicit ratings of communicatively significant behaviors by individuals who have had opportunities to observe and interact with the child being assessed. Formal tests have been developed including the Test of Pragmatic Skills (Shulman, 1986), the Let's Talk Inventory for Children (Bray & Wiig, 1987), and the Interpersonal Language Skills Assessment (Blagden & McConnell, 1985).

Communication intervention procedures

Communication intervention procedures have been heavily influenced by the social skill intervention literature, a literature which has grown rapidly in the last 20 years. The prominent theories in the social skill intervention literature are operant theory, social learning theory, and cognitive-behavioral theory. These theories focus on observable behavior, antecedent and consequent events, mediational processes and the relationships between problem-solving skills and observable behaviors. The instructional procedures derived from them include modeling, role-playing, self-instructions, reinforcement, coaching, and problem-solving strategies (see Asher, 1985, for review). All of these approaches have been incorporated, to some degree, into communication intervention, or pragmatic language intervention, as it is sometimes termed. Michelson et al. (1983) have summarized the following major assumptions underlying the current social skill intervention literature:

(1) Social skills are primarily specific verbal and nonverbal behaviors.
(2) Social skills involve initiation and responding behaviors.
(3) Social skills are influenced by the contexts in which the behaviors occur.
(4) Social skills are learned primarily through observation, modeling, performance, rehearsal, and feedback (i.e. learning principles).

Although models of social interactional competence differ, they all contain three basic components, at various levels of specification, for both encoding and decoding social interactions. These components are *goals*, the objective of the interaction; *behaviors*, the observable means by which the selected goal is pursued; and *evaluation*, the means by which the impact of the behaviors enacted and goals selected on the ongoing interaction is assessed. Gresham & Elliott (1984) have described problems within each of these types of components of social knowledge as indicating "acquisition deficits," problems suggesting that the requisite skills have not been learned, or "performance deficits," problems suggesting that the skills, although observable in the child's behavioral repertoire, are not being used at expected frequencies or at the appropriate times. Research with language disordered children is just beginning to explore questions regarding the components and types of difficulty most frequently observed within subgroups of this population.

Communication intervention strategies addressing acquisition and performance deficits within each of these components of social knowledge as they relate to communication behaviors include: teaching communicative alternatives for specific socially penalizing behaviors; using event based learning and scripts to facilitate socially appropriate communication; and, manipulating antecedent and consequent events.

Communicative alternatives to socially penalizing behaviors

The influence of the social skill intervention literature on communication intervention programs has been most apparent in their incorporation of direct instructional techniques. Formulaic utterances and memorized sequences, once devalued and considered counterproductive from the perspective of advancing generative grammatical knowledge, are being incorporated into programs as compensatory or coping strategies for dealing with interactionally problematic social situations for children.

As Goldstein & Gallagher (1992) have suggested, observing language disordered children's peer interactions and soliciting specific descriptive statements from communication partners about language disordered children are effective means for highlighting communicative behaviors that are socially negative or particularly socially penalizing and alienating. Gallagher & Craig (1984) used this type of identification procedure to study a 4-year-old specifically language impaired boy's highly frequent use of the phrase "It's gone." The boy, Clark, continued to use the phrase even though his peers responded negatively to it and said things like, "Why do you always say, 'It's gone'?" and "Don't say, 'It's gone' any more." Other children would look confused, walk away, turn their backs when Clark approached, or in other ways express their desire not to interact with Clark. Despite this feedback, Clark continued to use the phrase frequently. After studying his use of "It's gone," Gallagher & Craig (1984) concluded that Clark was using the phrase as a play access strategy and that it was probably an inappropriate extension of an early mother–child routine, the "appearance-disappearance game" (Ratner & Bruner, 1978; Snow, 1978).

Brinton & Fujiki (1993) shared a similar example of a young language disordered child who used the word "liar" to mean "You made a mistake" or "I disagree with you" (p. 196). This atypical use of the term continually offended his peers. Tomblin & Liljigreen (1985) identified similar problems with a 12-year-old language impaired child.

In each of these cases, the intervention program would target the penalizing communicative behavior, identify the interactional need the behavior is attempting to meet, select a communicative behavior that is functionally equivalent but more socially acceptable, and teach the latter behavior to the child as a memorized whole. If the functional analysis was correct, the selected alternative serves the same function, and the selected alternative is more acceptable to peers, establishing the alternative communicative behavior should be readily accomplished and the negative behavior need not be directly addressed. Direct instructional techniques similar to those that can be used to increase vocabulary are efficient means for achieving the intervention goal. Success is determined by the child's increased use of the alternative communicative behavior and consequent decreased use of the communicatively penalizing behavior. Examples include substitution of the phrase "Let's play" for "It's gone" in the first example as a more socially acceptable means of inviting peers to play, and substitution of the phrase "That's wrong" for "liar" in the second example.

Direct instructional techniques include: coaching; direct verbal instruction; providing explicit models of targeted language use; providing opportunities to rehearse targeted patterns; and providing feedback on performance. Modeling can involve role-playing, filmed segments, or videotaped interactions highlighting problematic behaviors and alternatives used by other children. These techniques are often used with acquisition deficits.

Event based learning and scripts

Direct instructional techniques also have been incorporated into communication intervention programs dealing with more general communicative interactional behaviors than those discussed above. Use of the terms "event based learning" or "scripts," to some extent, reflects the degree of directness employed in teaching the requisite communication skills, with the former being more instructionally indirect than the latter.

Event based learning strategies are based upon a rich child development literature (e.g. Bruner & Sherwood, 1976; Nelson & Seidman, 1984) that emphasizes the role of repetitive interactional routines in facilitating children's understanding of conversational structures, rhythms, rules, and the processes of joint referencing. Data from these studies suggests that children's conversational interactions are enhanced when they share event knowledge and mutual expectations.

An example of this approach is the intervention program developed by Snyder-McLean et al. (1984). Their program incorporated language structural intervention into familiar activities that were repeated as routines to facilitate the children's development of appropriate conversational use as a component of their language learning. These repetitive activities included food preparation, story telling, and so on. Snyder-McClean et al. reported that children enrolled in this program improved both communication skills and levels of peer interaction.

Communication intervention incorporating script learning also is organized around events but the language to be used is more directly prescribed and taught. Goldstein et al. (1988) have used this intervention strategy with preschoolers. Children were taught scripts around familiar events like ordering food at a restaurant. Roles were assigned, and the children were encouraged to maintain role-related behaviors in play with peers through clinician prompting and role modeling. Roles were exchanged periodically and elaborations of the script encouraged once the children performed well within the basic script structure. Goldstein et al. reported that using scripts in language intervention not only improved language skills but also improved the children's rate of social interactions with peers.

Manipulating antecedent and consequent events

Strategies that are designed to manipulate antecedent and consequent events are usually employed after the children have gained control over the desired communicative behavior, or when the children's behaviors suggest that their problems reflect performance deficits. The goal of manipulating antecedent events is to increase the number of opportunities to display and practice socially positive communicative behaviors. Analog situations can be used that enable particular interactive situations to occur at much higher frequencies than they would normally. Within these situations, prompting and cuing can be used to encourage the children to use their newly acquired or more effective communicative behaviors. The children also can be taught self-prompting rules or self-instruction strategies to guide their own behavior during social interactions.

The goal of manipulating consequent events is to increase the salience of the relationships between the child's behaviors and the impacts they have on interactive partners and also to increase the frequencies and explicitness of positive outcomes resulting from using particular communicative behaviors. This increases the reinforcement effects of positive outcomes and in so doing strengthens the targeted communicative behaviors and helps the child develop self-evaluative and self-monitoring skills.

PILOT DATA

Several of the strategies described above were incorporated into a 10-week communication intervention program offered by the Speech Foundation of Ontario Toronto Children's Centre under the direction of Deborah Hayden. The program was a receptive and expressive language structural intervention program that was delivered within the overall framework of event based learning. Familiar themes such as grooming, shopping, food preparation, and show-and-tell were the principal events incorporated into the intervention program which included receptive and expressive syntactic goals, and conversational goals such as turn-taking, and topic maintenance. Some key social phrases were presented repetitively but the program was designed to scaffold the children's performance by providing as little intrusion into the naturalness of the interactions as was needed to support the children's success levels and accomplish the intended goals. The program was designed to facilitate the development of functional communication skills in an environment that provided the children with the necessary motivation for communication to occur. The thematic approach provided children with the opportunities to learn and practice language forms, concepts, and interactional skills (see Chapter 20 for more details).

Within a pilot study funded by Fonds de la recherche en santé du Québec, Gallagher (1994) examined the longitudinal relationships among improvements in expressive and receptive language performance following the 10-week communication intervention program offered by the Speech Foundation of Ontario Toronto Children's Centre and changes in adaptability and social skills performance levels. The subjects were a group of preschool SLI children who were experiencing language and social behavior problems at clinically significant levels as determined by standardized tests. Specifically, the study examined the relationships among improvements in the children's language skills and changes in their social behavioral skills after the 10-week communication intervention program compared to changes that occurred following a subsequent 10-week nursery school program. The nursery school program included children without language or social behavioral difficulties and provided opportunities for general stimulation, pre-academic instruction, small group activities and peer social interaction. Children participated in the communication intervention program for $1\frac{1}{2}$ hours two days a week. They participated in the nursery school program 3 to 5 half-days each week. The goal of the pilot study was to explore hypotheses regarding the nature of the correlative effects of improvements in language and social skills in a population where problems with both sets of skills had reached clinically significant levels.

The subjects were four 4-year-old (SLI) children. Language assessment indicated that the SLI children had expressive and receptive syntactic language difficulties (performance more than 1.5 SD below age level on standardized language tests). Their vocabulary and speech skills were within the normal range for their age. The SLI children also were experiencing social interactional difficulties as determined by parent report and performance on standardized rating scales indicating significantly lower than expected adaptability and social skills (performance T score less than 40). Children who participated in the study were referred to the Centre for language intervention but could not be immediately accommodated within their ongoing treatment programs and had been placed on a waiting list. The children's participation in the study did not prejudice their access to inclusion in the Centre's ongoing programs, once space became available.

A group of three children who were developing language normally, and who were comparable to the SLI children in age, nonverbal intelligence, speech intelligibility, and social behavioral difficulties (as determined by the same tests), served as a comparison group. Changes in the social behavioral status of the latter group, following a 10-week nursery school program, were compared to those of the SLI group after each 10-week program in which they participated.

The results of the pilot study indicated that the SLI children's expressive and receptive language performance improved following the communication intervention program, and that these language improvements covaried with improvements in the children's social behavioral ratings on standardized rating scales. Parallel improvements were also noted in their peer interaction profiles within videotaped dyadic, peer play sessions. The results indicated that although the degree to which the SLI children and the comparison children differed from expected age levels on social behavioral scales were comparable at the beginning of the study (mean $=0.27$ SD and 0.26 SD above clinical thresholds, respectively), social behavioral changes for the SLI group, following the communication intervention program, were greater than those for the comparison group following the nursery school program (mean improvement $=0.15$ SD and 0.02 SD, respectively). Social behavioral improvements also were observed in the SLI children's dyadic peer interactions. The mean percentage of time that the SLI children spent interacting with peers during play increased from 28% to 53%.

During the 10-week period subsequent to the communication intervention program, two of the SLI children participated in the nursery school program and did not receive further language intervention during that time. The two other SLI children were able to obtain ongoing language intervention and did not participate in this phase of the pilot study. Further data was collected from the two SLI children who continued in the nursery school program. Results indicated that the social behavioral gains these children had made during the communication intervention program were maintained but no further improvements were noted (0.0 SD and 0.0 SD for each child, respectively).

The results of the pilot study suggest that communication intervention programs that incorporate language structural goals into an event based framework can result in improvements in children's language and social skills, even when those problems are clinically significant. This type of early language intervention may be the most efficient course of treatment for SLI children experiencing social behavioral problems since it addresses their language difficulties while resolving at least some of their social behavioral problems. Confidence in these data is limited, however, by the small number of children studied thus far. Further research is needed to explore the generalizability of the results obtained and the long-term preventative and/or ameliorative effects that may result on later mental health problems for which these children are at risk.

THE ROLE OF PEERS IN COMMUNICATION INTERVENTION

All of the communication intervention strategies discussed above can be implemented by professionals. There is an increasing awareness, however, that peers play a primary role in children's social worlds and that peer involvement in intervention may be essential to achieving effective communication goals. Price & Dodge's (1989) reciprocal influence model of peer interaction provides important insights into why this may be true. Within the model, both the behaviors of the children having social interactional problems and peer behaviors contribute to the maintenance of those problems.

According to the model, children who are socially inept contribute to their lower peer status by exhibiting higher frequencies of negative or socially ineffectual behaviors (Coie & Kupersmidt, 1983; Dodge, 1983). Since peers can not attend to all of the inputs within social interactions, they use processing strategies such as perceptual readiness and selective attention to manage the interactionally relevant information. Over time, schemas about other children, stereotypes, reputations, and so on, are established. Schemas are a natural strategy that develops to aid perceptual processing efficiency. They work to the disadvantage of socially unpopular children, however, because once they are established, schemas support processing biases that maintain the stability of reputations.

Data from Dodge (1980) and Hymel (1986) support the reciprocal influence model. They both found that when ambiguous behaviors were presented to peers they were more likely to be interpreted as negative if they were attributed to a disliked child than if they were attributed to a liked child. Children's reputations biased their perceptions of behaviors.

The model would predict that since peers are more likely to interpret the behaviors of disliked children negatively, they would be more likely to direct negative behaviors toward disliked children than toward other children. The peers' contributions to the negative interactions that would result can be seen as setting up a self-fulfilling prophecy that would only serve to reinforce negative biases.

In this way, both peers' perceptions and behaviors that they direct toward disliked children can function as precipitating and maintaining factors for social interactional problems. An example of these types of interactive effects was reported by Dodge & Frame (1982). They found that peers directed aggressive behaviors more frequently toward those children that they perceived to be aggressive.

Finally, social interactions may be further complicated by the fact that children with social interactional difficulties may not be as accurate as their peers in interpreting peer intentions and predicting probable consequences of interactive behaviors. Several studies suggesting that these children have difficulty evaluating and monitoring social interactions were reviewed above. The probability that a disproportionate number of negative peer behaviors may be directed toward them can only exacerbate these problems. One of the implications of this model is that peers need to be involved in the change process in order for interventions to be efficient and maximally effective. The goals of intervention must include behavioral and perceptual changes by both the targeted children and their peers.

The following summarizes the various roles peers can play in communication intervention.

Peer models

Peers have been used to model appropriate communicative behaviors for language disordered children either through direct observation, by including them as peer partners within intervention sessions to role-play target behaviors, or indirectly, through the use of films or videotape. Inclusion of peer input is an important component of selecting age-appropriate target behaviors since adult intuitions about social appropriateness throughout the developmental age range need to be validated within the children's peer culture. Child social perspectives develop through predictable stages (see Gallagher, 1993, for review) and are observable but not directly accessible to adults. For example, Cartledge, Frew, & Zaharias (1985) studied the perceptions of children and teachers regarding the types of social skills that learning disabled children would need to be successful in mainstreamed classrooms. Children rated most highly those social skills that the teachers rated as least important.

The inclusion of popular children within the intervention program can serve two purposes. First, they can provide examples of skilled behaviors that have contributed to their positive social status among peers. Second, their involvement with and interest in their language disordered partners can change earlier negative perceptions. As highly valued peers in the children's social context these children can serve as effective role models for other children's interactions with and interpretations of the behaviors of language disordered children. Although little systematic research of these issues relative to language disordered children is available to date, several studies in the social skill intervention literature have reported these types of positive consequences of peer involvement (see Furman & Gavin, 1989, for review).

Peer confederates

After new behaviors have been learned, peers can be included in intervention programs as a means of manipulating antecedent and consequent events for target children's behaviors, and as a means of providing increased opportunities to practice new language skills. Peers can be trained to elicit and reinforce the use of new behaviors in the children's natural interpersonal contexts.

Within social skill intervention studies, peer confederates have been trained to increase their frequencies of social initiations toward targeted children, including the frequencies with which they ask them to play, share toys or offer assistance. Others have been successfully included in intervention programs as reinforcement agents who provide positive attention and praise for using specific new behaviors within classroom settings (e.g., Guralnick, 1976; Strain, Shores & Timm, 1977).

Goldstein and his colleagues have adapted these techniques to the communicative interactions of preschool children (Goldstein & Wickstrom, 1986; Goldstein & Ferrell, 1987). Strategies they have taught peers include establishing eye contact and joint focus of attention with language disordered children, initiating joint play with them, prompting requests from them, and responding to them by repeating or expanding their utterances or by requesting clarification of their utterances when needed. The language disordered children included in these studies had moderate to severe developmental disabilities. The results indicated that the use of these strategies by peer partners increased other children's interaction rates with the language disordered children overall, particularly their response rates from other children.

Goldstein & Kaczmarek (1992) share the following cautions about the use of peer facilitative strategies. They recommend that the strategies chosen should not place language disordered children in subservient roles, should have a high probability of leading to sustained interaction, and should optimize the language disordered children's capabilities. They further suggest that sensitizing peers to nonverbal communicative behaviors can help them maintain their interactive roles even though the language disordered child may not be responding as they would typically expect. Goldstein and Kaczmarek found that peers were more persistent in their communicative interactions with language disordered children if they were able to interpret nonverbal behaviors, such as smiling, touching, handing the peer a toy, and so on, as communicative turns on the part of the language disordered child. This increased the peers' satisfaction with the interactions.

Peers may require prompting by adults to encourage their use of the strategies, particularly in the initial stages of transfer to classroom or playroom environments. This prompting needs to be as unobtrusive as possible so the naturalness of the ongoing interaction is minimally disrupted. In the above cited studies, Goldstein and colleagues used a variety of techniques to remind peers to use the strategies they had learned, including gestural cues and signs.

Again, using peer confederates can also help change those peers' perceptions of target children because the peers' attention is being directed toward the children's positive social behaviors. This is an effective means of changing perceptual biases that may exist.

Promoting positive peer interactions

Simply increasing the rate of interactions among peers may not positively affect peer perceptions of language disordered children, unless those interactions are positive. One of the ambiguities in the social skill intervention literature is the often implied assumption that increased rates of interaction are by definition helpful. Increased interaction rates can exacerbate children's social problems unless care is taken to ensure positive outcomes. If the interactions among target children and peers confirm peers' negative biases, their increased frequencies will only strengthen those biases.

One of the means that has been used to encourage positive peer interactions has been the use of cooperative group experiences (Furman & Garvin, 1989). Cooperative group experiences are small group activities that have the following characteristics: the goal of the activity is a group goal; the reward is a group reward; each child has a specialized task; the group's reward depends upon the successful contribution of each member; each child can competently perform the task assigned to him or her; and the activity elicits positive interactions among children. Successful participation in these types of activities can increase language disordered children's self-confidence and help to establish more positive perceptions of them by their peers.

These types of activities are more easily incorporated into ongoing classroom or playroom routines than the kinds of activities required for the establishment of new behaviors. Cooperative group experiences conform to the major characteristics that have been noted for teacher acceptance of classroom interventions. These are that the interventions are positive; that the activity utilizes minimal resources; that the activity does not result in negative consequences for any of the children; and that the activity benefits all of the children, not just the target children (see Elliott, 1988, for review).

SUMMARY

A great deal of treatment efficacy research will be needed to clarify and qualify the utility of social-interactional approaches to communication intervention with language disordered children. That work is just beginning and promises to continue for some time. Progress to date has already been encouraging, however. Intervention agents have been expanded to include teachers and peers, procedures have been expanded to include the full continuum of instruction from direct instruction to facilitation, and manipulations of antecedent and consequent events have extended from individually designed therapies to naturally occurring social contingencies. The promise is that we will be able to help children who are experiencing language and social difficulties in the most efficient and effective manner possible and that potential mental health problems will be prevented or significantly ameliorated as a consequence.

ACKNOWLEDGMENTS

This work was supported in part by a grant from the Fonds de la Recherche en Santé du Québec, Program 14 en recherche en santé mentale, dossier 930658-104, and in part by National Multipurpose Research and Training Center Grant DC-01409 from the National Institute on Deafness and Other Communication Disorders.

REFERENCES

Aram, D., Ekelman, B., & Nation, J. (1984). Preschoolers with language disorders: 10 years later. *Journal of Speech and Hearing Research, 27*, 232–244.

Asher, S. (1985). An evolving paradigm in social skill training research with children. In B. Schneider, K. Rubin, & J. Ledingham (eds) *Children's Peer Relations: Issues in Assessment and Intervention.* New York: Springer-Verlag (pp. 157–171).

Baker, L. & Cantwell, D. (1982). Developmental, social and behavioural characteristics of speech and language disordered children. *Child Psychiatry and Human Development, 12*, 195–206.

Baker, L. & Cantwell, D. (1987). A prospective psychiatric follow-up of children with speech/language disorders. *Journal of the American Academy of Child and Adolescent Psychiatry, 26*, 546–553.

Bates, E. (1976). *Language in Context.* New York: Academic Press.

Beitchman, J., Hood, J., & Inglis, A. (1990). Psychiatric risk in children with speech and language disorders. *Journal of Abnormal Child Psychology, 18*, 283–296.

Beitchman, J., Nair, R., Clegg, M., Ferguson, B., & Patel, P. (1986). Prevalence of psychiatry disorders in children with speech and language disorders. *Journal of the American Academy of Child Psychiatry, 25*, 528–553.

Blagden, C. & McConnell, N. (1985). *Interpersonal language skills assessment.* Moline, IL: LinguiSystems.

Bray, C. & Wiig, E. (1987). *Let's Talk Inventory for Children.* San Antonio, TX: Psychological Corp.

Brinton, B. & Fujiki, M. (1982). A comparison of request-response sequences in the discourse of normal and language-disordered children. *Journal of Speech and Hearing Disorders,* 47, 57–62.

Brinton, B. & Fujiki, M. (1993). Language, social skills, and socioemotional behavior. *Language, Speech, and Hearing Services in Schools,* 24, 194–198.

Brinton, B., Fujiki, M., Winkler, E., & Loeb, D. (1986). Responses to requests for clarification in linguistically normal and language-impaired children. *Journal of Speech and Hearing Disorders,* 51, 370–378.

Bruner, J. & Sherwood, V. (1976). Early rule structure: the case of peekaboo. In J. Bruner, A. Jolly, & K. Sylva (eds) *Play: Its Role in Evolution and Development.* New York: Penguin (pp. 277–285).

Camarata, S., Hughes, C., & Ruhl, K. (1988). Mild/moderate behaviourally-disordered students: A population at risk for language disorders. *Language Speech and Hearing Services in the Schools,* 19, 191–200.

Cartledge, G., Frew, T., & Zaharias, J. (1985). Social skill needs of mainstreamed students: peer and teacher perceptions. *Journal of Learning Disabilities,* 5, 484–488.

Coie, J. & Kupersmidt, J. (1983). A behavioral analysis of emerging social status in boys' groups. *Child Development,* 54, 1400–1416.

Craig, H. (1983). Applications of pragmatic language models for intervention. In T. Gallagher & C. Prutting (eds) *Pragmatic Assessment and Intervention Issues in Language.* San Diego, CA: College-Hill Press (pp. 65–82).

Craig, H. & Evans, J. (1989). Turn exchange characteristics of SLI children's simultaneous and nonsimultaneous speech. *Journal of Speech and Hearing Disorders,* 54, 334–347.

Craig, H. & Gallagher, T. (1986). Interactive play: the frequency of related verbal responses. *Journal of Speech and Hearing Research,* 29, 375–383.

Craig, H. & Washington, J. (1986). Children's turn-taking behaviors: Social-linguistic interaction. *Journal of Pragmatics,* 10, 173–197.

Craig, H. & Washington, J. (1993). Access behaviors of children with specific language impairment. *Journal of Speech and Hearing Research,* 36, 322–337.

Dodge, K. (1980). Social cognition and children's aggressive behavior. *Child Development,* 51, 162–170.

Dodge, K. (1983). Behavioral antecedents of peer social status. *Child Development,* 54, 1386–1399.

Dodge, K. & Frame, C. (1982). Social cognitive biases and deficits in aggressive boys. *Child Development,* 53, 620–635.

Elliott, S. (1988). Acceptability of behavioral treatments in educational settings. In J. Witt, S. Elliott, & F. Gresham (eds) *Handbook of Behavior Therapy in Education.* New York: Plenum (pp. 121–150).

Fujiki, M. & Brinton, B. (1991). The verbal noncommunicator: a case study. *Language, Speech, Hearing Services in Schools,* 22, 322–333.

Furman, W. & Garvin, L. (1989). Peers' influence on adjustment and development. In T. Berndt & G. Ladd (eds) *Peer relationships in child development.* New York: John Wiley (pp. 319–340).

Gallagher, T. (1983). Pre-assessment: a procedure for accommodating language use variability. In T. Gallagher & C. Prutting (eds) *Pragmatic Assessment and Intervention Issues in Language*. San Diego, CA: College-Hill Press (pp. 1–28).

Gallagher, T. (1991). A retrospective look at clinical pragmatics. In T. Gallagher (ed.) *Pragmatics of Language: Clinical Practice Issues*. San Diego, CA: Singular Publishing Group (pp. 1–9).

Gallagher, T. (1993). Language skill and the development of social competence in school-aged children. *Language, Speech and Hearing Services in the Schools*, 24, 199–205.

Gallagher, T. (1994). Language treatment outcomes as predictive indices of social-emotional status. Fonds de la Recherche en Santé du Québec, Program No. 14 en recherche en santé mentale, dossier 930658-104.

Gallagher, T. & Craig, H. (1984). Adult-child discourse: The conversational relevance of pauses. *Journal of Pragmatics*, 7, 347–360.

Gallagher, T. & Darton, B. (1978). Conversational aspects of the speech of language disordered children: Revision behaviours. *Journal of Speech and Hearing Research*, 21, 103–117.

Goldstein, H. & Gallagher, T. (1992). Strategies for promoting the social-communicative competence of young children with specific language impairment. In S. Odom, S. McConnell, & M. McEvoy (eds) *Social Competence of Young Children with Disabilities*. Baltimore, MD: Paul H. Brookes (pp. 189–214).

Goldstein, H. & Ferrell, D. (1987). Augmenting communicative interaction between handicapped and nonhandicapped preschoolers. *Journal of Speech and Hearing Disorders*, 16, 200–211.

Goldstein, H. & Kaczmarek, L. (1992). Promoting communicative interaction among children in integrated intervention settings. In S. Warren & J. Reichle (eds) *Causes and Effects in Communication and Language Intervention*. Baltimore, MD: Paul H. Brookes (pp. 81–111).

Goldstein, H., Wickstrom, S., Hoyson, M., Jamieson, B., & Odom, S. (1988). Effects of sociodramatic play training on social and communicative interaction. *Education and Treatment of Children*, 11, 97–117.

Goldstein, H. & Wickstrom, S. (1986). Peer intervention effects on communicative-interaction among handicapped and nonhandicapped preschoolers. *Journal of Applied Behavior Analysis*, 19, 209–214.

Gresham, F. & Elliott, S. (1984). Assessment and classification of children's social skills: a review of methods and issues. *School Psychology Review*, 13, 292–301.

Gualtieri, C., Koriath, U., Van Bourgondien, M., & Saleeby, N. (1983). Language disorders in children referred for psychiatric services. *Journal of the American Academy of Child Psychiatry*, 22, 165–171.

Guralnick, M. (1976). The value of integrating handicapped and nonhandicapped preschool children. *American Journal of Orthopsychiatry*, 42, 236–245.

Hadley, P. & Rice, M. (1991). Conversational responsiveness of speech- and language-impaired preschoolers. *Journal of Speech and Hearing Research*, 34, 1308–1317.

Hartup, W. (1983). Peer interaction and the behavioral development of the individual child. In W. Damon (ed.) *Social Personality Development: Essays on the Growth of the Child*. New York: W.W. Norton (pp. 220–233).

Hazen, N. & Black, B. (1989). Preschool peer communication skills: the role of social status and interaction context. *Child Development*, 60, 867–876.

Hymel, S., (1986). Interpretation of peer behavior: Affective bias in childhood and adolescence. *Child Development*, 57, 431–445.

Loucks, Y. & Gallagher, T. (1988). Dispute initiations among SLI and normal language preschoolers. Paper presented at the American Speech-Language-Hearing Association Convention, November, St Louis, MO.

Lund, N. & Duchan, J. (1988). *Assessing Children's Language in Naturalistic Contexts.* Englewood Cliffs, NJ: Prentice-Hall.

Mack, A. & Warr-Leeper, G. (1992). Language abilities in boys with chronic behaviour disorders. *Language Speech and Hearing Services in the Schools,* 23, 214–223.

Michelson, L., Sugai, D., Wood, R., & Kazdin, A. (1983). *Social Skills Assessment and Training with Children: An Empirically Based Approach.* New York, NY: Plenum Press.

Nelson, K. & Seidman, S. (1984). Playing with scripts. In I. Bretherton (ed.) *Symbolic Play: The Development of Social Understanding.* Orlando, FL: Academic Press (pp. 45–71).

Parker, J. & Gottman, J. (1989). Social and emotional development in a relational context. In T. Bernt & G. Ladd (eds) *Peer Relationships in Child Development.* New York: John Wiley (pp. 95–131).

Penn, C. (1988). The profiling of syntax and pragmatics in aphasia. *Clinical Linguistics & Phonetics,* 2, 179–207.

Price, J. & Dodge, K. (1989). Peers' contributions to children's social maladjustment. In T. Bernt & G. Ladd (eds) *Peer Relationships in Child Development.* New York: John Wiley.

Prutting, C. & Kirchner, D. (1983). Applied pragmatics. In T. Gallagher & C. Prutting (eds) *Pragmatic Assessment and Intervention Issues in Language.* San Diego, CA: College-Hill Press (pp. 29–64).

Prutting, C. & Kirchner, D. (1987). A clinical appraisal of the pragmatic aspects of language. *Journal of Speech and Hearing Disorders,* 52, 105–119.

Ratner, N. & Bruner, J. (1978). Games, social exchange and the acquisition of language. *Journal of Child Language,* 5, 391–401.

Roth, F. & Spekman, N. (1984). Assessing the pragmatic abilities of children: Part I. Organizational framework and assessment parameters. *Journal of Speech and Hearing Disorders,* 49, 2–11.

Schery, T. (1985). Correlates of language development in language disordered children. *Journal of Speech and Hearing Disorders,* 50, 73–83.

Searle, J. (1969). *Speech Acts.* Cambridge MA: Harvard University Press.

Shulman, B. (1986). *Test of Pragmatic Skills.* Arizona: Communication Skill Builders.

Silva, P., Williams, S., & McGee, R. (1987). A longitudinal study of children with developmental language delay at age three: later intelligence, reading, and behavior problems. *Developmental Medicine and Child Neurology,* 29, 630–640.

Snow, C. (1978). The conversational context of language acquisition. In R. Campbell & P. Smith (eds) *Recent Advances in the Psychology of Language: Language Development and Mother–Child Interaction.* New York, NY: Plenum (pp. 253–269).

Snyder-McClean, L., Solomonson. B., McClean, J., & Sack, S. (1984). Structuring joint action routines: a strategy for facilitating communication and language development in the classroom. *Seminars in Speech and Language,* 5, 213–228.

Strain, P., Shores, R., & Timm, M. (1977). Effects of peer social initiations on the behavior of withdrawn preschool children. *Journal of Applied Behavior Analysis,* 10, 289–298.

Tallal, P. (1988). Developmental language disorders. In J.F. Kavanaugh & T.J. Truss, Jr. (eds) *Learning disabilities: Proceedings of the National Conference.* Parkton, MD: York Press.

Tallal, P., Townsend, J., Curtiss, S., & Wulfeck, P. (1991). Phenotypic profiles of language-impaired children based on genetic/family history. *Brain and Language,* **41**, 81–95.

Tomblin, J. & Liljigreen, S. (1985). The identification of socially significant communication needs in older language impaired children: a case example. In D. Ripich & F. Spinelli (eds) *School Discourse Problems.* San Diego, CA: College-Hill Press (pp. 219–230).

20 Language intervention programming for preschool children with social and pragmatic disorders

DEBORAH A. HAYDEN AND MARGIT PUKONEN

This chapter will describe an approach to intervention programming used at the Speech Foundation of Ontario, Toronto Children's Centre, for preschool children assessed as having an expressive subtype of specific language impairment (SLI). The intent of this chapter will be to first outline the confusion inherent in the definition of SLI and to argue for the necessity to subgroup the various syndromes identified within the larger category. Further, the development of a group treatment program designed to address the underlying nature of a subtype, expressive disorder, will be discussed and the theoretical basis and general procedures detailed. An intervention protocol that provides information on grouping and programming guidelines, will be illustrated by examples and a case study and, finally, future research directions will be discussed.

DEFINING THE DISORDER

Understanding the child with specific language impairment (SLI) and the effects of this disorder has been problematic (Menyuk, 1964; Leonard, 1972; 1987; Leonard & Fey, 1991). The central issues in this debate have revolved primarily around the difficulties in discerning either a causative factor or a particular course of treatment.

As one might expect, questions about the underlying nature and defining characteristics of the impairment have been numerous. Some have theorized that the cause of the disorder is social-emotional (Rutter, Izeard, & Read, 1986). Others have postulated that a cognitive deficit related to both language and social-emotional behaviors is the causative factor (Pearl, 1987) and finally, that language disorders themselves may lead to both cognitive or social-emotional disruptions in the child's development (Baker & Cantwell, 1987).

Children with SLI, have been defined as those who demonstrate poor expressive or receptive language skills in the absence of clinically significant neurological impairment, hearing loss, emotional problems, or sensori-motor defects with non-verbal intelligence in the normal range (Stark & Tallal, 1981). Diagnostic criteria for specific language impairment requires a significant discrepancy of one to two standard deviations between nonverbal cognitive testing and expressive or receptive scores.

It has become increasingly accepted that the children who make up this group constitute a heterogeneous population (Leonard, 1972; Strominger & Bashier, 1977; Bloom & Lahey, 1978; Weiner, 1980; Aram, Ekelman, & Nation, 1984; Aram, Morris, & Hall, 1993; Stark et al., 1984). Recent attempts have been made to define subtypes or subgroups of this heterogeneous disorder (Aram & Nation, 1975; Rapin & Allen, 1983; Fey, 1986; Craig & Evans, 1993).

Rapin and Allen (1983) have proposed four major subtypes with the predominant being an expressive disorder. Within the expressive disorder they have further identified four subgroups: (1) the phonologic-syntactic, (2) the severe expressive with good comprehension, (3) the syntactic-pragmatic, and (4) the semantic-pragmatic without autism. The last two groups may best represent the children discussed in this chapter. Rapin and Allen described these children as impaired in comprehension and syntax development and severely limited in the pragmatic use of language. These children may name pictures, objects and give and follow simple commands but have difficulty formulating or responding to wh- questions or in conversational language. They may demonstrate difficulty considering the prior knowledge and information needs of the listener. They may also have difficulty grasping the full intent of questions and may focus on single words or short phrases and pursue tangentially related topics of their own. These children may often have difficulty with peer relationships and interactions.

Our efforts to define subgroups of children with specific language disability may be at best premature, but the need to define specific profiles of these children so that programs can be devised to accommodate their strengths and address their weakness are desperately needed.

LANGUAGE CHARACTERISTICS THAT DEFINE SLI CHILDREN

Children identified as specific language impaired have been examined on a multitude of tasks in multiple domains. A growing body of information on the pragmatic use of these children's language has especially become of interest. This literature highlights the difficulties these children have in integration of rule systems, that is, communication functions that underlie the selection of linguistic structures (MacNamara, 1972; Halliday, 1975; Bates, 1976; Bates & MacWhinney, 1979).

The general research findings discussed below are also representative of the clinical population discussed in this chapter. This population is aligned with an SLI expressive disorder subgroup. While they are clearly competent, albeit delayed, in the comprehension and acquisition of basic language forms, they have difficulty with complex linguistic reasoning and use. Of the areas investigated only the ones that have revealed significant differences between them and same-aged, normal language peers, are presented. The language difficulties experienced by this subgroup, and as defined by the literature, form part of the basis for the group intervention protocol discussed in later sections.

Pragmatic systems

Recently, the nature of SLI has been viewed from a pragmatic perspective (Gallagher, 1983, 1991; Craig, 1991, 1993; Leonard & Fey, 1991). In this perspective researchers have been primarily interested in how the language system and its form are used to communicate, in other words, the integration of rule systems and linguistic forms to develop speaker-listener interactions. This critical communication skill is often at risk or is poorly developed in the child with language impairment, and may cause difficulty with developing normal social interaction and peer relationships. The ability to integrate linguistic forms and subtle meanings inherent in social language interaction is essential to communication. Certain subgroups of SLI children appear to have more difficulty with this aspect of language (Fey, 1986; Leonard & Fey, 1991). It is not yet certain if the linguistic skills needed for negotiating complex interactions are at fault or if the conceptual demands, that is, their hierarchical planning and understanding of causal relationships may be poorly developed. One thing is certain, that conceptual, linguistic and pragmatic factors all need to be addressed in the SLI child. The following section discusses the linguistic areas where SLI children have shown deficiencies. Even with this research data the nature of the exact relationship between linguistic form and its use remains convoluted. This interrelation is explored throughout the chapter and the premise that is put forward is that social and pragmatic skills can be developed through language intervention strategies based on the integration of cognitive, linguistic, and pragmatic systems using a natural or event related content.

Linguistic form difficulties in the expression of language functions by SLI children

Difficulties with linguistic form have been developed and reported by many researchers for the general SLI population. While they may be observed in the general population, they are especially problematic for children in the expressive disorder subgroup. These difficulties have shown up in the functions of language that related to language form and have been examined primarily within dialogue and narrative discourse. Craig (1991) has been especially interested in how these difficulties interfere with children's abilities to use language in social relationships. A summary of this information and how it may affect interaction is presented.

Commenting and requesting

In two categories of intention, *imperative performance*, which get the listener to act, and *declarative performance*, which attempt to inform or focus the listener's attention, SLI children were found to have more difficulty than their same-aged peers (Craig, 1991). The SLI children tended to use more nonlinguistic signals, gestures, or comments to convey their message and tended to form less grammatically complete sentences. While in general the children appeared to have the ability to initiate and use various language structures, they often failed to use these structural resources in ways that were appropriate or clearly communicated their intent.

Understanding background information

Presuppositions refer to the speaker's awareness of background and foreground information that is important when providing information to the listener. In general, studies have shown that children with SLI demonstrate basic presuppositional knowledge. However, and in contrast to same-aged peers beyond a one-word stage, some language disordered children express presuppositions in a manner that is not typical of the structural level of their language.

Turn-taking

The ability to continue for the purpose of sharing and regulating information is critical to conversation. Information from several studies investigating successful turn-taking negotiation have implied that children with SLI differed significantly from those with normal language. They differed in producing significantly less other-directed speech, using fewer multi-utterance turns and in timing turns less tightly than their age-mates. Instead, the SLI children tended to produce significantly more responses and more adjacent speech than even the younger normal children. Overall, these children appeared to understand the idea of turns and to be able to regulate the turn-taking process. Their receptive and expressive difficulties, however, often complicated this process. Slow processing speed may affect comprehension and the ability to formulate semantically elaborate responses (Stark & Tallal, 1981).

Appropriateness of responding

Several areas have been investigated with regard to SLI children's ability to use response strategies within conversation (Gallagher & Darnton, 1978; Brinton & Fujiki, 1982; Leonard et al., 1982; Brinton et al., 1986; Craig & Gallagher, 1988). Overall, these areas suggest a multitude of difficulties for SLI children. However, the most important appears to be that children with

SLI, although recognizing the pragmatic obligation to respond, seem to have difficulty tailoring the linguistic structure of their responses to conversational demands. This deficit is thought to be partly due to inadequate linguistic resources and the children's inability to use the linguistic structures they do have to meet their pragmatic needs in varied conversational ways. Studies also supported the premise that these children may have additional difficulties in naming or using referents.

Story retelling

Another area to reveal problems is narratives or the ability to retell a story, either from original story generation, books, television, or movies. There is little doubt that even in children with normal language development this task is difficult, but the narrative produced by children with SLI differ in linguistically important ways. Their narratives are less complete, exhibit more breakdowns, and more incomplete and erroneous cohesive ties (Sleight & Prinz, 1985; Liles, 1987; MacLachlan & Chapman, 1988). Although SLI children produce narrative discourse and demonstrate knowledge of the basic discourse feature, they differ in the comprehensiveness of their stories and the manner in which they organize sentence relationships.

Conceptual developmental difficulties

Conceptual developmental difficulties have also been suspected by some investigators (Johnston, 1989). These areas relate to the high-level cognitive functions of which language is a part and include symbolic play, hierarchical planning and understanding causal relationships. These difficulties in SLI children have been found to often interfere with their ability to engage in pretend play or to use more advanced play schemes. These children also appear to be limited in the understanding and production of language forms used to denote time and space for organizing events, responding or in their narratives. Their ideas of cause and effect relationships, sequencing, and predictability have also been found to be significantly reduced compared to same-aged peers.

Whether these conceptually related deficits are part of the overall deficit or whether inadequate linguistic development contributes to the conceptual deficit is still very much debated. One thing is certain both of these areas are connected through language, and promote further growth of cognitive and social development.

In summary, children with SLI expressive disorder, although often delayed in language acquisition, operate much like their normal peers in their basic knowledge of simple information. Unlike their normal peers, however, they show difficulties in translating complex conceptual information into forms that provide a basis for interaction and social language use. This mix of problems has made these children often difficult to recognize as language impaired. Often these children are seen more as behaviorally disturbed or as unable to form cooperative peer relationships. While several researchers have recognized this problem (Craig, 1991, 1993; Gallagher, 1993; Fey, 1986; Johnston, 1989), few have designated intervention programs to address the specific nature of the SLI expressive disorder issues.

GROUP INTERVENTION MODELS FOR CHILDREN WITH SLI

The history of group intervention language programs developed, especially for children with SLI expressive disorder, is meagre. Recently, there has been some published information on programs designed to assess the effectiveness of different treatment approaches used with language impaired children. These have, however, not been designed especially to intervene with the type of children discussed in this chapter. In general, there are three types of group program models currently in use for children with language impairment. They are parent information and intervention models, integrated preschool models and integrated pre-school peer mentoring models. Each of these models is described briefly below.

Parent information and intervention models

An example of this type of program is the Language Interaction Intervention Program (LIIP) (Weistuch & Lewis, 1985, 1986; Weistuch & Byers-Brown, 1987). The program was designed to teach parents of preschool language delayed children to elicit language in natural, play-like, environments. The three components of the program were: group parent information sessions, where strategies for encouraging language development were taught; group children language stimulation sessions with a clinician while the parents received their training; and after-group child and parent simultaneous sessions. For this component, parents were placed with their children to practice the skills they had been taught while feedback was given to clinicians. Results from the original demonstration project indicated that parents who attended the program were successful in changing their use of language strategies with their children relative to matched controls (Weistuch & Lewis, 1985, 1986; Weistuch & Byers-Brown, 1987). Further to this project, a replication study was conducted where the LIIP program was taught to speech-language pathologists in various school districts to examine whether they could train parents and effectively change parent language style. The main areas examined for change were the parents' expansions and extensions. Results did not indicate a significant change in these areas, however, qualitative changes were suggested in other areas of parent–child communication. Other parent–child intervention models of this type have been described including one by Tannock & Girolametto (1992).

Integrated preschool models

An example of this type of model is the Language Acquisition Preschool Program (LAP) run by the Department of Speech-Language-Hearing at the University of Kansas (Rice & Wilcox, 1991). This demonstration project combines an integrated service delivery model for language stimulation with a preschool programming emphasis on language "enhancement" and direct intervention for children aged from 3 to 5 years (Bunce & Watkins, in press). The demonstration program is based on cognitive/social learning theory and uses a half-day preschool format. The program has developed a curriculum based on both semester and weekly themes that: (a) enhance the children's development of functional language and (b) facilitate interaction in a child centered environment where parent participation is encouraged. Six normal language learning children are fully integrated with six SLI children and six English as a Second Language (ESL) children. The LAP staff include a teacher with early childhood experience and extensive speech-language training, speech-pathology interns, ESL interpreters, parent services coordinator and support staff. Two groups of 18 children each attend per day, one in the morning and another in the afternoon. The program runs on a semester system, with two 16-week sessions and one 8-week session. Preliminary data have suggested that language and social communication is improved with this model and that, without intervention, "about 40% of preschool or kindergarten children identified with speech/language impairments do not stay with their kindergarten cohort in subsequent academic placement" (Rice, 1993, p. 6).

Integrated preschool peer mentoring

Sometimes referred to as "peer confederate" interventions, these efforts involve asking normal language children to help their classmates with disabilities (Goldstein, 1992). The normal peers are taught to use language strategies to initiate social or play behaviors with the language impaired children. Strategies for peer mediated approaches have included: (a) establishing eye contact, (b) initiating joint play, (c) self or other directed talk, (d) repeating, responding or expansion of utterances or repair strategies (Goldstein & Ferrell, 1987). One of the main purposes of this type of model is that it reduces the adult, prompt-dependent, interaction children with SLI often come to depend on and encourages facilitative strategies for social communication. Results have suggested that language impaired children appear to learn the new strategies from their normal peer partners and may eventually use them to monitor their own communication behaviors with other children.

Another purpose of this type of model is that it allows for more naturalistic language interaction and encourages, ultimately, pragmatic and social language skills that will be useful later in the child's life. While peer mentoring approaches may not be able to teach all of the sub-skills necessary for language development, that is, semantics and syntax, they appear to provide a cost effective way to change SLI children's use of language in social situations.

THE SPEECH FOUNDATION OF ONTARIO GROUP INTERVENTION PROGRAM

In addition to the programs outlined above, a program that incorporates these methods but develops its goals in the context of small homogeneous groups of children with comparable presenting SLI expressive difficulties has been carried out by the Speech Foundation of Ontario, Toronto Children's Centre. First, a general overview of the Centre's programs will be outlined and then a more specific focus on the SLI expressive subgroup intervention approach will be detailed.

The Speech Foundation of Ontario, Toronto Children's Centre has developed several intervention programs based exclusively on a group model. The program, mandated to treat children with specific speech/language impairments, has been in operation for 12 years. On a Speech-Language Pathologist's referral, children aged from 3 to 10 years are accepted into the program, if they meet the following two criteria: (1) a *relatively normal to mild* difficulty in hearing, nonverbal cognition, motor control and emotional/behavioral aspects of development and (2) a *significant* delay or disorder in language or expressive speech/language production relative to overall developmental level.

The Centre offers seven different group interventions, each with two or three levels of complexity, designed to focus on a different aspect or level of speech and language need. Some groups, for instance, speech, are more didactic and activity based, whereas others, for example, language, are more interactive and theme based. All groups run for a treatment block of 10 weeks, twice a week, for a total of 20 sessions. Children may be seen for up to four treatment blocks, thus may be eligible for 80 sessions of treatment.

Obtaining child profiles: assessment

Assessment protocols are used primarily for (a) identifying the child's strengths and weaknesses *across* the cognitive, linguistic, social and motor domains, (b) clarifying *within-domain* difficulties, and (c) selecting information that will allow for a homogeneous grouping.

The development of a communication profile on each child permits subgrouping those children, identified in earlier sections, needing intervention, especially in the areas of social and pragmatic language. The profile consists of the following formal and informal assessment information.

Communicative functions

Using a formalized observation procedure, in a play-like setting, the following functions are evaluated: (a) *range of functions* and use of specific functions, that is, requesting, objecting, protesting, calling; showing and commenting; (b) *joint attention*, that is, communicative acts used to direct another's attention; (c) *topic maintenance* and; (d) *repair strategies* or persistence in communication measured by repetition of a previous communicative act when a goal is not achieved.

Social-emotional and behavioral

Within this area the child's ability to cooperate, to use appropriate assertion to initiate interaction by showing responsibility for communication and for property, to use empathy by showing concern or respect for others and to evidence self-control in stressful or conflicting communicative interaction are assessed using observational and behavioral checklists. At the Centre, the parent and teacher rating scales are used to gather information about the child's observable positive (adaptive) and negative (clinical) behaviors. The information gained on these scales helps to identify the behaviors associated with the child's communication problem and may be useful for evaluating the changes by language intervention. Examples of the types of checklists used are: the Social Skills Rating System – Parent Scale and Teacher Scale (Gresham & Elliott, 1989). The Conners' Parent Rating Scales and Conners' Teacher Rating Scales (Conners, 1989) and the Behavior Assessment System for Children (BASC), (Reynolds & Kamphaus, 1992). Each of the three instruments may be administered in a relatively short time (10 to 20 minutes), have norms based on large representative samples and provide information on various behavioral difficulties. Different scales are employed for children with different presenting problems.

Linguistic profile

For children over four years of age, the following are administered routinely; the Test for Auditory Comprehension of Language – Revised (TACL-R) (Carrow-Woolfolk, 1985), the Peabody Picture Vocabulary Test – Revised (PPVT-R) (Dunn & Dunn, 1981), the Computer Analysis of Phonological Deviations (CAPD) (Hodson, 1985), the Expressive One Word Picture Vocabulary Test (Gardiner, 1979) and the Structured Photographic Expressive Language Test-II (Werner & Kresheck, 1983). As well, Mean Length of Utterance (MLU) (Miller & Chapman, 1981), is calculated using a language sample of 50 utterances obtained during a story-telling task and using pictures for elicitation. If sufficient qualitative and quantitative information can not be collected from the child on the above tests the following may be administered as an alternative: the Reynell Developmental Language Scales – Receptive and Expressive (Reynell, 1989).

Additional testing

Hearing, vision and intelligence testing are also necessary to determine if the child's characteristics comply with the Centre's entrance criteria, and are assessed before the child is admitted to program. If not already available from other assessments, hearing will be rescreened and an Arthur Adaptation of the Leiter International Performance Scales (Arthur, 1952) may be required to clarify nonverbal cognitive ability.

GROUPING CHILDREN

The group context has the potential to be a very rich therapeutic environment as the group element facilitates the development of a much broader range of communication skills than is possible through individual treatment (Fawcus, 1992). Children at the Centre are subgrouped and matched according to developmental level and primary area of speech/language need. Normally developing age-matched peers are not included in the groups due to the nature of the tertiary level service provided. Although the current trend in the literature (Goldstein & Kaczmarek, 1992; Rice, 1993), is towards integrating SLI children with their normal peers, the Centre group model has application as a compliment or adjunct to the child's regular preschool or school program. Within the matched groups, the SLI child has the opportunity to acquire social routines and language for interacting with peers through the guided interactions and scaffolding provided by the clinician. By participating in a small group of three to four, the SLI children develop familiarity with routines and expectations, which will help them participate more successfully in other group settings they encounter in their social and academic lives. Since groups naturally create a communication context, intervention activities are planned to integrate linguistic, cognitive, and social aspects. This increases the probability that language skills will generalize to other contexts and thus maximizes the effectiveness of therapy. Children are grouped according to profiles that have been developed for each group type. Children in the SLI expressive disorder subgroup tend to demonstrate the following characteristics; (a) be between 4 and 5 years of age; (b) have a nonverbal cognitive level low average to average; (c) have social language skills moderately/severely disordered; (d) have a receptive language moderately delayed to mildly delayed; (e) have an expressive language moderately delayed to mildly delayed; (f) have phonological skills that are low average to average.

THEORETICAL FRAMEWORK OF THE PROGRAM

Models for learning in the design of group programs

The underlying framework used at the Centre in the design of a group model for children with SLI, is based on language learning constructs. These constructs combine aspects of cognitive-linguistic and social language theory. This unique developmental approach integrates cognitive theory (Piaget, 1952, 1962), "event knowledge" (Nelson, 1986), the notion of a "zone of proximal development" (Vygotsky, 1978) and "scaffolding" (Bruner, 1983), to form a framework for intervention programming. What follows is a brief review of these theoretical positions.

Cognitive development

Piaget believed that all children follow the same developmental pattern in achieving awareness of self from others, and move from sensori-motor, to concrete, and to abstract reasoning. His work is vast and complex (for more detailed information see Brainerd (1978)). In brief, Piaget's view is that cognition precedes and influences language, although at later stages (pre-operational-operational) language may further cognition. Piaget derived his model from a biological framework and used the concepts "accommodation" and "assimilation" to imply that the organism must constantly adjust and learn from his environment and concurrently assimilate the new information into his cognitive structures. Piaget felt all children progress through the same stages in order to think "symbolically" and develop true language and thought. His stages include the sensori-motor from birth to approximately age 2, the pre-operational from approximately age 2 to 7, the concrete-operational from approximately age 7 to 11 and the formal-operational from approximately 11 through adulthood. Briefly, the sensori-motor stage is characterized by an absence of internalized (symbolic) thought. At this stage development of cognitive structures can only be expressed through physical action on the environment. The pre-operational stage is the beginning of internalized thought that arose from the earlier overt action schemes. During the concrete-operational stage the child is said to lose his/her intuitive character and begin more rigorous and logical mental operations which, however, are still based on observables. In the last stage, formal-operations, the child uses fully abstract, logical thinking.

Event knowledge

The basis of this theoretical approach is that children's knowledge of everyday experiences forms the initial content of their mental representations and therefore sets the groundwork for "thinking, talking and acting." Nelson

(1986) and her colleagues feel that early events or routines of daily living such as dressing, eating, bathing, or shopping constitute "sets" that free up mental energy. By using these routines children learn vocabulary, sequences of actions, predictable language, and social interactions. By engaging in familiar and predictable routines, the child's information processing may be enhanced and at the same time the social contexts for interaction and communication are realized. The role of "mother" or facilitator is critical in this approach as she is the catalyst for the child's successful interactions. In this role mothers must be aware of the child's communication attempts, acknowledge and expand the child's linguistic structures, and provide a further context for the child to continue the interchange. When both the adult and child process and share event knowledge, the interactions may form the link between cognitive and social learning.

Scaffolding

Scaffolding is a term and procedure developed by Bruner (1983) to further define transactional learning. The process of scaffolding language requires (a) providing a basic level of talk, (b) capitalizing on familar "routine events" or formats. Formats contain a sequential structure, clearly marked roles and scripts for the accompanying communication. Van Kleeck & Richardson (1988) have summed up these procedures for both the adult's role and the child's role into four stages. These stages will be covered in our discussion of goals of intervention below.

A zone of proximal development

Zone of proximal development is the main premise behind Vygotskian theory as the social basis of transactional learning. This premise states that there are two planes in the child's cultural development, the social and the psychological; and that all functions are learned first on one, the interpsychological, and then the other, the intrapsychological. The process allows the child to move from other-regulated behavior to self-regulated behavior, and to eventual independent thought. The adult is the "bridge" for helping the child go from one developmental level to the next. The adult's task is to determine the child's correct developmental level and how modifiable the child's behavior is with support from the adult. In this context Vygotsky feels that all individual psychological learning, including language, is acquired through social interaction with a more experienced and competent member of the culture.

By utilizing the above constructs, the Centre has developed group program formats that: (1) assess the level of the child's developmental and construct activities and procedures that are at the child's level or lead to an increase in developmental function, (2) incorporate the child's developmental level while building on the child's knowledge of events/routines as a basis for planning, (3) use adult modeling and support to develop activities that engage and promote the child's ongoing communication and (4) use procedures that create a context for the child to (a) become involved, familiar with and learn to anticipate the events, (b) learn target responses, (c) stabilize responses, gain control and interchange roles, and (d) begin to verbally plan, self-monitor, and generalize behaviors to new contexts. The intervention program described next is an example of how developments in research and the literature have been incorporated and applied in our specific clinical setting.

GOALS OF INTERVENTION

At the pre-school level oral language is considered to be one of the most important means of developing social relationships and for learning about the world. This automatically places children with SLI at a disadvantage since their social-pragmatic, linguistic and conceptual difficulties affect the quantity and quality of their interactions. Since knowledge about the world and language is acquired through interaction with more mature language users, SLI children's opportunities for learning are also compromised. Rienke & Lewis (1984) summarize the impact that language difficulties have on the SLI child in the school: "the child who does not readily engage in communicative exchange, seeks out information and maintains attention is not able to take full advantage of the language learning opportunities available in the school environment."

The primary purpose of intervention in the Speech Foundation of Ontario, Toronto Children's Centre (SFO-TCC) program is to help SLI children develop social-pragmatic skills, linguistic skills and cognitive-social knowledge which will enable them to participate more successfully in their subsequent social interactions and their academic environment. Specifically, emphasis is placed on facilitation of: (a) verbal expression of a full range of communicative intents, using more mature language forms than available in the child's repertoire; (b) augmenting social conversational skills; and (3) enhancing cognitive and social knowledge.

Developing expression of communicative intents

As discussed earlier in this chapter, Craig (1983) summarized the research on the pragmatic and linguistic characteristics of children with SLI. She concluded that children with SLI have difficulty integrating linguistic forms with discourse functions, that is, they do not use their linguistic forms to clearly express their communicative intents. In the SFO-TCC intervention program, linguistic goals which help the children communicate their intents more successfully are targeted. A variety of language forms are facilitated in therapy. Declarative sentences are used to express a variety of intents such as responding, commenting, sharing experiences, and so on. Morphological and grammatical forms such as plurals, verb tenses, pronouns, negatives are typically emphasized to help children express their ideas more accurately and clearly. Question forms are used to request objects and information to satisfy personal needs as well as for social purposes such as initiating interaction, maintaining a topic, or repairing conversational breakdown. Both "wh" questions and yes/no (is it...and do you...) questions are developed. Complex sentences are developed in order to relate longer and more complex ideas and experiences. Sentences using the conjunctions "and" "because" are most frequently targeted.

Developing social-conversational skills

Brinton & Fujiki (1989) describe normal development of three basic aspects of conversation: turn-taking, topic manipulation, and conversational repair. They also discuss the types of difficulties children with SLI experience in these areas and present a variety of intervention procedures. The three aspects of conversation which are readily addressed in our intervention program include:

(1) *Turn-taking:* This encompasses prerequisite behaviors such as attending to the speaker, waiting for a turn, responding either non-verbally or verbally during a turn as well as initiating turns. Strategies which are developed include establishing joint attention by calling the name of the person, touching their arm or making eye contact, requesting items or turns and waiting for a turn.

(2) *Topic maintenance/manipulation:* Maintaining topic includes skills such as responding to questions, commenting on a topic, adding relevant information, or asking relevant questions.

(3) *Conversational repair:* This area includes developing the children's awareness of where they have not communicated successfully, as well as helping them indicate when they have not understood someone else's communication. Strategies emphasized include encouraging children to respond to requests for clarification as well as helping them indicate when they have not understood or remembered information (e.g. "what?," "say it again," "I don't remember").

Developing cognitive and social knowledge

Guralnick (1994) states that "unless a child and his or her peers have shared understanding of the task or activities at hand, a common awareness of prevailing social rules and agreed upon patterns of interaction, coherent, connected, and relevant exchanges are not likely to occur." There is a need, therefore, to develop the children's organization and understanding of their world so that they can interact more successfully in it (Nelson, 1986;

Snyder-McLean et al., 1984). In the SFO-TCC intervention program the following group routines and scripts of familiar events are used to develop children's understanding of: (a) sequences of events wichin a routine or script; (b) the roles of participants; and (c) the relevant vocabulary and concepts.

Specific goals within each language area are selected according to the needs of the children in the group. The various language goals are then addressed within the context of group routines and theme related activities, which incorporate scripts. This creates a meaningful context in which language learning can occur.

PLANNING INTERVENTION ACTIVITIES

An activity, as defined at the SFO-TCC, is a unit which has a beginning and an end and is linked to other units over a specified period. The content of each activity is related to the content of the other activities (see Table 20.1 for a sample lesson plan). Therapy activities for each session are based on a theme which is developmentally appropriate for the group. Most activities include a script or a joint action routine (JAR) which is defined by Snyder-McLean et al. (1984) as "a ritualized interaction pattern involving joint action, unified by a specific theme or goal, which follows a logical sequence, each participant plays a recognized role with specific response expectancies." The JAR scripts are used extensively in the program because they integrate a range of language skills. They create a context within which children can practice new vocabulary, concepts, and linguistic forms within a meaningful social interaction to convey a range of communicative intents. The children also gain experience with conversational turn-taking and topic maintenance. Once the children are familiar with the sequence of events and the language, the JAR script creates the scaffold for learning new information as well as providing a base from which children can extend the topic and incorporate their own ideas into the interaction.

Activities are sequenced within the therapy session to create a predictable daily routine for the children. The session begins with daily routines such as attendance and show and tell. Specific roles and response expectancies are developed to facilitate turn-taking skills, asking questions for information or permission ("where did you get it?," "May I see it?"), responding to questions, sharing information ("I watch Sesame Street," "I have that at home") and for negotiating ("May I see it? You can see my toy").

The preparatory activity in the session serves to introduce the theme and to prepare the children to participate more successfully within JAR scripts. Snyder-McLean et al. (1984) call these activities "cooperative turn-taking games" and describe them as a type of JAR which helps children who have never participated in interactive group situations develop the essential skills participating in any JAR script. Turn-taking rules, listening, and responding to the speaker are emphasized during this activity. Theme related vocabulary,

Table 20.1. *Elaborated lesson plan for Session 1*

Activity	Goals	Sample scripts	Procedures for language development	Procedures for script acquisition	Materials
Daily routines:	For all 3 routines:				Children's show and tell items:
Show and tell routine	1. Social conversational skills • attend to speaker • wait for turn • respond on topic 2. Verbal expression of intents • responding, commenting, requesting information and turns • focus on negative forms "is/is not"	Show and tell script: Cl: Who has something for show and tell? Ch: I do Cl: What is it? Ch: It's a . . . Cl: Where did you get it? Ch: . . . Cl: May I see it? Comment on it	Nonverbal cues to encourage initiation and responding • establish eye contact • pause and wait for children to initiate Verbal techniques • model key vocabulary words and target phrases and forms • exaggerate new information using change in volume/pitch • model more complete forms	Cl. assumes more of "director" role to introduce script Model questions and responses, request children to imitate as appropriate As necessary, direct children when to listen, respond, take a turn	Clinician's show and tell item: picnic basket
Attendance routine	• "wh" questions and "May I see?" 3. Cognitive and social knowledge • introduce sequence of routines, roles and scripts • introduce vocabulary and concepts associated with routines, e.g. names of children, nouns, verbs, adjectives related to toys, weather, prepositions on, beside	Attendance script: Cl: Who is here today? Ch: I am/. . . is. Cl: Where will you put your picture? Ch: On the board/beside. . . (repeat) Cl: Everyone is here today. (. . . is not here today. Where is he/she? Ch: generate ideas or Cl. gives alternatives)	of children's spontaneous responses • elicit responses by asking "wh" and choice questions and sentence completions		Photographs of children Attendance board

(continued)

451

Table 20.1 (*cont.*)

Activity	Goals	Sample scripts	Procedures for language development	Procedures for script acquisition	Materials
Daily routines:	For all 3 routines:				Children's show and tell items:
Weather routine		Weather script: Cl: Look out the window. What is the weather like today? Ch: … Cl: (review options) it is/is not (snowy, rainy, sunny, cloudy).			Pictographs of sun, clouds, snow, rain
Preparatory activity:					
Place pictures related to a picnic on the park mural	1. Cognitive and social knowledge • introduce vocabulary associated with picnic: basket, blanket, sandwiches, juice, cups, napkins concepts: in, on 2. Social conversational skills • turntaking • waiting for turn • responding on topic 3. Expression on intents • request: my turn • direct: put it there • label pictures	Cl: Whose turn is it? Ch: My turn Cl: Pick one, don't peek. What is it? Ch: labels, comments Cl: Where will you put it? Ch: specifies location	Same as for daily routine activities Also, provide phonemic cues and/or choice questions to facilitate labeling	Same as for daily routines	Pictures of basket, blanket, juice, cups, sandwiches, napkins, turned upside down on the floor Large park mural on wall

452

Main activity:

| Making sandwiches for a picnic

Pack sandwiches, juice, cups, napkins in basket

Go for a "walk" around room and find a good spot for a picnic

Lay blanket on floor and have snack | 1. Expressing intents
• requesting: I want...
• protesting: I don't want...
• directing: spread it on the bread, wrap it up, put it in the basket

2. Social conversational skills
• turntaking
• maintaining topic

3. Cognitive and social knowledge
• vocabulary and concepts: bread, peanut butter, jam, spread, wrap, on, in | Clinician engages in self talk while making sandwich
Cl: Who wants to make a sandwich?
Ch: me/I do
Cl: What do you want on your sandwich?
Ch: responds (all have turn)
Cl: Let's go on a picnic. Who will carry the...?
or What do you want to carry?
Ch: responds
Cl: Let's go. (walk) is this a good spot?
Ch: respond yes/no
If yes, put blanket down, if no keep walking and ask same question, continue until find a good spot
Cl: I'm hungry. I want to eat. I want a sandwich.
Pause and wait to see whether children will request sandwich.
Cl: I'm thirsty. I want juice.
I need a cup.
Pour juice in cup.
Pause and wait for children to request.
If children do not request, ask someone if they want juice.
Start to pour juice in air and see whether they request cup.
If children don't respond, model for them. | Same as for daily routine activities | Same as for daily routine activities

Bread, peanut butter, jam, knife, wax paper

Basket, blanket, juice, cups, napkins |

(continued)

Table 20.1 (cont.)

Activity	Goals	Sample scripts	Procedures for language development	Procedures for script acquisition	Materials
Snack:					
Eat sandwiches made in main activity	1. Verbal expression of intents • requesting snack items • protesting • commenting 2. Social conversation skills • turntaking • initiating conversation • responding on topic	See script in main activity	Nonverbal cues to encourage initiation and responding • establish eye contact • pause and wait for children to initiate or respond • give children incorrect item Verbal techniques: • model key words and phrases • model more complete forms of children's productions • elicit responses by giving choices	Same as for daily routines	Same as for main activity
Story:					
	1. Cognitive and social knowledge • vocabulary and concepts for picnic, breakfast, lunch, dinner, snack, food items	No script Discuss pictures, read story	Verbal techniques: • model simple language forms appropriate to story • elicit responses through sentence completion, "why" questions, misleading items	Same as for daily routines	*Feed Little Bunny* by Harriet Ziefert
Free play:	1. Social conversation skills • initiating • responding on topic • turntaking	None	Cl. observes children in their spontaneous interactions and responds to what they are doing in ways which will promote/support interaction	Not applicable	Blanket and picnic basket filled with toy food

2. Expressions of intent
- responding
- requesting
- protesting

Verbal techniques:
- as necessary Cl. uses self talk to initiate or extend play and models language appropriate to what is happening or in response to children's initiations
- models language which can be used in peer interactions to request, protest, respond
- may direct children to ask each other for toys
- redirects children's comments and questions from self to peer

Nonverbal techniques: Cl. may hide key items (e.g. basket), place items out of reach or give more toys to one child than the other children to encourage requesting/initiating concepts, and linguistic forms are also introduced. Examples of such activities include cooperatively completing theme-related puzzles or uniset scenes, playing lotto games, pulling props out of a bag and talking about them, setting up the scene for the JAR (e.g. store, restaurant) or making props to be used in the JAR (e.g. sandwiches for a picnic, a menu for a restaurant).

The "main" activity for the session is a JAR/script associated with a theme. Themes range from daily routines with which the children have concrete experience, for example, grooming, feeding to those which the children may have had less experience with, for instance, shopping, picnic, McDonald's, doctor. A variety of semantic and linguistic goals relevant to the theme are incorporated into the script so that children have the opportunity to learn and practice new forms in a meaningful context. A theme is carried out over two sessions to increase the children's familiarity with the event so that they can participate more fully. Once the children have grasped the basic script, it can be expanded on the second day by introducing new vocabulary, additional steps to a sequence or extending it to related events (e.g. shopping at a toy store, then at a clothing store).

A snack routine is included in each therapy session. Its function within the session may vary from day to day. Some days it is the final step of a food preparation activity or part of the JAR (picnic, restaurant). On other occasions it may be used to facilitate the development of social interaction and conversational skills. Children are assigned roles where they have the opportunity to request food items or offer them to their peers (e.g., "I want a cookie," "Do you want some juice?"). Snack time is also a time for developing conversational skills around topics which the children initiate.

A story related to the theme is included in every therapy session. The story may be used for a variety of reasons, ranging from introducing or reviewing the theme, establishing and/or expanding on the JAR/script, emphasizing specific concepts, including new vocabulary or linguistic forms or providing a context for conversation. The inclusion of a story also promotes the development of literacy skills, since it is selected to represent an event which the children have experienced during the therapy session.

A free play period is included at the end of most therapy sessions. Toys and materials from the session and/or new materials related to the theme may be provided for the children to play with. Children have the opportunity to develop peer interaction skills in more spontaneous, naturalistic ways and to use the vocabulary, concepts, and linguistic forms introduced in the session. The clinician is available to model more appropriate or complex play, more appropriate language and to support peer interaction.

PROCEDURES USED IN INTERVENTION

The challenges of designing effective group therapy include meeting individual needs while ensuring that all group members are participating and having opportunities to experience events and to practice various language skills. In order to accomplish this, procedures for three different aspects of group intervention need to be considered. These include general procedures for facilitating language learning, procedures for developing group routines/scripts, and procedures for developing peer interaction skills.

Procedures to facilitate language development

Fey (1986) identifies three main approaches used in facilitating language learning: clinician/trainer oriented, child-oriented, and hybrid. The approaches differ in terms of who controls the learning environment, the naturalness of the learning environment, and the techniques used for facilitating language development. In clinician-oriented approaches, the clinician controls the intervention session and determines the goals of intervention, the presentation of stimuli and reinforcement. He/she also elicits the responses and determines whether they are correct or incorrect. In child-oriented approaches, the clinician or significant adult responds to children's behaviors in a manner that is assumed to facilitate language development. Clinicians expand, explain, recast what the child has said. They may have general language goals in mind, but do not generally focus on specific language structures. The hybrid approach, which best describes the SFO-TCC intervention program, is a blend of clinician and child-oriented approaches. The clinician selects specific goals and plans activities and materials that are highly conducive to the spontaneous attainment of these goals within a naturalistic, communicative context. The clinician responds to the children's initiations but also emphasizes specific language forms. The clinician creates the scaffold to allow the children to use more mature linguistic forms or conversational skills. Both nonverbal and verbal techniques are used to model and achieve various language goals.

Nonverbal procedures are most frequently used to encourage children to initiate and maintain interaction or to signal that a response is required. Nonverbal cues include establishing and maintaining eye contact, moving closer to a child or touching his/her arm, manipulating the environment so that children need to request items or indicate that something is missing or has gone wrong (e.g., by placing a toy out of reach, "forgetting" to give someone juice, and giving a child the object he did not request).

Verbal techniques are primarily employed to facilitate the use of more appropriate or mature linguistic forms. These techniques can be divided into modeling and eliciting strategies. Modeling provides children with information on what they could say in a specific situation to convey their intentions more clearly. Partial, complete or expanded models may be provided depending on the information the clinician wishes the children to focus on. Specific vocabulary or linguistic forms can also be highlighted for the children by decreasing rate of speech and utilizing changes in volume or intonation and stress for emphasis.

Eliciting strategies are used to encourage children to use specific vocabulary or linguistic forms. Some of the strategies utilized include sentence completion ("He ate the..."), asking "wh" questions ("what did he eat?"), choice questions ("Did he eat the cookie or the apple?"), questions to request clarification ("He ate what?") or questions to expand thinking ("What else do you think he ate?").

Procedures to facilitate script acquisition

As already discussed, routines and scripts are an important part of the intervention program. The acquisition of scripts is a dynamic process and the clinician's role and the degree of structure shifts in response to the children's development and knowledge of the routine/script. The change in clinician role corresponds to the stages in transactional learning described by Van Kleek & Richardson (1988) and is described more specifically in the context of socio-dramatic script training by Goldstein & Strain (1988). Initially, the clinician assumes a more directive role in order to establish group routines and group expectations. The clinician may model one of the roles and/or direct the children in their roles. The clinician initially assumes the responsibility for modeling responses, requesting direct imitation and indicating turns. As the children develop the schema for the activity and the associated language, the clinician uses fewer and less explicit cues to elicit responses. The children gradually assume control of the activity. They ask each other questions, respond to or direct each other and may even expand on the script. At this stage the clinician becomes a facilitator rather than a director and is available to support the children, as necessary.

Procedures to facilitate peer interaction

Peer interaction is promoted through the use of JARs/scripts. It is also facilitated by capitalizing on spontaneous incidents which arise during intervention sessions. Opportunities often arise where children can be encouraged to verbally request or negotiate for objects or turns or to express their feelings. In appropriate situations, the clinician may either direct, model or encourage a child on what to say or do in order to facilitate successful communication.

PRESENTATION

There are three basic principles clinicians should be aware of when working with a small group of children in a focused language intervention session which is greater than one hour in length. These principles assist the clinician in maintaining the attention and participation of the group so that all can participate and benefit from the intervention program. The three principles are as follows.

Establishing basic group/social interaction rules

The most common rules which need to be developed and reinforced are that one person speaks at a time, one must wait for their turn, and one must request items or turns from others (rather than grabbing). These rules ensure that all children have the opportunity to participate in the activities and express themselves. It is often necessary to make the "rules" explicit since the children in this type of group often have difficulty understanding indirect or implicit information. These rules also reinforce the basic conversation skills mentioned in the goals section.

All children must be able to participate in the activity

Children vary in the length of time they can assume an "observer" role and attend to what others are saying or doing. If they are not actively involved, they quickly lose interest and engage in behaviors that may disrupt the group. It is essential to organize the activity and materials so that *all* children have opportunities to participate directly in the activity. Active participation can be accomplished in a variety of ways. Children may be asked to hold or manipulate materials, direct other children, monitor the responses of other children and be ready to help them generate ideas of what might be done next or share personal experiences and feelings.

Be responsive to the children's interest and fatigue levels

The clinician must constantly evaluate the children's participation in activities and respond in ways which will maximize participation. Children's participation can often be extended by acknowledging their ideas and interests and incorporating them into the activity whenever possible. The clinician can also utilize pacing and timing of presentation of activities as well as affect to establish, maintain or regain children's participation (Kounin, 1970).

Pacing refers to the tempo of the activity, that is, how quickly the activity develops and how quickly turns are taken. For example, if the children's interest begins to wane, the tempo can be picked up by moving on to the next step in the activity, leaving out steps, reducing response expectation or speeding up the rate at which children have turns. Clinicians should also resist rushing through an activity when the children are interested in persisting with a particular aspect of it. Children do not usually attend to new information when their focus is on what they would rather be doing.

Timing involves knowing when to end an activity or introduce a new one. When children are losing interest in an activity, it may be best to abandon it. It is also important to know which activity to introduce next in order to recapture the children's interest. It is sometimes necessary to modify the preplanned therapy sequence and respond to the children's interests or needs for physical movement or change.

Affect is generated by the children's use of voice, facial expressions, and body language and can be used to create a mood for an activity. The clinician can generate excitement and suspense or calm the children and help them refocus their attention on a specific aspect of an activity by varying vocal volume, and pitch, and facial and body movements.

MATERIALS

The materials are the tangible aspect of an activity which the children can act upon. Materials capture the children's interest and often elicit language from them. When selecting materials for an intervention session, there are two major factors to consider, select materials appropriate to the developmental level of the children in the group, and consider how interesting the children will find the materials.

The developmental level of the children will determine the representational level of the materials which can be used. Some children may require objects and materials whereas other children may be able to relate to pictures and representational objects and participate in pretend play. Children at younger developmental levels will not be able to engage in an activity if they do not understand what the materials represent or if they are not ready to participate in pretend play. For example, the developmental level of the children in the group will determine the type of materials necessary to make a bus for a "Going on the Bus" routine. For children functioning at a younger developmental level, the clinician may need to make a large bus out of cardboard and mount it to a row of chairs in order for children to understand they are going on a bus ride. For higher level children, a row of chairs may suffice while for others the verbal explanation of "Let's pretend we're on a bus" may be enough to engage them in the bus routine.

It is also important to consider whether the materials may be so stimulating or interesting that they will detract from the language interaction that hopefully will be generated by the materials. If materials are too interesting, the children's focus will be on playing with them rather than talking about them or using them as a prop in a script. It is also important to keep materials to a minimum since too many objects or pieces may be overstimulating or confusing for the children.

CASE STUDY: IMPLICATIONS

In a demonstration project, to evaluate whether children with SLI, expressive disorder who display behavioral and social difficulties would benefit from intervention with the group language program outlined above, eight children were seen over a 10-week treatment period. Both groups were tested three times throughout the study; before treatment, once at the start of treatment and at the end of treatment. Normal peer partners participated in play sessions with the subjects in all three time periods. These sessions were taped for analysis, however, group results will not be elaborated upon here. A case presentation will be offered to illustrate the program application.

Laura was referred to the project at age 4 years 11 months. In parent reports she was described as a child who was frustrated, would "act out" frequently by grabbing, hitting and stamping her feet. On a parent questionnaire her mother indicated that, aside from her speech and language concern, she was concerned about Laura's ability to interact with others. The mother felt that Laura's problematic behavior was "likely" to be due to her speech and language delays but felt confused about the "source" of Laura's frustration, whether it was due to her difficulties in comprehension or in formulation. Pregnancy and birth history were not significant and motor milestones were achieved within normal limits, as was Laura's hearing.

At the time of initial assessment Laura experienced severe difficulty with selectively attending and maintaining joint focus, responding to questions and instructions, and in transferring her focus of attention from one activity to the next. Within a group context, she was noted to be very impulsive in her responses, and to easily mimic any uncooperative behavior displayed by other children. Initial testing results indicated that Laura was operating in the moderate to severe range on formalized tests of receptive language, while achieving low normal, nonverbal cognitive and speech production scores. On the Behaviour Assessment for Children (BASC) parent and teacher scales she had quite high scores in the areas of hyperactivity, aggression, attention, and social skills adaption. On the Conners' Parent and Teacher Rating Scales conduct and hyperactivity were significant. During final testing, these same areas were identified by both the parent and teacher as considerably improved. In some cases, raw score data showed changes of over 14 points. Results of final language testing also showed improvement, especially in raw score data related to the Test for Auditory Comprehension of Language–Revised (TACL-R) and the Structured Photographic Expressive Language Test–II (SPELT-II). Areas that appeared especially sensitive to change on the TACL-R were grammatical morphemes and elaborated sentences. Anecdotal clinical reports revealed that, after the 10-week session, Laura's overall attention greatly improved and that group routines and structured activities appeared to provide Laura with the predictable and clearly defined framework that she needed for language learning and social interaction. Laura also began to use spontaneous verbal means to interact and negotiate with her peers. In addition, the skills were reported to have generalized in the home environment during interactions with her sibling. Overall, Laura's interactions were now much more socially appropriate and she was able to use the language skills she had gained to negotiate and interact with her family and peer group.

SUMMARY AND FUTURE DIRECTIONS

In this chapter the broad definition and underlying causative nature of SLI has been questioned and a position was put forward that would support the necessity for subgrouping of children who have specific speech-language impairment. A SLI subgroup with expressive disorder, as loosely defined by Rapin & Allen (1983), Fey (1986), and Craig & Evans (1993), was discussed in terms of its conceptual, pragmatic, and linguistic characteristics and needs. The premise put forward was that small group language intervention programming may prove to be the most successful way for children in this subgroup to improve their pragmatic and social communication skills and, as a result, decrease their asocial and nonadaptive behaviors. Group programming was put forward as an optimal method for achieving positive results with this subgroup. Different group models that are currently in use such as parent–child modeling, integrated preschool models and integrated peer mentoring were also discussed. All of these models have advantages for the child with SLI expressive disorder, but none has been specifically designed to deal with this particular population.

The intervention approach designed at the Speech Foundation, Toronto Children's Centre, for the SLI expressive subgroup, was then reviewed and the group program designed for children with this disorder, detailed. This program, while incorporating many of the advantages of the other models uses a small, closely matched group design and a cognitive/social perspective to develop goals and intervention procedures for linguistic, social, and pragmatic development. The design of the group treatment process was explored and the key aspects of its organization described such as goals, theoretical approach, activities, procedures, presentation and materials. An example in the form of a single case study of a child treated with this approach was presented. Implications were that such a language intervention approach may be a powerful tool for social and pragmatic growth in children with SLI expressive disorder. This case study, part of a demonstration project, needs replication with a larger group of subjects before more information about the underlying nature of these children's social and pragmatic deficits as well as approaches effective in remediation can be decided upon.

REFERENCES

Aram, D.M., Ekelman, B.L., & Nation, J.E. (1984). Preschoolers with language disorders: 10 years later. *Journal of Speech and Hearing Research*, **27**, 232–244.

Aram, D.M. & Nation, J.E. (1975). Patterns of language of behavior in children with developmental language disorders. *Journal of Speech and Hearing Research,* **18**, 229–241.

Aram, D.M., Morris, R., & Hall, N.E. (1993). Clinical and research congruence in identifying children with specific language impairment. *Journal of Speech and Hearing Research,* **36**, 580–591.

Arthur, G. (1952). *The Arthur Adaptation of the Leiter International Performance Scale.* Washington, DC: Psychology Service Center Press.

Baker, L. & Cantwell, D.P. (1987). A prospective psychiatric follow-up of children with speech/language disorders. *Journal of the American Academy of Child and Adolescent Psychiatry,* **26**, 546–553.

Bashier, A.S., Wiig, E.H., & Abrahams, J.C. (1987). Language disorders in childhood and adolescence; implications for learning and socialization. *Paediatric Annals,* **16**, 145–156.

Bates, E. (1976). *Language and Context: The Acquisition of Pragmatics.* New York: Academic Press.

Bates, E. & MacWhinney, B. (1979). A functionalist approach to the acquisition of grammar. In D. Morehead & A. Morehead (eds) *Language Deficiency in Children: Selected Readings.* Baltimore, MD: University Park Press.

Block, J. & Block, J. (1980). *The California Child Q-Set.* Palo Alto, CA: Consulting Psychologists Press.

Bloom, L. & Lahey, M. (1978). *Language Development and Language Disorders.* New York: John Wiley.

Brainerd, C.J. (1978). *Piaget's Theory of Intelligence.* Englewood Cliffs, NJ: Prentice-Hall.

Brinton, B. & Fujiki, M. (1982). A comparison of request-response sequences in the discourse of normal and language disordered children. *Journal of Speech and Hearing Disorders,* **47**, 57–62.

Brinton, B. & Fujiki, M. (1989). *Conversational Management with Language Impaired Children: Pragmatic Assessment and Intervention.* Rockville: Aspen.

Brinton, B., Fujiki, M., Winkler, E., & Loeb, D. (1986). Responses to requests for clarification in linguistically normal and language-impaired children. *Journal of Speech and Hearing Disorders,* **5**(1), 370–378.

Bruner, J. (1983). *Childs Talk: Learning to Use Language.* New York: Norton.

Bunce, B.H. & Watkins, R.V. (in press). Language intervention within a pre-school classroom: implementing a language focused curriculum. In N. Rice & Wilcox (eds) *Language Acquisition Preschool.* Baltimore, MD: Paul Brooks.

Carrow-Woolfolk, E. (1985). *Test for Auditory Comprehension of Language Revised Edition.* Allen, TX: DLM Teaching Resources.

Conners, C.K. (1989). *Conners' Parent Rating Scale.* North Tonawonda, NY: Multi-Health Systems.

Craig, H.K. (1983). Applications of pragmatic language models for intervention. In T.M. Gallagher & C.A. Prutting (eds) *Pragmatic Assessment and Intervention Issues in Language.* San Diego, CA: College-Hill Press (pp. 101–128).

Craig, H.K. & Gallagher, T.M. (1988). The development of pragmatic connectives: 4- and 6-year-old comparisons. *Journal of Pragmatics,* **12**, 175–183.

Craig, H.K. (1991). Pragmatic characteristics of the child with specific language impairment: an interactionist perspective. In T.M. Gallagher (ed.) *Pragmatics of Language Clinical Practice Issues.* San Diego, CA: Singular Publishing (pp. 163–199).

Craig, H.K. & Evans, J.L. (1993). Pragmatics and SLI: within-group variations in discourse behaviors. *Journal of Speech and Hearing Research*, **36**, 777–789.

Dunn, L. & Dunn, L. (1981). *Picture Vocabulary Test – Revised*. Circle Pines, MN: American Guidance Service.

Fawcus, M. (1992). *Group Encounters in Speech and Language Therapy*. Great Britain: Far Communications.

Fey, M.B. (1986). *Language Intervention with Young Children*. Needham, MA: Allyn & Bacon.

Gallagher, T.M. & Darnton, B. (1978). Conversational aspects of the speech of language-disordered children: revision behaviors. *Journal of Speech and Hearing Research*, **21**, 118–135.

Gallagher, T.M. & Prutting, C.A. (1983). *Pragmatic Assessment and Intervention Issues in Language*. San Diego, CA: College-Hill Press.

Gallagher, T.M. (1991). *Pragmatics of Language Clinical Practice Issues*. San Diego, CA: Singular Publishing Group.

Gallagher, T.M. (1993). Social implications of specific language impairment. Paper presented at Spring symposium, University of Kansas, Kansas City, Kansas.

Gardiner, M.F. (1979). *Expressive One Word Picture Vocabulary Test*. Novata, CA: Academic Therapy Publications.

Goldstein, H. & Strain, P.S. (1988). Peers as communication intervention agents: some new strategies and research findings. *Topics in Language Disorders*, **9**, 44–57.

Goldstein, H. & Kaczmarek, L. (1992). Promoting Communicative Interaction among children in integrated intervention settings. In S.F. Warren & J. Reichle (eds) *Causes and Effects in Communication and Language Intervention*. Baltimore, MD: Paul Brooks (pp. 81–113).

Goldstein, H. & Ferrell, D.R. (1987). Augmenting communicative interaction between handicapped and non-handicapped preschoolers. *Journal of Speech and Hearing Disorders*, **19**, 200–211.

Gresham, F. & Elliott, S. (1989). *Social Skills Rating System*. Circle Pines, MN: American Guidance Service.

Guralnick, M.J. (1994). You can play … but you can't: a workshop on peer-related social competence. Paper presented at The Hanen Program Workshop. February, Toronto, Canada.

Halliday, M.A.K. (1975). Learning how to mean. In E. Lenneberg & E. Lenneberg (eds) *Foundations of Language Development: A Multidisciplinary Approach*. New York: Academic Press (pp. 239–265).

Hodson, B. (1985). *Computer Analysis of Phonological Deviations (CAPD)*. Stonington, IL: Phonocomp.

Hresko, W. & Brown, L. (1984). *Test of Early Socio-emotional Development*. Austin, TX: Pro-Ed Publishers.

Johnston, J. (1989). Specific language disorders in the child. In N. Lass (ed.) *Handbook of Speech-Language and Hearing Pathology*. Burlington, Ont: B.C. Decker (pp. 685–716).

Kounin, J. (1970). *Discipline and Group Management in Classrooms*. New York: Holt, Rinehart & Winston.

Leonard, L.B. (1972). What is deviant language? *Journal of Speech and Hearing Disorders*, **37**, 427–446.

Leonard, L.B. & Fey, M.E. (1991). Facilitating grammatical development: the contributions of pragmatics. In T.M. Gallagher (ed.) *Pragmatics of Language: Clinical Practice Issues*. San Diego, CA: Singular Publishing Group (pp. 333–355).

Leonard, L.B. (1987). Is specific language impairment a useful construct? In S. Rosenberg (ed.) *Advances in Applied Psycholinguistics: Disorders of First Language Acquisition, Vol. 1*. New York: Cambridge University Press (pp. 1–39).

Leonard, L., Camarata, S., Rowan, L., & Chapman, K. (1982). The communicative functions of lexical usage by language-impaired children. *Applied Psycholinguistics,* **3**, 109–125.

Liles, B. (1987). Episode organization and cohesive conjunctives in narratives of children with and without language disorder. *Journal of Speech and Hearing Research,* **30**, 185–196.

MacLachlan, B. & Chapman, R. (1988). Communication breakdowns in normal and language learning-disabled children's conversation and narration. *Journal of Speech and Hearing Disorders,* **53**, 2–7.

MacNamara, J. (1972). Cognitive basis of language learning in infants. *Psychological Review,* **79**, pp. 1–13.

Martin, R. (1988). *Martin Temperament Assessment Battery*. Brandon, VT: Clinical Psychology Publishing.

Menyuk, P. (1964). Comparison of grammar children with functionally deviant and normal speech. *Journal of Speech and Hearing Research,* **7**, 109–121.

Miller, J.F. & Chapman, R.S. (1981). The relation between age and mean length of utterance in morphemes. *Journal of Speech and Hearing Research,* **24**, 154–161.

Nelson, K. (1986). *Event Knowledge: Structure and Function in Development*. Hillsdale, NJ: Lawrence Erlbaum.

Pearl, R. (1987). Social Cognitive Factors in Learning – Disabled Children's Social Problems. In S. Ceci (ed.) *Handbook of Cognitive, Social and Neuropsychological Aspects of Learning Disabilities*. Hillsdale, NJ: Lawrence Erlbaum.

Piaget, J. (1952). *The Origins of Intelligence in Childhood*. New York: Norton.

Piaget, J. (1962). *The Language of Thought of the Child*. London: Kegan & Paul.

Rapin, I. & Allen, D.A. (1983). Developmental language disorders: Nosologic consideration. In U. Kirk (ed.) *Neuropsychology of Language, Reading and Spelling*. Orlando, FL: Academic Press (pp. 155–184).

Reynolds, C. & Kamphaus, R. (1992). *Behavior Assessment System for Children*. Toronto: Psycan.

Rice, M.L. & Wilcox, K.A. (1991). *Language Acquisition Pre-School Curriculum: Development and Implementation*. Department of Speech-Language-Hearing, University of Kansas, Lawrence.

Rice, M.L. (1993). Classroom-based pre-school language intervention: function, fun, effective, and follow-up. Paper presented at Advances in Paediatric Disorders Conference, Henry Ford Hospital, May, Detroit.

Rienke, J.A. & Lewis, J. (1984). Preschool intervention strategies: the communication base. *Topics in Language Disorders,* **5**, 41–57.

Reynell, J. (1989). *Reynell Developmental Language Scales, rev*. Windsor, NFER.

Reynolds, C.R. & Kamphaus, R.W. (1992). *Behaviour Assessment Systems for Children*. Cline Pines, MN: American Guidance Service.

Rutter, M., Izeard, C., & Read, P. (1986). *Depression in Young People*. New York, NY: Guilford Press.

Sleight, C. & Prinz, P. (1985). Use of abstracts, orientations, and codas in narration by language-disordered and nondisordered children. *Journal of Speech and Hearing Disorders,* **50,** 361–371.

Snyder-McLean, L., Solomonson, B., McLean, J., & Sack, S. (1984). Structuring joint action routines: a strategy for facilitating communication and language development in the classroom. *Seminars in Speech and Language,* **5,** No. 3.

Stark, R.E., Bernstein, L.E., Condino, R., Bender, M., Tallal, P., & Catts, H. (1984). Four year follow-up study of language impaired children. *Annals of Dyslexia,* **34,** 49–68.

Stark, R.E. & Tallal, P. (1981). Selection of children with specific language deficits. *Journal of Speech and Hearing Disorders,* **46,** 114–122.

Strominger, A.Z. & Bashier, A.S. (1977). Longitudinal study of language delayed children. Paper presented at the Annual Convention of The American Speech-Language-Hearing Association, November, Chicago, IL.

Tannock, R. & Girolametto, L. (1992). Reassessing parent-focused language intervention programs. In S.F. Warren & J. Reichle (eds) *Causes and Effects in Communication and Language Intervention, Vol. 1.* Baltimore, MD, Paul Brooks (pp. 49–81).

Van Kleek, A. & Richardson, A. (1988). Language delay in the child. In N. Lass, L.V. McReynolds, J.L. Northern, & D.E. Yoder (eds) *Handbook of Speech-Language Pathology and Audiology.* Philadelphia, PA: B.C. Decker (pp. 655–685).

Vygotsky, L.S. (1978). *Mind in Society: the Development of Higher Psychological Processes.* Cambridge: Harvard University Press.

Weiner, B. (1980). The role of affect in rational (attributional) approaches to human motivation. *Educational Research,* **9,** 4–11.

Weistuch, L. & Byers-Brown, B. (1987). Motherese as therapy: a program and its dissemination. *Child Language Teaching and Therapy,* **3**(1), 57–71.

Weistuch, L. & Lewis, M. (1985). The Language Intervention Project. *Analysis and Intervention in Developmental Disabilities,* **5,** 97–106.

Weistuch, L. & Lewis, M. (1986). Effect of maternal language intervention strategies on the language abilities of delayed two- to four-year-olds. Paper presented at the meeting of the Eastern Psychological Association, New York.

Werner, E.O. & Kresheck, J.D. (1983). *Structured Photographic Expressive Language Test-II.* Illinois: Janelle Publications.

21 Communication training approaches in autistic disorder

M. MARY KONSTANTAREAS

That language impairment is part of autistic disorder (AD) has been recognized from the outset (Kanner, 1943) but its central role was particularly stressed after the mid-1960s when language and communication were thought to underlie all other deficits and, if correctly addressed, to result in salutary changes in the children's overall functioning (Lovaas, et al., 1966). Although a more balanced view, emphasizing equally the cognitive and social deficits (Konstantareas, Homatidis, & Busch, 1989; Rutter & Schopler, 1987) currently prevails, it is still the case that no account of the nature of impairment of AD and particularly of treatment fails to address the area of language. The DSM-IV includes the following four symptoms under the cluster of communication deviance: (1) delay or total lack of the development of language; (2) in individuals with adequate speech, a marked inability to initiate or sustain conversation with others; (3) stereotypical or idiosyncratic language use, and (4) lack of varied and spontaneous make-believe play, appropriate to developmental level (APA, 1994).

The DSM-IV criteria by no means capture the full range of linguistic difficulties displayed by the highly heterogeneous AD population. Resnick & Rapin (1991), for example, view AD as a spectrum disorder coexisting and overlapping with the equally heterogeneous "developmental dysphasia." They argue that, although it more closely resembles the "semantic-pragmatic" type of language disorder, AD can also coexist with verbal auditory agnosia, phonologic-syntactic disorder and occasionally even lexical syntactic deficit disorder. This view is consistent with the following facts that argue in favor of AD's heterogeneity: (a) at least 50% of AD children are nonverbal at first assessment and most remain so at follow-up (Konstantareas, 1986), (b) as many as 50% of AD individuals have IQs that are roughly estimated not to exceed 50 (DeMyer, Hingtgen, & Jackson, 1981), (c) the nonverbal children tend to be among the lower-functioning, although not invariably so (Konstantareas, 1993), (d) there is considerable individual variation in symptom expression (Bishop, 1989), and (e) there is developmental progression in the symptomatology, with "no mode of communication" being mainly evident only in very young AD children or the very few who function at the level of profound retardation.

In view of these facts, it should appear that a single treatment strategy in general, or a strategy that pertains to communication acquisition in particular, may not be appropriate for all AD individuals. This chapter's aim is to critically review available evidence on language intervention strategies and their effectiveness with subgroups of AD children. In the process, issues requiring additional systematic work will be highlighted. The chapter will conclude with an attempt to document an apparent trend towards convergence of the two main paradigms of communication intervention to be discussed with this population.

THEORETICAL POSITIONS AND CORRESPONDING INTERVENTIONS

Two broad epistemological lines are relevant to communication intervention efforts in AD: behavioral functionalism and cognitive functionalism. Crossing these two general views are two modes of intervention, one emphasizing speech and the other the simultaneous use of sign and speech.

Behavioral functionalism

Basing their premises on Skinner's (1957) *Verbal Behavior*, behavioral functionalists reduced communication to speech and its modification by judiciously ordering the consequences of vocalization and speech production. At its inception, proponents of this view were suspicious of any mentalistic efforts such as those of psycholinguist Chomsky (1959), and certainly were not interested in clarifying language development or its pathology. Instead, the behaviorists' aim was to create a technology and a methodology for aiding language acquisition. For sheer continuity and concentration of application the best known group among the behavioral functionalists is that of Lovaas and his collaborators. Their work, spanning approximately three decades, can be divided into three periods: (i) the application of behavioral principles regardless of client characteristics; (ii) an attempt at early intervention; (iii) an effort to clarify effectiveness through long-term follow-up.

The first period

During the approach's initial phase, for the mute children, a two-stage sequence was followed. Phonemes were taught in the first stage through the process of imitation, shaping, chaining, and differential reinforcement. This was followed by training in morphemes and single words, out of context. Once these language forms were acquired, the second stage, involving the acquisition of functionally employed words, was introduced. For the echolalic children who were able to produce verbal labels, albeit out of context, training began with the second phase and proceeded to phrase and sentence introduction

(Lovaas et al., 1966). Although this approach may appear stilted, viewed in the context of the times, it represented a major breakthrough in a field dominated by a pessimistic stance toward AD children's chances to ever communicate, since it provided a well-articulated and laboratory based alternative.

The group's original effort was evaluated in a follow-up study (Lovaas et al., 1973), in which the following points were demonstrated that: (a) stimulus and response generalization and gain maintenance were not automatic but required explicit treatment attention; (b) the children's presenting characteristics bore a relationship to their amenability to speech training, as well as to gain generalization and maintenance (thus, if the children could verbalize at program onset, they were more likely to speak). (c) Once speech was acquired, it was not spontaneously and flexibly employed by the AD children in their daily contexts, despite the considerable vocabulary that had become available to them.

The second period

The Young Autism Project constituted the new version of the intervention. In describing it, Lovaas (1987) stressed the following points:

(1) In the original work, the children's relatively older age might have been responsible for the fact that their gains, as he states: "were specific to the particular environment in which they were treated, substantial relapse has been observed at follow-up, and no client has been reported recovered" (p. 3).

(2) If one started early, with children younger than 4 years of age, and intervened very intensively, relapses could be prevented and gains maintained across environments and responses. Lovaas believed that this could be achieved by treating the children for most of their waking hours for many years, in every setting in which they found themselves, involving all significant people in their lives. Others have also noted that younger children are more likely to benefit (e.g., Howlin & Yates, 1989).

(3) The chances for successful mainstreaming would be enhanced if the children were younger, were not labeled as handicapped, and were treated as other children their age.

The project's design and results have been reported at some length (Lovaas, 1987; Lovaas & Smith, 1988). In brief, three groups of children younger than 46 months were included:

(1) An experimental group, exposed to an intensive intervention aimed at language, social and behavioral remediation for 40 hours per week, for a period of two or more years. The therapy took place in all daily contexts to enhance generalization and was carried out by parents and knowledgeable therapists.

(2) Control group 1, that consisted of children comparable to the experimental in most ways, but exposed to the intervention for fewer than 10 hours per week, for the same total duration. This group was employed to control for spontaneous recovery, independent of the intervention.

(3) Control group 2 was comparable to the other two groups but was not exposed to any intervention. It was employed to guard against possible selection bias, favoring the experimental group. For practical reasons, no random assignment was used, an important methodological constraint that has been used to question the generalizability of the findings.

Results were compelling: as many as 47% of the experimental children achieved normal educational and intellectual levels and were functioning adequately in a regular grade 1 class; another 40% were mildly retarded and were assigned to special classes in regular schools; and only 10% were profoundly retarded and were assigned to classes for autistic and retarded children. By contrast, children in control group 1 managed far worse at follow-up: only 2% achieved normal functioning; as many as 45% were mildly retarded and placed accordingly, while the remaining 53% were severely retarded and placed in classes for the retarded and autistic. Children in control group 2 were not significantly different from those of control group 1.

These findings were offered as overwhelming evidence in favor of the intensive, early behavioral intervention. Lovaas (1987) conceded that it was possible that "on closer psychological assessment, particularly as these children grow older, certain deficits may remain" (p. 9). In a commentary and critique of these findings, Schopler, Short, & Mesibov (1987) have argued that one cannot interpret the results of the project because of three methodological shortcomings: (a) inappropriate choice of outcome measures, (b) subject selection bias, engendered by the lack of randomization, and (c) inadequate control groups.

The third period: long-term outcome of the behavioral approach

More recently, McEachin, Smith, & Lovaas (1993) followed-up the original group of children approximately 4.5 years after treatment termination. They attempted to determine if the gains of the nine children who had been classified as normal upon the first study's termination, continued to be normal on more intensive scrutiny at 13, and how they fared vis-à-vis the children in the original control group. A comprehensive test battery was administered that included items from standardized tests but also other items addressing symptomatology and diagnosis. Once again, results were apparently most encouraging: (a) the experimental group's IQ had increased by a mean of 30 points, on average, compared to the IQ of the control group children; (b) they showed significantly higher levels of adaptive functioning; and (c) of the nine best outcome subjects of the original study, eight continued to show average intelligence and good adaptive functioning. Furthermore, the intellectual profiles of these eight children did not show the unevenness that usually characterizes the profiles of AD individuals, and on clinical examination by blind raters, these profiles could not be distinguished from the profiles of typical children. None of the AD children in the control group, by contrast, were deemed to function normally either upon formal testing or after clinical assessment. The team emphasized the methodological soundness of their study and speculated that a possible explanation for the successful outcome may reside in the plasticity of the brains of young organisms, quoting research on lower animals to substantiate their point.

Lovaas, Calouri and Jada (1989) went a step further arguing that on the basis of the young project findings, withholding this form of treatment from AD children may not be merely unwise but outright unethical. Commentators, however, have varied in their reactions to these striking findings. Some have rejoiced, minimizing such problems as the non-random subject assignment (Baer, 1993) while others were more guarded, arguing that, for the effects to be convincing, they ought to be independently replicated (Foxx, 1993; Kazdin, 1993). Still others (Mesibov, 1993; Mundy, 1993), expressed concern about the claim that the AD children became "normal" as opposed to being merely "high functioning" AD individuals. Mundy (1993) has argued, for example, that results from the cognitive, personality, and social testing through the Personality Inventory for Children and the Vineland Social Maturity Scale tend to tap externalizing and not the more common internalizing difficulties high functioning AD children usually present. It is therefore possible that subtle difficulties, odd thought processes, obsessional preoccupations and worries, and so on, were not in fact picked up by the testing. Along comparable lines, Mesibov (1993) argued that, although the gains should be heartening to parents, the McEachin et al. (1993) report gives us no information as to the students' social interactions, friendships, and social communication, among other problems, that are so central to the AD syndrome. Hence we do not know if they are still AD. One could counter-argue, of course, that these and other more subtle problems should have been picked up by the "blind" clinicians who examined the children and, in a rejoinder, Smith, McEachin, & Lovaas (1993) have also pointed this out.

Needless to say that, despite the methodological problems, the reported outcome is sufficiently compelling that its significance should not be quibbled with nor minimized, particularly for the higher-functioning children. There is no systematic evidence on large scale successful treatment outcome studies with AD children, regardless of level of cognitive functioning to date. Indeed, we have very little comparable, systematically evaluated work on intervention, even though many treatment programs exist (e.g. Miller & Eller-Miller, 1989). For the lower functioning group exposed to simultaneous communication there is only one study (Konstantareas, 1987) but the follow-up period considered was, at most, 4 years. The Lovaas group's effort should therefore be seen as a major accomplishment and a challenge for others to replicate. Some of the obvious research and intervention issues to consider in such attempts should include the following: (a) If only a subgroup of AD children respond to the intensive intervention, what are their characteristics? Why only half of the experimental group responded so well and not all? A number of people have suggested that cognitive ability and ability at verbal imitation are good predictors of outcome with any intervention (Howlin & Yates, 1989) while others have argued that lack of verbal imitation and lower cognitive ability may necessitate other types of intervention (Carr, 1985; Konstantareas, 1993). If true, would mute children with IQs in the moderate to severe range become "normal" after intensive intervention? That cognitive ability at intervention's onset may be a key outcome variable not only makes intuitive sense but has also been found to discriminate successful from unsuccessful outcomes with other populations of language impaired children (cf. Conant et al., 1984; Elliott, Hall, & Soper, 1991; Konstantareas, 1987). Recent evidence from histologic examinations of AD individuals, varying in levels of cognitive ability prior to death, supports this view since it shows that alterations in the cell formation of key subcortical areas are less deviant for the higher functioning (Bauman, 1995). (b) How treatment elements and the profile of the children's competencies and deficits interact also seems worthy of careful scrutiny. Cognitive developmental theory and research suggest that readiness to profit from input should be a key element for successful outcome (cf. Miller & Eller-Miller 1989). (c) It would also be important to examine the characteristics of parents and teachers whose children do well. This is an obvious point to make and one borne out in previous work where parental motivation and willingness to implement therapeutic strategies were found to be the key variables associated with a positive outcome (Lovaas et al., 1973; Konstantareas, 1987). (d) Finally, it would be important to know more precisely what treatment elements out of the total "package" contribute to a successful outcome and others that may have little relevance for it.

What might be difficult to achieve, under present stringent ethical guidelines, is random subject assignment. Other studies evaluating intervention efforts have also found this requirement difficult to meet (Conant et al., 1984; Harris et al., 1990). It is encouraging, however, that concurrent validity has been addressed in some form, thanks to the fact that these studies have also reported that some young AD children have responded dramatically to intervention, showing improvements in IQ and overall functioning. A follow-up of these children will provide much needed additional information on the long-term prospects of those interventions. Once again, however, the randomization requirement has yet to be imposed. Using a waiting group control is also difficult since, for the intervention to succeed, it has to begin early. Ethics committees will therefore find it difficult to approve such a design.

The cognitive functionalist position

In contrast to the behaviorists' emphasis on structure and form, and on the role of the environment rather than the actor in determining the meaning of communication, the cognitive functionalists (Schuler & Prizant, 1985; Duchan, 1986) have based their theoretical and intervention efforts on the "speech act" approach of the early psycholinguists (Austin, 1962; Halliday, 1975). They have also borrowed from the work on normal language acquisition (Bruner, 1975; Bates, 1976). Although comparable in their views on the critical role of cognition, there are two camps within this group that differ from each other in some critical respects, although hitherto no formal labels have been attached to them. For one of the two, "communicative intent" is central, with intents being expressed through the communicator's "speech acts." For this group emphasis during assessment is given to analyzing samples of dysfunctional children's communications, including their echolalia, in an effort to understand the meaning or intent of each communication. In carrying out their assessments, they stress the necessity for many different tools and approaches to be employed. Once data have been collected, clinicians of this group proceed to provide programmatic principles for intervention rather than a detailed sequence of steps or a manual to be followed (Prizant & Schuler, 1987). They leave it to the people directly engaged with the children's training to apply the suggestions provided in the form of incidental language intervention in the children's natural environment. They acknowledge that level of cognitive functioning should be taken into account, advocating that higher-functioning individuals should be encouraged to move from a holistic and gestalt mode, that capitalizes on the situational recall of whole utterances for a limited set of communication purposes, to a more flexible and analytic mode. For the lower-functioning, they recommend that training for "a cued response style" may be more in keeping with the AD children's processing capabilities. They also argue against the nonanalyzed and memorized phrase training aimed at teaching language forms, the approach favored by the behaviorists.

Although it shares the previous group's general perspective, a second group of cognitive functionalists, who could be called the "ecological functionalists," tend to emphasize the communication's context (Donnellan, Meszaros, & Anderson, 1984; Frankel, Leary, & Kilman, 1987). Members of this group place less emphasis on communicative intent and more on: (a) parents and community agents rather than professionals being the therapists; (b) providing learning environments that are age and skills-appropriate; (c) using audio and video recordings as assessment techniques for microanalyzing sequences of behavior that occur infrequently and for discovering subtleties of communication that may pass unnoticed with real-time observation methods (Frankel, 1982); and (d) placing less emphasis on the communicator's intents, and greater weight on the ascription of meaning by the communicator's social group, by means of what they call "strategic contextualization." Thus, for example, a child's movement of the head towards an object may be interpreted as expressive of his desire for it, despite the fact that no objective evidence for the validity of this assumption is available (Frankel et al., 1987). In this position then not only spoken utterances but also posture, gesture, proximity, facial expression, and eye movements are considered basic competencies upon which more complex social interactions can be built.

In evaluating their collective position one is struck by the fact that, despite both groups' many objections to the behavioral paradigm, careful appraisal of their position reveals that they do share some of their principles. These include placing stress on a reinforcing and positive context, arguing against diagnosis prior to intervention, subscribing to the discovery and building on competencies, and targeting skills likely to lead to later independence. They also emphasize full community integration. Missing from the cognitive functionalists' model are: (a) some consideration of individual differences among AD children, this being particularly true of the second group; (b) the possibility that at least some of the individual's behaviors to which communicative intents are ascribed, may be devoid of such intents; (c) ways of validly determining the presence of such intentions in attempts at what they call "strategic contextualizatioan"; (d) clearly stated and sequentially presented intervention plans for improving the relevance, complexity and flexibility of the AD children's communication; and (e) interest in systematically demonstrating the effectiveness of their suggestions to parents and community agents. If one were to sum up the epistemological flavor of the two camps, one would be forced to conclude that while the behaviorists might appear too structured, mechanistic, and stilted, the cognitive functionalists tend to be too relaxed on structure and sequencing of interventions, and on evaluating their intervention's effectiveness.

On the positive side, aspects of this approach, particularly that of the first subgroup, have a distinct appeal, and many had in fact been employed in programming alternatives to the strictly behavioral position as early as the early 1970s (cf. Creedon, 1973; Konstantareas, Oxman, & Webster, 1977). They are also employed currently, albeit in the context of a broader conceptual base, which allows for diagnosis and for the contribution of psychological and developmental data to inform programming (Howlin & Yates, 1989; Miller & Eller-Miller, 1989; Watson et al., 1989; Harris et al., 1990).

MODALITIES OF INTERVENTION

As indicated earlier, as many as 50% of AD individuals may never gain useful speech, despite all efforts at training them toward vocal production. This reality has led to the development of "augmentative and alternative" communication training systems. They include natural languages, such as American Sign Language (ASL) or other sign languages employed by deaf communities and their derivatives such as signed English, and formally constructed communication systems such as the Bliss, the Rebus or the Pick symbols, all three of which constitute man-made or "artificial" languages. Workers in communication intervention with the AD, and indeed other severely dysfunctional populations, have not been equally sensitive to the need for these alternatives to speech training. Among the behaviorists, for example, only few have employed such alternatives (e.g., Goetz, Schuler, & Sailor, 1979; Carr, 1985), the majority preferring to exclusively emphasize speech. More recently, workers in the broader field of language impairment have been supportive of visually based systems such as sign language, especially for those subgroups of children who present with verbal dyspraxia or mixed expressive-receptive disorder, with or without concurrent AD (e.g., Resnick & Rapin, 1991).

Simultaneous communication training

The simultaneous use of speech and signs strategy emerged partly because early speech-only training was found ineffective with a large number of AD children (Creedon, 1973; Bonvillian & Nelson, 1978; Mack, Webster, & Goksen, 1980) and partly adventitiously, in the context of implementing the speech-only strategy. In the Webster et al. (1973) study, for example, videotaped samples of speech training revealed that an AD child tended to respond to the therapists' body movements and gestures rather than to their spoken utterances during training in speech acquisition. At around the same time Creedon (1973) also reported a successful outcome using a more formal approach that relied on a natural language, namely AMS or Signed English that allows for word order to be maintained. This approach was subsequently independently and successfully employed by workers in other centers, either in single-subject designs or with small groups. Because of its relative effectiveness, particularly with those AD children who were mute, this type of communication training has come to be considered as the main alternative to speech-only interventions, not only with AD but also with other populations of severely communication-impaired children (Konstantareas, 1993).

Why signs as opposed to words prove to be relatively effective with usually, but not always, the lower-functioning children, has been presented in some detail elsewhere (Konstantareas, 1986). Briefly, the reasons that have since emerged to be relevant are as follows. First, the AD children's greater difficulties with sequential auditory processing and better skills at visuospacial decoding as well as processing visuomotor and kinaesthetic information. The difficulties appear to be greater for the lower-functioning subgroup (Hermelin & O'Connor, 1970). The possibility that ear infections, with concomitant periodic hearing loss, may be related to this greater difficulty was raised in one of our studies where only the lower-functioning AD subgroup had suffered repeated ear infections during the first two years of life (Konstantareas & Homatidis, 1987). Condon's (1975) work on interactional dyssynchrony for auditory but not visual input in dysfunctional populations, particularly the AD, is consistent with this view. Upon microkinetic analysis he found that AD children displayed multiple entrainment to sound, that is, their body responded more than once to a single sound in a reverberatory fashion. They also showed a motor response delay of up to 24 frames of regular speed film, that is, a full second.

Another factor seems to be the lower-functioning children's lower readiness to process spoken language and their relatively better ability to understand and produce gestures, simple signs, and iconic signs for concrete objects. A 10-year-old's mental age of 12 months, for example, may place her below the cognitive ability for the production of spoken words, something that some communication therapists appear to largely ignore. Their argument is that AD children are untestable by conventional psychometric instruments (Frankel et al., 1987; Lovaas & Smith, 1988), contrary to evidence against this view (Frith, 1989; Lansing, 1989). When suitable instruments, sensitive and careful interaction with the child, and spaced assessments are attempted, AD children have been found to perform at all levels of cognitive ability. Hence their performance falls along a normal curve, although the overall curve would be shifted to the left and lower end of that for the typical population. In fact our own assessments have shown that a few mute AD children have nonverbal IQs in the bright normal or even the superior range. The correspondence between language and cognitive development is so compelling in typical children (Ingram, 1978), that we can hardly afford to ignore the child's nonverbal cognitive level in our intervention plans. Data on language acquisition and the central relevance of action and gesture as the building blocks in the evolution of spoken language (Locke, 1978) should serve as guides to our efforts. Some cultural anthropologists have in fact argued that sign languages may have emerged phylogenetically earlier than spoken languages (Hewes, 1973), hence it might be argued that they might be protolanguages that are easier to understand and be employed by neurologically constrained organisms, such as the AD children. With them emphasis may have to be placed in such prelinguistic skills development as shared attention and reference, turn-taking and imitation rather than speech production. Indeed, in our clinic these have been the approaches we are recommending that parents follow when the children function at the level of the sensorimotor period.

A third factor lies in motivational considerations and preferred mode of action. Most of the lower-functioning AD children appear to satisfy need states by goal-directed body movements aimed at securing the coveted object or accessing a desired activity. Such goal-directed actions can, and have been, capitalized upon to build corresponding signs, such as the signs for "come," "give," "go," "cookie," and so on, something not readily achievable through words. As well, these children tend to be highly impatient when confronted with small visual details as those required for academically demanding desk work, and tend to be highly motoric and active. Thus, at least in early intervention, efforts can be more successful if they capitalize upon and take into account the children's natural proclivities. Sign language lends itself well to the children's action-oriented body movements.

Finally, features of sign language render it particularly relevant to the information processing and special characteristics of the AD children. This allows for a suitable goodness of fit between communication system and its user. Iconic signs, for example, have been shown to be far easier for these children to acquire than noniconic (Konstantareas, Oxman, & Webster, 1978). Clearly, the concrete and "here and now" needs of the children are better served by a system that reduces processing effort. The slower presentation of sign language in deaf communication which is apparently half as rapid as that of speech, is another characteristic that makes signs easier to process (Bellugi & Fisher, 1972). Redundancy of signs, with one sign conveying information for more than one concept, for example, chair and sitting being represented by the same sign, also allows for a more economical and less taxing processing with the lower-functioning AD children. Lastly, signs can be taught through direct hand and body manipulation, while the body parts relevant to the production of speech such as the tongue, lips, mouth and oral cavity are less amenable to direct molding and shaping into speech sounds. Interestingly, the sounds which can be produced through some manipulation of the lips, such as "mh," "oh," and "bah," were among the first to be introduced in training mute children to vocalize (Lovaas et al., 1973).

Effectiveness of simultaneous communication training

Although simultaneous communication was initially responded to with suspicion, it is now adopted as a viable alternative to speech-only intervention, particularly with mute children. Since its first implementation in 1973, at least 30 studies on its use have appeared in the literature, mainly in the form of descriptive case presentations or reports on small groups of children. Bonvillian & Nelson (1978) and Konstantareas (1986), have provided reviews of this work. Insofar as the communication training is only one area of emphasis in programming, it is difficult to argue that gains in other areas of functioning can be attributed to it, but they have certainly been reported by most workers in the field.

Very little systematic research on the deployment of simultaneous communication training has been undertaken. Konstantareas, Webster, & Oxman (1979) found that sign acquisition, both receptive and expressive, was a function of the children's cognitive abilities. Also, although the children varied as to the aspect of the sign-word presentation they responded to – some responding to the words, others to the signs and others to the combination – all were able to acquire a large enough number of signs to allow them to communicate their basic needs. Moreover, 50% of the children became able to vocalize or speak by program termination a year later. As to the effects of communication acquisition on other areas of the children's functioning we found that, although the intensive programming reduced inappropriate and stereotypical behavior it had virtually no effect on spontaneous social interaction. The children reverted to their isolated or self-stimulatory behavior, once the therapists left the treatment room. Oxman, Konstantareas, & Leibovitz-Bojm (1979) examined vocalization levels of an experimental group exposed to simultaneous communication training and a control group who were matched on age and developmental functioning level and were exposed to conventional, though not intensive, programming relying on speech only. Although the experimental children's vocalization levels were lower, albeit not significantly so, at program onset, they were found to be higher at termination. Thus, at the very least, the children were unlikely to have been adversely influenced by exposure to signs. Indeed, as indicated earlier, the opposite turned out to have been the case in our own systematic study on communication acquisition (Konstantareas et al., 1979) and in a number of other studies (Creedon, 1973), where as many as 50% of the children were able to acquire speech as a result of exposure to this approach. Exposure to signs for severely language impaired children continues to be advocated by many workers (cf. Resnick & Rapin, 1991). Konstantareas & Lelbovitz (1981) examined whether single modality training (signing and mouthing), where auditory input was completely eliminated, would prove superior to two-modality training (signing and speaking), where both visual and auditory input is given, in view of concerns as to AD children's difficulties with auditory processing. The two-modality approach proved superior, although there is no clear explanation for the superiority.

Only the older, mute or minimally verbal AD children have thus far been exposed to simultaneous communication training. This is not because the younger and more verbal cannot benefit. On the contrary, Barrera & Sulzer-Azaroff (1983) showed that, not surprising in view of our previous discussion, young eholalic AD children were better able to acquire verbal labels through simultaneous communication than through speech-only training. Van Wagenen et al. (1985) also strongly recommend the use of simultaneous communication with the verbal and not merely the mute AD children, basing the recommendation on comparable findings. However parents, teachers, and some professionals continue to be less than enthusiastic about the use of signs. In fact, in the only available follow-up study on gain maintenance and generalization of simultaneous communication training, Konstantareas (1987) found some disconcerting results. Despite the group's excellent recall and use of signs, one to five years after exposure to intensive simultaneous communication training, parents and teachers employed words only to communicate with the children. This was true even for the totally mute children. It ought to be remembered as well that, in almost all cases in the past, mute AD children were first exposed to speech and, only after many years of failure and at an older age were they exposed to simultaneous communication. It is therefore still unclear what the outcome of an early intervention using this approach might be.

Simultaneous communication has been shown its promise with populations of children other than the AD such as the mentally retarded and the severely language impaired (Paul & Cohen, 1984). We have found, for example, that the superimposition of signs on omitted functors in the telegraphic speech of dysphasic children helped them to acquire the missing functors once the signs were removed (Konstantareas & Lelbovitz, 1981). It has also been used to teach a blind, AD girl to communicate meaningfully (Konstantareas, Hunter, & Sloman, 1992), even though sign language is viewed as a visual system. The mediating modalities were the tactile-kinaesthetic and the auditory, both apparently well known to teachers of the deaf and blind.

In summary, there are alternatives to speech training with those AD children who are either completely mute and unlikely to ever acquire spoken language as well as those who may have a few spoken words but do not employ them systematically and functionally. The beginnings have been made of classifying children's language competencies and deficits independent of their AD symptomatology (Bishop, 1989; Resnick & Rapin, 1991). Decisions as to how to best assign children to training modalities, and how to change modality on the basis of changes in the children's needs diachronically may have to await further clarity as they relate to presenting characteristics and intervention needs. We need, for example, to overcome the reluctance of parents to expose their children to simultaneous communication in favor of speech. To accomplish this, research into early intervention comparing the relative effectiveness of the two approaches with children of varying functioning levels will be necessary.

Other augmentative communication strategies

Three approaches can be considered here for which evidence as to efficacy is chiefly anecdotal: (a) systems employed with those AD children who, for whatever reason, cannot benefit from speech or simultaneous communication training, (b) interventions meant to be employed with other populations, which have also been attempted for their possible utility with AD children, and (c) augmentative strategies that rely on other people's contribution.

In order of degree of decoding complexity, formal picture boards, simple familiar object boards and photograph boards fall in the first category. These devices that are considered to be "aided," in comparison to sign language (Wilbur, 1985), are employed with AD children who appear not to respond to speech or to simultaneous communication training. A factor potentially responsible may lie on the children's fine motor control difficulties, which can considerably restrict the number of signs they can produce. Even when the pointing response is lacking, however, the children can touch the symbol, drawing or photograph corresponding to a desired object or activity, to make their needs known. In some instances these augmentative strategies are also employed in conjunction with simultaneous communication, in an effort to further reinforce the concepts introduced and taught through that medium. This has sometimes been referred to as "Total Communication." It is important to alert the reader to the fact that such systems are more likely to be relevant to the few AD individuals who suffer from concurrent neuro-muscular difficulties that make the planful use of hands either difficult or impossible. Individuals with Rett syndrome, with an inability to use their hands purposefully as one of the key symptoms, or those suffering from paraplegia or quadriplegia are cases in point. For such children other alternatives may also be sought, however, particularly for those who cannot rely on head or trunk movements as substitutes for touching by hand. There is little information on the effectiveness of these systems or on the characteristics of those who can benefit from their use.

Under the second category fall such augmentative systems as the Rebus and the Bliss Symbol Systems. Although the Rebus may be of relevance to the higher-functioning AD children, particularly in teaching them to read, the Bliss may be far too advanced for most. Bliss's pictographic alphabet, developed originally for cross-cultural communication, has been successfully targeted at those with neuromuscular disorders and intact cognitive structures. It is a rather abstract system that can be quite taxing to the processing abilities of most AD children. In one of the few studies available on its use, Hurlbut, Inata, & Green (1982) compared Bliss symbols to an iconic picture drawing system with three adolescents with Cerebral Palsy who had severe physical and mental disabilities and were non-ambulatory. No mention is made as to whether they were comorbid for AD but they were certainly mentally handicapped. Probe trials were conducted to assess stimulus and response generalization, response maintenance and spontaneous use of each system. Results revealed that all three adolescents required four times as many trials to acquire the Bliss symbols as the iconic signs. Compared to the Bliss symbols, furthermore, that required retraining for retention, all of the iconic drawings were recalled without additional training. This outcome ought not to come as a surprise to workers in this field, and it is consistent with the results of the previously reviewed study on the iconicity of signs with AD children (Konstantareas et al., 1978).

Finally, in the last four years there has been a heated debate around the use of facilitated communication (FC), an augmentative communication strategy that relies on the manual support of the communicator's hand or arm by another individual, the facilitator. Originating in Australia more than a decade ago (Crossley & McDonald, 1980), and employed initially with individuals with neuromuscular impairments, the technique was disseminated in North America by Biklen (1990). Biklen has argued that facilitation allows nonverbal AD individuals to access centrally available information that could not otherwise be expressed because of problems in "praxis." By this poorly defined term he appears to mean interference in motor expression by difficulties of unspecified origin. Thus he brings to the forefront once again the issue of AD's etiology. Providing strikingly rich and largely difficult to credit descriptive accounts of facilitated communications produced by AD individuals, Biklen (1990) questioned prevailing views on the competence levels of these individuals. He asked that views on etiology be revised in view of this evidence based on qualitative research methodology. He also asked facilitators to follow two precepts: (a) to assume the communicator's independence, and (b) to assume competence, since not to assume it, would feed into the AD individual's already low self-concept and sense of failure.

In trying to understand FC's emergence as a new fad, one has to link the phenomenon to two important contemporary movements regarding developmental disabilities: (a) the rule of the "Least Restrictive Alternative," and (b) the rule of "Full Community Integration." In light of the philosophical premises underlying both, it appears natural that questions about communicator independence, couched in the healthy scepticism of scientific scrutiny could be interpreted by FC's proponents as nonsupportive, if not outrightly callous, to those with special needs. The two rules are not far removed from explanations based on the notion of "strategic contextualization" discussed earlier. Only recently have efforts begun to systematically examine the validity of facilitated communication, prompted in part by concerns from its use in allegations of sexual abuse (Konstantareas, 1993). All available evidence to date points to facilitator influence (Wheeler et al., 1993). Gravelle & Konstantareas (1993) examined the contribution of three key aspects of facilitator support: emotional, physical, and mental with 13 AD children and young adults who had been exposed to this technique for at least two years. Although performance reached asymptotic levels on a variety of tasks, ranging in degree of decoding and encoding complexity, it did not exceed chance levels when only emotional support was provided and mental support, in the form of the facilitator knowing the correct answer, was withdrawn. This occurred despite the fact that the response requirement remained constant throughout, that is, the communication user was required to point only. This study, along with those mentioned earlier, places under serious doubt the presumed independence of facilitated communication from facilitator influence. Certainly, as others have argued (Cummins & Prior, 1992), the results of research on independence place the burden of proof as to the technique's validity on its proponents' camp. When highly private and sensitive communications of a personal nature, such as allegations of abuse or decisions of great import to the individual are involved, it is crucial that attempts at independent validation be made. This is not to argue that some, perhaps very few, mute AD individuals may not in fact possess literacy, since a few have nonverbal intelligence well above the prerequisite level for it. However, if they do, they should be able to display it, when conditions appropriate for demonstrating this ability are sensitively set. After all, AD children are quite capable of responding to items of formal psychometric and language tests, once conditions are suitably arranged. Further proof of the validity of this statement is the fact that over the years we have found that competencies obtained through direct psychological assessment are very rarely different from those obtained through parental and teacher interviews.

SUMMARY AND APPRAISAL OF RECENT TRENDS

Current trends can be summarized along the following lines:

(1) There is convergence on the importance of combining naturalistic with more formal, analogue-type instruction (Carr, 1985; Howlin & Yates, 1989; Lovaas et al., 1989), although we are far from clear as to how to best achieve this. Thus, although some behaviorists, for instance, Carr (1985), favor analogue training first, to be followed by naturalistic efforts; others such as Elliott et al. (1991), who compared the two types of training, have concluded in favor of natural language only training. However, the Elliott et al. study design was such that it did not allow for conclusive answers to be reached.

(2) There is also apparent agreement that not all AD children are good candidates for vocal communication, despite its obvious merits (Carr, 1985; Bishop, 1989; Haracopos, 1989; Howlin & Yates, 1989; Harris et al. 1990; Resnick & Rapin, 1991). Yet it is still the case that exposure to alternatives is viewed as a strategy of last resort. Perhaps because of this, they have not been given the careful research attention they deserve. To our knowledge, with the exception of our own research and research by Carr (1985), there is little information on parameters of relevance to sign implementation or of the other systems discussed. It is unclear, for example, which of the augmentative communication strategies outlined above is best suited to children with different characteristics and at different stages of their development. Helmer, Layton, & Wolf (1982) have offered a typology of child characteristics that may render them responsive to signs, words, or prelingual training. Yet thus far no effort has been made to test the validity of this typology's predictions. This is particularly disconcerting in view of the dramatic increase in the use of these systems, particularly of signs, with the severely impaired (Bonvillian & Orlansky, 1984). How motor deficits factor into the whole picture is also unclear. Bryen & Joyce (1986) have argued, for example, that although sign language can bypass speech

mechanisms, it cannot bypass required motor abilities. Yet our knowledge of motor deficits in AD individuals is extremely limited.

(3) There is increased acceptance of the fact that assessment is a key prerequisite to intervention, even by staunch advocates of the uselessness of testing (Lovaas et al., 1989). However, there is as yet little consensus as to what to include in such an evaluation for children of different ages and abilities. There is also no research as to different instruments' predictive power, although some, such as the Leiter test for assessing nonverbal IQ, tend to be favored more than others such as the Binet. Which linguistic scales should be employed for assessment has also not been agreed upon.

(4) The need to arrive at curricular items that correspond to a given child's developmental stage is another point of convergence across clinical investigators. Data on normal language acquisition have begun to appeal to some behaviorists for the wealth of information they hold. Carr (1985), for example, discusses the issue of the options we have for selecting the best method for teaching abstract concepts, that is, whether to use multiple exemplars or prototypes, which are thought to be better instances of certain concept classes. Research on this issue with AD children will be quite useful for better curricular development.

(5) There is also convergence of opinion on the need to achieve generalization in the most efficient manner possible, but divergence as to how to best achieve it. The behaviorists advocate as best the method of multiple exemplars, used comparably but with new materials in as many settings as possible. The cognitive functionalists, by contrast, argue that, to the extent that language is employed in context, there is no need to plan its generalization since it will occur automatically (Schuler & Prizant, 1985). Systematic evaluation of the two camps' conflicting claims has yet to be undertaken.

(6) There is also agreement that the language acquired through training should be used for communication, ideally for spontaneous communication. Once again, the cognitive functionalists feel that their approach *ipso facto* emphasizes learning that occurs spontaneously in the context of ongoing activity. The behaviorists consider the AD children's lack of spontaneity a reflection of a social reinforcement deficit, and attempt to address it accordingly (Carr, 1985).

(7) There is also increased interest in examining the issue of how integration might facilitate language acquisition (Harris et al., 1990). Thus far this issue has been given insufficient attention, however, in so far as it is charged with emotional overtones. To some professionals integration is a right rather than an alternative to be selected if it is shown to be beneficial to that particular child at that particular point in his/her development. Only dispassionate efforts at evaluating the

relative advantages and disadvantages of integration or rather of degree of integration, since a minimal level of integration is accepted by most as potentially fruitful. The little available research is not conclusive. Harris et al. (1990), for example, found that a segregated setting was preferable to an integrated one for AD children with severe behavioral problems. For those with less severe problems and the same functioning level, both approaches turned out to be equally effective.

(8) Finally, the microsoftware revolution has yet to be fully taken advantage of in efforts at augmentative communication training among the AD as it has been for cerebral palsied and retarded children. There have been attempts to employ video modeling to teach conversational speech to autistic children with some success, both in groups (Creedon, 1973; Miller & Eller-Miller, 1989) and using an operant paradigm (Charlop & Milstein, 1989), and more work along these lines may be anticipated in the future.

REFERENCES

American Psychiatric Association (APA) (1994). *Diagnostic and Statistical Manual of Mental Disorders, IV Ed.* Washington, DC: APA.

Austin, J. (1962). *Social Interaction.* London: Methuen.

Baer, D.M. (1993). Quasi-random assignment can be as convincing as random assignment. *American Journal of Mental Retardation,* **97**, 359–372.

Barrera, R.D. & Sulzer-Azaroff, B. (1983). An alternating treatment comparison of oral and total communication training programs with echolalic autistic children. *Journal of Applied Behavior Analysis,* **16**, 379–394.

Bates, E. (1976). *Language and Context. The Acquisition of Pragmatics.* New York: Academic Press.

Bauman, M. (1995). *The Neurodevelopmental basis of Autism.* Presentation at the Hospital for Sick Children, Toronto.

Bellugi, U. & Fisher, S. (1972). A comparison of sign language and spoken language. *Cognition,* **1**, 173–199.

Biklen, D. (1990). Communication unbound: autism and praxis. *Harvard Educational Review,* **60**, 291–314.

Bishop, D. (1989). Autism, Asperger's syndrome and the semantic-pragmatic disorder: Where are the boundaries? *British Journal of Disorders of Communication,* **24**, 107–121.

Bonvillian, J.D. & Nelson, K.E. (1978). Development of sign language in autistic children and other language-handicapped individuals. In P. Siple (ed.) *Understanding Language Through Sign Language Research.* New York: Academic Press (pp. 187–212).

Bonvillian, J.D. & Orlansky, M.D. (1984). Sign language acquisition: early steps. *Communication Outlook,* **6**, 10–12.

Bruner, J. (1975). The ontogenesis of speech acts. *Journal of Child Language,* **2**, 1–19.

Bryen, D. & Joyce, D. (1986). Sign language and the severely handicapped. *Journal of Special Education,* **20**, 183–194.

Carr, E. (1985). Behavioral approaches to language and communication. In E. Schopler

& G.B. Mesibov (eds), *Communication Problems in Autism*. New York: Plenum (pp. 37–57).

Charlop, M.H. & Milstein, J.P. (1989). Teaching autistic children conversational speech using video modeling. *Journal of Applied Behavior Analysis*, **22**, 275–285.

Chomsky, N. (1959). "Verbal Behavior" by B.F. Skinner. *Language*, **35**, 26–58.

Conant, S., Budoff, M., Height, B., & Morse, R. (1984). Language intervention: a pragmatic approach. *Journal of Autism and Developmental Disorders*, **14**, 301–312.

Condon, W. S. (1975). Multiple response to sound in dysfunctional children. *Journal of Autism and Childhood Schizophrenia*, **5**, 37–56.

Creedon, M.P. (1973). *Language Development in Nonverbal Autistic Children Using a Simultaneous Communication System*. Paper presented at the Society for Research in Child Development Meeting, Philadelphia, PA.

Crossley, R. & McDonald, A. (1980). *Annie's Coming Out*. New York: Penguin.

Cummins, R.A. & Prior, M.P. (1992). Autism and facilitated communication: a reply to Biklen. *Harvard Educational Review*, **62**, 228–241.

DeMyer, M.K., Hingtgen, J.N., & Jackson, R.K. (1981). Infantile autism reviewed: a decade of research. *Schizophrenia Bulletin*, **7**, 388–451.

Donnellan, A. M., Mezaros, R.A., & Anderson, J.L. (1984). Teaching students with autism in natural environments: What educators need from researchers. *Journal of Special Education*, **18**, 505–522.

Duchan, J.F. (1986). Language intervention through sensemaking and finetuning. In R. Schiefelbusch (ed.) *Communicative Competence: Assessment and Language Intervention*. Baltimore, MD: University Park Press (pp. 703–707).

Elliott, R.O., Hall, K., & Soper, H.V. (1991). Analog language teaching versus natural language teaching: generalization and retention of language learning for adults with autism and mental retardation. *Journal of Autism and Developmental Disorders*, **21**, 443–447.

Foxx, R. (1993). R.M. Sapid effects awaiting replication. *American Journal of Mental Retardation*, **97**, 375–376.

Frankel, R.M. (1982). Autism for all practical purposes: A microinteractional view. *Topics in Language Disorders*, **3**, 33–42.

Frankel, R.M., Leary, M., & Kilman, B. (1987). Building social skills through pragmatic analysis: assessment and treatment implications for children with autism. In D.J. Cohen, A. Donnellan, & R. Paul (eds) *Handbook of Autism and Pervasive Developmental Disorders*. New York: Wiley (pp. 333–359).

Frith, U. (1989). *Autism: Explaining the Enigma*. London: Blackwell.

Goetz, L., Schuler, A.L., & Sailor, W. (1979). Teaching functional speech to the severely handicapped: current issues. *Journal of Autism and Developmental Disorders*, **9**, 325–343.

Gravelle, G. & Konstantareas, M.M. (1993). Facilitated Communication: A controlled examination of the phenomenon. Invited symposium address at the 3rd International Conference in Autism, Toronto.

Halliday, M.A.K. (1975). *Learning How to Mean: Explorations in the Development of Language*. London: Edward Arnold.

Haracopos, D. (1989). Comprehensive treatment program for autistic children and adults in Denmark. In C. Gillberg (ed.) *Diagnosis and Treatment of Autism*. New York: Plenum (pp. 251–284).

Harris, S.L., Handelman, J.S., Kristoff, B. Bass, L., & Gordon, R. (1990). Changes in language development among autistic and peer children in segregated and integrated preschool settings. *Journal of Autism and Developmental Disorders*, **20**, 23–31.

Helmer, S., Layton, T., & Wolf, A. (1982). *Patterns of Language Behavior in Autistic Children*. Paper presented at the American Speech-Language-Hearing Association Annual Convention, Toronto.

Hermelin, B. & O'Connor, N. (1970). *Psychological Experiments with Autistic Children*. Oxford: Pergamon Press.

Hewes, G.H. (1973). Primate communication and the gestural origin of language. *Current Anthropology*, **14**, 5–24.

Howlin, P. & Yates, P. (1989). Treating autistic children at home: a London based programme. In C. Giliber (ed.) *Diagnosis and Treatment of Autism*. New York: Plenum (pp. 307–322).

Hurlbut, B.I., Inata, B.A., & Green, J.D. (1982). Nonvocal language acquisition in adolescents with severe physical disabilities: bliss symbol versus iconic stimulus formats. *Journal of Applied Behavior Analysis*, **15**, 241–258.

Ingram, D. (1978). Sensori-motor intelligence and language development. In A. Lock (ed.) *Action Gesture and Symbol: The Emergence of Language*. London: Academic Press (pp. 261–290).

Kanner, L. (1943). Autistic disturbances of affective contact. *Nervous Child*, **2**, 217–250.

Kazdin, A.E. (1993). Replication and extension of behavior treatment of autistic disorder. *American Journal of Mental Retardation*, **97**, 377–379.

Konstantareas, M.M. (1986). Manual language: its relevance to communication acquisition in autistic children. In H.T.A. Whiting & M.G. Wade (eds) *Themes in Motor Development*. Dordrecht: Martinus Nijhoff (pp. 159–179).

Konstantareas, M.M. (1987). Autistic children exposed to simultaneous communication training: a follow-up. *Journal of Autism and Developmental Disorders*, **17**, 115–131.

Konstantareas, M.M. (1993). Language and communicative behavior in childhood psychosis. In G. Blanken, J. Dittman, H. Grimm, J. Marshall J.,.& C.W. Wallesch (eds) *Linguistic Disorders and Pathologies: An International Handbook*. Berlin: Walter de Gruyter (pp. 804–824).

Konstantareas, M.M. & Homatidis, S. (1987). Brief report: ear infections in autistic and normal children. *Journal of Autism and Developmental Disorders*, **17**, 585–594.

Konstantareas, M.M., Homatidis, S., & Busch, J. (1989). Cognitive, communication, and social differences between autistic boys and girls. *Journal of Applied Developmental Psychology*, **10**, 411–424.

Konstantareas, M.M., Hunter, D., & Sloman, L. (1982). Training a blind autistic child to communicate through signs. *Journal of Autism and Developmental Disorders*, **12**, 11–17.

Konstantareas, M.M. & Lelbovitz, S.F. (1981). Early communication acquisition by autistic children: Signing and mouthing versus signing and speaking. *Sign Language Studies*, **31**, 135–154.

Konstantareas, M.M., Oxman, J., & Webster, C.D. (1977). Simultaneous communication with autistic and other severely dysfunctional nonverbal children. *Journal of Communication Disorders*, **10**, 267–282.

Konstantareas, M.M., Oxman, J., & Webster, C.D. (1978). Iconicity: effects on the acquisition of sign language by autistic and other severely dysfunctional children. In P. Siple (ed.) *Understanding language through sign language research*. New York: Academic Press (pp. 213–237).

Konstantareas, M.M., Webster, C.D., & Oxman, J. (1979). Manual language acquisition and its influence on other areas of functioning in autistic and autistic-like children. *Journal of Child Psychology and Psychiatry*, **20**, 337–350.

Lansing, M.D. (1989). Educational Evaluation. In C. Gillberg (ed.) *Diagnosis and Treatment of Autism*. New York: Plenum (pp. 151–166).

Locke, A. (1978). The emergence of language. In A. Locke (ed.) *Action, Gesture and Symbol: The Emergence of Language*. London: Academic Press (pp. 3–20).

Lovaas, O.I. (1987). Behavior treatment and normal educational and intellectual functioning in young autistic children. *Journal of Consulting and Clinical Psychology*, **55**, 3–9.

Lovaas, O.I., Calouri, K., & Jada, J. (1989). The nature of behavioral treatment and research with young autistic persons. In C. Gillberg (ed.) *Diagnosis and Treatment of Autism*. New York: Plenum (pp. 285–306).

Lovaas, O.I., Berberich, J.P., Perloff, B.F., & Schaeffer, B. (1966). Acquisition of imitative speech by schizophrenic children. *Science*, **151**, 705–707.

Lovaas, O.I., Koegel, R., Simmons, J., & Long, J.S. (1973). Some generalization and follow-up measures on autistic children in behavior therapy. *Journal of Applied Behavior Analysis*, **6**, 131–166.

Lovaas, O.I. & Smith, T. (1988). Intensive behavioral treatment for young autistic children. In B.B. Lahey & A.E. Kazdln (eds) *Advances in Clinical Psychology*, Vol. II. New York: Plenum (pp. 285–324).

Mack, J.E., Webster, C.D., & Goksen, I. (1980). Where are they now and how are they faring: follow-up of 51 severely handicapped speech-deficient children four years after an operant-based program. In C.D. Webster, M.M. Konstantareas, J. Oxman, & J.E. Mack (eds) *Autism: New Directions in Research and Education*. New York: Pergamon (pp. 349–367).

McEachin, J.J., Smith, T., & Lovaas, O.I. (1993). Long-term outcome for children with autism who received early intensive behavioral treatment. *American Journal of Mental Retardation*, **97**, 359–372.

Mesibov, G.B. (1993). Treatment outcome is encouraging. *American Journal of Mental Retardation*, **97**, 379–380.

Miller, A. & Eller-Miller, E. (1989). *From Ritual to Repertoire – A Cognitive Developmental Systems Approach with Behavior-Disordered Children*. New York: Wiley.

Mundy, P. (1993). Normal versus high-functioning status in children with autism. *American Journal of Mental Retardation*, **97**, 381–384.

Oxman, J., Konstantareas, M.M., & Lelbovitz-Bojm, S.F. (1979). Simultaneous communication training and vocal responding in nonverbal autistic-like children. *International Journal of Rehabilitation Research*, **2**, 394–396.

Paul, R. & Cohen, D.J. (1984). Outcomes of severe disorders of language acquisition. *Journal of Autism and Developmental Disorders*, **14**, 405–421.

Prizant, B. & Schuler, A.L. (1987). Facilitating communication: theoretical foundations. In D. Cohen, A. Donnellan, & R. Paul (eds) *Handbook of Autism and Pervasive Developmental Disorders*. New York: Wiley (pp. 289–300).

Resnick, T.J. & Rapin, I. (1991). Language disorders in childhood. *Psychiatric Annals*, **21**, 709–716.

Rutter, M. & Schopler, E. (1987). Autism and pervasive developmental disorders: concepts and diagnostic issues. *Journal of Autism and Developmental Disorders*, **17**, 159–186.

Schopler, E., Short, A., & Mesibov, B. (1987). Relation of behavior treatment to "normal functioning": comment on Lovaas. *Journal of Consulting and Clinical Psychology*, **57**, 162–164.

Schuler, A.L. & Prizant, B.M. (1985). Echolalia. In E. Schopler & G. Mesibov (eds) *Communication Problems in Autism*. New York: Plenum (pp. 163–184).

Siegel, B. (1991). Toward DSM-IV: a developmental approach to autistic disorder. In M.M. Konstantareas & J.H. Beitchman (eds) *Pervasive Developmental Disorders*. Psychiatric Clinics of North America. New York: Saunders (pp. 113–124).

Skinner, B.F. (1957). *Verbal Behavior*. New York: Appleton-Century-Crofts.

Smith, T., McEachin, J.J., & Lovaas, O.I. (1993). Comments on replication and evaluation of outcome. *American Journal of Mental Retardation*, **97**, 385–391.

Van Wagenen, L., Jensen, W.R., Worsham, N., & Petersen, B.P. (1985). The use of simultaneous communication to teach difficult verbal discriminations to an autistic and developmentally disabled child. *Australian Journal of Human Communication Disorders*, **13**, 143–152.

Watson, L., Lord, C., Schafer, B., & Schopler, E. (1989). *Teaching Spontaneous Communication to Autistic and Developmentally Handicapped Children*. New York: Irvington.

Webster, C.D., McPherson, H., Sloman, L., Evans, M.A., & Kuchar, E. (1973). Communicating with an autistic boy by gestures. *Journal of Autism and Childhood Schizophrenia*, **3**, 337–346.

Wheeler, D.L., Jacobson, J.W., Pagileri, R.A., & Schwartz, A.A. (1993). Experimental assessment of facilitated communication. *Mental Retardation*, **31**, 49–60.

Wilbur, R.B. (1985). Sign language and autism. In E. Schopler & G.B. Mesibov (eds) *Communication Problems in Autism*. New York: Plenum (pp. 229–253).

PART VI
OUTCOME STUDIES

Introduction

M. MARY KONSTANTAREAS

The four chapters in this part deal with issues on the long-term outcome of
children with speech and language disorders. They address a crucial aspect
of the entire area since they examine how early difficulties in speech/language
development impact on later academic, social, and personality adjustment.
Unless we are cognizant of the long-term implications of a developmental
deviation, we cannot fully appreciate its severity, complexity, and pervasive-
ness or the variables most likely to impact and influence its course and
long-term prognosis. The longitudinal designs relied upon in all four chapters
offer the best methodology to study these processes, despite their associated
high costs. In such designs the same individuals are examined across time,
frequently more than once. Thus any discontinuities that may occur in the
course of development are more likely to be captured and critically examined
if the same rather than different individuals are studied. Furthermore,
longitudinal designs allow for intrapersonal, interpersonal and broader social
ecology variables to be critically examined diachronically in their complex
transactions, particularly when advance statistical techniques are employed
for the data analyses.

Part VI commences with Chapter 22 and the Ottawa Longitudinal Study.
This epidemiological investigation began when the children were 5, and
involved 142 children deemed to meet criteria for speech/language disorders
out of a much larger sample. They were re-evaluated at a mean age of 12.5.
Data from that follow-up are employed by Beitchman, Brownlie, & Wilson
to address four key hypotheses proposed as to the possible links between
language and psychiatric difficulties. Their first, on whether speech/language
difficulties lead directly to psychiatric disorder, is answered, overall, in
the negative. Their findings revealed that, although these difficulties had an
independent effect on psychiatric disorder, other variables such as the
mothers' mental health and marital adjustment, were also predictive of an
adverse outcome. The data provided support for the second hypothesis that
speech/language difficulties predispose to learning disabilities upon school

entry, which may in turn lead to psychiatric disorder. However the authors caution that not all children with speech/language disorders in their follow-up suffered from learning disabilities, hence, once again, other factors may also be at work. Finally, the authors propose and systematically explore their last and most intriguing hypothesis, namely that neurodevelopmental immaturity may underlie and account for symptom overlap between speech/language impairment and ADHD, and perhaps also verbal deficits and other disorders.

Chapter 23 by Schachter offers a critical review of evidence on the association between speech/language impairment and academic performance, relying on follow-up work in this general area. The author begins by discussing the relationship between speech/language difficulties and reading underachievement, and presents and critically discusses some of the disagreements in the literature as to what constitutes learning disabilities and academic underachievement. In the process, she touches upon an issue that recurs in the other chapters in this section, namely the question as to how one is to factor IQ into underachievement, reading problems (cf. Williams & McGee), or speech/language problems (cf. Beitchman et al.). After reviewing clinic based studies, Schachter concludes that children with speech/language difficulties are at risk for developing academic problems as they progress through school. As to what mediates this difficulty, however, she informs us, the literature is not consistent since it points to different factors as potentially responsible. Turning to the community based investigations, the author finds that language, intellectual ability, socioeconomic status, and mother's education were the best predictors of academic achievement at follow-up. Thus she concludes that speech/language difficulties are only one of a number of other predictors of academic achievement, a not unexpected but certainly important finding since it can inform on etiological factors and possible remediation efforts in this area.

Chapter 24 by Williams & McGee addresses the topic of reading achievement and its relationship to personality functioning in later life. Considering the direction of effect, the authors argue in favor of the view that in childhood the predominant causal direction is from reading failure to disruptive behavior, and not the reverse. Williams & McGee then describe the Dunedin, New Zealand, longitudinal study of the health and development of a cohort of children born between 1972 and 1973 examined first at 3-years-of-age, and every two years thereafter, until the age of 21 years, thus far. Considering the data from three time points, upon entry to school, at 15 and at 18, and using structural equation modeling, they examined the causal relationships among a group of variables they considered to be relevant to reading difficulties and subsequent mental health. Surprisingly, for both boys and girls, they found no direct causal path between reading disability and antisocial behavior in adolescence or reading disability and antisocial behavior in adulthood. The authors conclude that any influence early problems might have on later adjustment may be indirect, mostly mediated by reading difficulties and antisocial and other behavior problems in childhood. The only outcome variable that was directly associated with literacy at age 18 was personal disadvantage for men but not women. The results of this large-scale study lead the authors to suggest that intervention in the area of reading should be undertaken very early, particularly for children coming from disadvantaged households.

Finally, in Chapter 25, Musselman, MacKay, Trehub, & Eagle examine the relationship between deafness and psychosocial functioning, drawing from a follow-up study of deaf children first assessed during the preschool period and followed-up in adolescence, 10 years later. The deaf children were subdivided into a group first exposed to an auditory/oral (A/O) system and then, because of difficulties in its utilization, to total communication (TC) and another, higher functioning group, exposed to an A/O communication system throughout. The groups were compared to typical children at both time points, using a battery of linguistic, cognitive, developmental, and personality instruments. Musselman et al. report that, when examined in childhood, the social profiles of the deaf children, regardless of mode of communication used, were not different from normative data. For both deaf subgroups, social development was related to the primary mode of communication used, that is, receptive sign/speech for the TC and speech for the A/O. In adolescence, although the A/O group fared better in overall communication, both deaf subgroups presented with skills that were insufficient for the demands of even secondary school education. As well, although the A/O adolescents exhibited patterns similar to those of hearing adolescents, those exposed to TC exhibited symptoms at the clinical or borderline-clinical range. The authors attribute this difference to the disruption in the pattern of communication as the children switched from the A/O to the TC system, and anticipate improvement as the deaf TC adolescents find their niche as adults in the deaf community.

22 Linguistic impairment and psychiatric disorder: pathways to outcome

JOSEPH H. BEITCHMAN, E.B. BROWNLIE,
AND BETH WILSON

INTRODUCTION

Speech/language impairment represents one of the most common types of childhood disorders and is associated with considerable psychiatric morbidity. Children with speech/language impairment have been found to show increased rates of psychiatric disorders compared to children with normal speech/language functioning. This increased risk for psychiatric disorder raises questions about the nature of the association between speech/language impairment and psychiatric disorders. One group of questions concerns the possible etiologic relation between speech/language impairment and psychiatric disorder. Does speech/language impairment cause psychiatric disorders? Do they arise independently? Or, are they both due to some underlying antecedent condition? A second group of questions concerns the possible mechanisms or pathways by which speech/language impairment could result in psychiatric disorder. Can we identify any pathways or mechanisms by which the effects of speech/language impairment are mediated? Can different effects be realized based on the specific speech/language functions affected? Or, is their relation due to some associated variables or to some antecedent underlying neurodevelopmental problem? These questions can be restated in the form of the following four hypotheses.

First, speech/language impairment may lead to psychiatric disorder through its effects on social and peer relations. Difficulties in comprehension and expression experienced by the speech/language impaired child may lead to frustration or lack of self-confidence. Given the centrality of communication in the social world, it would not be surprising that these children would suffer emotional and behavioral problems. Impaired communication may lead to poor peer relationships. Peer rejection and scapegoating may initiate a negative social spiral (Rice, 1993) that could contribute to later psychiatric impairment.

The impact of speech/language impairment on later psychiatric disorder may partly depend on the type of speech/language problem the child shows. Speech/language impairment is composed of separable skills and whether psychiatric disorder results and the kind of disorder that emerges may be a function of the specific type of linguistic skill affected. Some linguistic deficits are more likely than others to have serious effects on social relationships.

Second, since speech/language impaired young people are at high risk for learning disabilities, behavioral problems may develop as a result of difficulties experienced in academic settings, such as reading failure (Lynam et al., 1993). Under these circumstances, behavioral problems would not become evident until after the child was in school and had developed learning disabilities. This is one means by which speech/language impairment may affect psychiatric disorder, although they may develop somewhat independently from each other.

Third, it is possible that related variables may fully or partially account for the association between speech/language impairment and psychiatric disorder. In other words, psychiatric disorder among speech/language impaired children may be a function of concomitant variables such as social class, parental marital discord, and other related variables. Speech/language impairment is an insufficient explanation of behavior problems since not all speech/language impaired children develop behavior problems. The impact of additional variables may account for the association between speech/language and psychiatric disorder. If so, once these other variables are controlled or accounted for statistically, the association between speech/language impairment and psychiatric disorder would be reduced. In the most extreme case, in which additional factors fully account for the association between speech/language impairment and psychiatric disorder, the association would be considered spurious.

Fourth, an underlying factor may result in both speech/language impairment and psychiatric disorder, at least in some cases. Researchers have speculated that maturational lag (Bishop & Edmundson, 1987a) may explain the speech/language delay and similarly, that neurodevelopmental immaturity or deficits (Beitchman, 1985a; Beitchman et al., 1989b; Tallal, Dukette, & Curtiss, 1989; Locke, 1994) represent this underlying factor. For some children, therefore, speech/language impairment may be an expression of neurodevelopmental deficits or immaturity; if so, these young people should show behavioral and developmental problems secondary to these neurodevelopmental deficits or immaturities, as well as problems more directly attributable to difficulties with speech and language. Furthermore, evidence of these deficits or immaturities should be apparent among speech/language impaired children with behavioral disorders.

Utilizing data from the Ottawa follow-up study of 5-year-old speech/language impaired children, we will consider these four central ideas on the relation between speech/language impairment and psychiatric disorders. We will briefly describe the Ottawa Longitudinal Study and consider the evidence available on the merits of these four hypotheses.

THE OTTAWA LONGITUDINAL STUDY

Methods

The first study

A one-in-three random representative sample of all 5-year-old English speaking children from the Ottawa–Carleton region in Ontario, Canada were given the first stage of a three stage screening procedure. Each stage consisted of a battery of standardized tests. Stage I was a 30-minute language-screening interview. Children falling below the identified cutoff points received intensive testing by speech/language pathologists at stage II. One hundred and forty-two children scoring below the stage II cutoff points were identified as speech/language impaired and were selected for stage III testing. A control sample of 142 children matched for age and sex, and taken from the same classroom or school was selected and given the same stage III procedures as the speech/language impaired group. The parents of each of the stage III children were interviewed to determine the birth, medical, and developmental history of their children. Intelligence and audiological tests were given to the children. Finally, several measures of behavioral/psychiatric dysfunction were used: Achenbach's Child Behaviour Checklist (CBCL), Conners' Teacher Rating Scale (CTRS), and the Children's Self-Report Questionnaire (CSRQ). Semi-structured psychiatric interviews were also conducted with 85 of the children.

Approximately 19% of the children had speech/language disorders and of those children with speech/language disorders, 49% had a diagnosable psychiatric disorder. Thirty percent of the speech/language impaired children were diagnosed with ADHD and a further 12.5% had an internalizing disorder of anxiety or depression. The rate of these psychiatric disorders was significantly greater than the rate of psychiatric disorders in the control group. Diagnoses were made blind to the child's speech/language status and were based on standardized, semi-structured interviews with the parent and child. (For further details regarding the results of these studies, see Beitchman et al., 1986a; 1986b; and Beitchman, Hood, & Inglis, 1990.)

In an attempt to identify linguistic subtypes, cluster analysis was employed to classify these children at age 5. Based on the children's scores on measures of articulation, expressive and receptive language, and tests of auditory comprehension and auditory memory, four clusters were identified, of which three represent children with speech/language impairments. Each speech/language impaired cluster was labeled according to the dominant linguistic characteristics which emerged from this analysis: poor articulation, poor comprehension, and low overall. Differences among these groups according to cognitive, developmental, audiometric and behavioral variables were found (Beitchman et al., 1989a, 1989b).

The second study

The children from the first study were followed up in a second study conducted in 1989–90, when the children were on average 12.5-years-of-age. Of the 284 time 1 participants in the initial study, 266 (93.6%) were successfully recontacted. Of these 266 children, 244 (91.7%) agreed to participate in the follow-up study. This yielded an overall response rate of 85.9%, a loss to follow-up rate of 6.3% and a refusal rate of 7.8%.

As in the first wave, comprehensive testing of speech, language, cognitive, and academic competence was completed. In addition, detailed interviews with the child's parent, semi-structured diagnostic child psychiatric interviews, and teacher and parent behavioral rating scales were completed. Once again, the assessments were conducted blind to the child's speech/language status based on interviews with the parent and child. The same tests and procedures utilized at time 1 were used at time 2 unless there was a more current version of the previously used test.

Due to concerns over rater-dependent assessments of psychiatric disorder, we developed a comprehensive measure of psychiatric functioning – the psychiatric composite. The psychiatric composite variable was created to incorporate multiple perspectives on the child into a single dimensional measure of psychiatric functioning. The psychiatric composite is comprised of ratings from three sources: Mother (Achenbach CBCL Sum T), teacher (Achenbach CBCL Sum T), and psychiatrist (DSM-III Axis V Global Assessment Scale; GAS). The psychiatric composite variable is the sum of the standard scores for each of the three psychiatric outcomes, with higher scores reflecting greater psychopathology.

Speech/language impairment, psychiatric disorder and social relationships

Sufficient data demonstrate that speech and language impaired children are at increased risk for developing psychiatric disorders of all kinds (Chess & Rosenburg, 1974; Stevenson & Richman, 1976; Cantwell & Baker, 1977; Grinnell et al., 1983; Gualtieri et al., 1983; Cantwell & Baker, 1985; Baker & Cantwell, 1987; Beitchman et al., 1986b; Cantwell & Baker, 1991; Kotsopoulis & Boodoosingh, 1987). Whether one samples from a psychiatric population or a language-impaired population, it is clear that language impairment and psychiatric disorders occur together.

In the Ottawa Longitudinal Study, speech/language impaired children had higher scores on measures of psychopathology (and lower scores on measures of adjustment) according to multiple raters. These findings are shown in Table 22.1. Mothers' CBCL Sum T scores, teachers' TRF Sum T scores and CSRQ self-report clinical probability ratings were significantly higher at follow-up for the speech/language impaired group. Psychiatrists' GAS ratings were

Table 22.1. *Psychiatric outcome, social competence and adaptive functioning measures at age 12.5 by speech/language status at age 5*

	Speech/language impaired (N = 111)	Controls (N = 130)	p value
Mothers' CBCL Sum T[1]	57.60	53.60	0.006
Teachers' TRF Sum T[1]	55.90	51.60	0.002
CSRQ clinical probability[1]	0.36	0.32	0.05
Psychiatrists' GAS (adjustment)[2]	72.30	79.90	0.0001
Psychiatric composite[1]	0.85	−0.44	0.00
Mothers' CBCL social competence[2]	42.21	46.79	0.003
Teachers' TRF adaptive functioning[2]	45.52	49.44	0.004

Note: Due to missing data, some cell N's vary. [1] Higher scores indicate greater psychopathology. [2] Higher scores indicate better functioning.

significantly lower for the speech/language impaired group, indicating poorer adjustment. The psychiatric composite scores were significantly higher for the speech/language impaired group than for the controls.

One mechanism by which early speech/language impairment may lead to later psychiatric disorders is through difficulties with social relationships. The CBCL social competence scale and the TRF adaptive functioning scale were used to assess the children's social and coping skills at follow-up. Speech/language impaired children had lower scores on both mother-rated social competence and teacher-rated adaptive functioning (see Table 22.1). These findings support the idea that difficulties in social and peer relationships experienced by speech/language impaired children may be a factor in the development of psychiatric disorders.

The evidence presented above provides strong support for an association between speech/language impairment and elevated levels of psychopathology, according to multiple raters. However, this does not address the specific mechanisms or potential pathways through which the linguistic impairment may lead to psychiatric disorder. To answer this question, more precise delineation of the specific speech/language function affected is needed. We consider this issue in the section that follows – an exploration of the potential effects of specific linguistic factors on social relations.

Speech/language subtypes and psychiatric disorders

In addition to the data supporting an association between speech/language impairment and psychiatric disorder in general, specific speech/language deficits have been shown to be related to differential psychiatric outcome.

The practice of using undifferentiated, heterogeneous samples of speech/ language impaired children, common to most follow-up studies, undoubtedly obscures possible relationships between specific speech/language deficiencies and outcomes. Verbal deficits do not constitute a homogeneous entity and may include auditory comprehension deficits, expressive language problems, and articulation problems. General statements regarding verbal deficits may mask important differences regarding specific linguistic functions that apply to some but not to other subgroups of children.

However, few research efforts have focused on the classification of speech/language impaired children such that their course or prognosis could be predicted on the basis of some identifiable characteristic(s) common to the group as a whole. While broad classifications of speech/language impairment into categories such as syntactic-phonologic or semantic-pragmatic types have been described (Bishop & Rosenbloom, 1987), these typologies have not been empirically grounded, raising questions about the validity of these distinctions. Furthermore, the association of these typologies to psychiatric disorders has not been examined. It may be that different mechanisms or pathways explain the link to psychiatric disorder depending on the specific linguistic typology. For instance, evidence suggests that disorders of speech production carry a less serious prognosis than disorders of language (Baker & Cantwell, 1987).

Surprisingly few attempts have been made to assess the stability of speech/language subtypes from preschool to school age, and results of existing studies are mixed. In particular, most studies of subtype stability within *early* childhood have reported that distinct patterns of language functioning persist over time and are differentially related to outcome (e.g., Silva et al., 1983; Bishop & Edmundson, 1987b; Bishop & Adams, 1990). Tallal (1988), however, reported that subgroups identified at 4-years-of-age lost distinctiveness at follow-up four years later.

Utilizing a representative community sample of 5-year-old children, we have previously described four speech/language profiles or clusters: High overall, low overall, poor comprehension and poor articulation (Beitchman et al., 1989a; Beitchman et al., 1989b). When children in these clusters were followed to age 12.5, associations between the speech/language cluster and specific types of psychiatric problems were discovered. For example, 5-year-old children who originally comprised the low overall profile were found to show both increased rates of emotional disorders and externalizing disorders at follow-up (Beitchman et al., in press a). Children in the poor auditory comprehension cluster, in comparison with other speech/language profiles, showed increased levels of teacher-rated hyperactivity at follow-up. This was the only group to have shown an increase in hyperactivity symptoms. Boys among this group also showed high levels of aggressive behaviors.

This association between symptoms of distractibility/hyperactivity and auditory discrimination/comprehension has also been reported by Cook et al.

(1993). Classroom instruction, particularly with young children, often includes some circle or story time activity. At these times teachers may read a story to their students while the students are expected to sit quietly and listen. A comparable phenomenon occurs with older children: the teacher will lecture or provide some form of oral instruction while the students are expected to sit quietly and attend to the teacher. It seems plausible that the child or older student who has difficulty comprehending the orally based material will soon lose interest in the story or lecture and appear distracted, day dream, perhaps fidget, or even try to interact with other students. Such a student will quickly come to the attention of the teacher and may be labeled hyperactive or disruptive.

With reference to the Ottawa Longitudinal Study, it is also of interest that the boys with poor auditory comprehension showed higher levels of aggressive symptoms than boys in the other speech/language groups. According to teachers' ratings on the Teacher Report Form (TRF), boys with comprehension problems at age 5 showed significantly elevated levels of aggression at age 12.5. There is scant literature available in which this association has previously been described. As we shall discuss, interpersonal problem solving deficits may contribute to the behavioral problems of these boys.

Why should boys with comprehension problems in early childhood show pronounced levels of aggression in later childhood? We have found that children with early childhood auditory comprehension deficits tended to remain disadvantaged in terms of linguistic proficiency, cognitive abilities and academic performance at follow-up (Beitchman et al., in press b). Due to their auditory comprehension deficits, these boys may feel inept or out of step with their peers. Situations in which they believe themselves to be subject to ridicule or criticism are likely to be more common than among boys with adequate auditory comprehension. Consequently, they may be exposed to more conflicts in which coping strategies involving aggressive acts may be used to defend against real or imagined attacks on their self-esteem. Aggressive behavior may represent attempts to act out their frustration and sense of inequity in the face of real and perceived public ridicule. Studies of preschool children with deficits in auditory comprehension suggest that this may be one mechanism behind the link between poor auditory comprehension and aggressive behavior (Beitchman, 1985b).

The social cognition literature offers support for this point of view. Aggression in children has also been associated with a variety of interpersonal problem-solving deficits. Aggressive children are poor at taking the perspective of others and understanding their thoughts and feelings (Chandler, 1973; Chandler et al., 1974). This may explain why these children are also more likely to attribute aggressive intent to the interactions of others, and to suggest more aggressive solutions (Dodge, 1991; Rubin, Bream, & Rose-Krasnor, 1991). It is plausible that children with auditory comprehension difficulties in early childhood will be more vulnerable to the development of interpersonal problem-solving deficits. If deficits are present, they may also be more resistant to modification. It is simply not known to what extent auditory comprehension problems contribute to deficits in social cognition.

While interpersonal problem-solving deficits may partly explain why boys with a history of poor auditory comprehension act more aggressively than their male peers, further factors must also contribute to this behavior. Like boys from the poor comprehension cluster, boys from the low overall cluster also experienced auditory comprehension deficits in early childhood. In addition, boys from both the poor comprehension and low overall clusters showed difficulties with peer relationships as evidenced by lower mothers' ratings of social competence compared to boys without early speech/language impairment (post hoc test: $p < 0.01$). However, boys from the low overall cluster did not show increased levels of aggressive behavior.

Two possible explanations for this phenomenon should be considered. The difference in the expression of aggression could be related to expressive language skills, which were average or near average among the poor comprehension boys and poor among the low overall boys. Stronger expressive language skills may have facilitated the expression of aggression among boys in the poor comprehension group and/or weaker expressive language skills may have inhibited the expression of aggression among boys in the low overall group. Alternatively, other factors among the low overall group, such as the presence of more broadly based developmental problems, may lead instead to forms of symptom expression more readily identifiable as immature behavior, thereby mitigating or interfering with the development or expression of aggressive behavior. If so, behavior problems evident in early childhood but secondary to neurodevelopmental delays would in later childhood be identifiable as behavioral immaturity. We explore some of these ideas in a later section.

Verbal deficits, reading disabilities and psychiatric disorders

While early speech/language deficits are strongly associated with the development of psychiatric disorders, mediating factors such as academic performance must be taken into consideration. A large literature provides strong empirical support for an association between verbal deficits and psychiatric disorders. Studies on the role of academic difficulties in the development of psychiatric disorders have focused on externalizing disorders, specifically antisocial behavior. Researchers differ on the importance of academic difficulties, and specifically reading failure, in the development of antisocial outcomes.

One theory posits that verbal learning deficits produce antisocial behavior through the medium of school failure (Hirschi & Hindelang, 1977; Buikhuisen, 1987). Support for this hypothesis was found in a sample of black

12- and 13-year-old boys (Lynam et al., 1993). However, the relationship between verbal deficits and antisocial behavior among white boys in this study was not found to be mediated by school failure. While an important finding, these results are not generalizable to girls or to boys from other racial groups. Little additional evidence to support this hypothesis exists in current literature.

A second theory is that disruptive (externalizing) behavior at school entry precedes reading failure. Later delinquency is perhaps a consequence of the continuation of antisocial behavior into adolescence rather than a consequence of reading failure *per se* (Patterson et al., 1989). This view, strongly held by some (Patterson et al., 1989) was offered some support by Williams & McGee (1994) who found that poor reading was not associated with delinquent behavior in adolescence when prior history of externalizing behaviors was controlled. The path led from disruptive behavior at school entry to later delinquency. However, this finding is at odds with much of the theory posited in previous literature regarding this issue (e.g., Wadsworth, 1979; Maughan, Gray, & Rutter, 1985).

Given that reading disabilities are central to school progress and academic achievement, it is reasonable to suppose that internalizing disorders as well as externalizing disorders would be a potential consequence of reading disabilities. Differential manifestation of psychiatric disorders may be due to temperamental disposition and/or socialization. There are few studies in which children at risk for reading disabilities have been assessed at school entry prior to the identification of reading disabilities and then after the identification (and exposure to the consequences) of reading disability. We considered the rate of psychiatric disorders before and after a diagnosis of a learning disability in a group of children who at school entry did not show evidence of psychiatric disorder. In addition, we examined the rate of learning disabilities in children who at school entry showed evidence of psychiatric disorder. These findings are discussed below.

Table 22.2 shows the Time 2 outcomes of children who at Time 1 were speech/language (S/L) impaired but did not have a psychiatric disorder. Among the children who developed a psychiatric disorder at Time 2, 57.1% showed learning disabilities (LD) in reading decoding, whereas only 14.8% of children with no history of psychiatric disorder at Time 1 or Time 2 showed learning disabilities in reading decoding.

These results lend support to the idea that the rate of psychiatric disorders increases as a response to reading difficulties. It is possible that other factors, such as low SES, contributed to the high rate of psychiatric disorders among the LD subgroup presented above but these data do not allow exploration of these issues. It is nevertheless striking that among children with a prior history of speech/language impairment, with psychiatric disability emerging after school entry, more than half had a reading disorder. This raises critical

Table 22.2. *Time 2 psychiatric status by Time 2 LD (reading decoding) in Time 1 S/L impaired children without Time 1 psychiatric disorder*

	Time 2 LD – Reading decoding	
Time 2 psychiatric status	LD (%)	Not LD (%)
Psychiatric disorder	57.1	42.9
No psychiatric disorder	14.8	85.2

Note: N = 41, p < 0.0074.

issues for educators, clinicians and therapists in terms of prevention and treatment, for this high risk group.

Often children with learning disabilities are thought to be at increased risk for externalizing disorders, such as antisocial behavior. In order to test this hypothesis, we examined the proportion of children with internalizing versus externalizing disorders. Among learning disabled children with psychiatric disorders, approximately 62.5% were diagnosed with externalizing disorders and the remaining 37.5% were diagnosed with internalizing disorders. It is apparent from these numbers that concerns regarding the potential adverse effects of academic failure cannot be restricted to externalizing disorders alone.

We also tested the theory that a prior history of behavior disorders results in learning disabilities. We examined the proportion of children with and without behavior disorders at school entry to see if there were differences in the rate of learning disabilities seven years later. These results are shown below in Table 22.3.

Among children with speech/language impairment at age 5, no differences were found in the rate of reading disabilities at age 12.5 between children with and without evidence of psychiatric disorder at age 5. For a large proportion of children with a prior history of speech/language impairment, newly emergent psychiatric disorders co-occur with reading disabilities. From this sample, it does not appear that a prior history of behavior disorders increases the risk of reading disabilities at age 12.5.

It is also apparent that learning disabilities cannot be the entire explanation for the association between speech/language impairment and psychiatric disorders since not all the speech/language impaired children with psychiatric disorders had learning disabilities. What additional factors account for the development of psychiatric disorders among these speech/language impaired children? These ideas will be explored in the following section.

Table 22.3. *Percent Time 2 LD (reading decoding) in children with and without Time 1 psychiatric disorder*

	Time 2 LD – Reading decoding	
Time 1 psychiatric status	LD (%)	Not LD (%)
Psychiatric disorder	19.5	80.5
No psychiatric disorder	17.2	82.8

Note: N = 193, p = n.s.

Speech/language impairment, psychiatric disorders and associated variables

The relative importance of speech/language variables, in comparison with other associated variables, in accounting for psychiatric disorder has been examined in only a limited number of studies. Some information can be gleaned from studies by Silva, Williams, & McGee (1987) and Benasich, Curtiss, & Tallal (1993). These investigators found a significant association between speech/language function and behavior problems, even after family disadvantage was controlled. Benasich and colleagues found that change in nonverbal IQ was associated with psychiatric disorder and that the severity of early speech/language impairment was not related to later outcome. These two studies represent the only known attempt to examine the relation of speech/language impairment to later psychiatric disorder controlling for other variables. However, the Benasich study only followed children to age 8 and the Silva study did not provide a comprehensive examination of psychiatric outcome at follow-up.

In the Ottawa Longitudinal Study, we examined the relation of speech/language impairment to a dimensional measure of general psychopathology – the psychiatric composite. This multi-rater scale combined three standard scores: mothers' CBCL Sum T, teachers' TRF Sum T, and Psychiatrists' Global Assessment Scale (GAS). Children with speech/language impairment at age 5 had significantly higher (more severe) scores on the psychiatric composite at age 12.5 than control children (p < 0.01).

With this measure of general psychopathology we were able to examine the relative importance of other variables in accounting for the variance in the psychiatric composite among speech/language impaired children. It should be noted that considerably fewer speech/language impaired children (N = 56) than the entire sample of speech/language impaired children from the time 1 study (N = 142) were included in the analysis. Twenty-nine speech/language impaired children failed to participate in the follow-up study, 41 had insufficient psychiatric data at follow-up to calculate psychiatric composite scores, and an additional 16 were missing data on some of the Time

1 predictors. The subsample of 56 speech/language impaired children were not different from speech/language impaired children not included in the analysis in terms of SES and percentage of single versus dual parent families. The subsample had higher Bankson percentiles (M = 42.7) than remaining speech/language impaired children (M = 31.1) (p < 0.05). The subsample also had slightly higher time 1 IQ scores (M = 104.2) than remaining speech/language impaired children (M = 99.0) (p < 0.05). Based on these differences, it appears that the subsample is a somewhat less impaired subset of the original speech/language impaired sample.

Time 1 variables from language/cognition, demographics, child mental health, developmental/medical and parent mental health domains were considered as possible predictor variables of Time 2 psychiatric composite scores. Table 22.4 shows the adjusted R^2 and beta weights for the regression model which best predicted Time 2 outcome. Adjusted R^2, listed cumulatively, is the percentage of variance that can be accounted for by the variables entered into the regression model. The beta weights represent the relative importance of each variable in the model in predicting psychiatric composite at follow-up. Each beta weight indicates the amount of change that is produced in the dependent variable by one standardized change in each independent variable when the other independent variables are controlled.

What do these findings mean? First, using these 1982 predictors, it is possible to account for more than 50% of the variance in the 1990 psychiatric outcomes, as measured by the psychiatric composite. The list of predictors reveals a balancing of environmental constitutional, and family variables in relation to outcome seven years later. If only one variable could be used to predict outcome at age 12.5, it would be the mother's adversity variable. This composite variable is comprised of mothers' ratings of depression, anxiety, and marital adjustment and discord, if applicable. The importance of the adversity variable should not be surprising. It is known that mothers who are depressed or anxious, or involved in discordant marital relationships, will report that their children show higher levels of behavioral disturbance than mothers with lower levels of adversity (Rutter, 1989). Typically, however, this finding is based on concurrent, not longitudinal data. This finding is important because it shows that a mother's adversity score when the child was 5-years-of-age is predictive of the child's disturbance seven years later. It is possible that a mother's mental health and marital adjustment (where applicable) has a direct impact on her child's mental health, which carries forward in time.

The Bankson Language Screening Test (BLST), which taps expressive language, proved to be the next most important predictor of psychiatric outcome at age 12.5. This variable contributed an additional 15% of explained variance after the mother's adversity variable had been entered. A 20th percentile cutoff for BLST scores was used. When this variable was entered as a continuous function, it did not remain in the equation. Clearly, this

Table 22.4. *Age 5 predictors of psychiatric composite scores in S/L impaired 12.5-year-old children (N = 56)*

1982 predictor*	Adjusted R^2	Beta weights
Mother's adversity	0.23	0.26
Bankson (20th percentile)	0.38	−0.20
Health composite	0.47	0.34
Mother's CBCL sum T score	0.52	0.26
CTRS (square root)	0.56	0.23
SES group	0.59	−0.20

* See text for definition of terms.

screening instrument is important in predicting psychiatric disturbance, but it appears that its importance is not equal across its full range. Its maximum predictive power emerged when children scoring at the 20th percentile point or less were distinguished from children scoring higher.

The health composite variable is an interesting combination of child health and maternal perceptions of child health. This variable contributed the largest increase to explained variance after the BLST. In comparison with the other variables, it has the most direct effect on psychiatric outcome, and its unique variance is the largest, having the least overlap with the other predictors. The health composite consists of five items: mother's reports of prenatal stress, perinatal intensive care, child not in excellent health at age 5 and extended infant hospitalization, and audiometry failure. When hospital birth records were consulted for a subsample of cases, intensive care could not be confirmed. However, the children whose mothers endorsed this item had lower mean birth weights than other children. Although the maternal reports could not be confirmed, it appears that they reflect genuine difficulties and health concerns. Present health difficulties and/or the mother's perceptions that her child is not in excellent health or her belief that something was wrong with her child at the time of birth, was related to the child's progress seven years later. In other words, it is not simply that the child had something wrong with him or her, or that the mother believed that something was wrong with him or her, it is these two in combination.

Teachers' and mothers' 1982 ratings of the children's behavioral disturbance were predictive of 1990 psychiatric composite scores. These variables combined, however, only accounted for a reduction in unexplained variance of 11%, suggesting that prior history of disorder may be relevant to later outcome but that other variables are better predictors. It is also noteworthy that the Conners Teacher Rating Scale, compared to the mother's behavior ratings (Sum T), are equally predictive of outcome at 12.5 years of age, however, they explain non-overlapping variance in psychiatric composite scores. This provides support for the importance of multiple behavioral ratings, since although both ratings are equally predictive of psychiatric outcome, they tend to identify different children, or different aspects of the same children with behavior problems.

SES factors were last to enter the equation, contributing an additional 4% of explained variance. Issues of social class have been commonly associated with psychiatric disorder, consequently its inclusion is not surprising. Perhaps one may wonder why it added only 4% additional explained variance. This can probably be explained by the fact that SES is correlated with the other variables that entered the regression equation. This means that portions of the variance attributable to SES are already accounted for by these other variables.

In sum these findings suggest that expressive language at age 5, as measured by the BLST, captures 15% of the variance in psychiatric outcome at age 12.5 in a speech/language impaired sample. Not surprisingly, mother's mental health and marital adjustment accounted for the largest share of explained variance. It is also of interest that IQ (whether entered as full scale, verbal or performance IQ) did not enter the equation for the speech/language impaired sample, although Full Scale IQ was an important predictor of outcome among the entire sample of speech/language impaired and control children. It appears that the BLST replaces IQ in relation to predicting outcome in the speech/language impaired sample. Because IQ and speech/language functioning are highly correlated, the effects of the IQ variable are likely subsumed within the language variable.

It is clear that early speech/language impairment is one of a number of factors which are associated with later psychiatric disorder. Speech/language impairment remains an important predictor of psychiatric disorder, even when associated variables are taken into account. Although the impact of speech/language impairment may occur through mediating factors such as peer relationships and school performance for some children, for other children underlying antecedent variables may lead to both speech/language impairment and psychiatric disorder. We will explore the possible role of neurodevelopmental immaturity as an underlying antecedent factor leading to global impairments in the following section.

Speech/language impairment and neurodevelopmental immaturity/deficits

Severe forms of neurodevelopmental deficits can be found in children considered to be autistic. Here the social and behavioral problems of the children extend beyond anything that could be attributed solely to the child's language difficulties. Clearly, underlying neurodevelopmental problems are experienced by these children although their precise mechanisms are not well understood. Are there other syndromes experienced by speech/language impaired children in which behavioral problems could be ascribed to some underlying neurodevelopmental problems? Cantwell, Baker, & Rutter (1978) have described a group of children with developmental dysphasias who were considered socially awkward at follow-up. It is possible that their behavioral difficulties are not entirely attributable to their language deficits. Instead, neurodevelopmental problems may have accounted for both their language and social difficulties.

The nature of these neurodevelopmental deficits is not known and at this time must be considered speculative. However, it may be appropriate to think of these neurodevelopmental deficits under two categories: (1) as specific deficits affecting certain areas of the brain and nervous system and; (2) as general deficits affecting the child in global ways. There has been considerable interest in executive functions and the possible role of frontal lobe functioning as a factor in such behavioral disorders as attention deficit hyperactivity disorder (ADHD). Although this remains a controversial idea, it may help to explain the symptom overlap common to speech/language impaired children and children with ADHD. Given that children with ADHD are thought to have difficulties with self-control, tend to be impulsive, have problems planning and are prone to behavioral outbursts, and given that some speech/language impaired children show similar characteristics, it is germane to ask whether these behavioral problems could be explained by underlying executive function deficits. The answer to this question is not known, but it is an intriguing speculation worthy of research inquiry.

Another possibility is that the speech/language impairment may reflect a more general or broader neurodevelopmental dysfunction or delay. Locke (1994) has used the term neuromaturational delay in reference to speech/language impaired children. Locke believes that children with speech/language disorders experience an abnormally slow rate of brain development and as a consequence, exhibit many behaviors that distinguish them from their linguistically normal peers. These behaviors include inferior tactile and visual perception (Johnston et al., 1981), and clumsiness in motor tasks (Powell & Bishop, 1992), among others. Whether there would be corresponding delays in social and emotional development has not been systematically addressed but would seem to be a natural consequence of delayed brain maturation. Furthermore, the form of this delayed brain development could manifest itself differently at different ages. In other words, while children with such delays may show different kinds of specific behavioral problems at different developmental stages, a consistent thread of behaviors typical of chronologically younger children would be apparent throughout.

We have postulated elsewhere (Beitchman, 1985a) that antecedent underlying neurodevelopmental immaturity is responsible for the co-occurrence of speech/language impairment and hyperactivity. Similarly, Boudreault et al. (1988) have reported an association between pervasive attention deficit disorders and verbal deficits. Rutter (1989) believes that there may be a distinct syndrome of pervasive hyperactivity/inattention which tends to be associated

Table 22.5. *Mean Time 2 CBCL mother's immaturity factor T scores by Time 1 S/L and CTRS hyperactivity status: boys (N = 132)*

		Time 1 S/L Status	
		S/L Impaired	Controls
Time 1 CTRS	Hyperactive	69.5^a	59.25^b
	Not Hyperactive	61.16^c	59.4^d

Note: p < 0.001, a > b, c, d (p < 0.01).

with neurodevelopmental delays with an onset in the preschool years. To date there is little available literature on the later behavioral outcome of these so-called developmentally immature children. If the behavioral and linguistic problems these speech/language impaired hyperactive children show arise from, or are expressions of, neurodevelopmental immaturity, these children should continue to reveal evidence of immaturity in later childhood. Evidence for immaturity might appear in the form of behaviors judged to be more appropriate for chronologically younger children; other forms of delayed development, such as poor visual motor skills, might appear as well. We examine some of these issues below.

Table 22.5 shows the relationship between Time 2 mother-rated immaturity factor T scores and Time 1 teacher-rated hyperactivity status among boys from the speech/language impaired and control groups. Study data revealed that boys who, at age 5, were classified as both hyperactive and speech/language impaired had higher immaturity scores than other boys at age 12.5. The individual items thought to reflect immaturity included: acts too young for his age, clings to adults or too dependent, demands a lot of attention, and prefers playing with younger children.

Utilizing visual-motor skills as another measure of developmental progress we compared the level of visual motor skills among the same four groups to see if there was any other evidence of the postulated immaturity of the speech/language impaired hyperactive boys at age 12.5. These results are shown in Table 22.6 below.

The overall F test was highly significant, but the *post hoc* test failed to identify the source of significance. Nevertheless, these results provide additional support for the notion that significant differences can be found on variables measuring maturity of developmental function when hyperactive speech/language impaired boys are compared to non-hyperactive and control boys. It is pertinent to note, however, that boys identified at age 5 as speech/language impaired and hyperactive when followed to age 12.5 continued to show evidence of immature behavior and immature visual motor

Table 22.6. *Mean Time 2 VMI standard scores by Time 1 S/L and CTRS hyperactivity status: boys (N = 132)*

		Time 1 S/L Status	
		S/L Impaired	Controls
Time 1 CTRS	Hyperactive	95.8	101.7
	Not Hyperactive	99.3	108.1

Note: p < 0.002.

development. This is consistent with the idea of a general delay in brain development. Presumably, delays in more specific aspects of brain development would be reflected in lags in the development of more specific functions. That is, delays may affect one specific area and not another. For example, differential lags may be reflected in impaired executive control but visual-motor skills may be normal. Further research examining executive function tasks must be conducted to explore the role of specific delays in brain development among speech/language impaired children.

CONCLUSION

The association between speech/language impairment and psychiatric disorder is complex and the effects of speech/language impairment are manifested through the operation of many different factors. The process by which children with a history of speech/language impairment develop psychiatric disorders can best be understood through a number of causal pathways. The heterogeneity of speech/language impairments and psychiatric symptoms experienced by these children cannot be adequately explained by any one process.

Our first hypothesis considered the effects of early childhood speech/language impairment on social and peer relations and the subsequent development of psychiatric disorders. Most studies concurred that speech/language impairment is one variable of many associated with psychiatric disorders. In the Ottawa Longitudinal Study, speech/language impairment was one of the most important variables in predicting psychiatric outcome at seven year follow-up. Children with early speech/language impairment scored higher on ratings of psychopathology and lower on ratings of global functioning at age 12.5. Speech/language impaired children also had poorer scores on social competence and adaptive functioning, lending support to the possibility that poor social skills mediate the association between speech/language impairment and psychiatric disorders, at least for some children.

The examination of speech/language clusters allowed us to identify particular speech/language deficits that may be involved in the development of psychiatric disorders through their effects on social relations. In comparison to other speech/language impaired children and normal controls, children with auditory comprehension deficits had high rates of hyperactivity. Boys with auditory comprehension deficits also showed elevated levels of aggression compared to boys in the other groups. Some of the psychiatric consequences of auditory comprehension deficits may be mediated by poor social skills. Other mediating factors, in addition to poor social skills, may also affect the nature of this association.

Our second hypothesis considered the mediating effects of school failure, specifically learning disabilities, on the association between speech/language deficits and psychiatric disorder. Some support for this hypothesis was found in the work of Lynam et al. (1993) who found that the association between speech/language deficits and antisocial behavior at follow-up was mediated by school failure among black boys. However, school failure was not a mediating factor for white boys in this study. The issue of race requires further exploration for our understanding of the mechanisms involved in the development of psychiatric disorder among speech/language impaired young people. Evidence against the pathway through reading disabilities was found in a study by Williams & McGee (1994), in which poor reading was not associated with delinquent behavior in adolescence when prior history of externalizing behaviors was controlled. Data from the Ottawa Longitudinal Study showed that learning disabilities and psychiatric disorders measured at follow-up co-occurred among children with a history of speech/language impairment who did *not* have psychiatric symptoms at age 5. These findings suggest that school failure and learning disabilities play a role in the development of psychiatric disorders among some children. However, further research is required to better understand this association and the specific subgroups of children affected in order to design effective interventions for children most at risk for psychiatric disorder through this pathway.

Our third hypothesis examined the effect of related factors on the association between early childhood speech/language deficits and the development of psychiatric disorders. In the Ottawa longitudinal study, a multiple regression analysis revealed that the mother's adversity and SES were strong predictors of scores on a comprehensive measure of global psychopathology among speech/language impaired children seven years later. Maternal reports of the child's health history was another strong predictor. However, children's behavioral and language measures also accounted for considerable variance in this measure of psychopathology. In other words, this study revealed that health and environmental factors may partially contribute to this association. However, they cannot account for the entirety of this phenomenon. Impaired language function at age 5 independently predicts psychiatric disorder at age 12.

It is most likely that high rates of psychiatric disorders among speech/language impaired children are due, in part, to the concomitant variables with which speech/language impairment is associated. In this way the combination of speech/language impairment and associated variables leads to a cumulative risk model of psychiatric disorder. It is not known whether interactions between speech/language variables and other concomitant risk variables increase the risk for psychiatric disorders among some groups but not others.

Preliminary data suggests that this does indeed occur. For instance, the combination of delayed visual motor development and single-parent households was associated with substantially increased risk of psychiatric disorders among children in the Ottawa Longitudinal Study. It will be important to explore specific types of interactions between speech/language impairment and other environmental risk factors to identify the paths through which psychiatric disorder develops and the specific groups at increased risk.

Our fourth hypothesis considered the role of neurodevelopmental immaturity as an antecedent variable responsible for the co-occurrence of psychiatric disorders and speech/language impairment. For some children, the connection between speech/language impairment and psychiatric disorder may depend more on antecedent conditions than on speech/language deficits themselves. Speech/language impairment may be a proxy for underlying neurodevelopmental deficits. Research among autistic children lends support to this hypothesis. In this chapter, this notion was most clearly supported in the association found between speech/language impairment and hyperactivity in the Ottawa Longitudinal Study. Evidence in support of this hypothesis emerged in the form of significantly higher ratings of both immature behaviors and delayed visual motor development among a subgroup of boys previously identified as speech/language impaired and hyperactive. It is unclear from this data how possible neurodevelopmental deficits impact on girls. Investigators have yet to give this area the research attention it deserves.

Other considerations have not been explored in this brief overview of some pathways to psychiatric disorder. Cognitive impairments based on speech/language deficits may act to limit children's abilities to use language to modulate emotions, express feelings and ideas, delay action and control their own and other people's behavior. Verbal mediation is a key factor in self-regulation (Hogan & Quay, 1984). Verbal deficits may prohibit children from developing internal verbally based means of inhibiting antisocial impulses (Yeudall, 1980; Tarter et al., 1984). Under these circumstances, speech/language impaired children will be prone to behavioral outbursts, on the one hand and withdrawal on the other. According to this hypothesis, behavioral problems arise due to cognitive deficits that increase the child's vulnerability to psychiatric disorder. Improvements in verbal competence may improve the child's ability to utilize verbal mediation strategies to delay action, to self-regulate and to modulate his or her own emotions. These are important concepts that require careful scrutiny and further investigation.

REFERENCES

Baker, L. & Cantwell, D.P. (1987). A prospective psychiatric follow-up of children with speech/language disorders. *Journal of the American Academy of Child and Adolescent Psychiatry*, **26**, 546–553.

Beitchman, J.H. (1985a). Speech and language impairment and psychiatric risk: Toward a model of neurodevelopmental immaturity. *Psychiatric Clinics of North America*, **8**, 721–735.

Beitchman, J.H. (1985b). Therapeutic considerations with the language impaired preschool child. *Canadian Journal of Psychiatry*, **30**, 609–613.

Beitchman, J.H., Nair, R., Clegg, M., Ferguson, B., & Patel, P.G. (1986a). Prevalence of speech and language disorders in 5-year-old kindergarten children in the Ottawa-Carleton region. *Journal of Speech and Hearing Disorders*, **51**, 98–110.

Beitchman, J.H., Nair, R., Clegg, M., Ferguson, B., & Patel, P.G. (1986b). Prevalence of psychiatric disorders in children with speech and language disorders. *Journal of the American Academy of Child Psychiatry*, **25**(4), 528–535.

Beitchman, J.H., Hood, J., & Inglis, A. (1990). Psychiatric risk in children with speech and language disorders. *Journal of Abnormal Child Psychology*, **18**(3), 283–296.

Beitchman, J.H., Hood, J., Rochon, J., Peterson, M., Mantini, T., & Majumdar, S. (1989a). Empirical classification of speech/language impairment in children: I. Identification of speech/language categories. *Journal of the American Academy of Child and Adolescent Psychiatry*, **28**, 112–117.

Beitchman, J.H., Hood, J., Rochon, J., & Peterson, M. (1989b). Empirical classification of speech/language impairment in children: II. Behavioral Characteristics. *Journal of the American Academy of Child and Adolescent Psychiatry*, **28**, 118–123.

Beitchman, J.H., Wilson, B., Brownlie, E.B., Walters, H., Inglis, A., & Lancee, W. (in press a). Long-term consistency in speech/language profiles: behavioral, emotional and social outcomes. *Journal of the American Academy of Child and Adolescent Psychiatry*.

Beitchman, J.H., Wilson, B., Brownlie, E.B., Walters, H., & Lancee, W. (in press b). Long-term consistency in speech/language profiles: developmental and academic outcomes. *Journal of the American Academy of Child and Adolescent Psychiatry*.

Benasich, A.A., Curtiss, S., & Tallal, P. (1993). Language, learning and behavioral disturbances in childhood: a longitudinal perspective. *Journal of the American Academy of Child and Adolescent Psychiatry*, **32**, 585–593.

Bishop, D.V.M. & Adams, C. (1990). A prospective study of the relationship between specific language impairment, phonological disorders, and reading retardation. *Journal of Child Psychology and Psychiatry*, **31**, 1027–1050.

Bishop, D.V.M. & Edmundson, A. (1987a). Specific language impairment as a maturational lag: Evidence from longitudinal data on language and motor development. *Developmental Medicine and Child Neurology*, **29**, 442–459.

Bishop, D.V.M. & Edmundson, A. (1987b). Language-impaired 4-year-olds: Distinguishing transient from persistent impairment. *Journal of Speech and Hearing Research*, **52**, 156–173.

Bishop, D.V.M. & Rosenbloom, L. (1987). Childhood language disorders: Classification and overview. In W. Yule & M. Rutter (eds) *Language Development and Disorders.* Oxford: MacKeith Press (pp. 16–41).

Boudreault, M., Thivierge, J., Cote, R., Boutin, Y., Julien, Y., & Bergeron, S. (1988). Cognitive development and reading achievement in pervasive-ADD, situational-ADD and control children. *Journal of Child Psychology and Psychiatry, 29,* 611–619.

Buikhuisen, W. (1987). Cerebral dysfunctions and persistent juvenile delinquency. In S.A. Mednick and T.E. Moffitt (eds) *The Causes of Crime: New Biological Approaches.* New York: Cambridge University Press (pp. 168–184).

Cantwell, D.P. & Baker, L. (1991). Association between attention deficit-hyperactivity disorder and learning disorders. *Journal of Learning Disabilities,* 24(2), 88–95.

Cantwell, D.P. & Baker, L. (1985). Psychiatric and learning disorders in children with communication disorders. Part II: Methodological approach and findings. In K.D. Gadow (ed.) *Advances in Learning and Behavioral Disabilities* Vol. 4. Greenwich, CT: JAI (pp. 29–47).

Cantwell, D.P. & Baker, L. (1977). Psychiatric disorder in children with speech and language retardation: a critical review. *Archives of General Psychiatry,* 34, 583–591.

Cantwell, D.P., Baker, L., & Rutter, M. (1978). A comparative study of infantile autism and specific developmental receptive language disorder. IV. Analysis of syntax and language function. *Journal of Child Psychology and Psychiatry,* 19, 351–362.

Chandler, M.J. (1973). Egocentrism and antisocial behaviour: The assessment and training of social perspective-taking skills. *Developmental Psychology,* 9, 326–332.

Chandler, M.J., Greenspan, S., & Barenboim, C. (1974). Assessment and training of role-taking and referential communication skills in institutionalized emotionally disturbed children. *Developmental Psychology,* 10, 546–553.

Chess, S. & Rosenburg, M. (1974). Clinical differentiation among children with initial language complaints. *Journal of Autism and Childhood Schizophrenia,* 4, 99–109.

Cook, J.R., Mausbach, T., Burd, L., Generoso, G., Slotnick, H., et al. (1993). A preliminary study of the relationship between central auditory processing disorder and attention deficit disorder. *Journal of Psychiatry and Neuroscience,* 18, 130–137.

Dodge, K.A. (1991). The structure and function of reactive and pro-active aggression. In D.J. Pepler & K.H. Rubin (eds) *The Development and Treatment of Childhood Aggression.* Hillsdale, NJ: Lawrence Erlbaum (pp. 201–218).

Grinnell, S.W., Scott-Hartnet, D., & Glasier, J.L. (1983). Language disorders (Letter to the Editor). *Journal of the American Academy of Child and Adolescent Psychiatry,* 22, 580–581.

Gualtieri, C.T., Koriath, W., Van Bourgondien, M., & Saleeby, N. (1983). Language disorders in children referred for psychiatric services. *Journal of the American Academy of Child and Adolescent Psychiatry,* 22, 165–171.

Hirschi, T. & Hindelang, M.J. (1977). Intelligence and delinquency: a revisionist review. *American Sociological Review,* 42, 571–587.

Hogan, A.E. & Quay, H.C. (1984). Cognition in child and adolescent behavior disorders. In B.B. Lahey & A.E. Kazdin (eds) *Advances in Clinical Child Psychology,* Vol. 7. New York: Plenum Press (pp. 1–34).

Johnston, R.B., Stark, R.E., Mellits, E.D., & Tallal, P. (1981). Neurological status of language-impaired and normal children. *Annals of Neurology,* 10, 159–163.

Kotsopoulis, A. & Boodoosingh, L. (1987). Language and speech disorders in children attending a day psychiatric programme. *British Journal of Disorders of Communication*, **22**, 227–236.

Locke, J.L. (1994). Gradual emergence of developmental language disorders. *Journal of Speech and Hearing Research*, **37**, 608–616.

Lynam, D., Moffitt, T., & Stouthamer-Loeber, M. (1993). Explaining the relation between IQ and delinquency: class, race, test motivation, school failure, or self-control? *Journal of Abnormal Psychology*, **102**, 187–196.

Maughan, B., Gray, G., & Rutter, M. (1985). Reading retardation and antisocial behaviour: a follow-up into employment. *Journal of Child Psychology and Psychiatry*, **49**, 226–238.

Patterson, G.R., DeBaryshe, B.D., & Ramsey, E. (1989). A developmental perspective on antisocial behavior. *American Psychologist*, **44**, 329–335.

Powell, R.P. & Bishop, D.V.M. (1992). Clumsiness and perceptual problems in children with specific language impairment. *Developmental Medicine and Child Neurology*, **34**, 755–765.

Rice, M. (1993). Don't talk to him; he's weird: a social consequences account of language and social interactions. In A.P. Kaiser & D.B. Gray (eds) *Enhancing Children's Communication: Research Foundations for Intervention*. Baltimore, MD: Brookes (pp. 139–158).

Rubin, K.H., Bream, L.A., & Rose-Krasnor, L. (1991). Social problem solving and aggression in childhood. In D.J. Pepler & K.H. Rubin (eds) *The Development and Treatment of Childhood Aggression*. Hillsdale, NJ: Lawrence Erlbaum (pp. 219–248).

Rutter, M. (1989). Isle of Wight revisited: Twenty-five years of child psychiatric epidemiology. *Journal of the American Academy of Child and Adolescent Psychiatry*, **28**, 633–653.

Silva, P.A., McGee, R.O., & Williams, S.M. (1983). Developmental language delay from three to seven years and its significance for low intelligence and reading difficulties at age seven. *Developmental Medicine and Child Neurology*, **25**, 783–793.

Silva, P.A., Williams, S.M., & McGee, R.O. (1987). A longitudinal study of children with developmental language delay at age three: later intelligence, reading and behaviour problems. *Developmental Medicine and Child Neurology*, **29**, 630–640.

Stevenson, J. & Richman, N. (1976). The prevalence of language delay in a population of three year old children and its association with general retardation. *Developmental Medicine and Child Neurology*, **18**, 431–441.

Tallal, P. (1988). Developmental language disorders. In J.F. Kavanagh & T.J. Truss, Jr. (eds) *Learning Disabilities: Proceedings of the National Conference*. Parkton, M.D.: York Press (pp. 181–272).

Tallal, P., Dukette, D., & Curtiss, S. (1989). Behavioral/emotional profiles of preschool language impaired children. *Developmental Psychopathology*, **1**, 51–67.

Tarter, R.E., Hegedus, A.M., Winsten, N.E., & Alterman, A.I. (1984). Neuropsychological, personality, and familial characteristics of physically abused delinquents. *Journal of the American Academy of Child Psychiatry*, **23**, 668–674.

Wadsworth, M. (1979). *Roots of Delinquency*. Oxford: Martin Robertson.

Williams, S. & McGee, R. (1994). Reading attainment and juvenile delinquency. *Journal of Child Psychology and Psychiatry*, **35**(3), 441–459.

Yeudall, L.T. (1980). A neuropsychological perspective of persistent juvenile delinquency and criminal behavior. *Annals of the New York Academy of Science*, **347**, 349–355.

23 Academic performance in children with speech and language impairment: a review of follow-up research

DEBBIE CAROL SCHACHTER

INTRODUCTION

Academic or school related problems can occur in the individual subjects of reading, spelling or mathematics or in several subjects. Academic under-achievement may occur as a result of low intelligence, inadequate schooling, poor motivation, emotional problems, or the presence of specific learning disabilities. Specific learning disabilities are defined as underachievement in acquiring reading, spelling, or arithmetic skills with the delays not explained by lower intellectual potential, sensory impairments, or environmental deprivation (Fletcher & Morris, 1986). The precise causal mechanisms for the development of specific learning disabilities is unclear. Reading and spelling disabilities are often conceptualized as having either a language based deficit or a deficit in visual-perceptual domains (Maughan & Yule, 1993). The core deficit among many reading disabled children is believed to be a problem with phonological processing (Wagner, 1986; Shaywitz, Fletcher, & Shaywitz, 1996). In contrast, mathematical disabilities have been less well studied. Rourke & Finlayson (1978) believe children with deficits in mathematics alone have primarily visual spatial skills deficits in contrast to those with reading and spelling difficulties whom they believe have an underlying language disorder.

If reading disabilities are primarily language based (Mann & Brady, 1988) one would expect children with language problems to be at increased risk of developing language based reading disabilities, and spelling and writing difficulties. In fact, children with speech and language impairments develop more problems in academic subjects than controls and are at an increased risk for developing learning problems (Cantwell & Baker, 1985). This observation, however, has several explanations. First, the presence of speech and language problems may make academic problems more likely to occur because much of what is learned in school is transmitted verbally. Second, if there is a problem with verbal communication particularly in its comprehension, it may make the acquisition of new material more difficult. Thus, speech and language problems would be risk factors for the development of a wide variety of academic problems, the risk being mediated through the faulty communication of these children. Alternatively, whatever causes children to be impaired in their oral language development may make them more likely to have reading difficulties. In fact, phonological processing is believed to play a causal role in the acquisition of reading skills. Deficits in phonological processing are commonly observed among reading disabled subjects (Wagner, 1986; Wagner & Torgesen, 1987).

If speech or language impairment were specific risk factors for academic underachievement then one would expect the following statements to be true. First, academic problems should be more common among speech/language impaired children than controls. Second, the speech or language problems should be present prior to the development of the academic problems. Third, children with more severe speech or language impairments should have more severe academic problems than those with less severe language problems. Fourth, the association between speech and language impairments and academic problems would not be explained by other confounding variables. Finally, the effect of speech and language impairments on academic problems would be specific. That is speech and language impairments would lead to a specific academic problem. For example, one would expect difficulties primarily in one subject exclusively although any subject that depended on speech/language skills would be affected.

While cross-sectional studies support the association between speech and language disorders and academic problems, they do not help us understand causality and do not address whether the presence of speech and language disorders poses an increased risk on the development of academic problems. The best method to examine the strength of the association between speech and language impairments and academic underachievement is through longitudinal studies. Longitudinal studies of children with speech and language delays provide a unique opportunity to examine the empirical evidence for the association between language delays and learning problems by obtaining children with language problems and children without language problems and observing their academic development. Thus, one can examine whether there is an increased risk of academic difficulties among children with speech and language impairment. In addition, the characteristics of children that may predispose them to developing academic problems can also be examined. This Chapter reviews the available longitudinal studies of children with speech and language disorders.

Prior to reviewing the literature, however, it is important to clarify the terms to be used in this review. Language refers to oral communication and encompasses both expressed language (speech and the production and articulation of words) and receptive language (the understanding of language). Children can exhibit difficulties with either expressive language, receptive language or both. This may be a reflection of a delay in language development or a specific language impairment. By definition, to have a specific language disorder, however, there should be a discrepancy between the child's measured language competence and the child's nonverbal intellectual potential with the child's language ability significantly lower than the child's nonverbal intellectual potential. However, the magnitude of the discrepancy varies between investigators. Depending on the cut off chosen, different children will be identified as speech and/or language delayed.

In this chapter, academic outcome will be used to refer to a variety of terms including school class placement, highest level of education completed, scores on standardized measure of achievement and presence of learning disabilities. Adding further complexity to the varied measures of outcome is the diversity with which the individual outcome measures are ascertained. For example, schools may have different educational programs, different criteria for special classes. Tests used to measure achievement can also vary between settings and studies. Some tests measure reading decoding, whereas others assess reading comprehension. Similarly, some tests measure mathematics comprehension and/or computation whereas others assess both.

Perhaps the most problematic outcome measure is that of specific learning disabilities. Specific learning disabilities refer to a heterogeneous group of difficulties or impairments in reading, spelling or mathematics that are not explained by intellectual level, sensory impairments or social deprivation (Fletcher & Morris, 1986).

Operationally, there are two major approaches to defining learning disabilities. The first defines a learning disability as achievement below that expected for chronological age and may or may not use an IQ cutoff. The second defines a learning disability to be achievement in an academic subject significantly below intellectual potential. However, the discrepancy varies from one to two standard deviations depending on the investigator. Adding further complexity to this issue Shaywitz et al. (1996) have recently postulated that reading disabilities may not be a disorder *per se*, but rather represent the lower end of a continuum of reading ability.

Therefore, when the literature in this field is being reviewed it is critical to examine the definitions used to describe the initial language difficulty of the children and the measure of academic achievement. For example, if children whose language delay is the result of a general intellectual delay or deficiency are included in the sample it is likely that these children will continue to be delayed in reading, spelling or mathematics when they are older, reflecting the effects of the intellectual deficit rather than the language delay. If these children were excluded from the sample, the outcome would reflect that of children with language delay alone. The outcome might be expected to be better than if children with lower overall intellectual potential were included in the sample.

It is also important to consider how the sample being studied was selected as this affects the representativeness of the sample and the ability to draw generalizations from the study. Most of the studies' samples were ascertained through specialized settings where children with speech and language impairment are being evaluated or through community samples.

The initial longitudinal studies examined the academic outcome of children who were sampled from speech/language clinics. Many of these studies had significant methodological weakness including a low response rate and an absence of control groups.

CLINIC BASED STUDIES

One of the earliest (King, Jones, & Lasky, 1982), was a retrospective 15-year follow-up study of 50 children seen at a university speech and hearing clinic. The children were initially seen between ages 3 to 6. Only 60 of the original sample of 150 children were contacted and of these, only 50 participated in the study. Thus, there may be respondent bias and the generalizability of the results is clearly questionable. Furthermore, follow-up was conducted through telephone interviews, with no direct assessment of children's abilities. Nevertheless, according to parent reports, 52% of subjects had difficulty in reading, mathematics or English, and 28% of the sample had received tutoring. Thus, children had a variety of academic difficulties. In summary, while this study showed many subjects experienced academic difficulties, there were significant methodological weaknesses including the low response rate, the lack of direct assessment of the children, and the absence of a control group. More important, however, was the absence of clear description of the speech/language children in terms of other characteristics which may have also predisposed them to poor school performance. For example, it is unclear whether or not these children were of average intelligence. If children of below average intellectual ability were included in the sample, it might explain the below average academic achievement.

Another early study was a 13 to 20 year retrospective follow-up study of 18 language impaired and 18 articulation impaired children who attended a speech and hearing clinic (Hall & Tomblin, 1978). Subjects had normal auditory acuity and an intelligence quotient of at least 80. Thus, children whose language delay was secondary to a general cognitive impairment or intellectual deficiency were excluded. Language impaired subjects had two of the following criteria: (1) a clinical diagnosis of speech or language retardation, (2) a spread of at least 20 points between performance and verbal measures of intelligence, (3) a vocabulary score at least one year below that expected for chronological age, and (4) scores on language tests 1 standard deviation or more below expected. The articulation impaired subjects had articulation scores below that expected for age, they showed no evidence of language impairment and they had a clinical diagnosis of an articulation disorder. At follow-up, the average age of language impaired subjects was 22.3 years and that of the articulation impaired subjects was 23 years. The investigators studied only 36 out of a possible sample of 281 children, thereby leading to questions regarding the generalizability of the findings. Follow-up information was gathered from parents and in addition, from school records containing standardized test results. At the time of follow-up, the subjects had finished or were finishing their secondary school education.

The investigators noted that the outcome among the language impaired children was worse than among the articulation impaired children. Fewer language impaired children compared to articulation impaired children progressed beyond high school. This study also had significant methodological weaknesses including the low response rate, the lack of direct assessment of the children, and the absence of a control group. However, this study was important because it was among the first to compare the outcome among children with different types of speech and language impairments and for its use of explicit criteria to define speech or language disorders.

This study suggested that language impairment is a more important risk factor for poor school achievement than articulation impairment. This observation is plausible in that disorders in the production or understanding of language might be expected to be more central to language than simple pronunciation difficulties. Furthermore, if poor school performance was language based one would expect children with language based disorders to have more learning problems than those with articulation problems. However, in this study it was unclear whether the language impaired children were more disadvantaged intellectually or socially than the articulation impaired children. If the children in the two groups were not matched for these factors or this was not controlled for statistically in the analyses of the data, then it is unclear if differences observed between language impaired and articulation impaired children reflect the effects of the speech and language status or were attributed to these other factors. Class differences might contribute to or interact with the lower rate of completion of high school rather than the language impairment *per se*.

Aram & Nation (1980) conducted a five-year retrospective follow-up of children originally seen as preschoolers at the Cleveland Hearing and Speech Center. Of 515 eligible children, 115 were contacted and 63 children participated in the study, again raising questions regarding the generalizability of findings and possible respondent bias. At follow-up, the average age of the subjects was 7.11 years, and information was obtained from parent and teacher questionnaires. At follow-up, only 59% of subjects were studying in regular classes. According to teachers, approximately 30% of subjects had difficulties in mathematics, spelling, or reading. Approximately 40% of subjects were below grade level in mathematics and reading while 24% were underchieving in spelling. Preschool measures of language comprehension, formulation, phonology, syntax, semantics and speech production correlated with outcome. There was, however, no association between duration of preschool speech therapy and academic abilities. Other difficulties with this study included the heterogeneity of the initial sample, the lack of description of the characteristics of the children, particularly their social class, intelligence, and their psychosocial characteristics, all of which could contribute to outcome. Again this study had significant weaknesses including the low response rate and the lack of a control group. However, its significance lies in its demonstration that various aspects of language were associated with outcome.

Aram, Ekelman, & Nation (1984) conducted a 10-year prospective study of language impaired preschoolers originally seen at a hearing and speech clinic. Twenty of 47 preschoolers who were diagnosed as language disordered by a speech/language pathologist were studied at follow-up. Subjects were excluded if they had neurological or craniofacial abnormalities. Subjects were initially administered several language tasks and tests of language function in addition to non-language measures such as a measure of intelligence, socioeconomic measure, race and sex and a measure of selective attention. At follow-up, subjects had an average age of 14 years 10 months, and were administered widely used measures of academic abilities, intelligence and speech and language development. Over half the sample scored below the 25th percentile on standardized academic tests. Even when children with mental retardation were excluded from the sample, 50%, 56%, and 75% of adolescents scored below the 25th percentile in reading, spelling, and mathematics respectively. Initial measures of intelligence and phonological formulation independently predicted follow-up reading ability and class placement in this sample. However, after multivariate analyses only intelligence was significantly associated with follow-up reading performance (Aram et al., 1984). Thus, this study suggested that intelligence confounded the association between speech and language impairment and academic achievement. That is, underlying differences in the intellectual levels of the speech and language and control children could explain the differences in academic outcome between the two groups.

Stark et al. (1984) conducted a prospective $3\frac{1}{2}$ to 4-year follow-up study of 29 children with speech and language impairment and 14 control children between the ages of 4 and 8. This was one of the first studies to use both an explicit definition of speech or language impairment and a control group. In addition, at follow-up subjects were administered standardized tests of reading, intelligence, speech, and language. All subjects had nonverbal intelligence scores within the normal range and lacked evidence of neurologic deficits. The language impaired subjects had a language age at least one year below their chronological age, a receptive language at least six months below performance mental age and expressive language at least one year below performance mental age. Normal controls had an overall language score no more than six months below age. At follow-up all language impaired children had reading scores an average of two years below expected or chronological age, whereas controls were on average two years ahead of expectation. However, initially all the 7 to 8-year-old language impaired children were also having reading difficulties. When a reading disability was defined as performance in reading comprehension and/or vocabulary at least two grades below age level, 90% of language impaired children had a reading disability compared to none of the control children. The few language impaired children who were not defined as reading disabled were classified as having normal or mildly impaired language skills at follow-up.

Baker & Cantwell (1987) conducted a 4 to 5-year prospective study of 300 children initially seen through a community speech and language clinic. These children were diagnosed initially as having a speech or language disorder, although the specific criteria used were not detailed (Cantwell, Baker, & Mattison, 1979). These children were the first 300 of 500 who responded to a mailing, again raising the question of respondent bias. The mean age of the children at the initial assessment was 5.7 years (range 2.0 to 15.9 years) and at follow-up was 9.1 years. The group had an average intellectual level. Approximately 25% of subjects developed a learning disability during the follow-up period. The children with initial language disorders were likely to have learning disabilities. Again, this study lacked a control group and the definition of learning disability in this study is unclear.

Rissman, Curtiss, & Tallal (1990) evaluated the five-year outcome for specifically language impaired 4-year-old children. The language impaired subjects were defined as having nonverbal intelligence scores of at least 85, a language age at least one year below performance IQ and chronological age, normal hearing, no autism, and neurological disorder. Twenty-two of 67 subjects were lost to follow-up. After following subjects for five years, the investigators examined the predictive ability of IQ, socioeconomic status, sex and language measures on prediction of subsequent school placement. Three language measures, socioeconomic status and IQ correctly classified 78.6% of children in special day classes and 50% of children in regular or pull-out classroom situations. The best predictor of school placement was, however, receptive language skills at age 4. At age 8, intelligence and socioeconomic status also predicted long-term outcome, but were less successful at predicting withdrawal or regular class placement. By the fifth year of the study, 40% of children were in pull-out programs and 37% were in regular class placements.

In summary, these studies suggest many of these children develop academic difficulties as they progress through school, with language skills linked to academic placement. However, one study suggests that the association is explained by differences between the intellectual level of speech/language impaired children and controls (Aram et al., 1984) and another study suggests that differences in socioeconomic status may explain the association (Rissman et al., 1990). The studies may also suffer from selection bias in that the samples were obtained through clinics and specialized settings. The children who were referred to these centers or who attended them may not represent the larger population of speech/language impaired children.

If the children seen in these specialized settings differed from the larger population of language and speech impaired children on characteristics associated with academic outcome then the results of these studies would not apply to the larger population. For example, if these children seen in treatment settings were more likely to come from higher socioeconomic classes the outcome might be more favorable than it would otherwise be. Alternatively, children referred to specialized settings may have more severe language impairments or other coexisting problems such as behavior problems, both of which might be expected to adversely affect academic performance. For these reasons it is preferable to examine the association in community ascertained samples which are potentially free of possible selection bias. Typically, however, community studies are more expensive and frequently rely on group testing rather than individually administered tests. In addition, they tend to use statistical rather than clinical definitions of disability.

COMMUNITY STUDIES

The few available community studies also support the association between speech and language impairment and an adverse academic outcome. Menyuk et al. (1991) prospectively studied 130 children with an average age of 5, prior to beginning kindergarten. These children were classified into three groups; those with a specific language impairment, those who had a history of a language delay and had outgrown it, and those who where born prematurely. The language impaired children had receptive language skills six months below expected on the basis of their chronological age and an expressive language age one year below chronological age. Those with a history of language delay were only six months behind on language tests or in the past had some language therapy, and it was recommended they be re-evaluated. All subjects had normal performance intelligence. Children were evaluated after three years. At follow-up language impaired children had more reading problems (50%), than premature children (31%), or children with a history of a language delay (33%). They concluded that childrens' early abilities to retrieve letter names and make phonic word segments were related to later reading ability.

Sheridan & Peckham (1975, 1978) studied children in the British National Child Development Study, a longitudinal study of a representative cohort of children born in one week in March 1958 in England, Wales, and Scotland. The study examined the academic outcome for 215 children identified at age 7 as having marked speech difficulties despite normal hearing. Children were identified by both physicians and teachers as suffering from speech difficulties. However, these children did not undergo a more detailed speech or language assessment by a qualified speech/language pathologist and thus the validity of these diagnoses is in question. It is, however, likely that children at age 7 who experienced marked speech problems also had language problems as well. At age 7, 15% of the cohort of 215 were receiving some special education. At age 11, data on 190 children (88% of original sample) indicated that 35% were receiving some special education. At age 11, 180 or 84% of the original sample were contacted, 30% of these subjects were in special schools. At follow-up children were administered tests of reading and mathematics. Reading and mathematics scores of the speech impaired cohort were lower than controls independent of whether or not the speech impairment had improved at follow-up. Thus this study demonstrates that, within a representative population, children with early history of speech difficulties have an increased likelihood of having a poorer academic outcome than children free of speech difficulties. However, the study results would have had greater validity if the method of identifying speech difficulties had been validated and if the intellectual level had been controlled for or examined. The finding of lower reading and mathematics scores independent of speech at follow-up suggests that it is not the presence of speech problem at follow-up that results in school problems but the early speech problems. It is likely that the early speech difficulty is a marker for children of lower intelligence, or those with language delays, particularly receptive delays.

One of the best studies reported to date is probably the prospective community study of a birth cohort of New Zealand children (Silva, 1980; Silva, Williams, & McGee, 1987; Silva, McGee, & Williams, 1983). These children were administered developmental language tests at ages 3 and 5, intellectual tests at age 7, and reading tests at ages 7 and 11. Language delay was defined as a score below the fifth percentile of the cohort. Scores were defined as one, two and three years below the mean for 7-year-olds, 9-year-olds and 11-year-olds respectively. The reading scores for children with comprehension delay, expressive delay, or general language delay increased more slowly than those of the nonlanguage impaired between the ages of 7 to 11 and were similar to scores of children two or more years below their chronological age. These results, therefore support the previous data, that early language delays lead to reading problems. However, these children also had other differences than the remainder of the sample. Significantly more children with general comprehension delay came from a disadvantaged social class and all language groups had lower intellectual potential than the rest of the cohort. Both of these factors may explain or confound the association observed. In this study language delay was defined as a score below the fifth percentile. It is unclear whether children with milder delays would also experience the same outcome. The population studied, however, was slightly advantaged socially and a more adverse outcome may have been obtained with a more disadvantaged and possibly representative population. Thus despite methodological weakness, the conclusions of the studies reviewed above are similar, language delays appear to lead to academic delays. Causality, however, is not clearly demonstrated.

A major problem with this study and the earlier studies is that few if any, have controlled for variables which may potentially confound the association between speech and language impairment and academic outcome. For example, children with speech/language impairment have other characteristics which distinguish them from nonspeech/language impaired children. They often have lower levels of intelligence, lower socioeconomic status, more behavior, psychiatric and familial problems than non speech/language impaired children (Beitchman et al., 1986; Beitchman, Peterson, & Clegg, 1988). Preschoolers with language delay also have lower intelligence and more behavior problems reported through to age 11 than nonlanguage impaired children (Silva, Williams, & McGee, 1987). Several of these factors, particularly intelligence, lower socioeconomic status and attentional factors predict later academic achievement (Aram et al., 1984; Tramontana, Hooper, & Selzer, 1988). McGee and Share (1988) reviewed some of the evidence related to whether attention deficit disorder leads to learning difficulties and concluded that the question cannot be as yet adequately answered. They noted their own work failed to find an association between mothers' reports of difficulty managing a 3-year-old and the later development of a reading disability at ages 7, 9 and 11.

Because many of the correlates of speech/language impairment are also correlates of poor academic achievement and/or learning disabilities, it is important to examine whether these variables confound the association between speech/language disorders and academic problems. To address these questions, prospective controlled studies are required. Furthermore, the studies need to be designed using matched groups with controls matched to cases for potential confounding variables or through the use of appropriate statistical analyses to control for these potential confounding variables.

Recently a prospective longitudinal community study involving 142 control children and 142 speech/language impaired children has been completed (Beitchman et al., 1993). The children were initially identified through a community survey. The speech/language cohort was defined as 5-year-old children whose scores were at least one standard deviation below expected on standard language tests or those having speech difficulties. Control children scored normally on these measures. Although the children were administered tests of intelligence, the measure of intelligence was not used to classify the children. In addition to these measures, a wide variety of other behavioral, demographic, and cognitive characteristics of the children were determined. Perceptual motor skills were determined using the Berry Test of Visual Motor Integration. Initially, the speech/language impaired children were more likely to have more behavior problems than controls, and to be more likely to come from lower socioeconomic classes (Beitchman, Peterson, & Clegg, 1988).

At follow-up seven years later, 244 of the 284 cases participated. Subjects were individually administered standard measures of achievement in reading, spelling, and mathematics, and were also administered intellectual and language tests. Learning disabilities were more common among speech/language impaired children than among control although the rates varied depending on the definition of learning disability adopted (Beitchman et al., 1993). For example, when learning disability was defined as achievement one year below current grade level, 40% of speech/language impaired children had a learning disability on a measure of overall achievement compared to 10% of controls, for a relative risk of 4.0 (Beitchman et al., 1993). For reading 42% of speech/language impaired children had a disability compared to 8% of controls, for spelling 41% versus 18% and for mathematics, 46% versus 9% when achievement was defined as one year below current grade level (Beitchman et al., 1993).

Through the use of multivariate statistics the investigators noted that children with speech and/or language impairments, those of lower intelligence, children whose mothers had lower levels of education, or whose parents initially had lower socioeconomic status based on occupation had lower achievement scores at follow-up. Intelligence was the strongest predictor of achievement on the battery composite, followed by mother's education, the child's initial language status as impaired or not, and then socioeconomic status. Other behavioral and cognitive measures were not associated with outcome in multivariate analyses suggesting a less important role than language, intelligence, socioeconomic status, and mother's education when all these factors are examined jointly.

To address the question of whether there is a gradient in effect, that is whether children with more severe language impairments have more academic difficulties than those without, a second regression was analyzed. Initial scores on the Bankson Language Screening Test, a screening test of expressive language, independently predicted almost half the variation in achievement scores on the battery composite. Furthermore, scores on the Bankson Language Screening Test added to the prediction of achievement compared to prediction based on whether a child was language impaired or control alone.

In these models behavioral measures did not predict overall achievement whereas intelligence and mother's education were associated with achievement scores. Hinshaw (1992) reviewed the association between the behavioral measures of inattention as well as externalizing behavior and academic achievement. Hinshaw (1992) noted that causality was not established and suggested the association might be mediated through verbal deficits. Tramontana et al. (1988) also noted that behavioral measures were less important than cognitive measures in predicting academic achievement. Thus, this finding seems to be in agreement with other studies.

CONCLUSION

To conclude, there appears to be a consensus in the literature with all studies of speech and language impaired children showing higher rates of academic underachievement than controls. The underachievement has been measured through high school completion, records, parent and teacher reports, and standardized tests. In addition, presence of learning disabilities and placement in special education classes have also been used to assess academic outcome.

Furthermore, the underachievement appears to be in all academic subjects. Nevertheless, many methodological problems limit the conclusions that can be drawn from these studies, particularly the fact that most did not control for potentially confounding variables such as social class or intelligence. In those studies in which there was an attempt to statistically control for the effect of these variables, two of the studies continued to observe an independent effect of speech/language status on achievement, while one did not. These findings support the literature on the preschool predictors of academic achievement. Tramontana et al. (1988) in a review of this field noted that IQ was among the best predictors of achievement as were language measures. Lower social class was associated with a lower achievement in several studies (Tramontana et al., 1988).

All the studies reviewed have observed an increased rate of poor academic achievement among children with speech and/or language impairments compared to controls.

In summary, the literature supports the association between speech and language impairment and academic underachievement. Most longitudinal studies show more academic problems among speech and language impaired children than controls thereby satisfying the first requirements for an association. Second, the results of longitudinal studies of language impaired or language delayed children suggest that many develop delays in school work and poorer academic skills than nonlanguage delayed children. Thus, the presence of the language delay or impairment antedates the academic difficulty leading to further support for a causal mechanism. However, some of the delay in academic skills noted among samples of language impaired children is probably explained by other characteristics of language impaired children such as their tendency to have lower levels of intelligence or to come from more socially disadvantaged backgrounds. In addition to these mediating variables, there is probably some specific contribution of speech and language impairment on the acquisition of academic skills. Preliminary analyses of these data suggest a gradient in effect, with children who have more severe speech and/or language problems developing more severe learning problems.

Finally, while it is a fairly consistent finding that speech and language problems lead to academic underachievement, there is not sufficient data to support the specificity of this effect. Examinations of the predictors of achievement in the individual spheres of reading, spelling, and mathematics should provide further data on this. One difficulty, however, in achieving this end would arise as the speech/language impaired cohort is a heterogeneous group. Therefore, to better understand the association it is probably necessary to examine subgroups of speech/language impaired children and to see within which groups the risk or assocation with academic difficulties is most striking. Beitchman et al. (1989) classified children in their cohort into four groups on the basis of their scores on language tests. These groups were described as high overall, low overall, poor auditory comprehension, and poor articulation. One might hypothesize that children in the low overall cluster or group would have lower performance in all subject areas than those in other groups, whereas children with poor auditory comprehension would have difficulty primarily with reading and spelling skills. Furthermore, when assessing mathematics skills in older children, language skills might be expected to influence mathematics achievement as mathematics more often involves complex word problems.

In addition, further support for this association would be achieved by demonstrating that speech and language impaired children develop a specific language based learning disability. Nevertheless, to summarize, the literature reviewed does support the association between speech and language impairment and academic problems with some of the effect mediated through other characteristics of children with speech or language delays. The other characteristics that have been identified as important in predicting academic outcome within the speech and language impaired cohort include intelligence of the child, the socioeconomic status, the mother's education, and the severity of the child's language disorder.

REFERENCES

Aram, D.M., Ekelman, B.L., & Nation, J.E. (1984). Preschoolers with language disorders: 10 years later. *Journal of Speech and Hearing Research*, **27**, 232–244.
Aram, D.M. & Nation, J.E. (1980). Preschool language disorders and subsequent language and academic difficulties. *Journal of Communication Disorders*, **13**, 159–170.
Baker, L. & Cantwell, D.P. (1987). A prospective psychiatric follow-up of children with speech/language disorders. *Journal of the American Academy of Child and Adolescent Psychiatry*, **26**(4), 546–553.
Beitchman, J.H., Ferguson, B., Schachter, D., Brownlie, E.B., Inglis, A., Wild, J., Lancee, W., Kroll, R., Mathews, R., Brunshaw, J., Walters, H., & Martin, S. (1993). A seven year follow-up study of speech/language impaired and control children. Final Report. Health and Welfare Canada. Grant No. 6606-3812-42.
Beitchman, J.H., Peterson, M., & Clegg, M. (1988). Speech and language impairment and psychiatric disorder: the relevance of family demographic variables. *Child Psychiatry and Human Development*, **18**(4), 191–207.
Beitchman, J.H., Hood, J., Rochon, J., Peterson, M., Mantini, T., & Majumdar, S. (1989). Empirical classification of speech/language impairment in children. Identification of Speech/Language Categories. *Journal of the American Academy of Child and Adolescent Psychiatry*, **28**, 112–117.
Beitchman, J.H., Nair, R., Clegg, M., & Patel, P.G. (1986). Prevalence of speech and language disorders in 5-year-old kindergarten children in the Ottawa-Carleton region. *Journal of Speech and Hearing Disorders*, **51**, 98–110.

Cantwell, D.P. & Baker, L. (1985). Speech and language: development and disorders. In M. Rutter & L. Herson (eds) *Child and Adolescent Psychiatry: Modern Approaches*, 2nd edn. London: Blackwell Scientific (pp. 526–544).

Cantwell, O.P., Baker, L., & Mattison, R.E. (1979). The prevalence of psychiatric disorder in children with speech & language disorder: An epidemiological study. *Journal of the American Academy of Child Psychiatry*, **18**, 450–461.

Fletcher, J.M. & Morris, R. (1986). Classification of disabled learners: beyond exclusionary definitions. In C. Ceci (ed.) *Handbook of Cognitive, Social and Neuropsychology Aspects of Learning Disabilities*. Hillsdale, NJ: Lawrence Erlbaum (pp. 55–79).

Hall, P.K. & Tomblin, J.B. (1978). A follow-up study of children with articulation and language disorders. *Journal of Speech and Hearing Disorders*, **43**, 227–241.

Hinshaw, S.P. (1992). Externalizing behavior problems and academic underachievement in childhood and adolescence: causal relationships and underlying mechanisms. *Psychological Bulletin*, **111**(1), 127–155.

King, R.R., Jones, C., & Lasky, E. (1982). In retrospect: a fifteen year follow-up. Report of speech-language-disordered children. *Language-Speech and Hearing Services in Schools*, **13**, 24–32.

Mann, V.A. & Brady, S. (1988). Reading disability: the role of language deficiencies. *Journal of Consulting and Clinical Psychology*, **56**(6), 811–816.

Maughan, B. & Yule, W. (1993). Reading and other learning disabilities. In M. Rutter, E. Taylor, & L. Hersove (eds) *Child and Adolescent Psychiatry: Modern approaches*, 3rd edn. London: Blackwell Scientific (pp. 647–655).

McGee, R. & Share, D.L. (1988). Attention deficit disorder – hyperactivity and academic failure: which comes first and what should be treated. *Journal of the American Academy of Child and Adolescent Psychiatry*, **27**(3), 318–325.

Menyuk, P., Chesnick, M., Liebergott, J.W., Korngold, B., D'Agostino, R., & Belanger, A. (1991). Predicting reading problems in at-risk children. *Journal of Speech and Hearing Research*, **34**, 893–903.

Rissman, M., Curtiss, S., & Tallal, P. (1990). School placement outcomes of young language impaired children. *Journal of Speech-Language Pathology and Audiology*, **14**(2), 49–58.

Rourke, B.P. & Finlayson, M.A.J. (1978). Neuropsychological significance of variations in patterns of academic performance: verbal and visual-spatial abilities. *Journal of Abnormal Child Psychology*, **6**(1), 121–133.

Shaywitz, S.E., Fletcher, J.M., & Shaywitz, B.A. (1996). A conceptual model and definition of dyslexia: findings emerging from the Connecticut Longitudinal Study (this volume, pp. 199–223).

Sheridan, M.D. & Peckham, C.S. (1978). Follow-up to 16 years of school children who had marked speech defects at 7 years. *Child Care, Health and Development*, **4**, 145–157.

Sheridan, M.D. & Peckham, C.S. (1975). Follow-up at 11 years of children who had marked speech defects at 7 years. *Child Care, Health and Development*, **1**, 157–166.

Silva, P.A., Williams, S., & McGee, R. (1987). A longitudinal study of children with developmental language delay at age three: later intelligence, reading and behavior problems. *Developmental Medicine and Child Neurology*, **29**, 630–640.

Silva, P., McGee, R., & Williams, S.M. (1983). Developmental language delay from three to seven years and its significance for low intelligence and reading difficulties at age seven. *Developmental Medicine and Child Neurology*, **25**, 783–793.

Silva, P. (1980). The prevalence, stability and significance of developmental language delay in preschool children. *Developmental Medicine and Child Neurology*, **22**, 768–777.

Stark, R.E., Bernstein, L.E., Condino, R., Bender, M., Tallal, P., & Catts III, P. (1984). Four-year follow-up study of language impaired children. *Annals of Dyslexia*, **34**, 49–68.

Tramontana, M.G., Hooper, S.R., & Selzer, S.C. (1988). Research on the preschool prediction of later academic achievement: a review. *Developmental Review*, **8**, 89–146.

Wagner, R.K. (1986). Phonological processing abilities and reading: implications for disabled readers. *Journal of Learning Disabilities*, **19**, 623–630.

Wagner, R.K. & Torgesen, J.K. (1987). The nature of phonological processing and its causal role in the acquisition of reading skills. *Psychological Bulletin*, **101**(2), 192–212.

24 Reading in childhood and mental health in early adulthood

SHEILA WILLIAMS AND ROB McGEE

READING AND DEVELOPMENT

Learning to read during the early school years is critical for a child's educational progress. Children who cannot read enter a cycle of continuing disadvantage from the time they begin school when compared with their reading peers. Poor reading leads to relatively slower increases in language ability from primary school to preadolescence (Share & Silva, 1988), together with a slower rise in intellectual ability during the early school years (Share, McGee, & Silva 1989). Stanovich (1986) has described this pattern of continuing disadvantage in terms of "the poor getting poorer," a pattern whereby more is given to those that have, while more is progressively taken away from those that have not. This ongoing disadvantage has perhaps been underestimated in discussions of reading disability, in part because its examination relies on longitudinal study of children over time. What evidence there is suggests that the development of further linguistic and cognitive processes during schooling is founded upon an ability to read; poor reading skills affect the efficiency and development of these other cognitive processes.

In more widespread fashion, poor reading influences the child's involvement in the educational process as a whole. Studies of attentional processes in the classroom suggest that attention changes moment by moment in response to what is occurring in class. Inattention is strongly predicted by errors made during oral reading, and children who become inattentive in the course of a reading lesson are less and less likely to resume being attentive (Imai et al., 1992). Thus, poor readers are likely to be trapped in a cycle of progressive inattention in the classroom because of their reading failure. Their inattention similarly interferes with further attempts to read (see also Rowe & Rowe, 1992). In the longer term, academic failure is associated with poor academic self-concept, a perception that personal success and failure are not under the individual's control, and poor expectations about future academic performance (Rogers & Saklofske, 1985). Findings from a longitudinal study of New Zealand children (the Dunedin Multidisciplinary Health and Development Study – DMHDS), suggest that by the time they are ready to enter high school, reading disabled children perceive themselves to be "below average" in their reading, spelling, and general school work. They are less attached to and involved with school, they find school less enjoyable, and they intend to leave school at an earlier age than their peers who can read (McGee et al., 1988a). This can only derive from a sense of frustration at being a daily captive in an environment where they cannot keep up with much of what is going on in the classroom, where some form of failure is probably an everyday occurrence, and where they recognize that other students and perhaps even the teacher have a low opinion of their abilities. By adolescence, children with reading disability in early schooling continue to show impaired reading performance and poor examination attainment (Watson, Watson, & Fredd 1982; Maughan et al., 1985; Williams & McGee, 1994). By the age of school leaving, and particularly at present in a time of high unemployment in many Western countries, poor reading skills seem to offer the prospect of limited work opportunities or no work at all.

READING AND BEHAVIOR IN CHILDHOOD

Given this cycle of disadvantage associated with poor reading skills, it seems reasonable to believe that the mental health of the child with reading disability would suffer both in the short and long term. Much of the work in this area derived originally from Burt's (1931) observations of the relationship between poor reading and delinquency and this relationship has been noted by subsequent researchers (see McGee et al., 1988a for a summary of this literature). However, a second line of research has derived from early observations of an association not only between reading disability and inattentive and hyperactive behaviors, but also from observations of emotional withdrawal and defeatism among those with poor reading skills (e.g., Blanchard, 1928; Gates, 1941). At least during the early school years, the critical issue for remediation is to describe the causal pathways between reading and behavior problems to identify what best to treat. Rutter, Tizard, & Whitmore (1970) propose three hypotheses describing the possible causal relationships between reading and behavioral or emotional problems. Reading failure may precede mental health problems which arise as a consequence of progressive school failure, subsequent low self-esteem and association with other disruptive peers. Alternatively, inattentive and disruptive behavior at age of school entry may interfere with the acquisition of early reading skills. A third hypothesis is that some other factor such as background social disadvantage, causes both disruptive behavior and reading failure. It is also feasible that some combination of these hypotheses is correct.

It is not our intention to fully review all the relevant research here. Nevertheless, we believe that the evidence tends to favor the view that the predominant causal direction is initially not from disruptive behavior to reading failure during the early school years. For example, preschool behavior characterized by problems of hyperactivity and distractibility does not seem of itself to predict subsequent reading disability to any great extent (McGee & Share, 1988). Studies of preschool children from clinic samples indicate a strong relationship between disruptive behavior and language difficulties (Beitchman, Tuckett, & Batth, 1987; Love & Thompson, 1988). That is, for many children disruptive behavior is already associated with poorer language skills during the preschool years and evidence from the DMHDS suggests that it is these associated language deficits which probably lead to poorer acquisition of reading skills among those with hyperactivity in the preschool period (McGee et al., 1991). The association between reading disability and behavior problems, particularly pervasive hyperactivity, seems to be most strongly evident at age of school entry (McGee, Williams, & Feehan, 1992). It may well be the case that for certain children these behavioral and literacy problems are so intertwined that disentangling which comes first is not possible. Research on the nature of attentional processes during reading lessons seems to suggest as much (Imai et al., 1992). On the other hand, subsequent rises in the level of other kinds of behavior problems, particularly antisocial behavior, among reading disabled boys and girls over the early school years suggest that a significant degree of behavioral disturbance derives from reading failure (McGee et al., 1988a). There does not appear to be a strong relationship between poor reading skills in childhood and the occurrence of depression (Kashani et al., 1983; McGee & Williams, 1988). However, there is some evidence that children with learning disabilities are perceived by their peers as shy, constantly help-seeking and as victims of bullying (Nabuzoka & Smith, 1993), and a lower level of reading skills in preadolescence seems to be related to anxiety at that age (McGee et al., 1988a; Williams et al., 1989).

READING AND MENTAL HEALTH IN LATE
ADOLESCENCE AND EARLY ADULTHOOD

As we have noted elsewhere (McGee et al., 1988a), there have been relatively few prospective longitudinal studies examining the significance of reading difficulties for later mental health, and what studies there are have been concerned almost exclusively with later antisocial offending. In the main, the evidence suggests somewhat surprisingly no significant relationship between reading problems and later delinquency (Maughan, Gray, & Rutter, 1985; Wadsworth, 1979). Similarly, studies based upon more general measures of school achievement provide little evidence for an association between poor academic achievement and later antisocial behavior (Elliott & Voss, 1974; Ensminger, Kellam, & Rubin, 1983; Olweus, 1983; Spreen, 1981). Using longitudinal data from the DMHDS we have recently examined the relationship between reading skills during the early school years and juvenile delinquency in adolescence (Williams & McGee, 1994). This research used structural equation modeling to address the question "do poor reading skills lead to later juvenile offending" from both a dimensional (cumulative score based) and categorical (classification based) perspective. In summary, models based upon the dimensional approach suggested that there was no direct causal path from early reading to later delinquency. Rather, any association between early reading and later delinquency was mediated by the association between early reading scores and early antisocial behavior as noted above. That is, poor reading skills placed the individual at risk for antisocial behavior during early schooling and it was this behavior which predicted future delinquency. Categorical models, on the other hand, which identified subgroups of children as reading disabled, suggested that for boys early reading disability may predict future conduct disorder at age 15.

Apart from antisocial behavior in adolescence and early adult, other mental health outcomes associated with poor reading have received little attention. Spreen (1987) found some evidence for higher levels of emotional maladjustment among learning disabled men and women in their twenties, and more recently, Klein and Manuzza (1993) have reported higher rates of alcoholism and drug related problems in a sample of 91 children with reading disorders followed into adulthood. Both these studies were based upon clinic samples, and there is a clear need for follow-up studies of children based upon samples from the general population. In the remainder of this chapter, we examine the long-term association between reading ability during early schooling and mental health problems at adolescence (age 15 years) and early adulthood (age 18 years) using data from the Dunedin longitudinal study of child development. Our aim was to develop some exploratory models of the relationships between early reading performance and later mental health using a structural equation modeling approach. This analytic technique seems ideally suited to explore relationships among constructs relating to literacy and mental health over time using both dimensional and categorical approaches to the data. A subsidiary aim was to examine the relationship between early literacy and subsequent educational and economic disadvantage in early adulthood.

THE DUNEDIN STUDY

The DMHDS is a longitudinal study of the health and development of a cohort born between 1 April 1972 and 31 March 1973, at Queen Mary Hospital, Dunedin. Silva (1990) has provided an overview of the study's aims, history and development. The children were first followed up at age 3 years (1975–76), and from a total of 1139 children known to be living in Otago (the province in which Dunedin is situated) at that time, 1037 children were enrolled in the study. They were generally representative of the original birth cohort in terms of perinatal problems, mode of delivery at birth, birth weight or neonatal problems. However, they were under-representative of both the highest and the lowest socioeconomic status (SES) levels, and proportionally fewer of the mothers of those enrolled were solo parents at the time of the child's birth. The sample has been assessed every two years thereafter to age 15 years (1987–88) with subsequent assessments at age 18 (1990–91) and at age 21 years (1993–94). A feature of the study has been a low rate of sample attrition. For example, 976 were contacted at age 15 and 988 at age 18 years, representing over 95% of those still alive. The research reported in this chapter is based on data collected at age 7 and 9 years, and again at 15 and 18 years. The analyses reported below were based upon the 349 boys and 319 girls for whom data for all relevant variables were available.

Measures during early schooling

Over the course of the DMHDS, information has been gathered on a variety of different aspects of each individual's development. Reading ability was assessed at ages 7 and 9 by the Burt Word Reading Test, a measure of word recognition skills (Scottish Council for Research in Education, 1976). In addition, at age 7, prose reading skills were assessed by a short story (Silva, 1981), and spelling was assessed at age 9 (Smith & Pearce, 1966). Reports of behavior problems from ages 5 to 9 years were obtained from the Rutter et al. (1970) Child Scales A and B for parents and teachers respectively. These scales list a variety of behavioral and emotional problems and a total score may be obtained from the sum of individual scores. An index of family disadvantage was formed at age 7 from several different measures including low SES, child of a solo parent, parental separations, maternal depression, low maternal mental ability, large family size, and low family social support (see McGee et al., 1985).

Measures at age 15 years

Reading was again assessed using the Burt test. A mental health interview included a modified version of the Diagnostic Interview Schedule for Children or DISC-C (Costello et al., 1982), a structured interview based upon DSM-III criteria for disorders of childhood and adolescence. The DISC-C allows identification of disorder as well as providing "dimensional" scores for different categories of disorder. The assessment of mental health and results at age 15 is provided by McGee et al. (1990). In the research to be reported here, we used four-dimensional measures based upon self-report of symptoms of attention deficit-hyperactivity, conduct problems (conduct and oppositional behaviors), anxiety (overanxious, separation anxious and phobic symptoms), and depression (major depressive episode and dysthymic symptoms). These broadly reflect the distinction between dimensions of externalizing and internalizing mental health problems. An index of family disadvantage at age 15 was formed using similar measures to that at age 7.

Measures at age 18

Outcome at early adulthood was based upon two broad assessments, one of mental health and the second of personal disadvantage experienced at age 18. A modified version of the Diagnostic Interview Schedule (DIS, version III, revised) was used to assess the presence of symptoms of the more common disorders of adulthood, according to DSM-III-R criteria (Robins et al., 1989). Four scores for dimensions of conduct problems, substance use, anxiety and depression were formed on the basis of self-report for the criterion symptoms. An index of personal disadvantage for age 18 was formed on the basis of self-report of the following: left school with less than three years of high school; having no school qualifications; perceived difficulty in supporting self; individual or partner having or expecting a dependent child; and being currently unemployed. Full details concerning the assessment of mental health and disadvantage at age 18 are given by Feehan et al. (1994).

Missing data

Differences were noted between those with complete data and those without for the prose reading test (a difference of 0.43 standard deviation units), teacher report of behavior problems at age 7 (0.24 SD units) and age 9 (0.26 SD units). Those with missing data had lower prose reading scores and higher teacher reported problem scores. At age 7, those with incomplete data scored 0.33 SD units higher on the measure of family disadvantage, and a similar difference of 0.21 SD units was noted at age 15. All other differences were nonsignificant, and the overall pattern of results suggested that differences between those with and without complete data were not especially large.

DESCRIPTIVE RESULTS

Sex differences

The means and standard deviations for the various measures for both boys and girls are shown in Table 24.1. There were statistically significant sex differences for many of the variables including reading and teacher rated behavior problems in childhood, and reading and a number of mental health variables in adolescence. For this reason, and because our earlier work suggested sex differences in the nature of the relationships among these variables, separate models were developed for males and females.

Correlations among the measures

Table 24.2 shows the correlation matrix for the various measures described above. Inspection of the table indicates the size of the correlations between

Table 24.1. *Means and standard deviations for the variables included in the model for both boys and girls*

Variable	Boys (n = 349)		Girls (n = 319)		t*	
	Mean	SD	Mean	SD		
Age 7						
Burt reading score	26.8	12.46	32.3	12.32	5.75	
Prose reading	78.5	11.92	82.2	6.12	5.15	
Behavior score (parent)	9.1	5.47	8.4	5.33	−1.61	NS
Behavior score (teacher)	4.2	4.65	3.2	4.17	−2.64	
Family disadvantage	0.8	0.99	0.8	0.94	−0.31	NS
Age 9						
Burt reading score	51.2	18.77	56.5	16.94	3.86	
Dunedin Spelling Test	9.1	6.04	11.6	5.63	5.62	
Behavior score (parent)	8.4	5.56	7.6	5.00	−2.14	NS
Behavior score (teacher)	4.6	5.19	3.1	4.09	−4.18	
Age 15						
Burt reading score	88.5	16.18	92.1	13.61	3.14	
Anxiety score	7.7	5.47	10.1	6.13	5.25	
Depression score	2.3	4.67	3.6	6.79	2.98	
Attention score	7.5	4.80	7.0	4.70	−1.34	NS
Conduct score	3.9	6.01	3.5	4.75	−0.91	NS
Family disadvantage	0.6	0.78	0.7	0.82	0.98	NS
Age 18						
Anxiety score	7.7	8.08	11.7	9.79	5.81	
Depression	4.5	8.94	8.5	11.43	5.02	
Conduct	1.9	3.18	0.8	1.90	−5.45	
Substance use	7.9	10.65	4.9	8.66	−3.93	
Personal disadvantage	0.5	0.89	0.5	0.89	−0.29	NS

*Statistically significant using the Bonferroni inequality to adjust for multiple tests (p < 0.05). NS, not significant.

the early reading scores and later mental health variables. Because of the large number of variables involved care should be taken in considering the statistical significance of these. For the most part the correlations between reading performance in childhood and mental health variables at ages 15 and 18 years were not significant. Among the girls, however, reading at age 7 was inversely related to attention problems at age 15 and anxiety at both ages. Among the boys, reading at 7 was also inversely related to attention problems at age 15. Among adolescent girls, reading at age 15 was inversely related to anxiety at age 18, while for the adolescent boys reading at age 15 was inversely related to conduct problems, substance use and anxiety. It is interesting to note that the correlations between many of the variables measured at both ages 7 and 9 years and personal disadvantage at 18 were relatively higher than most of the other correlations. Early reading, behavior problems and family

Table 24.2. *Correlation matrix for the variables included in the model (boys above the diagonal and girls below the diagonal)*

	1	2	3	4	5	6	7	8	9	10	11	12	13	14	15	16	17	18	19	20
Age 7																				
1. Burt reading score		0.65	−0.18	−0.28	−0.26	0.88	0.82	−0.22	−0.24	0.67	−0.11	0.11	−0.17	−0.05	−0.16	−0.10	0.02	−0.11	−0.04	−0.24
2. Prose reading	0.69		−0.21	−0.22	−0.19	0.58	0.55	−0.24	−0.23	0.54	−0.10	0.08	−0.15	0.03	−0.11	−0.05	0.00	−0.06	−0.05	−0.22
3. Behavior score (parent)	−0.18	−0.14		0.18	0.31	−0.12	−0.11	0.71	0.13	−0.18	0.16	0.00	0.13	0.08	0.16	0.06	−0.03	0.02	0.05	0.14
4. Behavior score (teacher)	−0.29	−0.32	0.13		0.20	−0.26	−0.30	0.24	0.44	−0.24	0.09	−0.01	0.16	0.21	0.07	0.11	0.01	0.14	0.06	0.24
5. Family disadvantage	−0.27	−0.16	0.24	0.13		−0.23	−0.20	0.27	0.15	−0.25	0.05	0.04	0.17	0.17	0.45	0.02	0.08	0.17	0.09	0.32
Age 9																				
6. Burt reading score	0.86	0.61	−0.17	−0.27	−0.23		0.87	−0.17	−0.26	0.72	−0.10	0.10	−0.15	−0.04	−0.14	−0.11	0.02	−0.09	−0.04	−0.23
7. Dunedin Spelling Test	0.82	0.64	−0.12	−0.26	−0.20	0.85		−0.18	−0.27	0.69	−0.09	0.11	−0.15	−0.09	−0.16	−0.16	0.01	−0.12	−0.06	−0.19
8. Behavior score (parent)	−0.20	−0.23	0.70	0.18	0.18	−0.23	−0.22		0.24	−0.17	0.21	0.03	0.19	0.17	0.19	0.15	0.04	0.08	0.11	0.23
8. Behavior score (teacher)	−0.29	−0.28	0.17	0.13	0.17	−0.27	−0.28	0.22		−0.28	0.19	0.09	0.13	0.18	0.05	0.13	0.13	0.19	0.17	0.22
Age 15																				
10. Burt reading score	0.67	0.62	−0.18	−0.34	−0.20	0.76	0.73	−0.29	−0.32		−0.17	0.03	−0.19	−0.19	−0.09	−0.14	−0.05	−0.25	−0.14	−0.19
11. Anxiety score	−0.19	−0.25	0.11	0.29	0.08	−0.17	−0.22	0.14	0.21	−0.24		0.27	0.44	0.11	0.07	0.35	0.14	0.04	0.03	0.06
12. Depression score	0.02	−0.02	−0.05	0.02	0.01	0.00	0.01	−0.03	0.09	0.07	0.31		0.27	0.20	0.09	0.27	0.22	0.12	0.16	0.13
13. Attention score	−0.16	−0.17	0.08	0.11	0.08	−0.12	−0.12	0.11	0.15	−0.13	0.36	0.34		0.52	0.21	0.32	0.23	0.30	0.34	0.31
14. Conduct score	−0.03	−0.02	0.07	−0.04	0.12	0.00	0.02	0.09	0.03	−0.00	0.13	0.41	0.55		0.21	0.27	0.26	0.49	0.54	0.57
15. Family disadvantage	−0.16	−0.03	0.24	0.08	0.48	−0.14	−0.07	0.17	−0.01	−0.12	0.06	0.03	0.03	0.13		0.08	0.04	0.22	0.17	0.16
Age 18																				
16. Anxiety score	−0.18	−0.12	0.13	0.05	0.08	−0.12	−0.15	0.05	0.03	−0.12	0.37	0.26	0.36	0.17	0.17		0.49	0.22	0.30	0.10
17. Depression	−0.03	−0.10	0.04	0.07	0.08	−0.10	−0.02	0.04	0.05	0.02	0.25	0.35	0.29	0.21	0.14	0.49		0.24	0.30	0.10
18. Conduct	0.06	−0.01	0.01	0.01	0.10	−0.07	0.07	0.05	−0.03	−0.07	0.13	0.27	0.30	0.29	0.23	0.26	0.27		0.67	0.39
19. Substance use	−0.08	−0.10	−0.03	0.02	0.10	−0.03	−0.07	−0.07	−0.03	−0.03	0.19	0.22	0.38	0.35	0.08	0.41	0.44	0.45		0.35
20. Personal disadvantage	−0.29	−0.25	0.26	0.18	0.33	−0.26	−0.24	0.22	0.26	−0.28	0.18	0.10	0.36	0.36	0.34	0.21	0.22	0.20	0.31	

disadvantage were all related to personal disadvantage in the early adult years. Among the girls early family disadvantage was particularly important. Although the magnitude of the correlations between early reading and personal disadvantage at 18 were similar for boys and girls, the correlation between reading at age 15 and subsequent personal disadvantage was higher for boys ($r = -0.39$) than girls ($r = -0.28$).

Reading disability and mental health

McGee et al. (1988a) identified 40 boys and 40 girls as reading disabled at both ages 7 and 9 years. At age 18, mental health interviews were carried out with 32 of the reading disabled boys, whose mean reading scores at ages 7 and 9 were 10.2 and 23.3 compared with 28.4 and 53.5 for the remainder of the sample and 36 of the reading disabled girls whose mean reading scores at ages 7 and 9 were 15.4 and 32.0 compared with 34.0 and 58.9 for the remainder of the sample. The overall rate of mental health disorder among those reading disabled as children was 44% compared with 36% of the comparison group at age 18, and the association between early reading status and mental health outcome at age 18 was nonsignificant, chi square (1 df) = 1.55, p > 0.05. Exploration of the relationship between reading status and type of disorder (i.e., externalizing, internalizing and mixed) also suggested no relationship between reading status and nature of mental health problems at age 18.

Early reading disability, however, was significantly associated with self-perceived disadvantage at age 18 years. If a score of 2 or more indicates high disadvantage, 28% of the 18-year-olds with early reading disability had a score of 2 or more, compared with 11% of the remainder, chi square (1 df) = 15.62, p < 0.001. This finding is in accord with the correlational results presented above.

DIMENSIONAL MODELS OF READING AND MENTAL HEALTH

Statistical analysis

Structural equation modeling is an analytic technique which can be used to examine the causal relationships among a group of variables by defining underlying constructs or so called "latent variables" measured by observed variables, and by subsequently exploring the associations among these constructs. In the present context, for example, a latent variable for the construct "literacy at age 7" can be measured by the word recognition and prose reading tests at that age. The correlations between these two reading variables and the underlying construct are the equivalent of factor loadings in a simple factor analysis. This part of the model constitutes a measurement model. The structural equation part of the model then examines the relationships among the latent variables. LISREL allows the parameters for the model to be fitted simultaneously and can be based either on the variance-covariance matrix or on a correlation matrix. Here, LISREL7 was used to model the longitudinal data (Jöreskog & Sörbom, 1989) based upon the covariance matrix and the model was estimated using the method of maximum likelihood.

Latent variables were derived for early literacy at age 7 using the word recognition and prose reading test scores, and at age 9 using the word recognition and spelling scores. At age 15, the single measure of word recognition was used in the model. Latent variables for behavior at ages 7 and 9 were based upon the parent and teacher reports. At ages 15 and 18 the latent variables for internalizing disorder were based upon the scores for depression and anxiety. The latent variable for externalizing disorder at age 15 was based upon scores for attention deficit-hyperactivity and conduct problems, and that at 18 years upon scores for substance use and conduct problems.

Assumptions in the models

The models to be described were based upon those which examined the association between early reading and later delinquency (Williams & McGee, 1994) and several of the initial assumptions in the models were the same. Probably the most contentious assumption we make here concerns the omission of IQ; reading and spelling scores in the models were not adjusted for IQ but were used as direct measures of reading skill. Reading ability, however, is frequently defined in the literature in terms of the discrepancy between the child's current level of reading skill and that predicted by his or her IQ. In this type of definition, IQ is a kind of unalterable proxy to identify the expected level of reading which the child is assumed to be capable of reaching. We have not adjusted for IQ in the dimensional models for several reasons. First, a strong case can be made that the difference between definitions of reading skill based upon scores unadjusted for IQ and scores adjusted for IQ are of little theoretical consequence (see, for example, the recent discussion of this topic by Stanovich, 1993). On the other hand, the practical significance may be that definitions of reading in terms of IQ discrepancy lead to the neglect of research on children with poor reading and low IQ. Second, as noted in the introduction, poor reading skills directly influence the child's cognitive and language skills so that any discrepancy between reading and IQ is not a simple reflection of the discrepancy between actual reading ability and the child's potential reading ability. Third, we found that the models for the relationship between reading and delinquency were essentially the same whether or not reading scores were adjusted for IQ at age of school entry

(Williams & McGee, 1994). We will take up the issue of IQ again in the discussion of our findings.

Second, the models were not designed to test the causal direction of the relationship between reading and behavior problems in early childhood. It is already apparent that reading is strongly related to behavior problems from an early age (McGee et al., 1988a; 1993) and as we argued above, the evidence tends to favor the hypothesis that antisocial behavior arises and continues to increase over the early school years as a function of early reading failure. We have therefore identified the causal paths as flowing from literacy to behavior at age 7 years. Third, Feehan (1993) found evidence for long-term associations between early measures of disadvantage and mental health at age 18, so a test of this possible relationship was included in the model. Further, it was hypothesized that literacy and the latent variable for externalizing disorder at age 15 were associated with personal disadvantage at age 18. While earlier studies have suggested that there was no association between internalizing disorder at 15 and personal disadvantage at 18 it was of interest to examine association. So that the models suggested by these hypotheses could be tested using LISREL7, the parameters for some paths were constrained to zero reflecting the lack of association expected between some pairs of variables.

Given these assumptions, a schematic representation of the proposed model is shown in Figure 24.1. Possible paths from family disadvantage were omitted in the interests of parsimony. Paths for the correlations between the errors in the measures repeated on two or more occasions have also been omitted from Figure 24.1 but were included in the analysis.

The model for males

In terms of the measurement aspects of the model, the parameters linking the observed variables with the latent variables indicate the size of the correlation between the observed variable and the underlying construct or latent variable, and these are reported separately in Table 24.3. It can be seen from the table that the loadings for those variables measuring literacy were higher than those measuring behavior problems, suggesting that the reading tests were better measures of the underlying latent variable called literacy than the parent and teacher Child Scales A and B were of the latent variable behavior problems. The loadings for the measures of attention deficit-hyperactivity and conduct at age 15, and substance use and conduct measured at 18 for the latent variables measuring externalizing behavior were both reasonably high. The loadings for anxiety and depression as indicators of internalizing disorder at age 15 were rather lower than those at 18, suggesting that the latent variable at 18 was a better measure of the underlying construct.

Figure 24.2 shows the model that was fitted for males, with the parameters expressed in standardized form. The parameters may be interpreted either as regression coefficients if they have a single arrow, or as correlations between

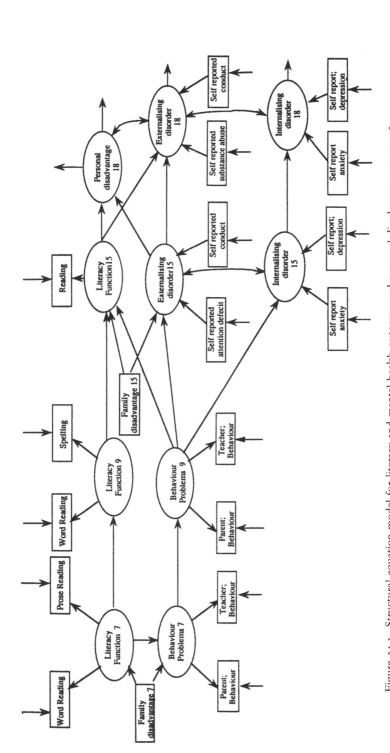

Figure 24.1. Structural equation model for literacy and mental health outcome and personal disadvantage at age 18.

Table 24.3. *Standardized factor loadings for the variables and error terms for the variables and the latent variables included in the model for both boys and girls*

	Boys (n = 349)		Girls (n = 319)	
	Factor loading	Error term	Factor loading	Error term
Literacy Function 7		0.93		0.94
Burt reading score	0.97	0.07	0.92	0.15
Prose reading	0.68	0.54	0.76	0.43
Behavior 7		0.58		0.66
Parent	0.44	0.81	0.34	0.88
Teacher	0.53	0.72	0.50	0.75
Literacy Function 9		0.15		0.15
Burt reading score	0.95	0.09	0.89	0.20
Dunedin Spelling Test	0.92	0.16	0.94	0.12
Behavior 9		0.28		0.06
Parent	0.53	0.71	0.42	0.81
Teacher	0.52	0.73	0.55	0.69
Literacy Function 15		0.39		0.35
Burt reading score	1.00		1.00	
Internalizing 15		0.91		1.00
Anxiety score	0.46	0.79	0.44	0.81
Depression score	0.50	0.75	0.67	0.55
Externalizing 15		0.82		1.00
Attention score	0.65	0.57	0.75	0.44
Conduct score	0.82	0.33	0.76	0.42
Internalizing 18		0.54		0.65
Anxiety score	0.77	0.41	0.67	0.55
Depression score	0.66	0.56	0.75	0.44
Externalizing 18		0.55		0.78
Conduct	0.78	0.40	0.58	0.66
Substance use	0.85	0.28	0.97	0.07
Personal disadvantage 18		0.66		0.70
Disadvantage	1.00		1.00	

pairs of latent variables if they have two arrows. The parameters in Figure 24.2 show that both literacy and behavior problems were relatively stable between ages 7 and 9 and that literacy at age 9 was a good predictor of literacy at age 15. However, there were no direct causal paths from early literacy to the later mental health. The latent variable for behavior problems at age 9 was inversely related to literacy at age 15 and predicted both the latent variables for internalizing and externalizing disorder at age 15 as well. Personal disadvantage at age 18 was predicted by literacy and externalizing disorder

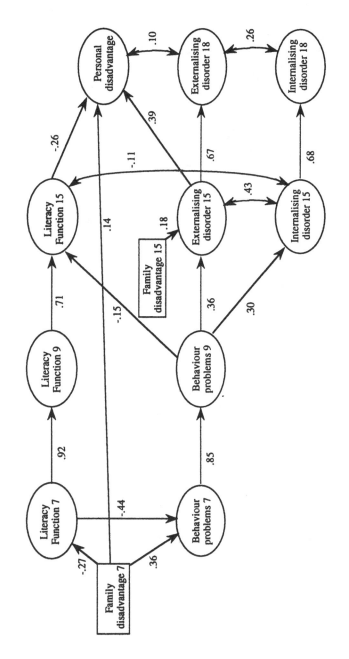

Figure 24.2. Structural equation model for boys.

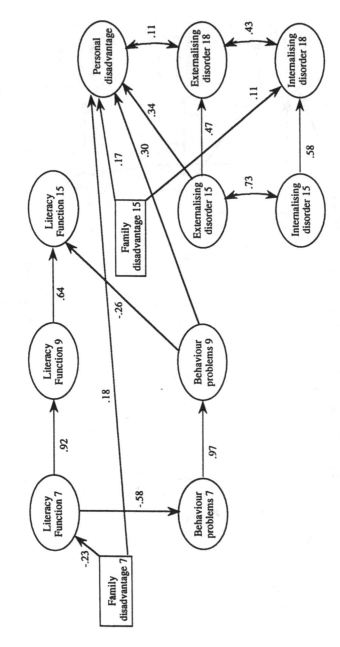

Figure 24.3. Structural equation model for girls.

at age 15 as well as by family disadvantage at age 7. At age 18 personal disadvantage was significantly correlated with the latent variable for externalizing disorder. There was no direct path from reading at age 15 to either of the latent variables for mental health at age 18.

The model for females

The model fitted to the covariance matrix for girls is shown in Figure 24.3. The results for the period of childhood are similar to those for the boys with both literacy and behavior showing high levels of stability between age 7 and 9 years. As was the case with the boys, there were no direct paths from early literacy to later mental health. The latent variable for behavior at 9 was inversely associated with literacy at age 15 and positively associated with personal disadvantage at age 18. Furthermore, personal disadvantage at 18 was predicted by family disadvantage at both 7 and 15 years. Literacy at age 15 was not a predictor of either later personal disadvantage or disorder among girls.

CATEGORICAL MODELS OF READING AND MENTAL HEALTH

Statistical analysis

In the following analyses, correlations among categorical variables (or polychoric correlations) allowed the use of a categorical approach to the data. Such a categorical approach may be contrasted with the dimensional approach used above to identify points of divergence and convergence in the models. The categorical models were based upon classification of groups of children who were described as having reading disability, as showing significant levels of behavior problems in childhood, and as having a mental health disorder in adolescence or early adulthood. The categorical analyses were based upon the 349 males and 319 females included in the dimensional analyses.

The categorical analyses used classifications derived from earlier research with the DMHDS sample. For example, the category "behavior problems in childhood" included those children identified from age 5 to 9 years as showing significant levels of problem behavior reported by both the parent and the teacher using the recommended cutoff scores for the Child Scale A and B (McGee et al., 1993). Those with pervasive problems are most likely to be identified by this method, and in a sense this is similar to using the parent and teacher scales to identify a latent variable in the dimensional analysis. The category reading disability included those children identified as reading disabled during the early school years (McGee et al., 1988a).

Mental health outcomes in the categorical models were limited to age 18 for the sake of parsimony in presenting the results. Elsewhere, we have suggested that greater impairment is associated with externalizing disorders such as conduct disorder or substance dependence, than with an internalizing disorder such as anxiety or depression, and impairment is greatest among those with disorders in both domains (Feehan et al., 1994). This being so, an ordinal variable was used to describe mental health disorder at age 18 years as follows. We have given those with both an internalizing and an externalizing disorder a rank of 3, those with an externalizing disorder a rank of 2 and those with an internalizing disorder a rank of 1.

The model for males

The model for males, fitted using weighted least squares, is depicted in Figure 24.4. The analysis suggested that early reading disability was a statistically significant predictor of both personal disadvantage and mental health disorder at age 18. Family disadvantage at age 7 predicted both reading disability and significant behavior problems in childhood as well as personal disadvantage at age 18. While the overall fit of the model was high, the amount of variance actually explained by the model was relatively low in comparison with the dimensional model above. The measurement error, indicated by the arrows in the diagram was relatively high, 0.93 for instance for both early behavior problems and later psychiatric diagnosis. This suggests that the model may

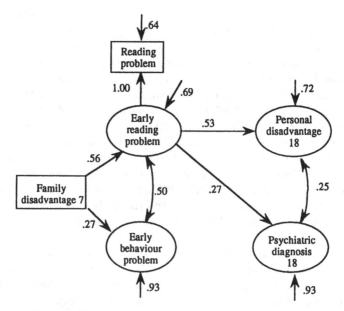

Figure 24.4. Structural equation model for mental health disorder and personal disadvantage at age 18 for boys based upon polychoric correlations.

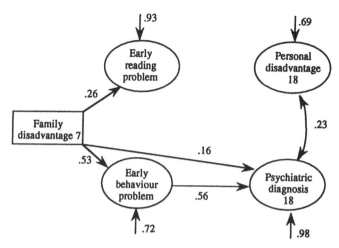

Figure 24.5. Structural equation model for mental health disorder and personal disadvantage at age 18 for girls based upon polychoric correlations.

not represent the original very well and that the regression coefficients should be interpreted with caution.

The model for females

A model for the women is shown in Figure 24.5, and in this case the mental health outcome at age 18 was predicted by having a significant behavior problem in childhood. Family disadvantage at age 7 predicted both reading and behavior problems in childhood as well as mental health disorder at age 18. In this case the correlation between reading disability and behavior problems was significant. Again the overall goodness of fit of the model was high. However, the unexplained variance in this model was also high suggesting that the estimates may be biased because too few explanatory variables were included in the model.

CONCLUSION

What do these findings tell us about the longer-term outcomes associated with early reading problems? In the first instance, it seems clear that there are long-term associations between reading performance in the early school years and reading in adolescence and early adulthood. This is consistent with findings from other research that reading problems do persist to some degree into adulthood (Maughan et al., 1985; Rodgers, 1986; Spreen, 1988). In the present study, the results from age 7 to 15 years as shown in Figures 24.2 and 24.3 suggest that the long-term associations between early and late reading skills are the same for males and females. However, it would be wrong to believe that early reading skills necessarily set low limits on an individual's level of literacy in adulthood. As Rodgers (1986) points out, the view that psychological development is concentrated in early life is a potent one, but is clearly not the full story. His longitudinal study of reading from age 15 to 26 years suggests that substantial improvements in reading might occur from adolescence to adulthood, and that there may be a corresponding decline in the prevalence of illiteracy over this period. Other research from the DMHDS (McGee et al., 1988b) indicates that some children with very poor levels of reading at age 7 do "catch up" with their peers by preadolescence. What is important, therefore, is to try to identify those factors which might predict better outcome in literacy. For example, we found that the reading ability of the mother was significantly higher among those poor readers with a better outcome at preadolescence. Level of literacy in the home and reading remediation at school may provide the child with the necessary skills to overcome any early setbacks in achieving literacy.

As noted in the introduction, there is strong evidence for an association between reading skills and problem behaviors during the early school years. Given this initial association, what are the mental health outcomes in adolescence and adulthood? The findings from the dimensional models depicted in Figures 24.2 and 24.3 indicate that for both boys and girls there was no direct causal path from early reading to mental health outcomes in adolescence, nor any path from reading in adolescence to mental health outcomes in early adulthood. This confirms and extends our earlier findings relating to reading and delinquency (Williams & McGee, 1994). Overall, the results from the DMHDS suggest that among the majority of school aged children, any influence early reading problems might have on later mental health is indirect, most likely operating via the association between reading and antisocial and other behavior problems during the early school years. Put another way, early difficulties in reading acquisition place the child at risk for behavior problems and these in turn enhance the risk of later mental health problems. These early onset behavior problems, however, have additional consequences. They appear to directly influence reading levels at adolescence for both boys and girls, and this is consistent with the findings of Fergusson and Horwood (1992) who reported that inattentive behaviors in preadolescence exerted a small but significant effect on later reading. Furthermore, among females, behavior problems at age 9 exert a direct influence on personal disadvantage at age 18 years.

In the dimensional models we made no concessions for a role of IQ in the relationship between literacy and mental health. As we outlined earlier, part of the reason for this was based upon our earlier observations that adjusting reading scores for IQ did little to alter the findings in the models of reading and delinquency (Williams & McGee, 1994). At the same time, we have argued that it makes little sense to define reading ability in terms of IQ-discrepant scores if in fact a consequence of poor reading ability is to drive down IQ (see Share, McGee, & Silva, 1989). To many, such a view may clearly border on heresy. However, we would argue that an emphasis on reading rather than IQ is appropriate in examining possible associations with behavior, and in particular changes in behavior problems during the early school years. Two findings from the DMHDS suggest that literacy may be more important than IQ in predicting early problem behavior. Stanton et al. (1990) used hierarchical regression procedures to examine the relative contributions of preschool IQ, school-aged IQ and reading ability on teacher rated problem behavior. While preschool IQ was predictive of behavior problems at age of school entry, subsequent changes in levels of problem behavior were not correlated with IQ once the effects of reading had been taken into account. McGee et al. (1988a; footnote 3) found no evidence for an increased rate of behavior problems among boys with low IQ (all less than 100 with a mean of 93.0) but with normal reading scores from ages 7 to 11. By contrast, a second group of boys with equivalent low IQ levels but markedly impaired reading showed high levels of behavior problems over the early school years.

The dimensional models suggest that the only outcome variable at age 18 years that was associated directly with literacy was personal disadvantage at age 18 among the young men. At age 18 years, the extent to which the individual experienced disadvantage was a function of the level of disadvantage experienced by his family during his childhood, and mental health problems and level of literacy in adolescence. Both mental health and literacy in adolescence, in turn, are a function of early behavior problems and reading skills. This model suggests a view of disadvantage in early adulthood as being determined by nominally separate but interacting forces. It remains to be seen just how damaging in turn this disadvantage will be to future development as these young men enter their twenties. Disadvantage among the young women was also a function of mental health at adolescence and family disadvantage at that time. Literacy, however, was not directly related to later personal disadvantage for the young women.

The presence of a relationship between early reading and later disadvantage in males but not females is of interest in that it parallels other similar sex differences. For example, at age 15 a global measure of self-perceived "strengths" or competencies was related to attachment to school among the boys but not the girls, while reading level at age 15 was more strongly correlated with strengths among the boys (Williams & McGee, 1991). While the possible mechanisms accounting for these sex differences are unclear, it may well be that the longer-term consequences of reading problems for males and females are different. Perhaps the most we can say at present is that these differences warrant further exploration.

Before comparing the findings from the dimensional and categorical models it is worth noting at the outset that the former describe relationships among continuous variables and reflect to a large extent what holds for the majority of the sample. Categorical models, on the other hand, describe what is happening at the margins of the sample. An analogy might be between methodologies based upon the whole population and those based upon a clinical sample. This being so, divergency in the models may not be unexpected. Despite problems with the measurement aspects of the categorical models, they suggest that reading disability in childhood is of more significance for boys than girls in that it predicts both personal disadvantage and mental health disorder at age 18. This finding confirms our earlier observation that reading disabled boys are at higher risk of conduct disorder at age 15 (Williams & McGee, 1994). The categorical models also emphasize the long-term effects of early disadvantage for both boys and girls. Comparison of the dimensional and categorical models, however, needs to be viewed with some degree of circumspection because of the extent of unexplained variation in the latter.

What is of particular note in our results is the extent to which the effects of early family disadvantage are pervasive and long lasting, predicting both early literacy and behavior problems in boys and girls, as well as personal disadvantage at age 18 among the young men. At a time when models of adult psychopathology and development often place considerable stress upon the potency of intra-individual variables (e.g., Humphreys & Rappaport, 1993), part of the reality seems to be that early events which are by and large beyond the control of the child may well set the scene for what will happen in the important period of transition from adolescence to early adulthood.

The results from the DMHDS on the long-term outcomes associated with differing levels of reading skills in childhood add to the growing literature emphasizing the importance of achieving early literacy. Children with poor reading skills clearly face some ongoing disadvantage in comparison with their reading peers. Furthermore, they are likely to come from disadvantaged family backgrounds where literacy levels in the home may also be poor (Share et al., 1983; McGee et al., 1988b). Early intervention is required to break this chain of disadvantage. What form such intervention takes may depend on the nature of the child's problems. Elsewhere (McGee & Share, 1988), we have argued strongly for the view that early successful intervention with reading alone has the potential to bring about both literacy and behavioral change, and there is some evidence for this in the literature (Arnold et al., 1977; Farkas, 1993). It may be the case that for some children, problems of reading and hyperactivity are so closely linked at age of school entry (McGee et al., 1993) that both reading remediation and techniques for addressing problem behavior will provide the best approach. Finally, if it is possible to carry out cross-tutoring reading programs in the home, both reading impaired parent and child may be able to enhance their reading skills.

ACKNOWLEDGMENTS

The DMHDS has been supported by the Health Research Council of New Zealand as well as by grant MH-45070 to Terrie Moffitt from Violence and

Traumatic Stress Branch of the United States National Institutes of Health. The authors are particularly indebted to the many people who contributed to the research effort involving the collection of mental health and literacy information described in this chapter. Finally, our thanks go to those enrolled in the DMHDS and to their parents for their long-term commitment to this important research.

TECHNICAL APPENDIX

The model for boys was based upon observed correlations for 20 variables and 57 parameters were estimated. The final chi square value was 256.6 with 150 degrees of freedom. The goodness of fit index, which can have a maximum of 1.0, was 0.93 with the adjusted value being 0.90. All the paths described in the model were statistically significant.

When the models using the continuous variable were fitted, provision was made for some of the error terms to be correlated to improve the fit of the models. For completeness sake these are reported here. The correlations between the error terms for the Burt reading tests and the parent and teacher measures of behavior for boys at age 7 and 9 which were statistically significant were 0.04, 0.51 and 0.21, respectively. The correlation of 0.14 between the error terms for the measures of anxiety at age 15 and 18 was also significant.

The model for girls was also based upon correlations from 20 variables and fitted 58 parameters. The final chi square value was 279.0 with 152 degrees of freedom. The goodness of fit index was 0.92, and the adjusted value was 0.89. All the paths described in the model were statistically significant. The correlations between the error terms for the word reading test, the parent and teacher behavior scores at age 7 and 9 for girls were significant They were 0.10, 0.56 and 0.24 respectively. Also correlated were the errors for the reading score at ages 9 and 15 which was 0.07 and the anxiety scores at age 15 and 18 which was 0.16.

REFERENCES

Arnold, L.E., Barneby, N., McManus, J., Smeltzer, D.J., Conrad, A. et al. (1977). Prevention by specific perceptual remediation for vulnerable first graders. *Archives of General Psychiatry*, **44**, 69–81.

Beitchman, J., Tuckett, M., & Batth, S. (1987). Language delay and hyperactivity in preschoolers: evidence for a distinct subgroup of hyperactives. *Canadian Journal of Psychiatry*, **32**, 683–687.

Blanchard, P. (1928). Reading disabilities in relation to maladjustment. *Mental Hygiene*, **12**, 772–788.

Burt, C. (1931). *The Young Delinquent*. London: University of London Press.

Costello, A., Edelbrock, C., Kalas, R., Kessler, M., & Klaric, S.A. (1982). *Diagnostic Interview Schedule for Children (DISC)*. Contract No. RFP-DB-81-0027. Bethesda, MD: National Institute of Mental Health.

Elliott, D.S. & Voss, H.L. (1974). *Delinquency and Dropout*. Lexington, KY: Lexington Books.

Ensminger, M.E., Kellam, S.G., & Rubin, B.R. (1983). School and family origins of delinquency: comparisons by sex. In K.T. van Dusen & S.A. Mednick (eds), *Prospective Studies of Crime and Delinquency*. Boston, MA: Kluwer Nijhoff.

Farkas, G. (1993). Structured tutoring for at risk children in the early years. *Applied Behavioral Science Review*, 1, 69–92.

Feehan, M. (1993). The continuity of mental health disorders from ages 15 to 18 years. Thesis submitted for the Degree of Doctor of Philosophy, University of Otago, Dunedin.

Feehan, M., McGee, R., Nada Raja, S., & Williams, S. (1994). DSM-III-R disorders in New Zealand 18-year-olds. *Australian and New Zealand Journal of Psychiatry*, 28, 87–99.

Fergusson, D.M. & Horwood, L.J. (1992). Attention deficit and reading achievement. *Journal of Child Psychology and Psychiatry*, 33, 375–385.

Gates, A.I. (1941). The role of personality maladjustment in reading. *Journal of Genetic Psychology*, 59, 77–83.

Humphreys, K. & Rappaport, J. (1993). From the community mental health movement to the war on drugs: a study in the definition of social problems. *American Psychologist*, 48, 892–901.

Imai, M., Anderson, R.C., Wilkinson, I.A.G., & Yi, H. (1992). Properties of attention during reading lessons. *Journal of Educational Psychology*, 84, 160–173.

Jöreskog, K.G. & Sörbom, D. (1988). *PRELIS A Program for Multivariate Data Screening and Data Summarization*. Mooresville, Indiana: Scientific Software.

Jöreskog, K.G. & Sörbom, D. (1989). *LISREL7 User's Reference Guide*. Mooresville, Indiana: Scientific Software.

Kashani, J.H., McGee, R., Clarkson, S.E., Anderson, J.C., Walton, L.A., et al. (1983). Depression in a sample of 9-year-old children: prevalence and associated characteristics. *Archives of General Psychiatry*, 40, 1217–1223.

Klein, R.G. & Manuzza, S. (1993). A 15-year follow-up of 91 children with pure reading disorders. Paper presented at the Society for Research in Child and Adolescent Psychopathology Annual Meeting, February 17–21, Santa Fe, New Mexico.

Love, A.J. & Thompson, M.G.G. (1988). Language disorders and attention deficit disorders in young children referred for psychiatric services. *American Journal of Orthopsychiatry*, 58, 52–64.

Maughan, B., Gray, G., & Rutter, M. (1985). Reading retardation and antisocial behavior: a follow-up into employment. *Journal of Child Psychology and Psychiatry*, 26, 741–758.

McGee, R., Feehan, M., Williams, S., Partridge, F., Silva, P.A., & Kelly, J. (1990). DSM-III disorders in a large sample of adolescents. *Journal of the American Academy of Child and Adolescent Psychiatry*, 29, 611–619.

McGee, R., Partridge, F., Williams, S., & Silva, P.A. (1991). A twelve year follow-up of preschool hyperactive children. *Journal of the American Academy of Child and Adolescent Psychiatry*, 30, 224–232.

McGee, R. & Share, D.L. (1988). Attention deficit disorder-hyperactivity and academic failure: which comes first and what should be treated? *Journal of the American Academy of Child and Adolescent Psychiatry*, 27, 318–325.

McGee, R., Share, D.L., Moffitt, T.E., Williams, S.M., & Silva, P.A. (1988a). Reading disability, behavior problems and juvenile delinquency. In D.H. Saklofske & S.G.B. Eysenck (eds) *Individual Differences in Children and Adolescents: International Perspectives.* London: Hodder & Stoughton (pp. 158–172).

McGee, R. & Williams, S. (1988). Childhood depression and reading disability: is there a relationship? *Journal of School Psychology,* **26**, 391–394.

McGee, R., Williams, S., Bradshaw, J., Chapel, J.L., Robins, A., & Silva, P.A. (1985). The Rutter scale for completion by teachers: factor structure and relationships with cognitive abilities and family adversity for a sample of New Zealand children. *Journal of Child Psychology and Psychiatry,* **26**, 727–739.

McGee, R., Williams, S., & Feehan, M. (1992). Attention deficit disorder and age of onset of problem behaviors. *Journal of Abnormal Child Psychology,* **20**, 487–502.

McGee, R., Williams, S., & Feehan, M. (1993). Behavior problems in New Zealand children. In P.R. Joyce, R.T. Mulder, M.A. Oakley-Browne, J.D. Sellman & W.G. Watkins (eds) *Development Personality and Psychopathology.* Christchurch (NZ): Department of Psychological Medicine, Christchurch School of Medicine.

McGee, R., Williams, S., & Silva, P.A. (1988b). Slow starters and long-term backward readers: a replication and extension. *British Journal of Educational Psychology,* **58**, 330–337.

Nabuzoka, D. & Smith, P.K. (1993). Sociometric status and social behavior of children with and without learning difficulties. *Journal of Child Psychology and Psychiatry,* **34**, 1435–1448.

Olweus, D. (1983). Low school achievement and aggressive behavior in adolescent boys. In D. Magnusson & V.L. Allen (eds) *Human Development: An Interactional Perspective.* New York: Academic Press (pp. 353–365).

Robins, L.N., Helzer, J.E., Cottler, L., & Goldring, E. (1989). *NIMH Diagnostic Interview Schedule: Version III Revised.* Written under contract to the National Institute of Mental Health.

Rodgers, B. (1986). Changes in the reading attainment of adults: a longitudinal study. *British Journal of Developmental Psychology,* **4**, 1–17.

Rogers, H. & Saklofske, D.H. (1985). Self-concepts, locus of control, and performance expectations of learning disabled children. *Journal of Learning Disabilities,* **18**, 273–278.

Rowe, K.J. & Rowe, K.S. (1992). The relationship between inattentiveness in the classroom and reading achievement: an exploratory study. *Journal of the American Academy of Child and Adolescent Psychiatry,* **31**, 357–368.

Rutter, M., Tizard, J., & Whitmore, K. (1970). *Education, Health and Behavior.* London: Longman.

Scottish Council for Research in Education (1976). *The Burt Word Reading Test – 1974 Revision.* London: Hodder & Stoughton.

Share, D.L., Jorm, A.F., Maclean, R., Matthews, R., & Waterman, B. (1983). Early reading achievement, oral language ability and a child's home background. *Australian Psychologist,* **18**, 75–87.

Share, D.L., McGee, R., & Silva, P.A. (1989). IQ and reading progress: a test of the capacity notion of IQ. *Journal of the American Academy of Child and Adolescent Psychiatry,* **28**, 97–100.

Share, D.L. & Silva, P.A. (1988). Language deficits and reading retardation: cause or effect? *British Journal of Disorders of Communication,* **22**, 219–226.

Silva, P.A. (1981). A simple prose reading test to identify seven-year-olds with reading problems. *National Education*, **9**, 36–38.

Silva, P.A. (1990). The Dunedin Multidisciplinary Health and Development Research Study: a fifteen-year longitudinal study. *Paediatric and Perinatal Epidemiology*, **4**, 96–127.

Smith, C.T.W. & Pearce, D.W. (1966). Testing spelling: attainment norms and comparison for pupils from 9 to 13 years. *National Education*, **1**, 117–120.

Spreen, O. (1981). The relationship between learning disability, neurological impairment and delinquency. *Journal of Nervous and Mental Disease*, **169**, 791–799.

Spreen, O. (1987). *Learning Disabled Children Growing Up*. Lisse, Netherlands: Swets & Zeitlinger.

Spreen, O. (1988). Prognosis of learning disability. *Journal of Consulting and Clinical Psychology*, **56**, 836–842.

Stanovich, K.E. (1986). Matthew effects in reading: some consequences of individual differences in the acquisition of literacy. *Reading Research Quarterly*, **21**, 360–406.

Stanovich, K.E. (1993). A model for studies of reading disability. *Developmental Review*, **13**, 225–245.

Stanton, W.R., Feehan, M., McGee, R., & Silva, P.A. (1990). The relative value of reading ability and IQ as predictors of teacher reported behavior problems. *Journal of Learning Disabilities*, **23**, 514–517.

Wadsworth, M. (1979). *Roots of Delinquency*. Oxford: Martin Robinson.

Watson, B.V., Watson, C.S., & Fredd, R. (1982). Follow-up studies of specific reading disability. *Journal of the American Academy of Child Psychiatry*, **21**, 376–382.

Williams, S. & McGee, R. (1991). Adolescents' self-perceptions of their strengths. *Journal of Youth Adolescence*, **20**, 325–337.

Williams, S. & McGee, R. (1994). Reading and juvenile delinquency. *Journal of Child Psychology and Psychiatry*, **35**, 441–459.

Williams, S., McGee, R., Anderson, J., & Silva, P.A. (1989). The structure and correlates of self-reported symptoms in 11-year-old children. *Journal of Abnormal Child Psychology*, **17**, 55–71.

25 Communicative competence and psychosocial development in deaf children and adolescents

CAROL MUSSELMAN, SHERRI MacKAY,
SANDRA E. TREHUB, AND RITA S. EAGLE

A number of investigators have identified links between language skill and psychosocial adjustment (e.g., Beitchman et al., 1986). The study of children with prelingual deafness provides a unique opportunity to investigate these relationships because their language difficulties arise from peripheral damage to the organ of hearing rather than from neurological disorders, generalized intellectual impairments, or primary impairments in social responsiveness.

DEAFNESS: LANGUAGE AND EDUCATIONAL ISSUES

The majority of children with severe or profound deafness fail to achieve intelligible speech (e.g., Jensema & Trybus, 1978; Musselman, 1990), mastery of English syntax (e.g., Quigley, Power, & Steinkamp, 1977), or age-appropriate communication skills (e.g., MacKay-Soroka, Trehub, & Thorpe, 1987; 1988; Brownell, Trehub, & Gartner, 1988). Thus it is not surprising that deaf children lag considerably behind hearing children in metalinguistic skills (e.g., Gartner, Trehub, & MacKay-Soroka, 1993), and that deaf adolescents and adults typically attain only a Grade 4 or 5 reading level (Reich [Musselman] & Reich, 1974; Allen, 1986).

One constant in the history of deaf education is continuing disagreement over the optimal approach to intervention (see Lane, 1984; Moores, 1987). Throughout the greater part of this century, most programs have been auditory-oral (A/O), an approach that emphasizes the development of spoken language through the provision of appropriate amplification, training of residual hearing and speechreading.

Total communication (TC), which first achieved prominence in the 1970s, is an alternative approach that supplements spoken English with visual systems of communication, including fingerspelling and manual gestures. The backbone of TC programs is simultaneous communication (SimCom), in which spoken English is coordinated with one of several invented systems of manually coded English (e.g., Signed English, Signing Exact English). These systems use signs borrowed from a natural sign language, such as American Sign Language, together with invented signs for the grammatical features of English (e.g., -ed, -ing) to provide a visual analog to the spoken message (Stokoe, 1975).

Most deaf children with deaf parents (about 10% of the population) are exposed from birth to a natural sign language such as American Sign Language (ASL) or Langue des Signes Québecoises (LSQ). Unlike the signed codes, sign languages differ syntactically from spoken languages (see Wilbur, 1987), capitalizing on some of the unique communication possibilities afforded by the visual modality (Hoffmeister, 1982). Deaf children of deaf parents follow the same timetable in acquiring ASL or LSQ as do hearing children acquiring English or French (Petitto, 1992), and generally surpass deaf children of hearing parents in language and academic development (Vernon & Koh, 1970; Balow & Brill, 1975). These findings have generated interest in the educational use of natural sign languages. Those who favor this approach consider deaf persons to belong to a cultural minority which has ASL (or LSQ) as its "native" language (e.g., Padden & Humphries, 1988; Sacks, 1989). A few programs are currently pursuing an English as a second language model rather than a special education model, systematically incorporating deaf language, role models and culture into the curriculum (Johnson, Liddell, & Erting, 1989).

Although there are as yet no comparative studies of bilingual/bicultural programs, numerous studies have compared students in A/O and TC programs. The results, however, are equivocal because A/O children typically have more hearing and are socioeconomically advantaged compared to TC children (e.g., Geers, Moog, & Schick, 1984). Furthermore, choice of program seems to contribute less to outcome than do the combined effects of hearing level, intellectual ability, and family environment (Bodner-Johnson, 1986; Musselman, Lindsay, & Wilson, 1988a).

DEAFNESS: PSYCHOSOCIAL ISSUES

The presence of a deaf child has considerable impact on a hearing family. Hearing mothers of deaf children report higher levels of stress (Lederberg & Mobley, 1990; Calderon & Greenberg, 1993) and dissatisfaction (Luterman, 1987) than do mothers with hearing children. As early as infancy, there are reports of disruption in the development of reciprocal interactions between hearing mothers and their deaf infants (e.g., Spencer & Gutfreund, 1990). Hearing mothers of deaf children and adolescents are more didactic and controlling than mothers of hearing children (Schlesinger & Meadow, 1972; Wedell-Monnig & Lumley, 1980; Gartner, 1993), and their deaf children show delayed development of social initiative, compliance, and play behavior (Schirmer, 1989; Cornelius & Hornett, 1990). A few investigators have found these differences to be minimal (Greenberg & Marvin, 1979; Lederberg & Mobley, 1990; van Ijzendoorn et al., 1992), but their findings are atypical.

Estimates of mental health problems in deaf children and adults vary considerably (for reviews, see Meadow & Trybus, 1979; Greenberg & Kusché, 1989). Although the incidence of major mental illness appears to be no different for deaf than for hearing individuals (Rainer, Altshuler, & Kallman, 1963), there are numerous reports of a substantially higher incidence of impulsiveness (e.g., Chess & Fernandez, 1980), emotional immaturity (Greenberg & Kusché, 1989), egocentricity (e.g., Bachara, Raphael, & Phelan, 1980), and depressive symptoms (e.g., Leigh et al., 1989) in deaf compared to hearing children, adolescents, and adults. The validity of these studies is compromised, however, by the use of instruments developed for and normed on hearing individuals, and failure to accommodate the language difficulties of deaf persons and their unique experiences and culture (Moores, 1987; Marschark, 1993).

To the extent that greater social and emotional difficulties exist, these may reflect problems in communication rather than deafness *per se.* Studies have shown that the quality of interaction between hearing mothers and their deaf children is related to communication ability; deaf mothers and their deaf children, who share an accessible communication system, have interactions which are similar to hearing dyads (Greenberg & Marvin, 1979; Meadow, Greenberg, & Erting, 1983; Leigh, 1987). Deaf children and adolescents in the mainstream have poorer social functioning than those placed with deaf peers, reportedly because of communication difficulties (e.g., Reich [Musselman], Hambleton, & Houldin, 1977; Foster, 1989).

OUR STUDY OF DEAF CHILDREN AND ADOLESCENTS

We had the opportunity of examining communication and psychosocial functioning in a sample of deaf individuals who were studied first in early childhood and subsequently in adolescence. For the purposes of this chapter, we posed the following questions: How does the development of communication and social skills differ in deaf and normally hearing individuals? To what extent do skills in early childhood predict skills in adolescence? What is the relation between communication skill and psychosocial adjustment in early childhood and adolescence? These questions were motivated by an attempt to understand how early childhood deafness influences the course of development, most particularly the interplay of language and psychosocial adjustment over the lifespan.

The original study population consisted of all 3- to 5-year-old children in the Province of Ontario who were enrolled in an educational program for deaf children. About 80% of the families agreed to participate, yielding a sample of 153 children. The present report is restricted to deaf children with hearing parents, who numbered 139 (61 boys, 78 girls) in the preschool period. The children had severe (≥ 70 dB) or profound (≥ 90 dB) deafness, with hearing thresholds averaging 99 dB (SD = 17.0). Almost all of the children were prelingually deaf, which means that they were either congenitally deaf or became deaf before 2 years of age. Performance IQ (Wechsler) averaged 108 (SD = 18.6). These children participated in a longitudinal study extending over the next four years. Information about the original sample and their early linguistic, academic, and social development are available elsewhere (Musselman, Lindsay, & Wilson, 1988a; Musselman, Lindsay, & Wilson, 1988b; Musselman, Wilson, & Lindsay, 1988). In adolescence, 64 of these students (19 male, 45 female)[1] agreed to participate in a further study. Their hearing loss (M = 100.6 dB) and Performance IQ (M = 108.4) did not differ significantly from the original sample, indicating that the adolescent sub-sample was representative of the original sample and of deaf students in general. The present report includes data from the final year of the early childhood phase (M = 6 years, 9 months) and from the adolescent phase (M = 16 years, 7 months) of the study.

In line with general practice at the time, over 90% of the original sample were enrolled in auditory-oral (A/O) programs soon after diagnosis. By the end of the preschool study, less than 60% were still being educated orally, declining to about 33% in adolescence. This dramatic shift primarily reflects the flow of students into total communication (TC) programs as academic demands increased, although it is possible we overestimated the shift due to greater difficulty in identifying mainstreamed A/O students. As in other studies, A/O and TC students differed in a number of respects; in the preschool years, A/O students typically had more hearing (94 vs 106 dB), higher Performance IQ (113 vs 101), better educated mothers, and more educational assistance from their parents. More importantly, they were generally students who had succeeded orally, in comparison to their peers who transferred to TC programs at different times after encountering difficulties.

To provide baseline data on our psychosocial measures, we recruited a sample of normally hearing adolescents from a subject pool at the University of Toronto (M = 15 years, 4 months). Not only were these adolescents somewhat younger than the deaf teens, but they also had a slightly higher family socioeconomic status (SES). Nevertheless, both groups included participants from a broad SES spectrum and had a mean SES just above the national average.

Communicative competence: early childhood

Measures of communicative competence in early childhood included an assessment of speech and of English language comprehension (spoken English or SimCom). The spoken English measure was derived from an oral language sample elicited with picture story cards. The results revealed extremely limited

---

[1] This imbalance between the sexes was due to a higher refusal rate on the part of deaf males.

spoken language. Although the mean number of intelligible words was 39.6, more than half of the children had no intelligible speech. The A/O children had significantly better spoken language ability than the TC children (60.6 vs 7.4 words), a difference that is not surprising in view of the aforementioned differences in hearing levels.

The Language Assessment Battery (Reich [Musselman], Keeton & Lindsay, 1981) was used to assess children's comprehension of English grammar. Words and sentences were presented in the modality used in the child's school (speech alone or SimCom), with children responding by manipulating objects in a doll's house. The test had been designed to assess structures that hearing children generally acquire by age 5 (Brown, 1973). Although the children showed considerable progress during the preschool period, their performance was still well below ceiling by the final phase of the early childhood study. The performance of children in A/O programs significantly exceeded that of children in TC programs. When multivariate analyses were performed with differences in hearing and Performance IQ partialed out, the TC children scored higher than the A/O children (see Musselman, Lindsay, & Wilson, 1988). This apparent advantage is striking in view of the differences in family background and the lack of continuity in educational programming that characterized the TC group. These findings suggest that the language development of the TC children was enhanced by the change in communication method.

Psychosocial development: early childhood

Most commonly used measures of psychosocial functioning are inappropriate for deaf children because they assume spoken language competence. We developed a structured parent interview by combining the Self-Help and Social subscales of Alpern and Boll's (1972) Developmental Profile with items based on the timetable of social development outlined by Gesell (1949). The resulting scale contained 144 items covering three broad areas of development: Self-Help (eating, toileting, dressing, bathing routines), Social Relations (sleep routines, play and pastimes, personhood, peer relations), and Social Comprehension (personal space, comprehension, responsibility, functional sequences). Statistical studies show that the scale has good psychometric properties.

Scores in each area systematically increased over the course of early childhood. In general, the scores of the deaf children did not differ from those expected by Alpern and Boll (1972) and by Gesell (1949) for hearing children. Although absolute scores of the A/O and TC children did not differ, TC children again scored higher when we partialed out differences in hearing and Performance IQ. Thus, deaf children, despite substantial delays in language, had social skills that were substantially similar to those of normally hearing children. The use of a communication mode that differed from that of society as a whole did not impede, and may even have facilitated, the acquisition of appropriate social skills in the TC group.

In further analyses, we explored the relations between communication and social development. Different patterns of findings reflected differences in communication mode. Within the A/O group, the communication measures (which were both administered in speech) were moderately correlated with Social Relations (spoken language: $r = 0.33$, $p = 0.002$; language comprehension: $r = 0.36$, $p = 0.001$) and Social Comprehension scores (spoken language: $r = 0.48$, $p = 0.000$; language comprehension: $r = 0.52$, $p = 0.000$), but not with Self-Help. Within the TC group, spoken language was unrelated to social development. Instead, we found moderate ($r = 0.46$, $p = 0.000$) to strong correlations ($r = 0.59$, $p = 0.000$) between the language comprehension measure (administered in SimCom) and all of the social development scores, including Self-Help. For A/O and TC children, then, social development was related to their primary mode of communication.

Communicative competence: adolescence

We assessed the communication proficiency of deaf adolescents in spoken English, simultaneous communication, and ASL, using an adaptation of the Sign Communication Proficiency Interview (Newell et al., 1983). The interview involves native speakers engaging the individual in spontaneous conversation using a flexible, but structured protocol. Following previous studies of deaf adolescents (Moores et al., 1987; Geers & Moog, 1989), each young person had three conversational partners: a hearing person who spoke, a hearing person using SimCom, and a deaf person using ASL. Language proficiency was rated on a 12-point scale: No Ability, Adaptive, Adaptive+, Novice, Novice+, Survival, Survival+, Intermediate, Intermediate+, Advanced, Advanced+, and Superior Ability. Independent ratings of 45 interviews yielded very high levels of inter-rater reliability for the speech ($r = 0.91$) and ASL ($r = 0.98$) interviews. Lower reliability for the SimCom interview ($r = 0.72$) reflected the use of different sign systems among educational programs (Akamatsu, Miller, & Musselman, 1994).

Adolescents in A/O programs achieved significantly higher overall levels of communication proficiency than TC adolescents, with mean scores at the Advanced level on the spoken language interviews. TC students averaged Intermediate+ on the SimCom interview, a level of performance matched by A/O adolescents who used their oral skills in that setting. TC students also averaged Intermediate+ on the ASL interviews. It is noteworthy that TC students communicated as effectively in ASL, a language in which they had received no formal instruction, as in SimCom, in which they had received extensive instruction. ASL scores were related to students' age, while spoken language and SimCom scores had plateaued.

We considered a score of Intermediate or higher to represent a level of proficiency adequate for everyday communication. Criteria for this skill level include the ability to use simple sentences and appropriate vocabulary to communicate about familiar, concrete topics. Using these criteria, most A/O and TC students demonstrated functional or better communication skills in their best interview. TC adolescents, however, had oral communication skills that were below the level of functional adequacy (Survival) and A/O adolescents had even lower ASL skills (Novice). Accordingly, these two groups would be limited to the most rudimentary interactions with one another. Furthermore, the average skill levels of TC adolescents on their best interview are likely insufficient for the demands of secondary and post-secondary education.

Although adolescent communication proficiency revealed considerable progress relative to skill levels observed in early childhood, considerable stability was evident. For the A/O group, spoken language and language comprehension scores from early childhood were highly correlated with adolescent oral proficiency, accounting for up to 60% of the variance. For the TC group, there were moderate correlations between spoken language measures over time ($r = 0.53$, $p = 0.000$) and between early childhood language comprehension and SimCom proficiency ($r = 0.38$, $p = 0.004$); a relation between language comprehension in early childhood and ASL proficiency in adolescence was evident but weaker ($r = 0.24$, $p = 0.05$). Relations within the TC group may have been higher had we restricted our comparisons to students who were in TC programs at both the early childhood phase and the adolescent phase. Nevertheless, despite the 10-year gap and changes in educational programming, there was remarkable stability in the relative communicative performance of these deaf children.

IQ measures

Because of the English language difficulties of many deaf children, researchers and clinicians generally use nonverbal measures of intelligence (Vernon, 1969). Nevertheless, recent research indicates that verbal IQ scales can be administered effectively by examiners who are fluent in sign (Sullivan & Schulte, 1992). There are indications, moreover, that verbal IQ, administered in deaf students' usual mode of communication, is a better predictor of academic achievement than are the nonverbal measures (Sullivan, 1990). In the present study, a hearing psychometrist who was also a sign language interpreter administered the Verbal and Performance sections of the WISC-III and WAIS-R tests (depending on age) in each deaf adolescent's preferred mode of communication (Nizzero, Musselman, & MacKay-Soroka, 1993). A/O and TC students did not differ on Performance IQ, scoring close to the expected value of 100. A/O adolescents, however, had significantly higher Verbal IQ (M = 84.9, SD = 11) than TC adolescents (M = 76.8, SD = 8.5), both groups scoring well below the mean for the normally hearing population. For both A/O and

TC adolescents, the highest score from the three interviews was strongly related to Verbal IQ (A/O: r = 0.76, p = 0.001; TC: r = 0.48, p = 0.002), but not to Performance IQ.

The measure of Verbal IQ provides another perspective on the language skills of the sample. Unlike the communication proficiency interviews which emphasize interpersonal communication, Verbal IQ assesses the ability to use language for thinking. The scores of the deaf adolescents suggest that they lack sufficient skill to use language as an effective educational tool, a suggestion which is consistent with their performance on the communication proficiency interviews.

Psychosocial measures: adolescence

We adapted the Youth Self Report (Achenbach, 1991) so that it could be administered effectively to deaf adolescents, regardless of their level of reading skill (MacKay-Soroka et al., 1993). The Youth Self Report (YSR) is a well-standardized and widely used measure of adolescent psychopathology with established reliability and validity. For the deaf sample, items were revised by substituting simpler vocabulary and syntactic structures than those in the original version (e.g., "If I do something wrong, I feel guilty" was substituted for "I don't feel guilty after doing something I shouldn't"), and equivalent versions were developed in both simultaneous communication and ASL. Reliability of the revised form (r = 0.87) was comparable to the one-week test-retest reliability of the original YSR (Achenbach, 1991).

The subgroups of deaf adolescents differed substantially from one another. TC adolescents had significantly higher scores on Total Behaviour Problems, Internalizing, and Externalizing scales than did A/O adolescents. TC adolescents also had significantly higher scores than A/O adolescents on a number of YSR subscales (somatic complaints, anxious/depressed, social problems, attention problems, and aggressive behavior). A/O deaf adolescents did not differ from their hearing counterparts aside from slightly higher scores on the withdrawn and social subscales. Approximately 36% of TC adolescents had Total Behavior Problem scores in the clinical range compared to 5% of the A/O teens and 17% of the normally hearing teens. A further 31% of the TC adolescents scored in the borderline clinical range compared to 10% of the A/O adolescents and 10% of the normally hearing teens.

The deaf adolescents in our sample who were experiencing clinically significant adjustment problems are best characterized as exhibiting mixed disorders exemplified by a variety of internalizing and externalizing symptomatology. In general, the subscales showing the highest elevations were social problems (e.g., teased, not liked) and withdrawn (e.g., "I refuse to communicate with people"). Unlike other researchers (e.g., Harris, 1978; Chess & Fernandez, 1980), we did not find that problems of impulse control were primary (i.e., delinquency, aggression). Indeed, the deaf sample as a whole did not differ from the hearing controls on these subscales, nor did the disproportionate number of females in the deaf sample account for the lack of differences.

Unexpectedly, for TC adolescents, neither their best communication proficiency scores, their SimCom scores, nor their ASL scores were significantly related to YSR scores. Even more surprising were the significant relations between TC students' scores on the speech interview and YSR scores (Total Problem Behaviors: $r = 0.38$, $p = 0.05$; Internalizing: $r = 0.39$, $p = 0.05$; anxious/depressed: $r = 0.44$, $p = 0.005$; attention problems: $r = 0.34$, $p = 0.05$), showing that students with better speech reported more symptoms.

For TC students, good speech relative to their TC peers may have generated uncertainty about their identity in the deaf and hearing worlds. Moreover, good speech may have been associated with a relatively late shift to TC programs. Those TC students with better speech likely remained in A/O programs longer than their deaf peers with poorer speech. These "late signers," aware of their failure in an oral program, would have faced a whole new set of communication and social adjustments when they changed programs. Indeed, we found the highest level of symptomatology in a group of late signers, many of whom likely lacked functional communication skills in early childhood.

It is not surprising to uncover relations between early language abilities and adolescent adjustment. Specifically, language comprehension scores in early childhood were significantly associated with Total Problem Behaviors ($r = -0.27$, $p = 0.041$), Internalizing ($r = -0.26$, $p = 0.047$) and Externalizing scores ($r = -0.31$, $p = 0.019$), as well as with a number of subscale scores. This confirms the view, noted at the outset, that early language difficulty impedes social development and may compromise long-term psychosocial adjustment. For A/O students, their relatively good language ability in early childhood (compared to that of TC students) may have contributed to their overall healthy adjustment in adolescence.

Although communication proficiency in adolescence failed to predict levels of symptomatology as expected, adolescent IQ was predictive. Within the sample as a whole, Verbal IQ was significantly related to the three summary scores and to several subscale scores, with no relation between Performance IQ and symptomatology. For the TC group, Verbal IQ was moderately associated with Total Behavior Problems ($r = -0.36$, $p = 0.025$) and Internalizing symptoms ($r = -0.35$, $p = 0.031$), as well as several subscale scores. For A/O adolescents, however, Verbal IQ was largely unrelated to YSR scores.

The overall pattern of findings confirms the predictive validity of Verbal IQ in a deaf population (Sullivan, 1990). Interestingly, Verbal IQ, with its basis in language, goes beyond elementary language skills (e.g., Vocabulary subscale) to include verbally based knowledge (e.g., Information) and verbal reasoning (e.g., Similarities and Comprehension). Although the skills measured on the Verbal IQ scale predict literacy (Nizzero et al., 1993), Verbal IQ scores would not be expected to predict psychosocial adjustment, at least not IQ scores within the normal range. The TC sample, however, included adolescents with Verbal and Performance IQs well below the population mean, individuals who may have had problems in addition to deafness (e.g., subtle problems associated with the etiologies of maternal rubella, low birth weight, meningitis). Thus this group may include individuals whose difficulties with verbally mediated cognitive skills are sufficient to compromise psychosocial adjustment as well as school success.

SUMMARY AND IMPLICATIONS

We have identified similarities and differences in the development of deaf children with hearing parents and normally hearing children, as well as between subgroups of deaf children. Deaf children's performance on measures of communication proficiency, both in early childhood and adolescence, showed severe delays. These delays were less severe for students in auditory/oral (A/O) than for those in total communications programs (TC). The development of social skills in early childhood seemed to follow a similar developmental course for deaf and hearing individuals. Even in adolescence, A/O students exhibited patterns of adjustment that were similar to those of hearing adolescents. TC students, however, differed substantially from both hearing adolescents and from A/O adolescents, exhibiting a profile of symptoms that placed many in the clinical or borderline-clinical range.

These differences between A/O and TC students in communication and psychosocial development cannot be solely attributed to their educational placement or mode of communication. As the program of choice, auditory/oral students tended to have more residual hearing and higher nonverbal intelligence, and to come from economically and educationally advantaged families. For example, although 33% of the A/O adolescents had hearing thresholds in the severe range (i.e., less than 90 dB), fewer than 10% of TC adolescents did so. Furthermore, almost all TC students had experienced a period of relative failure in an A/O program, varying from a few months to many years. Moving to a TC program as a second option, these students effectively started their education late, and were usually further hampered by their parents' and teachers' lack of proficient signing skills. Nevertheless, a number of TC students displayed communication skills and levels of psychosocial adjustment which equalled those of the best A/O students.

Although the two phases of the study were separated by 10 years and involved different measures, communication performance showed considerable stability over time. This was especially the case for A/O students, a finding that partly reflects continuity in their educational programming. This finding implies that deaf children who make poor progress in acquiring spoken language during early childhood are unlikely to significantly change their position in later years.

American Sign Language (ASL) proficiency followed a markedly different developmental course. A/O adolescents with the best spoken language tended not to learn ASL at all. For TC students, exposure to ASL was considerably later than for the other language modalities, resulting in greater proficiency among older than younger adolescents. Moreover, equivalent achievement in SimCom and ASL in the context of unequal exposure confirms the greater efficiency and learnability of ASL. Among TC youth, proficiency in ASL was positively related to proficiency in speech and SimCom, a finding which has been noted elsewhere (Hatfield, Caccamise, & Siple, 1978). We would expect the ASL skills of this group to continue developing throughout adolescence and adulthood as their movement into the Deaf community provides further exposure (Mayberry & Eichen, 1991).

While simultaneous communication might be expected to bridge skills in spoken language and ASL, it functioned differently within the two groups, showing strong relations with spoken language for A/O students and with ASL for TC students. Thus, what appears as a unified system, functions as two different systems, the auditory signal being primary for A/O students and the visual signal for TC students. It is noteworthy that the sensory channel overrides linguistic considerations in these relationships: thus, simultaneous communication, which follows English grammar, was more closely related to ASL for TC students than to spoken language.

As expected, communication proficiency and psychosocial adjustment were related, although not in a straightforward way. In early childhood, the level of communication proficiency, although severely delayed overall, seemed sufficient to support normal psychosocial development, a conclusion supported by several other studies (Lederberg, Rosenblatt, & Vandell, 1987; Lederberg & Mobley, 1990). It is likely that idiosyncratic gestural systems supplemented conventional communication skills, a phenomenon that has been documented for hearing (Accredolo & Goodwyn, 1988) as well as for deaf children (Goldin-Meadow & Mylander, 1985).

The adolescent picture differs substantially. Many of the TC adolescents were experiencing considerable adjustment problems, both intrapsychically as well as in their external relationships. Interestingly, levels of adolescent adjustment were related to communicative competence in early childhood, underscoring the importance of early communication skill in establishing a foundation for subsequent adjustment. Concurrently, psychosocial adjustment was most strongly related to verbal IQ, reflecting the increasing influence of language and cognition in the social realm.

The most immediate consequence of childhood deafness in hearing families is disruption in the normal pattern of interaction and communication. In early childhood, however, most families seem able to adjust to this unexpected situation, likely by supplementing the auditory channel with visual cues. As a result, psychosocial development proceeds normally, despite delayed language. By adolescence, however, the level of communication skill attained by many deaf individuals, while sufficient for simple social interactions, may be insufficient for more complex interactions and the demands of schooling. Moreover, asymmetries in the communication skills of parents, teachers and deaf adolescents may further impede the development of normal relationships, leading to the emergence of a variety of adjustment problems.

The deaf adolescent's communication and socioemotional difficulties may attenuate when they find their place in the deaf community as adults, their "home among strangers" (Schein, 1989). Low levels of literacy, however, will persist for many individuals and serve as life-long barriers to further learning (Stanovich, 1993) and occupational success (Reich [Musselman] & Reich, 1974).

We have shown that the relations between language and psychosocial adjustment are not straightforward, but vary with age, likely reflecting changes in the communication demands imposed by the social environment. Deaf persons without fluent spoken language inhabit two worlds: a hearing world – which is the locus of early family relationships, school and work – and a Deaf world which is the likely milieu of adult social and family life. In attempting to bridge these worlds for the majority of deaf persons, the evidence that we have presented suggests the importance of establishing an effective communication system early in life. This objective requires the early identification of children needing signed communication, and the development of adequate sign skills in their parents and teachers. Our data also support explorations in the use of natural sign languages to enhance the communication skills of deaf students and provide life-long learning opportunities for deaf adults.

ACKNOWLEDGMENTS

The preparation of this chapter was assisted by grants from the Ontario Ministry of Education and the Social Sciences and Humanities Research Council (to C. Musselman), the Ontario Ministry of Community and Social Services (to S. MacKay and S. E. Trehub), and the National Health Research and Development Program (to S. MacKay and S. E. Trehub). We are indebted to Susan Dickens, who ably managed our large data set, and to Adele Churchill, Lee Johnson, Nancy Dye, Cathy Lee Roarke, Ann Colquhoun, Phyllis Vazquez, Anne Miller, and Irene Nizerro for their skillful and sensitive work during the long and arduous process of data collection.

REFERENCES

Accredolo, L. & Goodwyn, S. (1988). Symbolic gesturing in normal infants. *Child Development,* **59**, 450–467.

Achenbach, T.M. (1991). *Manual for the Youth Self-Report and 1991 Profile.* Burlington, VT: University of Vermont.

Akamatsu, C.T., Miller, A., & Musselman, C. (1994). Using the Language/Communication Proficiency Interview as a form of dynamic assessment. Paper presented at the meeting of the American Educational Research Association, New Orleans.

Allen, T.E. (1986). Patterns of academic achievement among hearing impaired students: 1974–1983. In A.N. Schildroth & M.A. Karchmer (eds) *Deaf Children in America.* San Diego, CA: College-Hill Press (pp. 161–206).

Alpern, G.D. & Boll, T.J. (1972). *The Developmental Profile.* Indianapolis, IN: Psychological Developmental Publications.

Bachara, G.H., Raphael, J., & Phelan, W.J. (1980). Empathy development in deaf preadolescents. *American Annals of the Deaf,* **135,** 38–41.

Balow, I.H. & Brill, R.G. (1975). An evaluation of reading and academic achievement levels of 16 graduating classes of the California School for the Deaf, Riverside. *Volta Review,* **77,** 255–266.

Beitchman, J.H., Nair, R., Clegg, M., Ferguson, B., & Patel, P.G. (1986). Prevalence of psychiatric disorders in children with speech and language disorders. *Journal of the American Academy of Child Psychiatry,* **25,** 528–535.

Bodner-Johnson, B. (1986). The family environment and achievement of deaf students: a discriminant analysis. *Exceptional Children,* **52,** 443–449.

Brown, R. (1973). *A First Language: The Early Stages.* Cambridge, MA: Harvard University Press.

Brownell, M., Trehub, S.E., & Gartner, G. (1988). Children's understanding of referential messages by deaf and hearing speakers. *First Language,* **8,** 271–286.

Calderon, R. & Greenberg, M.T. (1993). Considerations in the adaptation of families with school-age deaf children. In M. Marschark & D. Clark (eds) *Psychological Perspectives on Deafness.* Hillsdale, NJ: Lawrence Erlbaum (pp. 27–47).

Cantwell, D.P. & Baker, L. (1987). *Developmental Speech and Language Disorders.* New York: Guilford Press.

Chess, S. & Fernandez, P. (1980). Do deaf children have a typical personality? *Journal of the American Academy of Child Psychiatry,* **19,** 654–664.

Cornelius, G. & Hornett, D. (1990). The play behavior of hearing-impaired kindergarten children. *American Annals of the Deaf,* **135,** 316–321.

Foster, S. (1989). Social alienation and peer identification: a study of the social construction of deafness. *Human Organization,* **48,** 226–235.

Gartner, G.M. (1993). Mother–child Interaction in Deaf-Child/Hearing-Mother Dyads: Maternal Directives on Nonverbal Tasks – Preschool to Adolescence. Unpublished doctoral dissertation, University of Toronto.

Gartner, G.M., Trehub, S.E., & MacKay-Soroka, S. (1993). Word awareness in hearing-impaired children. *Applied Psycholinguistics,* **14,** 61–73.

Geers, A. & Moog, J. (1989). Factors predictive of the development of literacy in profoundly hearing-impaired adolescents. *Volta Review,* **91,** 69–86.

Geers, A., Moog, J., & Schick, B. (1984). Acquisition of spoken and signed English by profoundly deaf children. *Journal of Speech and Hearing Disorders,* **49,** 378–388.

Gesell, A. (1949). *Child Development: An Introduction to the Study of Human Growth.* New York: Harper & Row.

Goldin-Meadow, S. & Mylander, C. (1985). Gestural communication in deaf children: the effects and non-effects of parental input on early language development. *Monograph of the Society of Research in Child Development Vol. 49.* Chicago: University of Chicago Press, for the Society for Research in Child Development.

Greenberg, M.T. & Kusché, C.A. (1989). Cognitive, personal, and social development of deaf children and adolescents. In M.C. Wang, M.C. Reynolds, & H.J. Wallberg (eds) *Handbook of Special Education: Research and Practice: Vol. 3. Low Incidence Conditions.* New York: Pergamon Press (pp. 95–129).

Greenberg, M.T. & Marvin, R.S. (1979). Attachment patterns in profoundly deaf preschool children. *Merrill-Palmer Quarterly, 25*(4), 265–279.

Harris, R.I. (1978). Impulse control in deaf children: research and clinical issues. In L.S. Liben (ed.) *Deaf Children: Developmental Perspectives.* New York: Academic Press (pp. 137–156).

Hatfield, N., Caccamise, F., & Siple, P. (1978). Deaf students' language competency: a bilingual perspective. *American Annals of the Deaf, 123,* 847–856.

Hoffmeister, R.J. (1982). Acquisition of signed languages by deaf children. In H. Hoemann & R. Wilbur (eds) *Interpersonal Communication and Deaf People.* Washington, DC: Gallaudet College Press.

Jensema, C.J. & Trybus, R.J. (1978). *Communication Patterns and Educational Achievement of Hearing Impaired Students.* Washington, DC: Gallaudet College Office of Demographic Studies.

Johnson, R., Liddell, S., & Erting, C. (1989). *Unlocking the Curriculum: Principles for Achieving Success in Deaf Education.* Gallaudet Research Institute Working Paper 89–3. Washington, DC: Gallaudet.

Lane, H. (ed.) (1984). *The Deaf Experience: Classics in Language and Education* (trans. F. Philip). Cambridge, MA: Harvard University Press.

Lederberg, A.R. & Mobley, C.E. (1990). The effect of hearing impairment on the quality of attachment and mother-toddler interaction. *Child Development, 61,* 1596–1604.

Lederberg, A.R., Rosenblatt, V., & Vandell, D.L. (1987). Temporary and long-term friendships in hearing and deaf preschoolers. *Merrill-Palmer Quarterly, 33,* 515–533.

Leigh, I.W. (1987). Parenting and the hearing impaired: attachment and coping. *Volta Review, 89,* 11–21.

Leigh, I.W., Robins, C.J., Welkowitz, J., & Bond, R.N. (1989). Toward a greater understanding of depression in deaf individuals. *American Annals of the Deaf, 134,* 249–254.

Luterman, D. (1987). *Deafness in the Family.* Boston, MA: College-Hill Press.

MacKay-Soroka, S.A., Trehub, S., Musselman, C., Dickens, S.E., Churchill, A., Vasquez, P., Miller, A., & Nizzero, I. (1993). Deaf adolescents' self-reported behavioral and emotional functioning. Paper presented at the meeting of the Canadian Psychological Association, Montreal.

MacKay-Soroka, S., Trehub, S., & Thorpe, L. (1987). Deaf children's referential messages to mother. *Child Development, 58,* 385–394.

MacKay-Soroka, S., Trehub, S., & Thorpe, L. (1988). Reception of mothers' referential messages by deaf and hearing children. *Developmental Psychology, 24,* 277–285.

Marschark, M. (1993). *Psychological Development of Deaf Children.* New York: Oxford University Press.

Mayberry, R.I. & Eichen, E.B. (1991). The long-lasting advantage of learning sign language in childhood: another look at the critical period for language acquisition. *Journal of Memory and Language,* **30,** 486–512.

Meadow, K.P., Greenberg, M.T., & Erting, C. (1983). Attachment behavior of deaf children with deaf parents. *Journal of the American Academy of Child Psychiatry,* **22,** 23–28.

Meadow, K.P. & Trybus, R.J. (1979). Behavioral and emotional problems of deaf children: An overview. In L.J. Bradford & W.G. Hardy (eds) *Hearing and Hearing Impairment.* New York: Grune & Stratton (pp. 395–403).

Moores, D.E. (1987). *Educating the Deaf: Psychology, Principles, and Practices,* 3rd edn. Dallas: Houghton Mifflin.

Moores, D., Thomas, K., Johnson, R., Cox, P., Blennerhassett, L., Kelly, L., Sweet, C., & Fields, L. (1987). *Factors Predictive of Literacy in Deaf Adolescents in Total Communication Programs.* Washington, DC: Gallaudet University Research Institute.

Musselman, C. (1990). The effect of hearing loss on the spoken language of preschool deaf children. *Journal of Childhood Communication Disorders,* **13,** 193–205.

Musselman, C., Lindsay, P.H., & Wilson, A.K. (1988a). An evaluation of recent trends in preschool programming for hearing-impaired children. *Journal of Speech and Hearing Disorders,* **53,** 71–88.

Musselman, C., Lindsay, P.H., & Wilson, A.K. (1988b). The effect of mothers' communication mode on language development in deaf children. *Applied Psycholinguistics,* **9,** 185–203.

Musselman, C., Wilson, A.K., & Lindsay, P.H. (1988). The effects of age of intervention, program intensity, and parent instruction on hearing impaired children. *Exceptional Children,* **55,** 222–234.

Newell, W., Caccamise, F., Boardman, K., & Holcomb, B.R. (1983). Adaptation of the Language Proficiency Interview (LPI) for assessing sign communicative competence. *Sign Language Studies,* **41,** 311–352.

Nizzero, I., Musselman, C., & MacKay-Soroka, S. (1993). Verbal and nonverbal intelligence as predictors of academic achievement in deaf teenagers. Paper presented at the meeting of Convention of American Instructors of the Deaf, Baltimore, MD.

Padden, C. & Humphries, T. (1988). *Deaf in America: Voices from a Culture.* Cambridge, MA: Harvard University Press.

Petitto, L.A. (1992). Modularity and constraints in early lexical acquisition: evidence from children's early language and gesture. In M.R. Gunnar & M. Maratsos (eds) *Modularity and Constraints in Language and Cognition. Minnesota Symposia on Child Psychology: Vol. 25.* Hillsdale, NJ: Lawrence Erlbaum (pp. 25–58).

Quigley, S.P., Power, D.J., & Steinkamp, M.W. (1977). The language structure of deaf children. *Volta Review,* **79,** 73–84.

Rainer, J.D., Altshuler, K.Z., & Kallman, F.J. (1963). *Family and Mental Health Problems in a Deaf Population.* New York: NY State Psychiatric Institute.

Reich [Musselman], C., Hambleton, D., & Houldin, B. (1977). The integration of hearing-impaired children in regular classrooms. *American Annals of the Deaf,* **122,** 534–543.

Reich [Musselman], C. & Reich, P.A. (1974). The occupational history of urban deaf adults. *Journal of the Rehabilitation of the Deaf,* **8,** 1–10.

Reich [Musselman] C., Keeton, A., & Lindsay, P. (1981). The Language Assessment Battery for Hearing Impaired Children. *The ACEHI Journal,* **7,** 155–163.

Sacks, O.W. (1989). *Seeing Voices: A Journey into the World of the Deaf.* Toronto: Stoddart.

Schein, J.D. (1989). *At Home Among Strangers.* Washington, DC: Gallaudet University Press.

Schirmer, B. (1989). Relationship between imaginative play and language development in hearing-impaired children. *American Annals of the Deaf,* **134**, 219–222.

Schlesinger, H.S. & Meadow, K.P. (1972). *Sound and Sign: Childhood Deafness and Mental Health.* Berkeley, CA: University of California Press.

Spencer, P. & Gutfreund, M.K. (1990). Directiveness in mother-infant interactions. In D. F. Moores & K.P. Meadow-Orlans (eds) *Educational and Developmental Aspects of Deafness.* Washington, DC: Gallaudet University Press (pp. 350–365).

Stanovich, K.E. (1993). Does reading make you smarter? Literacy and the development of verbal intelligence. In H.W. Reese (ed.) *Advances in Child Development and Behavior, Vol. 24.* San Diego: Academic Press (pp. 133–180).

Stokoe, W.C. (1975). The use of sign language in teaching English. *American Annals of the Deaf,* **120**, 417–421.

Sullivan, P.M. (1990). Mental Health Services to Deaf Youth. Paper presented at the meeting of the Tenth Annual Mental Health and Deafness Conference, Toronto.

Sullivan, P.M. & Schulte, L.E. (1992). Factor analysis of WISC-R with deaf and hard-of-hearing children. *Psychological Assessment,* **4**, 537–540.

Vernon, M. (1969). Sociological and psychological factors associated with hearing loss. *Journal of Speech and Hearing Research,* **12**, 541–563.

Vernon, M. & Koh, S.D. (1970). Early manual communication and deaf children's achievement. *American Annals of the Deaf,* **115**, 527–536.

Vygotsky, L. (1986). *Thought and Language* (trans. A. Kozulin). Cambridge, MA: MIT Press.

van Ijzendoorn, M.H., Goldberg, S., Kroonenberg, P.M., & Frenkel, O.J. (1992). The relative effects of maternal and child problems on the quality of attachment: a meta-analysis of attachment in clinical samples. *Child Development,* **63**, 840–858.

Wedell-Monnig, J. & Lumley, J.M. (1980). Child deafness and mother–child interaction. *Child Development,* **51**, 766–774.

Wilbur, R.B. (1987). *American Sign Language: Linguistic and Applied Dimensions.* Boston, MA: Little Brown.

Index